HEART DISEASE KILLS SOMEONE IN THE U.S. EVERY 33 SECONDS

HEART DISEASE KILLS TEN TIMES MORE WOMEN ANNUALLY THAN BREAST CANCER

Bearing those facts in mind, it's no wonder we have become increasingly aware of the relationship between high cholesterol and heart disease—and mindful of the importance of monitoring cholesterol intake. The revised sixth edition of *THE CHOLESTEROL COUNTER,* from Annette B. Natow and Jo-Ann Heslin—the nutrition experts you can trust—takes the guesswork out of healthy living.

Look inside to learn the difference between "good" and "bad" cholesterol and to find out whether your cholesterol intake is too high. Then consult *THE CHOLESTEROL COUNTER*'s up-to-date, comprehensive listings of over 20,000 foods and take control of the amount of cholesterol you eat each day.

THE CHOLESTEROL COUNTER

An essential reference for healthy living!

Books by Annette B. Natow and Jo-Ann Heslin

THE
CHOLESTEROL COUNTER

Sixth Edition

**Annette B. Natow, Ph.D., R.D.
and Jo-Ann Heslin, M.A., R.D.**

POCKET BOOKS

New York   London   Toronto   Sydney

POCKET BOOKS, a division of Simon & Schuster, Inc.
1230 Avenue of the Americas, New York, NY 10020

Copyright © 2004 by Annette B. Natow and Jo-Ann Heslin

An *Original* Publication of POCKET BOOKS

All rights reserved, including the right to reproduce
this book or portions thereof in any form whatsoever.
For information address Pocket Books, 1230 Avenue
of the Americas, New York, NY 10020

ISBN: 0-7434-6438-9

First Pocket Books printing February 2004

10 9 8 7 6 5 4

POCKET and colophon are registered trademarks of
Simon & Schuster, Inc.

Photo credit: FoodPix

Manufactured in the United States of America

For information regarding special discounts for bulk purchases,
please contact Simon & Schuster Special Sales at 1-800-456-6798 or
business@simonandschuster.com

*To our families who support us through every project:
Harry, Allen, Irene, Sarah, Meryl, Marty, Laura, George,
Emily, Steven, Joseph, Kristen, Brian, Karen, and John.*

ACKNOWLEDGMENTS

For graciously sharing their knowledge: Martin Lefkowitz, M.D., and Irene E. Rosenberg, M.D.

For all her support and help, our agent, Nancy Trichter.

For her suggestions and editing skills, Sara Clemence.

Without the tireless cooperation of Steven Natow, M.D., and Stephen Llano, *The Cholesterol Counter, sixth edition* would never have been completed.

A special thank you to our editor, Micki Nuding.

"If only half a dozen foods were available the matter would be quickly settled."

Mary Swartz Rose, Ph.D.
Feeding the Family
The MacMillan Company, 1919

CONTENTS

PART ONE

Brand Name, Nonbranded (Generic)
& Take-Out Foods

PART TWO

Restaurant Chains

INTRODUCTION

High cholesterol:

- is a major risk factor for heart attack
- is a major risk factor for stroke
- increases your risk of cancer
- increases your risk of dementia
- combined with high blood pressure, puts you at risk for hearing loss
- combined with a diet high in fat, puts you at risk for gallstones

Heart disease—or more correctly, cardiovascular disease (CVD)—is the leading cause of death in the U.S. It kills one person every 33 seconds. Heart attacks and strokes disable even more people than they kill; more than the number of people who die from all forms of cancer!

Research worldwide shows that high cholesterol levels are one of the most important risk factors for heart disease. The higher your cholesterol, the greater your risk. Lowering your cholesterol lowers your risk. For every 1% decrease in cholesterol, your risk for heart disease drops 3% to 4%.

Heart disease often gives you no warning signs. That's why prevention is so important.

You should know:

- In 48% of men and 63% of women who die suddenly from heart attack or stroke, there are no warning signs.
- Cardiovascular disease kills twice as many men as cancer.
- If your cholesterol level is 200 to 239, your risk of having a heart attack is twice that of someone whose cholesterol is 200 or less.
- More than half of all men over 20 have cholesterol levels over 200.
- Heart attacks kill 10 times more women every year than breast cancer.
- African American women are 2 to 3 times more likely to die from a heart attack than other women.
- Women's average cholesterol levels are higher than men's after age 55.
- 102.3 million Americans have cholesterol values of 200 or higher. Of these, 41.3 million have levels of 240 or above.

FINDING CHOLESTEROL

What is cholesterol?

Cholesterol, a white, waxy, fatlike substance, is part of every cell in your body. Cholesterol insulates nerve cells and helps skin cells retain moisture. Cholesterol makes up a major part of your brain. It's the main building block from which vitamin D and essential hormones, such as cortisone, estrogen, progesterone, and testosterone, are made. But having too much cholesterol in your blood is unhealthy. Some of the extra cholesterol can be deposited on your artery walls, narrowing them and interfering with normal blood flow.

Which foods have cholesterol?

You get some cholesterol every time you eat animal foods—such as meat, poultry, fish, eggs, milk, yogurt, cheese, and butter. Egg yolks are a major source of cholesterol; egg whites don't have any. Caviar and liver are also very high in cholesterol.

There is no cholesterol in any food that grows in the ground. Vegetables, fruits, nuts, seeds, cereals, and grains have none.

Cholesterol can also be made in the body by your liver. In fact, most people make three times more cholesterol than they eat in food.

Keep It Simple—

If a food grows in the ground, it has no cholesterol.
If a food has a face, it has cholesterol.

Using the "Keep It Simple" rule, which of the following foods have cholesterol?

FOOD	YES	NO
Cheddar cheese	X	
Chicken leg	X	
Egg	X	
Hamburger	X	
Lobster	X	
Milk	X	
Salmon	X	
Almonds		X
Apple		X
Avocado		X
Olive oil		X
Peanut butter		X
Tomato		X
Watermelon		X

The first 7 foods all contain cholesterol. Hamburger comes from a steer. Salmon and lobster are seafood. Chicken legs and eggs come from chickens. Cheddar cheese and milk come from cows. All of them have faces!

The rest are from plants that grow in the ground. They have no cholesterol. Almonds, avocado, olive oil, and peanut butter all have fat, but it's vegetable fat, so there is no cholesterol.

The Cholesterol Counter lists the amount of cholesterol in over 20,000 foods. Even if a food is not listed, you can still determine if it is a source of cholesterol by asking, "Does it have a face?"

MEASURING CHOLESTEROL

Blood cholesterol values are measured in milligrams (mg). The number of milligrams (mg) of cholesterol in 1 deciliter (dl), which is slightly less than half a cup, is the value used to describe how much cholesterol is in your blood. For example, 180 mg/dl = 180 milligrams of cholesterol per deciliter of blood. To make things simpler, your doctor may give you just the number, 180, rather than the more complete measurement.

Do you know your number?

The Centers for Disease Control and Prevention estimate that 73% of Americans know their cholesterol levels.

The National Cholesterol Education Program (NCEP) recommends that all adults over age 20 be screened for cholesterol at least once every 5 years. Those with higher than normal readings should be checked more often. A cholesterol screening can tell you a great deal. You'll find out your total cholesterol, HDL cholesterol, LDL cholesterol, and a "ratio."

Total cholesterol is just that: the overall amount of cholesterol in a given volume of blood. Ideally you want your levels to be below 200, to keep down your risk of heart disease.

But it's a little more complicated than that. Cholesterol, a fatlike substance, is coated with a protein so it can travel in your blood, which is mainly water. The combination of fat and protein is called a *lipoprotein*.

LDL (low-density lipoprotein) is the main cholesterol carrier. If too much LDL cholesterol circulates in the blood, it can stick to the walls of the arteries leading to the heart and brain. This could eventually form plaque—thick, hard deposits that can clog arteries. A clogged artery leading to the heart can cause a heart attack. A clogged artery leading to the brain can cause a stroke. This is why LDL cholesterol is often referred to as "bad" cholesterol. The lower your levels of LDL, the lower your risk of heart disease. Desirable levels of LDL are less than 100.

About one-third of the blood's cholesterol is carried by HDL (high-density lipoprotein). Experts believe HDL cholesterol carries cholesterol away from the arteries back to the liver, where it is broken down and removed from the body. Because this may slow the growth of plaque, HDL is referred to as "good" cholesterol. Levels under 40 are considered too low.

Having low LDL cholesterol and high HDL cholesterol reduces your risk of developing plaques and lowers your risk for heart disease.

Your "ratio" is determined by dividing HDL cholesterol into total cholesterol. For example: if your total cholesterol is 200 and your HDL cholesterol is 50, your ratio is 4:1. A ratio below 5:1 is good. The optimum is 3.5:1.

It's important to get a full lipid profile, because measuring just total cholesterol can be misleading. Some people may have normal or near-normal cholesterol values but high LDL (bad cholesterol) values.

ADULT BLOOD CHOLESTEROL LEVELS

Total Cholesterol

Desirable	under 200
Borderline high	200 to 239
High	240 or higher

LDL Cholesterol		HDL Cholesterol	
Optimal	under 100	Low	Less than 40
Near or above optimal	100 to 129	High	60 or higher
Borderline high	130 to 159		
High	160 to 189		
Very high	190 or higher		

National Cholesterol Education Program, *Third Report of the Expert Panel on Detection, Evaluation, and Treatment of High Blood Cholesterol in Adults (Adult Treatment Panel III)*, 2001.

CONTROLLING CHOLESTEROL

If my cholesterol is 220, what should I do?

Lifestyle changes should be the first step in lowering your cholesterol. Losing weight (even a small amount), exercising regularly, quitting smoking, eating less fat and cholesterol, and eating more fiber (more about that on pages 14 to 15) are all important strategies to help you lower total cholesterol and increase HDL. Even small changes, like losing 5 pounds or taking a walk every day, will make a difference.

Many foods that are high in cholesterol are also high in total fat and saturated fat. When you lower your cholesterol intake, you reduce your intake of other fats, too, lowering your overall risk for heart disease.

How much cholesterol should I eat each day?

The National Cholesterol Education Program recommends no more than 200 milligrams of cholesterol a day. The American Heart Association (AHA) recommends that you limit your average cholesterol intake to less than 300 milligrams a day; 200 milligrams a day if you have heart disease. On average, American men eat about 330 milligrams of cholesterol a day; women about 240.

Your daily cholesterol intake should be based on the results of your latest lipid profile. If your total cholesterol and LDL levels are within the desirable range, stay under 300 milligrams a day. If your numbers are up, reduce your intake to 200 milligrams a day.

To lower my cholesterol, do I have to stop eating steak and eggs?

All foods can fit into a low cholesterol diet, but some may need a little more negotiation than others. An egg has 213 milligrams of cholesterol. So having a scrambled egg for breakfast is no problem. But if you need to restrict your cholesterol to 200 milligrams a day, you'll need to make nonmeat, nondairy choices for lunch and dinner. If you are averaging 300 milligrams or less cholesterol a day, you still have some to spare.

Many of us enjoy an occasional steak. Three ounces of porterhouse steak has 70 milligrams of cholesterol. By keeping portion size moderate, you can enjoy a steak every now and then. The key is to consider choices for the day. If one choice is high in cholesterol, balance it with others that are low. If you stick with moderate portions, it's not that hard to do.

Can large meals make your cholesterol go up?

Some recent research shows that eating smaller, more frequent meals helps to lower cholesterol. The researchers think that larger meals may trigger extra cholesterol production in the body. Research subjects that ate 6 times a day had an average of 5% lower levels of cholesterol than those who ate 1 or 2 times a day. This may seems like a small difference, but small changes can add up to a significant impact on your cholesterol level and your ultimate risk for heart disease.

Is there a margarine on the market that lowers cholesterol?

Yes, there are two brands—*Benecol* and *Take Control*—that contain a food ingredient called plant stanols. Plant stanols keep your digestive tract from absorbing cholesterol. The result is lower blood levels of LDL (bad) cholesterol, with no effect on HDL (good) cholesterol. Stanol-containing margarines need to be eaten 2 or 3 times a day to be effective and they cost more than regular margarines. But the stanols are not absorbed into your body, so there are virtually no side effects from their use.

Coming soon—

Scientists at Cambridge University in Britain have developed a cheddar cheese containing plant stanols. Eating about 2 ounces a day can result in a 10% to 13% reduction in cholesterol.

Does drinking wine help lower cholesterol?

Alcohol in moderation, especially red wine, has been linked with higher HDL (good) cholesterol and an overall lower risk for heart disease. For those who don't drink alcohol, purple grape juice also provides a protective effect.

Can cholesterol ever be too low?

Very low cholesterol, below 100, may be a sign of malnutrition, an overactive thyroid, liver damage, or some types of cancer. When total cholesterol values fall below 180, there is an increased risk for hemorrhagic stroke, which is when a blood

Cholesterol Up

Drinking 5 or 6 cups of "French-pressed" coffee a day can increase cholesterol as much as 14%. Boiled European coffee increases cholesterol much more than the filtered drip coffee served in the U.S.

Cholesterol Down

Garlic, pecans, walnuts, almonds, green and black tea, and olive and canola oils all help lower LDL (bad) cholesterol.

vessel bursts instead of becoming clogged with plaque. Ischemic stroke, the clogged-artery type, accounts for 80% of all strokes. Having a cholesterol value between 180 and 200 may be best to avoid both types of stroke.

Why did my doctor give me a drug to lower my cholesterol?

Of the 65 million Americans who need to lower their cholesterol levels, about half should be able to do it by making lifestyle changes. The rest need medication in addition to lifestyle changes. You probably fall into the second half. The good news is that the medications available are very effective and will be even more effective if you exercise, lose weight, don't smoke, and eat well. The bad news is that many people often don't take their medication regularly and some stop taking it altogether. It is important to follow your doctor's instructions and take your medication every day.

COMMON CHOLESTEROL-LOWERING MEDICATIONS

STATINS	BILE ACID SEQUESTRANTS	FIBRIC ACIDS	NIACIN
Crestor	Colestid	gemfibrozil (generic)	Niacor
Lescol	Questran		Niaspin
Lipitor		Lopid	
Mevacor		Tricor	
Pravachol			
Zocor			

FACTS ON FIBER

*Diets rich in fiber can lower cholesterol levels
by 20% or more.*

Fiber is the part of plants your body cannot break down and use. Studies have shown that people who eat more fiber are less likely to have heart disease and type 2 diabetes. Having diabetes puts you at even greater risk of developing heart disease than those who don't have diabetes.

Whole grains, oat bran, beans, and psyllium will help lower cholesterol levels, but all food fibers offer benefits.

Your body uses cholesterol to make bile, which helps you digest fat. Most bile is recycled by the body. When you eat foods high in fiber, the fiber binds with bile and stops it from being recycled. As a result, your body uses up cholesterol to make more bile. If you continue to eat a fiber-rich diet interfering with bile recycling, your cholesterol goes down.

Though we eat a lot of carbohydrates, most people don't eat a lot of fiber. We eat more sugar (soda and candy) and refined carbohydrates (white flour and white bread), and too few fruits and vegetables. We should be eating about 25 grams of fiber a day, but most of us get 15 or less. To reach 25 grams of fiber, aim for 3 to 5 servings of whole grain breads and cereals, 3 servings of fruit, and 3 servings of vegetables a day.

Fiber can be divided into two types: dietary fiber, which is naturally present in foods, and added fiber, which is nondigestible carbohydrate used as a food ingredient. Both have beneficial effects in your body. They help prevent constipation, make you feel full with fewer calories, lower blood sugar levels, and lower blood cholesterol.

Add Some Fiber to Your Life

- Eat fruits and vegetables instead of drinking juice.

- Eat the fiber-rich skins of cucumbers, apples, pears, potatoes, and zucchini.

- Choose whole grains—brown rice, oatmeal, cracked wheat, and whole wheat spaghetti, cereal, and bread.

- Eat beans and lentils a few times a week.

- Try soybeans—soynuts, tofu, tempeh.

- Have vegetarian meals a few times a week.

- Eat dried fruits and raisins.

- Eat bran and wheat germ.

- In addition to food, you may want to try a fiber supplement.

Got Oatmeal?

75% of households have oatmeal in the cupboard. Eating oatmeal or another oat-based cereal, like Cheerios, every day can help lower total cholesterol and LDL (bad) cholesterol.

COUNTING CHOLESTEROL

If you are like most people, you didn't give a lot of thought to what you ate until your doctor told you to "watch your cholesterol." What does this really mean? A moderate cholesterol diet has no more than 300 milligrams of cholesterol a day. A low cholesterol diet has no more than 200 milligrams.

If your total cholesterol is close to 200, your LDL cholesterol is close to 100, and your HDL cholesterol is between 40 and 60, you can eat up to 300 milligrams of cholesterol a day. If any of your numbers are less than desirable, or if your doctor has prescribed a cholesterol-lowering medication, you should eat less than 200 milligrams a day.

Many of the foods listed below are made with whole milk, cheese, or butter, all of which add cholesterol. But there are alternatives that can help you keep your cholesterol down.

INSTEAD OF THIS:	TRY THIS:	MILLIGRAMS CHOLESTEROL SAVED
Cheesecake	Angelfood cake	155
Omelet, plain	Sunny-side-up egg	139
Burrito with beans, cheese, and beef	Burrito with beans	120
Rich vanilla ice cream	Ice pop	118

INSTEAD OF THIS:	TRY THIS:	MILLIGRAMS CHOLESTEROL SAVED
Pecan pie	Apple pie	106
Tossed salad and egg and cheese	Tossed salad	98
Zabaione	Baked custard	90
Potato salad	Mashed potatoes	84
Alfredo sauce	Marinara sauce	75
Chow mein, chicken	Chow mein, vegetable	75
Hamburger patty	Veggie burger patty	71
Pork skins	Popcorn	66
Pound cake	Pound cake, low fat	66
Chicken breast, battered and fried	Chicken breast, roasted	36
Creamed spinach	Leaf spinach	35
Latte with whole milk	Latte with skim milk	29
Roast beef sandwich, with cheese	Roast beef sandwich, plain	25
Blue cheese salad dressing	Italian salad dressing	20
Sour cream	Fat free sour cream	20
White toast with butter	Whole wheat toast with margarine	11

EASY STEPS TO LOWER CHOLESTEROL

- Use liquid vegetable oils—olive, canola, corn, soybean, sunflower, and safflower.
- Limit servings of meat, poultry, fish, and shellfish to 3- to 4-ounce portions.

- Use lean cuts of meat and trim off all visible fat.

- Eat poultry without the skin.

- Whenever possible, cook without adding fat.

- Bake, broil, or roast.

- Use more beans and vegetables to make up for smaller servings of meat, fish, and poultry.

- Limit eggs to four a week, including those used in cooking and desserts.

- Substitute two egg whites for one egg with yolk.

- Use lowfat or nonfat milk, cheese, yogurt, and ice cream, and fat free sour cream.

- Use margarine instead of butter.

- Use lowfat or fat free salad dressings and gravies.

- Eat fiber-rich foods—beans, whole grains, bran, brown rice, dried fruits, fruits, and vegetables.

Now it's your turn to track your cholesterol intake for one day. Based on your blood cholesterol values, decide if you should be eating less than 300 milligrams or less than 200 milligrams a day. Write down everything you eat and drink to get the most realistic picture of one day. Note the amount of fiber you're eating, too. You should do this daily, or at least a few times a week, to be sure you are meeting your cholesterol goals. In *The Cholesterol Counter* you'll find the cholesterol values for more than 20,000 foods, beginning on page 27.

DAILY CHOLESTEROL RECORD

Cholesterol: Aim for _____ mg/day
Fiber: Aim for 25 mg/day

	Cholesterol	Fiber
Breakfast		
Lunch		
Snack		
Dinner		
Snack		
Totals:		

Did your cholesterol total less than 300 milligrams for the day? Did you get enough fiber? If not, you need to start making wiser choices.

USING YOUR CHOLESTEROL COUNTER

The Cholesterol Counter lists the calories, portion size, cholesterol, and fiber of more than 20,000 foods. Now you can compare the values in your favorite foods and, when necessary, choose substitutes when you go out to shop or eat. This will save you time and help you decide what to buy.

With this information at your fingertips, you'll find it easy to eat healthy. A dash (—) appears in some entries. This means that no analysis was done for cholesterol or fiber in that food. It is not the same as a "0", which means there is no cholesterol or fiber in the food.

The counter section of the book is divided into 2 parts—Part 1: Brand Name, Nonbranded, and Take-Out Foods; and Part 2: Restaurant Chains. Each part lists foods or restaurant chains alphabetically.

In Part 1, for each category, you will find nonbranded (generic) foods listed first, in alphabetical order, followed by an alphabetical listing of brand name foods. The nonbranded listing will help you estimate the calorie, cholesterol, and fiber values for foods when you do not see your favorite. They can also help you to evaluate store brands. Large categories are divided into subcategories, such as canned, fresh, frozen, and ready-to-eat, to make it easier to find what you're looking for. Some categories have "see" and "see also" footnotes, to help you find related items.

Because we all eat out so often, we've listed more than 500 take-out foods in Part 1. These are found in the take-out sub-category in many categories throughout this section of the book. Look there for foods you take-out or order in, because these foods are not nutrition labeled.

Most foods are listed alphabetically. But in some cases, foods are grouped by category. For example, a tuna sandwich is found in the SANDWICH category. Other group categories include:

Asian Food   Page 33
    includes all types of Asian foods except
    egg rolls and sushi, which are found in
    separate categories

Deli Meats/Cold Cuts   Page 265
    includes all sandwich meats except
    chicken, ham, and turkey, which are
    found in separate categories

Dinner   Page 270
    includes all by brand name, except
    pasta dinners, which are found in a
    separate category

Liquor/Liqueur   Page 402
    includes all alcoholic beverages except
    beer, champagne, and wine, which are
    found in separate categories

Nutrition Supplements   Page 432
    includes all dieting aids, meal replacers,

and drinks, except energy bars and
energy drinks, which are found in
separate categories

Sandwiches   **Page 554**
includes popular sandwich choices

Spanish Food   **Page 618**
includes all types of Spanish and
Mexican foods except salsa and
tortillas, which are found in separate
categories

In Part 2, Restaurant Chains, we list 78 national and regional restaurant, candy, coffee, doughnut, ice cream, and sandwich chains.

With *The Cholesterol Counter* as your guide, you will never again wonder how much cholesterol is in the food you eat. You will always be able to tell if a food is high, moderate, or low in cholesterol.

DEFINITIONS

as prep (as prepared)—refers to food that has been prepared according to package directions

lean and fat—describes meat with some fat on its edges that is not cut away before cooking, or poultry prepared with skin and fat as purchased

lean only—refers to lean meat that is trimmed of all visible fat, or poultry without skin

shelf stable—refers to prepared products found on the supermarket shelf that are ready-to-eat or are ready to be heated, and do not require refrigeration

take-out—describes prepared dishes that you purchase ready-to-eat; those included serve as a guide to the calories, cholesterol, and fiber in products you may purchase.

ABBREVIATIONS

avg	=	average
diam	=	diameter
fl	=	fluid
frzn	=	frozen
g	=	gram
in	=	inch
lb	=	pound
lg	=	large
med	=	medium
mg	=	milligram
oz	=	ounce
pkg	=	package
pt	=	pint
prep	=	prepared
qt	=	quart
reg	=	regular
sec	=	second
serv	=	serving
sm	=	small
sq	=	square
tbsp	=	tablespoon
tr	=	trace
tsp	=	teaspoon
w/	=	with
w/o	=	without
<	=	less than

NOTES

Cals = Calories

Chol = Cholesterol
   All cholesterol values are given in milligrams (mg)

Fiber = Fiber
   All fiber values are given in grams (g)

tr (trace) = less than 1 mg of cholesterol or 1 gram of fiber

— (dash) indicates data was not available

0 (zero) indicates that there is no cholesterol or fiber in that food

Discrepancies in figures are due to rounding, product reformulation, and reevaluation. Labeling law allows rounding of values. Much of the data listed is analysis data, obtained directly from manufacturers, not from labels. Therefore, some values may differ from labels because they have not been rounded.

PART ONE

Brand Name, Nonbranded (Generic) and Take-Out Foods

Your goal is to pick low cholesterol foods
most of the time.

FOOD	PORTION	CALS	CHOL	FIBER
ABALONE				
fresh fried	3 oz	161	80	–
raw	3 oz	89	72	–
ACEROLA				
fresh	1	2	0	–
ACEROLA JUICE				
juice	1 cup	51	0	–
ADZUKI BEANS				
canned sweetened	1 cup	702	0	–
dried cooked	1 cup	294	0	–
yokan sliced	3¼ in slices	112	0	–
AKEE				
fresh	3.5 oz	223	0	–
ALE (see BEER AND ALE)				
ALFALFA				
sprouts	1 cup	40	0	–
sprouts	1 tbsp	1	0	–
ALLIGATOR				
cooked	3 oz	126	57	0
ALLSPICE				
ground	1 tsp	5	0	–
ALMONDS				
almond butter honey & cinnamon	1 tbsp	96	0	–
almond butter w/ salt	1 tbsp	101	0	–
almond butter w/o salt	1 tbsp	101	0	–
almond meal	1 oz	116	0	–
almond paste	1 oz	127	0	–
dried unblanched	1 oz	167	0	–
dry roasted unblanched	1 oz	167	0	–
dry roasted unblanched salted	1 oz	167	0	–

FOOD	PORTION	CALS	CHOL	FIBER
dry roasted w/ salt	24 nuts (1 oz)	170	0	3
jordan almonds	10 (1.4 oz)	190	0	1
oil roasted blanched	1 oz	174	0	3
oil roasted blanched salted	1 oz	174	0	—
oil roasted unblanched	1 oz	176	0	—
praline	17 pieces (1.4 oz)	210	0	3
toasted unblanched	1 oz	167	0	3
Lance				
Smoked	1 pkg (0.8 oz)	130	0	3
Maranatha				
Raw Almond Butter	2 tbsp	190	0	4
Roasted Almond Butter	2 tbsp	220	0	3
Tamari Almonds	¼ cup	160	0	3
Nutella				
Spread	1 tbsp (0.5 oz)	85	0	—
Planters				
Almonds	1 oz	170	0	3
Gold Measure Slivered	1 pkg (2 oz)	340	0	4
Honey Roasted	1 oz	160	0	2
AMARANTH				
uncooked	1 cup (6.8 oz)	729	0	30
ANISE				
seed	1 tsp	7	0	—
ANTELOPE				
roasted	3 oz	127	107	—
APPLE				
CANNED				
sliced sweetened	1 cup	136	0	—
Del Monte				
Fruit Pleasures Pie Spiced Apples	½ cup (4.1 oz)	70	0	1
Luck's				
Fried Apples	½ cup (4.7 oz)	130	0	2
DRIED				
cooked w/ sugar	½ cup	116	0	—
cooked w/o sugar	½ cup	172	0	—
rings	10	155	0	—

FOOD	PORTION	CALS	CHOL	FIBER
Sonoma				
Pieces	10–12 pieces (1.4 oz)	110	0	4
FRESH				
apple	1	81	0	3
w/o skin sliced	1 cup	62	0	2
w/o skin sliced & cooked	1 cup	91	0	–
w/o skin sliced & microwaved	1 cup	96	0	–
Chiquita				
Apple	1 med (5.4 oz)	80	0	5
Cool Cut				
Apples & Caramel Dip	1 pkg (4.25 oz)	180	5	3
Tastee				
Candy Apple	1 (3 oz)	160	0	4
Caramel Apple	1 (3 oz)	160	0	4
FROZEN				
sliced w/o sugar	½ cup	41	0	–
Stouffer's				
Escalloped	1 cup (6 oz)	180	0	3
TAKE-OUT				
baked	1 (5.3 oz)	126	0	3
baked no sugar	1 (5.9 oz)	82	0	3
APPLE JUICE				
frzn as prep	1 cup	111	0	–
frzn not prep	6 oz	349	0	–
juice	1 cup	116	0	tr
After The Fall				
Organic	1 bottle (10 oz)	110	0	–
Vermont Apple	1 bottle (10 oz)	110	0	–
Vermont Apple	1 bottle (8 oz)	90	0	–
Vermont Harvest Moon Sparkling Apple Cider	8 fl oz	110	0	–
Apple & Eve				
100% Juice	8 fl oz	110	0	–
Cider	8 fl oz	110	0	–
Eden				
Organic Juice	8 oz	80	0	0

FOOD	PORTION	CALS	CHOL	FIBER
Everfresh				
Apple Juice	1 can (8 oz)	110	0	0
Hansen's				
Junior Juice 100%	1 box (4.23 oz)	60	0	1
Hood				
Select Cider	1 cup (8 oz)	120	0	–
Mott's				
100% Juice	8 fl oz	120	0	0
100% Juice	1 box (8 oz)	120	0	–
100% Natural	8 fl oz	120	0	0
Nantucket Nectars				
100% Pressed	8 oz	100	0	–
NutraBalance				
Plus Fibre	1 pkg (8 oz)	120	0	10
Ocean Spray				
100% Juice	8 oz	110	0	0
Snapple				
Snapple Apple	8 fl oz	120	0	–
Swiss Miss				
Hot Apple Cider Mix	1 serv	84	0	1
Hot Apple Cider Mix Low Calorie	1 serv	14	0	0
Tropicana				
Season's Best	8 oz	110	0	–
Turkey Hill				
Herbal Cider w/ Chamomile & Lemongrass	1 cup	100	0	–
Veryfine				
100% Juice	1 bottle (10 oz)	150	0	0
Juice-Ups	8 fl oz	120	0	0
White House				
Juice	8 oz	120	0	–
APPLESAUCE				
sweetened	½ cup	97	0	2
unsweetened	½ cup	53	0	2
Eden				
Organic	½ cup	50	0	2
Organic Sweet Cinnamon	½ cup	50	0	4

FOOD	PORTION	CALS	CHOL	FIBER
Mott's				
Single-Serve Cinnamon	1 pkg (4 oz)	100	0	—
Single-Serve Natural	1 pkg (4 oz)	50	0	—
Single-Serve Original	1 pkg (4 oz)	100	0	—
White House				
Applesauce	½ cup (4.4 oz)	90	0	2
Chunky	½ cup (4.4 oz)	90	0	2
Cinnamon	½ cup (4.5 oz)	100	0	2
Natural Plus	½ cup (4.4 oz)	70	0	2
APRICOT JUICE				
nectar	1 cup	141	0	2
APRICOTS				
CANNED				
halves heavy syrup pack w/ skin	1 cup (9.1 oz)	214	0	—
halves water pack w/ skin	1 cup (8.5 oz)	65	0	—
halves water pack w/o skin	1 cup (8 oz)	51	0	—
heavy syrup w/ skin	3 halves	70	0	—
juice pack w/ skin	3 halves	40	0	—
light syrup w/ skin	3 halves	54	0	—
puree from heavy syrup pack w/ skin	¾ cup (9.1 oz)	214	0	—
puree from light pack w/ skin	¾ cup (8.9 oz)	160	0	—
puree from water pack w/ skin	¾ cup (8.5 oz)	65	0	—
puree juice pack w/skin	1 cup (8.7 oz)	119	0	—
water pack w/ skin	3 halves	22	0	—
water pack w/o skin	4 halves	20	0	—
Del Monte				
Halves Unpeeled Lite	½ cup (4.3 oz)	60	0	1
Orchard Select Halves Unpeeled	½ cup (4.4 oz)	80	0	1
DRIED				
halves	10	83	0	3

FOOD	PORTION	CALS	CHOL	FIBER
halves cooked w/o sugar	½ cup	106	0	–
Del Monte				
Sun Dried	⅓ cup (1.4 oz)	80	0	6
Sonoma				
Dried	10 pieces (1.4 oz)	120	0	1
FRESH				
apricots	3	51	0	–
Chiquita				
Apricots	3 med (4 oz)	60	0	1
FROZEN				
sweetened	½ cup	119	0	–
ARROWHEAD				
fresh boiled	1 med (⅓ oz)	9	0	–
ARROWROOT				
flour	1 cup (4.5 oz)	457	0	4
ARTICHOKE				
CANNED				
Progresso				
Hearts	2 pieces (2.9 oz)	30	0	1
Hearts Marinated	2 pieces (1.1 oz)	170	0	0
S&W				
Marinated Hearts	2 pieces (1 oz)	20	0	1
FRESH				
boiled	1 med (4 oz)	60	0	–
hearts cooked	½ cup	42	0	–
FROZEN				
cooked	1 pkg (9 oz)	108	0	–
Birds Eye				
Hearts	½ cup	40	0	6
ARUGULA				
fresh	½ cup	2	0	–
ASIAN FOOD (see also DINNER, EGG ROLLS, SUSHI)				
CANNED				
chow mein chicken	1 cup	95	8	–
Chun King				
Beef Pepper Oriental BiPack	1 cup (8.8 oz)	98	14	3

FOOD	PORTION	CALS	CHOL	FIBER
Chow Mein Beef BiPack	1 cup (8.6 oz)	78	6	3
Chow Mein BiPack Chicken	1 cup (8.8 oz)	98	6	3
Chow Mein Pork BiPack	1 cup (8.6 oz)	78	10	2
Hot & Spicy Chicken BiPack	1 cup (8.6 oz)	98	19	1
Sweet & Sour Chicken BiPack	1 cup (8.9 oz)	161	25	3
La Choy				
Beef Pepper Oriental BiPack	1 cup (8.8 oz)	98	14	3
Chow Mein Beef BiPack	1 cup (8.6 oz)	78	6	3
Chow Mein Chicken BiPack	1 cup (8.9 oz)	98	6	3
Chow Mein Shrimp BiPack	1 cup (8.6 oz)	52	4	3
Main Entree Chow Mein Chicken	1 cup (9.3 oz)	80	9	3
Oriental Beef w/ Noodles BiPack	1 cup (8.8 oz)	156	17	4
Oriental Chicken w/ Noodles BiPack	1 cup (8.7 oz)	154	23	2
Sweet & Sour Chicken BiPack	1 cup (8.9 oz)	161	25	3
Teriyaki Chicken BiPack	1 cup (8.6 oz)	109	20	3
FRESH				
wonton wrappers	1	23	1	–
Azumaya				
Round Wraps	10	160	10	1
Square Wraps	6	160	10	1
Wrappers Large Square	3	170	10	1
Nasoya				
Egg Roll Wrapper	3	170	10	1
Won Ton Wrappers	8	160	10	1
FROZEN				
Amy's				
Bowls Teriyaki	1 pkg (10 oz)	300	0	3

FOOD	PORTION	CALS	CHOL	FIBER
Skillet Meals Teriyaki Stir Fry	1 cup	320	0	4
Stir Fry Thai	1 pkg (9.5 oz)	270	0	2
Banquet				
Fried Rice w/ Chicken & Egg Rolls	1 meal (8.5 oz)	330	60	5
Birds Eye				
Easy Recipe Creations Oriental Lo Mein	2¼ cups	230	5	2
Easy Recipe Creations Sesame Ginger Teriyaki	2¼ cups	140	0	4
Easy Recipe Creations Spicy Szechuan Cashews	2¼ cups	180	0	4
Green Giant				
Create A Meal LoMein Stir Fry as prep	1¼ cups (10 oz)	320	60	4
Create A Meal Sweet & Sour Stir Fry as prep	1¼ cups (10 oz)	290	60	5
Create A Meal Szechuan Stir Fry as prep	1¼ cups (10 oz)	340	60	5
Create A Meal Teriyaki Stir Fry as prep	1¼ cups (10 oz)	240	55	4
La Choy				
Beef Pepper Oriental	1 cup (7.1 oz)	151	10	2
Chow Mein Vegetable	1 cup (8.9 oz)	108	0	5
Lean Cuisine				
Everyday Favorites Oriental Style Dumplings	1 pkg (9 oz)	300	20	2
Everyday Favorites Teriyaki Stir Fry	1 pkg (10 oz)	290	20	4
Luigino's				
Chicken & Almonds With Rice	1 pkg (8 oz)	250	20	3
Chop Suey Pork With Rice	1 pkg (8.5 oz)	210	15	2

FOOD	PORTION	CALS	CHOL	FIBER
Lo Mein Chicken	1 pkg (8 oz)	320	15	3
Lo Mein Shrimp	1 pkg (8 oz)	190	15	4
Oriental Beef & Peppers With Rice	1 pkg (8 oz)	230	10	2
Rice Gourmet				
Chicken Teriyaki Rice Bowl	1 bowl (10.9 oz)	430	25	1
Stouffer's				
Chicken Chow Mein w/ Rice	1 pkg (10.6 oz)	260	25	3
Tyson				
Chicken Fried Rice Kit w/ Sauce	1 pkg (14 oz)	440	30	5
Weight Watchers				
Smart Ones Chicken Chow Mein	1 pkg (9 oz)	200	25	3
Smart Ones Hunan Style Rice & Vegetables	1 pkg (10.34 oz)	280	0	5
Smart Ones King Pao Noodles & Vegetables	1 pkg (10 oz)	250	5	5
Smart Ones Spicy Szechaun Style Vegetables & Chicken	1 pkg (9 oz)	220	10	3
MIX				
Annie Chun's				
Chow Mein Noodles w/Garlic Scallion Sauce	1 serv	240	0	2
TAKE-OUT				
buddha's delight w/ cellophane noodles fat choi jai	1 serv (7.6 oz)	211	tr	2
cha siu bao steamed buns w/ chicken filling	1 (2.3 oz)	160	15	tr
chicken teriyaki	¾ cup	399	92	–
chicken teriyaki w/ rice	1 serv (11 oz)	430	25	1
chop suey w/ beef & pork	1 cup	300	68	–
chop suey w/ pork	1 cup	375	62	2

FOOD	PORTION	CALS	CHOL	FIBER
chow mein chicken	1 cup	255	75	–
chow mein pork	1 cup	425	89	3
chow mein shrimp	1 cup	221	55	3
chow mein vegetable	1 serv (8 oz)	90	0	4
filipino chicken adobo	1 serv (15 oz)	555	116	1
fried rice vegetable	1 cup	210	0	1
phad thai	1 serv (9.2 oz)	232	0	1
sesame seed paste bun	1 (2.5 oz)	220	0	2
shrimp chips	1¼ cups (1 oz)	140	0	0
shu mai chicken & vegetable dumplings	6 (3.6 oz)	160	35	1
sweet & sour pork	1 serv (8 oz)	250	30	2
sweet red bean bun	1 (2.5 oz)	130	0	2
szechuan chicken w/ lo mein	1 cup (5.3 oz)	190	5	0
wonton fried	½ cup (1 oz)	111	31	1
wonton soup	1 cup	205	89	1

ASPARAGUS
CANNED

FOOD	PORTION	CALS	CHOL	FIBER
spears	½ cup	24	0	–
Del Monte				
Cuts & Tips	½ cup (4.4 oz)	20	0	1
Spears Extra Long	½ cup (4.4 oz)	20	0	1
Spears Tender Young	½ cup (4.4 oz)	20	0	1
Tips Hand Selected	½ cup (4.4 oz)	20	0	1
Green Giant				
Cut Spears	½ cup (4.2 oz)	20	0	1
Cut Spears 50% Less Sodium	½ cup (4.2 oz)	20	0	1
Extra Long Spears	4.5 oz	20	0	1
Spears	4.5 oz	20	0	1
LeSueur				
Spears Extra Large	4.5 oz	20	0	1
Owatonna				
Spears Cut	½ cup	20	0	–
S&W				
Green	6 pieces (4.5 oz)	15	0	1
FRESH				
cooked	4 spears	14	0	–

FOOD	PORTION	CALS	CHOL	FIBER
cooked	½ cup	22	0	—
raw	½ cup	16	0	—
raw	4 spears	14	0	—
FROZEN				
cooked	4 spears	17	0	—
cooked	1 pkg (10 oz)	82	0	—
Birds Eye				
Cuts	½ cup	25	0	2
Jumbo Spears	3 oz	20	0	1
Green Giant				
Harvest Fresh Cuts	⅔ cup (3 oz)	25	0	1
AVOCADO				
fresh	1	324	0	—
fresh mashed	1 cup	370	0	—
Chiquita				
Fresh	⅓ med (1 oz)	55	0	3
TAKE-OUT				
guacamole	1 serv (2.2 oz)	105	0	2
BACON				
breakfast strips cooked	3 strips	156	36	0
pan fried	3 strips	109	16	0
Armour				
Star cooked	1 strip	38	6	—
Black Label				
Center Cut cooked	3 slices (0.5 oz)	70	15	0
Cooked	2 slices (0.5 oz)	80	15	0
Low Salt cooked	2 slices (0.5 oz)	80	15	0
Health Is Wealth				
Uncured Sliced	2 slices (0.5 oz)	70	10	—
Hormel				
Bacon Bits	1 tbsp (7 g)	30	5	0
Bacon Pieces	1 tbsp (7 g)	25	10	0
Microwave cooked	2 slices (0.5 oz)	70	15	0
Old Smokehouse				
Cooked	2 slices (0.5 oz)	80	15	0
Oscar Mayer				
Bacon Bits	1 tbsp (0.2 oz)	25	5	0
Bacon Pieces	1 tbsp (0.2 oz)	25	5	0
Center Cut cooked	2 slices (0.4 oz)	70	15	0

FOOD	PORTION	CALS	CHOL	FIBER
Cooked	2 slices (0.5 oz)	70	15	0
Lower Sodium cooked	2 slices (0.5 oz)	70	15	0
Thick Cut cooked	1 slice (0.4 oz)	60	10	0
Range Brand				
Cooked	2 slices (0.7 oz)	100	20	0
Ready Crisp				
Fully Cooked	3 slices (0.5 oz)	70	15	–
Red Label				
Cooked	2 slices (0.5 oz)	80	15	0
BACON SUBSTITUTES				
bacon substitute	1 strip	25	0	–
Bac-Os				
Chips or Bits	1½ tbsp (7 g)	30	0	0
Lightlife				
Fakin' Bacon Bits	1 tsp	45	0	0
Smart Bacon	2 strips (0.8 oz)	45	0	0
Louis Rich				
Turkey Bacon	1 slice (0.5 oz)	35	15	0
McCormick				
Bac'n Pieces	2 tsp	20	0	–
Morningstar Farms				
Breakfast Strips	2 (0.5 oz)	60	0	tr
Mr. Turkey				
Slice	1	25	10	–
Worthington				
Stripples	2 strips (0.5 oz)	60	0	tr
BAGEL				
cinnamon raisin	1 (3½ in)	194	0	–
cinnamon raisin toasted	1 (3½ in)	194	0	–
egg	1 (3½ in)	197	17	–
egg toasted	1 (3½ in)	197	17	–
mini onion	1 (1.4 oz)	100	0	1
oat bran	1 (3½ in)	181	0	–
oat bran toasted	1 (3½ in)	181	0	–
onion	1 (3½ in)	195	0	2
plain	1 (3½ in)	195	0	2
plain toasted	1 (3½ in)	195	0	2
poppy seed	1 (3½ in)	195	0	2

FOOD	PORTION	CALS	CHOL	FIBER
Alvarado St. Bakery				
Sprouted Wheat	1 (3.3 oz)	260	0	2
Sprouted Wheat Cinnamon/Raisin	1 (3.3 oz)	280	0	3
Sprouted Wheat Onion/Poppyseed	1 (3.3 oz)	320	0	2
Sprouted Wheat Sesame	1 (3.3 oz)	320	0	2
Otis Spunkmeyer				
Barnstormin' Blueberry	1 (3.6 oz)	250	0	3
Barnstormin' Cinnamon Raisin	1 (3.6 oz)	230	0	3
Barnstormin' Onion	1 (3.6 oz)	230	0	3
Barnstormin' Plain	1 (3.6 oz)	240	0	3
Pepperidge Farm				
Mini	1 (1.4 oz)	120	0	tr
Plain	1 (3.5 oz)	290	0	2
Sara Lee				
Blueberry	1 (2.8 oz)	210	0	2
Cinnamon Raisin	1 (2.8 oz)	220	0	3
Egg	1 (2.8 oz)	210	0	2
Oat Bran	1 (2.8 oz)	210	0	3
Onion	1 (2.8 oz)	210	0	2
Plain	1 (2.8 oz)	210	0	2
Poppy Seed	1 (2.8 oz)	210	0	2
Sesame Seed	1 (2.8 oz)	210	0	2
Thomas'				
Everything	1 (3.6 oz)	300	0	3
Multi-Grain	1 (3.6 oz)	280	0	4
Plain	1 (3.6 oz)	280	0	2
Uncle B's				
Plain	1 (2.8 oz)	210	0	2
Wonder				
Blueberry	1 (3 oz)	210	0	1
Cinnamon Raisin	1 (3 oz)	210	0	2
Onion	1 (3 oz)	210	0	1
Plain	1 (3 oz)	210	0	2
Rye	1 (3 oz)	220	0	2
Wheat	1 (3 oz)	210	0	2

FOOD	PORTION	CALS	CHOL	FIBER
BAKING POWDER				
baking powder	1 tsp	2	0	–
low sodium	1 tsp	5	0	–
Calumet				
Baking Powder	¼ tsp (1 g)	0	0	0
Watkins				
Baking Powder	¼ tsp (1 g)	0	0	0
BAKING SODA				
baking soda	1 tsp	0	0	–
BALSAM PEAR				
leafy tips cooked	½ cup	10	0	–
leafy tips raw	½ cup	7	0	–
pods cooked	½ cup	12	0	–
BAMBOO SHOOTS				
canned sliced	1 cup	25	0	–
fresh	½ cup	21	0	–
fresh cooked	½ cup	15	0	–
Chun King				
Bamboo Shoots	2 tbsp (0.8 oz)	3	0	tr
La Choy				
Bamboo Shoots	2 tbsp (0.8 oz)	3	0	tr
BANANA				
banana chips	1 oz	147	0	2
fresh	1	105	0	2
fresh mashed	1 cup	207	0	4
powder	1 tbsp	21	0	–
Chiquita				
Fresh	1 med (4.4 oz)	110	0	4
Rainforest Farms				
Slices Dried	5 slices (1.3 oz)	60	0	–
BARBECUE SAUCE				
barbecue	1 cup	188	0	–
Bull's Eye				
Original	2 tbsp	50	0	–
Healthy Choice				
Hickory	2 tbsp (1.1 oz)	26	0	tr
Hot & Spicy	2 tbsp (1.1 oz)	25	0	tr

FOOD	PORTION	CALS	CHOL	FIBER
Original	2 tbsp (1.1 oz)	25	0	tr
House Of Tsang				
Hong Kong	1 tbsp (0.6 oz)	10	0	0
Hunt's				
Bold Hickory	2 tbsp (1.2 oz)	47	0	1
Bold Original	2 tbsp (1.2 oz)	46	0	1
Hickory & Brown Sugar	2 tbsp (1.3 oz)	75	0	1
Honey Hickory	2 tbsp (1.2 oz)	54	0	1
Honey Mustard	2 tbsp (1.2 oz)	48	0	1
Hot & Spicy	2 tbsp (1.2 oz)	48	0	1
Light Original	2 tbsp (1.2 oz)	23	0	1
Mesquite	2 tbsp (1.2 oz)	40	0	1
Mild	2 tbsp (1.2 oz)	41	0	1
Mild Dijon	2 tbsp (1.2 oz)	39	0	tr
Open Range Original	2 tbsp (1.2 oz)	39	0	1
Open Range Premier	2 tbsp (1.3 oz)	56	0	1
Open Range Smokey	2 tbsp (1.2 oz)	37	0	1
Original	2 tbsp (1.2 oz)	40	0	1
Teriyaki	2 tbsp (1.2 oz)	46	0	1
Kraft				
Char-Grill	2 tbsp (1.3 oz)	60	0	0
Extra Rich Original	2 tbsp (1.2 oz)	50	0	0
Hickory Smoke	2 tbsp (1.2 oz)	40	0	0
Hickory Smoke Onion Bits	2 tbsp (1.2 oz)	45	0	0
Honey	2 tbsp (1.3 oz)	50	0	0
Honey Hickory	2 tbsp (1.3 oz)	60	0	0
Honey Mustard	2 tbsp (1.3 oz)	60	0	0
Hot	2 tbsp (1.2 oz)	40	0	0
Hot Hickory Smoke	2 tbsp (1.2 oz)	40	0	0
Kansas City Style	2 tbsp (1.2 oz)	50	0	0
Mesquite Smoke	2 tbsp (1.2 oz)	40	0	0
Molasses	2 tbsp (1.3 oz)	70	0	0
Onion Bits	2 tbsp (1.2 oz)	45	0	0
Original	2 tbsp (1.2 oz)	40	0	0
Roasted Garlic	2 tbsp (1.2 oz)	50	0	0
Spicy Honey	2 tbsp (1.3 oz)	60	0	0
Teriyaki	2 tbsp (1.3 oz)	60	0	0
Thick'N Spicy Brown Sugar	2 tbsp (1.2 oz)	60	0	0

FOOD	PORTION	CALS	CHOL	FIBER
Thick'N Spicy Hickory Bacon	2 tbsp (1.2 oz)	60	0	0
Thick'N Spicy Hickory Smoke	2 tbsp (1.2 oz)	50	0	0
Thick'N Spicy Hickory Smoke	2 tbsp (1.2 oz)	50	0	0
Thick'N Spicy Honey	2 tbsp (1.2 oz)	60	0	0
Thick'N Spicy Honey	2 tbsp (1.3 oz)	60	0	0
Thick'N Spicy Honey Mustard	2 tbsp (1.3 oz)	60	0	0
Thick'N Spicy Kansas City Style	2 tbsp (1.3 oz)	60	0	0
Thick'N Spicy Mesquite Smoke	2 tbsp (1.2 oz)	50	0	0
Thick'N Spicy Original	2 tbsp (1.2 oz)	50	0	0
Lawry's				
Dijon Honey	¼ cup	203	0	tr
McIlhenny				
Sauce	2 tbsp (1.1 oz)	70	0	tr
Muir Glen				
Garlic Mesquite	2 tbsp (1.3 oz)	40	0	tr
Hot & Smoky	2 tbsp (1.2 oz)	40	0	tr
Original	2 tbsp (1.2 oz)	40	0	tr
Red Wing				
"K" Sauce	2 tbsp (1.2 oz)	45	0	0
Watkins				
Bold	2 tsp (0.4 oz)	25	0	0
Honey	2 tsp (0.4 oz)	25	0	0
Mesquite	2 tsp (0.4 oz)	25	0	0
Original	2 tsp (0.4 oz)	25	0	0
Smokehouse	2 tsp (0.4 oz)	25	0	0
BARLEY				
flour	1 cup (5.2 oz)	511	0	15
malt flour	1 cup (5.7 oz)	585	0	12
pearled cooked	1 cup (5.5 oz)	193	0	6
pearled uncooked	1 cup (7 oz)	704	0	31
BARRACUDA				
fresh	3 oz	122	66	0

FOOD	PORTION	CALS	CHOL	FIBER
BASIL				
fresh chopped	2 tbsp	1	0	—
ground	1 tsp	4	0	—
leaves fresh	5	1	0	—
Watkins				
Liquid Spice	1 tbsp (0.5 oz)	120	0	0
BASS				
freshwater raw	3 oz	97	58	—
sea cooked	3 oz	105	45	—
sea raw	3 oz	82	35	—
striped baked	3 oz	105	87	—
BAY LEAF				
crumbled	1 tsp	2	0	—
Watkins				
Bay Leaves	¼ tsp (0.5 g)	0	0	0
BEAN SPROUTS (see ALFALFA, SPROUTS)				
BEANS (see also individual names)				
CANNED				
baked beans plain	½ cup	118	0	10
baked beans vegetarian	½ cup	118	0	10
baked beans w/ beef	½ cup	161	29	—
baked beans w/ franks	½ cup	182	8	9
baked beans w/ pork	½ cup	133	9	7
baked beans w/ pork & sweet sauce	½ cup	140	9	7
baked beans w/ pork & tomato sauce	½ cup	123	9	7
Amy's				
Vegetarian Baked	½ cup	120	0	6
B&M				
99% Fat Free Baked Beans	½ cup (4.6 oz)	160	0	7
Baked With Honey	½ cup (4.7 oz)	170	0	8
Barbeque Baked Beans	½ cup (4.6 oz)	210	0	9
Brick Oven Baked	½ cup (4.6 oz)	180	5	7
Extra Hearty Baked	½ cup (4.6 oz)	190	<5	8

FOOD	PORTION	CALS	CHOL	FIBER
Bush's				
Baked With Onions	½ cup (4.6 oz)	150	5	6
Barbecue	½ cup (4.6 oz)	160	0	6
Homestyle Baked	½ cup (4.6 oz)	160	5	8
Maple Cured Bacon	½ cup (4.6 oz)	150	0	7
Vegetarian	½ cup (4.6 oz)	130	0	6
Chi-Chi's				
Refried	½ cup (4.2 oz)	100	0	4
Refried Beans Fat Free	½ cup (4.2 oz)	120	0	4
Refried Beans Vegetarian	½ cup (4.2 oz)	100	0	4
Eden				
Organic Baked w/ Sorghum & Mustard	½ cup (4.6 oz)	150	0	7
Friend's				
Original Baked	½ cup (4.6 oz)	170	<5	7
Gebhardt				
Chili	½ cup (4.6 oz)	134	0	7
Refried Jalapeno	½ cup (4.5 oz)	105	1	6
Refried No Fat	½ cup (4.5 oz)	92	0	6
Refried Traditional	½ cup (4.5 oz)	109	1	6
Refried Vegetarian	½ cup (4.5 oz)	118	tr	7
Green Giant				
Pork And Beans w/ Tomato Sauce	½ cup (4.5 oz)	120	0	4
Spicy Chili	½ cup (4.5 oz)	110	0	5
Three Bean Salad	½ cup (4.2 oz)	90	0	4
Health Valley				
Honey Baked	½ cup	110	0	7
Honey Baked No Salt	½ cup	110	0	7
Heartland				
Iron Kettle Baked	½ cup (4.6 oz)	150	<5	5
Hormel				
Beans & Wieners	1 can (7.5 oz)	290	50	6
Hunt's				
Big John's Beans & Fixin's	½ cup (4.7 oz)	127	3	6
Homestyle Country Kettle	½ cup (4.6 oz)	152	1	7

FOOD	PORTION	CALS	CHOL	FIBER
Homestyle Special Recipe	½ cup (4.7 oz)	185	1	8
Mix & Serve	½ cup (4.7 oz)	125	1	8
Pork & Beans	½ cup (4.6 oz)	157	2	7
Pork & Beans	½ cup (4.5 oz)	130	tr	4
Kid's Kitchen				
Microwave Meals Beans & Weiners	1 cup (7.5 oz)	310	45	8
Old El Paso				
Mexe-Beans	½ cup (4.6 oz)	110	0	7
Refried	½ cup (4.2 oz)	110	<5	5
Refried Fat Free	½ cup (4.4 oz)	110	0	6
Refried Spicy	½ cup (4.3 oz)	140	<5	6
Refried Vegetarian	½ cup (4.1 oz)	100	0	6
Refried With Cheese	½ cup (4.2 oz)	130	5	6
Refried With Green Chilies	½ cup (4.3 oz)	110	<5	6
Refried With Sausage	½ cup (4.1 oz)	200	10	8
Open Range				
Ranch	½ cup (4.4 oz)	124	1	8
Pringles				
Vegetarian	1 cup (7.9 oz)	250	0	9
Rosarita				
3 Bean Recipe Bacon & Jalapeno	½ cup (4.6 oz)	117	1	5
3 Bean Recipe Chiles & Chicken	½ cup (4.6 oz)	115	1	4
3 Bean Recipe Chilies & Chorizo	½ cup (4.6 oz)	111	1	4
3 Bean Recipe Onions & Peppers	½ cup (4.6 oz)	104	1	5
Fiesta Beans Bacon & Jalapenos	½ cup (4.6 oz)	117	1	5
Fiesta Beans Chicken & Chilies	½ cup (4.6 oz)	115	1	4
Fiesta Beans Chilies & Chorizo	½ cup (4.6 oz)	110	1	4
Fiesta Beans Onions & Peppers	½ cup (4.6 oz)	104	1	5
Refried Bacon	½ cup (4.5 oz)	116	1	8

FOOD	PORTION	CALS	CHOL	FIBER
Refried Green Chile	½ cup (4.5 oz)	110	1	7
Refried Low Fat Black	½ cup (4.5 oz)	107	0	7
Refried Nacho Cheese	½ cup (4.5 oz)	108	2	6
Refried No Fat	½ cup (4.5 oz)	120	0	6
Refried No Fat Green Chiles & Lime	½ cup (4.5 oz)	101	0	8
Refried No Fat w/ Zesty Salsa	½ cup (4.5 oz)	105	0	6
Refried Onion	½ cup (4.5 oz)	114	1	6
Refried Spicy	½ cup (4.5 oz)	118	0	6
Refried Traditional	½ cup (4.5 oz)	108	0	5
Refried Vegetarian	½ cup (4.5 oz)	237	tr	13
S&W				
Barbecue Beans Ranch Recipe	½ cup (4.5 oz)	100	0	8
Taco Bell				
Home Originals Fat Free Refried Beans	½ cup (4.6 oz)	110	0	6
Home Originals Fat Free Refried Beans w/ Mild Chilies	½ cup (4.5 oz)	110	0	5
Home Originals Refried Beans	½ cup (4.7 oz)	140	0	7
Van Camp				
Baked Fat Free	½ cup (4.6 oz)	132	0	5
Baked Original	½ cup (4.7 oz)	143	1	6
Baked Southern Style Sauteed Onion	½ cup (4.8 oz)	145	1	8
Baked Sweet Hickory & Bacon	1 can (4.8 oz)	143	tr	6
Beanee Weenee BBQ	1 cup (7.7 oz)	290	35	7
Beanee Weenee Baked	1 cup (9.1 oz)	410	40	10
Beanee Weenee Microwave	1 cup (7.5 oz)	260	35	6
Beanee Weenee Original	1 cup (9.1 oz)	320	40	8
Beanee Weenee Zestful	1 cup (7.7 oz)	300	35	7
Brown Sugar	½ cup (4.6 oz)	170	5	6
Pork And Beans	½ cup (4.6 oz)	110	0	6
Vegetarian	½ cup (4.6 oz)	110	0	5

FOOD	PORTION	CALS	CHOL	FIBER
FROZEN				
Natural Touch				
Nine Bean Loaf	1 in slice (3 oz)	160	<5	5
MIX				
Melting Pot				
Terrazza Napoli Mixed Beans	1 cup	200	<5	2
TAKE-OUT				
baked beans	½ cup	190	6	–
barbecue beans	3.5 oz	120	0	–
four bean salad	3.5 oz	100	0	–
refried beans	½ cup	43	2	–
three bean salad	¾ cup	230	0	1
BEECHNUTS				
dried	1 oz	164	0	–
BEEF *(see also* BEEF DISHES, VEAL*)*				
CANNED				
corned beef	1 oz	71	24	–
Armour				
Chopped Beef	2 oz	170	40	0
Corned Beef	2 oz	120	50	0
Potted Meat	1 can (3 oz)	120	75	0
Tripe	3 oz	90	125	0
Hormel				
Corned Beef	2 oz	120	50	0
Cubed Beef	½ cup (4.9 oz)	130	60	0
Potted Meat	4 tbsp (2 oz)	100	50	0
Treet				
Luncheon Loaf	2 oz	130	50	0
Luncheon Loaf 50% Less Fat	2 oz	110	45	0
DRIED				
Armour				
Sliced	7 slices (1 oz)	60	25	0
Hormel				
Pillow Pack	10 slices (1 oz)	45	20	0
FRESH				
bottom round lean & fat trim 0 in Choice roasted	3 oz	172	66	–

FOOD	PORTION	CALS	CHOL	FIBER
bottom round lean & fat trim 0 in braised	3 oz	193	82	–
bottom round lean & fat trim ¼ in Choice braised	3 oz	241	81	–
bottom round lean & fat trim ¼ in Choice roasted	3 oz	221	68	–
brisket flat half lean & fat trim 0 in braised	3 oz	183	81	–
brisket flat half lean & fat trim ¼ in braised	3 oz	309	81	–
brisket point half lean & fat trim 0 in braised	3 oz	304	78	–
brisket point half lean & fat trim ¼ in braised	3 oz	343	79	–
brisket whole lean & fat trim 0 in braised	3 oz	247	79	–
brisket whole lean & fat trim ¼ in braised	3 oz	327	80	–
chuck arm pot roast lean & fat trim 0 in braised	3 oz	238	85	–
chuck arm pot roast lean & fat trim ¼ in braised	3 oz	282	85	–
chuck blade roast lean & fat trim 0 in braised	3 oz	284	88	–
chuck blade roast lean & fat trim ¼ in braised	3 oz	293	88	–
corned beef brisket cooked	3 oz	213	83	–
eye of round lean & fat trim 0 in Choice roasted	3 oz	153	59	–
eye of round lean & fat trim ¼ in Choice roasted	3 oz	205	62	–

FOOD	PORTION	CALS	CHOL	FIBER
flank lean & fat trim 0 in braised	3 oz	224	62	—
flank lean & fat trim 0 in broiled	3 oz	192	58	—
ground extra lean broiled medium	3 oz	217	71	—
ground extra lean broiled well done	3 oz	225	84	—
ground extra lean fried medium	3 oz	216	69	—
ground extra lean fried well done	3 oz	224	79	—
ground extra lean raw	4 oz	265	78	—
ground lean broiled medium	3 oz	231	74	—
ground lean broiled well done	3 oz	238	86	—
ground regular broiled medium	3 oz	246	76	—
ground regular broiled well done	3 oz	248	86	—
ground low-fat w/ carrageenan raw	4 oz	160	53	—
porterhouse steak lean & fat trim ¼ in Choice broiled	3 oz	260	70	—
porterhouse steak lean only trim ¼ in Prime broiled	3 oz	185	68	—
rib eye small end lean & fat trim 0 in Choice broiled	3 oz	261	70	—
rib large end lean & fat trim 0 in roasted	3 oz	300	72	—
rib large end lean & fat trim ¼ in broiled	3 oz	295	69	—
rib large end lean & fat trim ¼ in roasted	3 oz	310	72	—
rib small end lean & fat trim 0 in broiled	3 oz	252	70	—

FOOD	PORTION	CALS	CHOL	FIBER
rib small end lean & fat trim ¼ in broiled	3 oz	285	71	—
rib small end lean & fat trim ¼ in roasted	3 oz	295	71	—
rib whole lean & fat trim ¼ in Choice broiled	3 oz	306	70	—
rib whole lean & fat trim ¼ in Choice roasted	3 oz	320	72	—
rib whole lean & fat trim ¼ in Prime roasted	3 oz	348	72	—
shank crosscut lean & fat trim ¼ in Choice simmered	3 oz	224	68	—
short loin top loin lean & fat trim 0 in Choice broiled	3 oz	193	65	—
short loin top loin lean & fat trim 0 in Choice broiled	1 steak (5.4 oz)	353	119	—
short loin top loin lean & fat trim ¼ in Choice braised	3 oz	253	68	—
short loin top loin lean & fat trim ¼ in Choice broiled	1 steak (6.3 oz)	536	143	—
short loin top loin lean & fat trim ¼ in Prime broiled	1 steak (6.3 oz)	582	143	—
short loin top loin lean only trim 0 in Choice broiled	1 steak (5.2 oz)	311	113	—
short loin top loin lean only trim ¼ in Choice broiled	1 steak (5.2 oz)	314	112	—
shortribs lean & fat Choice braised	3 oz	400	80	—
t-bone steak lean & fat trim ¼ in Choice broiled	3 oz	253	70	—

FOOD	PORTION	CALS	CHOL	FIBER
t-bone steak lean only trim ¼ in Choice broiled	3 oz	182	68	—
tenderloin lean & fat trim ¼ in Choice broiled	3 oz	259	73	—
tenderloin lean & fat trim ¼ in Choice roasted	3 oz	288	73	—
tenderloin lean & fat trim ¼ in Choice broiled	3 oz	208	72	—
tenderloin lean & fat trim ¼ in Prime broiled	3 oz	270	73	—
tenderloin lean only trim ¼ in Choice broiled	3 oz	188	71	—
tip round lean & fat trim 0 in Choice roasted	3 oz	170	69	—
tip round lean & fat trim ¼ in Choice roasted	3 oz	210	70	—
tip round lean & fat trim ¼ in Prime roasted	3 oz	233	70	—
top round lean & fat trim 0 in Choice braised	3 oz	184	77	—
top round lean & fat trim ¼ in Choice braised	3 oz	221	77	—
top round lean & fat trim ¼ in Choice broiled	3 oz	190	72	—
top round lean & fat trim ¼ in Choice fried	3 oz	235	82	—

FOOD	PORTION	CALS	CHOL	FIBER
top round lean & fat trim ¼ in Prime broiled	3 oz	195	72	–
top sirloin lean & fat trim 0 in Choice broiled	3 oz	194	76	–
top sirloin lean & fat trim ¼ in Choice broiled	3 oz	228	76	–
top sirloin lean & fat trim ¼ in Choice fried	3 oz	277	83	–
tripe raw	4 oz	111	107	–
Healthy Choice				
Ground Extra Lean	4 oz	130	55	0
Laura's Lean				
Eye Of Round	4 oz	140	60	–
Flank Steak	4 oz	140	50	–
Ground 92% Lean	4 oz	160	60	–
Ground Round 94% Lean	4 oz	140	60	–
Ribeye Steak	4 oz	140	60	–
Sirloin Tip Round	4 oz	120	65	–
Sirloin Top Butt	4 oz	140	60	–
Strip Steak	4 oz	140	55	–
Tenderloins	4 oz	140	65	–
Top Round	4 oz	130	55	–
Maverick Ranch				
Ground Round Extra Lean	4 oz	130	60	–
Organic Valley				
Extra Lean Ground	3 oz	130	55	0
Extra Lean Patties	1 (3.2 oz)	130	60	0
FROZEN				
patties broiled medium	3 oz	240	80	–
READY-TO-EAT				
smoked beef cooked	1 sausage (1.4 oz)	134	29	–
Alpine Lace				
Roast Beef 97% Fat Free	2 oz	70	40	0

FOOD	PORTION	CALS	CHOL	FIBER
Boar's Head				
Corned Beef Brisket	2 oz	80	40	0
Eye Round Pepper Seasoned	2 oz	90	40	0
Italian Style Oven Roasted Top Round	2 oz	80	40	0
Roast Beef Cajun	2 oz	80	35	0
Top Round Deluxe	2 oz	90	30	0
Top Round Oven Roasted No Salt Added	2 oz	90	30	0
Healthy Choice				
Deli-Thin Roast Beef	6 slices (2 oz)	60	25	0
Fresh-Trak Roast Beef	1 slice (1 oz)	30	10	0
Jordan's				
Healthy Trim 97% Fat Free Roast Beef Medium	1 slice (1 oz)	30	20	0
Healthy Trim 97% Fat Free Roast Beef Rare	1 slice (1 oz)	30	20	0
Tyson				
Beef Strips Seasoned	1 serv (3 oz)	140	55	0
TAKE-OUT				
roast beef medium	2 oz	70	30	–
roast beef rare	2 oz	70	30	–
BEEF DISHES				
CANNED				
Armour				
Corned Beef Hash	1 cup (8.3 oz)	440	100	2
Corned Beef Hash w/ Peppers & Onions	1 cup (8.3 oz)	270	100	3
Roast Beef Hash	1 cup (8.4 oz)	400	95	3
Roast Beef In Gravy	½ cup (4.6 oz)	150	75	0
Stew	1 cup (8.6 oz)	220	30	2
Dinty Moore				
Meatball Stew	1 cup (8.4 oz)	250	40	2
Sliced Potatoes & Beef	1 can (7.5 oz)	230	35	4
Stew	1 cup (8.3 oz)	230	40	2
Stew	1 cup (8.2 oz)	230	40	2

FOOD	PORTION	CALS	CHOL	FIBER
Hormel				
Beef Goulash	1 can (7.5 oz)	230	50	3
Roast Beef With Gravy	2 oz	60	30	0
Mary Kitchen				
Corned Beef Hash	1 cup (8.3 oz)	410	80	2
Corned Beef Hash 50% Reduced Fat	1 cup (8.3 oz)	280	65	3
Roast Beef Hash	1 cup (8.3 oz)	390	70	2
Sausage Hash	1 cup (8.3 oz)	410	85	2
FROZEN				
Banquet				
Sandwich Toppers Creamed Chipped Beef	1 pkg (4 oz)	120	25	0
Sandwich Toppers Gravy & Salisbury Steak	1 pkg (5 oz)	210	25	2
Sandwich Toppers Gravy & Sliced Beef	1 pkg (4 oz)	70	25	0
Luigino's				
Creamed Sauce Shaved Cured Beef With Croutons	1 pkg (8 oz)	360	60	3
Egg Noodles Rich Gravy Swedish Meatballs	1 cup (7.5 oz)	280	70	3
Egg Noodles Rich Gravy Swedish Meatballs	1 pkg (9 oz)	340	80	3
MIX				
Casbah				
Gyro as prep	1 patty (2 oz)	145	63	tr
Hamburger Helper				
BBQ Beef as prep	1 cup	320	55	1
Beef Pasta as prep	1 cup	270	50	1
Beef Romanoff as prep	1 cup	280	50	0
Beef Stew as prep	1 cup	260	50	2
Beef Taco as prep	1 cup	280	50	2
Beef Teriyaki as prep	1 cup	290	50	2
Cheddar & Broccoli as prep	1 cup	350	60	0
Cheddar Melt as prep	1 cup	310	55	1

FOOD	PORTION	CALS	CHOL	FIBER
Cheddar'n Bacon as prep	1 cup	330	65	2
Cheeseburger Macaroni as prep	1 cup	360	65	1
Cheesy Hashbrowns as prep	1 cup	400	60	2
Cheesy Italian as prep	1 cup	320	60	1
Cheesy Shells as prep	1 cup	330	60	tr
Chili Macaroni as prep	1 cup	290	55	2
Fettuccine Alfredo as prep	1 cup	300	55	0
Four Cheese Lasagne as prep	1 cup	330	55	0
Italian Parmesan w/ Rigatoni as prep	1 cup	300	50	tr
Lasagne as prep	1 cup	270	50	2
Meat Loaf as prep	⅛ loaf	270	110	0
Meaty Spaghetti & Cheese as prep	1 cup	290	50	1
Mushroom & Wild Rice as prep	1 cup	310	55	2
Nacho Cheese as prep	1 cup	320	55	tr
Pizza Pasta w/ Cheese Topping as pre	1 cup	280	50	2
Pizzabake as prep	⅛ pie	270	45	tr
Potatoes Au Gratin as prep	1 cup	280	55	2
Potatoes Stroganoff as prep	1 cup	250	50	2
Reduced Sodium Cheddar Spirals as prep	1 cup	300	55	0
Reduced Sodium Italian Herby as prep	1 cup	270	50	2
Reduced Sodium Southwestern Beef as prep	1 cup	300	50	2
Rice Oriental as prep	1 cup	280	50	0
Salisbury as prep	1 cup	270	50	1

FOOD	PORTION	CALS	CHOL	FIBER
Spaghetti as prep	1 cup	270	50	1
Stroganoff as prep	1 cup	320	55	0
Swedish Meatballs as prep	1 cup	290	55	2
Three Cheeses as prep	1 cup	340	55	tr
Zesty Italian as prep	1 cup	300	50	2
Zesty Mexican as prep	1 cup	280	50	2
READY-TO-EAT				
Smithfield				
Beef Tips w/ Gravy	½ cup	170	50	tr
Thomas E. Wilson				
Roast Beef In Brown Gravy	1 serv + gravy (3.5 oz)	160	55	0
SHELF-STABLE				
Dinty Moore				
Microwave Cup Corned Beef Hash	1 pkg (7.5 oz)	350	60	2
Microwave Cup Hearty Burger Stew	1 pkg (7.5 oz)	240	40	3
Microwave Cup Stew	1 pkg (7.5 oz)	190	40	2
Hormel				
Microcup Meals Stew	1 cup (7.5 oz)	190	35	2
Lunch Bucket				
Beef Stew	1 pkg (7.5 oz)	170	25	2
TastyBite				
Beef Roganjosh	1 pkg (9.5 oz)	270	25	3
Meatballs Vindaloo	1 pkg (9.5 oz)	270	25	4
TAKE-OUT				
beef bouriguignon	1 serv (7 oz)	254	128	1
bulgoghi korean grilled beef	1 serv (5.2 oz)	256	67	tr
greek moussaka	1 serv (8.5 oz)	450	179	1
shepherds pie	1 serv (7 oz)	282	70	2
stew w/ vegetables	1 cup	220	71	—
stroganoff	¾ cup	260	69	—
swiss steak	4.6 oz	214	61	2
BEEFALO				
roasted	3 oz	160	49	—

FOOD	PORTION	CALS	CHOL	FIBER
BEER AND ALE				
beer light	12 oz can	100	0	—
beer regular	12 oz can	146	0	—
Amstel				
Light	12 oz	95	0	—
Anheuser Busch				
Natural Light	12 oz	110	0	—
Bud				
Light	12 oz	108	0	—
Guiness				
Kaliber nonalcholic	12 oz	43	0	—
Kingsbury				
Nonalcoholic	12 fl oz	60	0	—
Michelob				
Light	12 oz	134	0	—
Miller				
Lite	12 oz	96	0	—
Molson				
Light	12 oz	109	0	—
Piels				
Light	12 oz	136	0	—
Schmidts				
Light	12 oz	96	0	—
BEET JUICE				
juice	7 oz	72	0	
BEETS				
CANNED				
harvard	½ cup	89	0	—
pickled	½ cup	75	0	—
sliced	½ cup	27	0	—
Del Monte				
Pickled Crinkle Style Sliced	½ cup (4.5 oz)	80	0	2
Sliced	½ cup (4.3 oz)	35	0	2
Whole	½ cup (4.3 oz)	35	0	2
Green Giant				
Harvard	⅓ cup (3.1 oz)	60	0	2
Sliced	½ cup (4.2 oz)	35	0	2
Sliced No Salt Added	½ cup (4.2 oz)	35	0	2

FOOD	PORTION	CALS	CHOL	FIBER
Whole	½ cup (4.2 oz)	35	0	2
Greenwood				
Harvard	1 serv (4.4 oz)	100	0	1
Pickled	1 oz	25	0	0
LeSueur				
Baby Whole	½ cup (4.3 oz)	35	0	2
S&W				
Julienne	½ cup (4.3 oz)	30	0	1
Pickled Sliced	1 oz	15	0	1
Pickled Whole	1 oz	15	0	1
Sliced	½ cup (4.3 oz)	30	0	1
Whole Small	½ cup (4.3 oz)	30	0	1
Veg-All				
Small Sliced	½ cup	40	0	1
FRESH				
greens cooked	½ cup	20	0	—
greens raw	½ cup	4	0	—
greens raw chopped	½ cup	4	0	—
raw sliced	½ cup (2.4 oz)	29	0	—
sliced cooked	½ cup (3 oz)	38	0	—
whole cooked	2 (3.5 oz)	44	0	—
whole raw	2 (5.7 oz)	70	0	—

BEVERAGES (*see* BEER AND ALE, CHAMPAGNE, COFFEE, DRINK MIXERS, ENERGY DRINKS, FRUIT DRINKS, ICED TEA, LIQUOR/LIQUEUR, MALT, MILKSHAKE, SODA, TEA/HERBAL TEA, WATER, WINE)

BISCUIT
FROZEN

FOOD	PORTION	CALS	CHOL	FIBER
Jimmy Dean				
Chicken Twin	2 (3.2 oz)	280	25	2
Sausage Twin	2 (3.4 oz)	330	30	2
Steak Twin	2 (3.2 oz)	270	25	2
Rudy's Farm				
Ham Twin	2 (3 oz)	160	20	1
Sausage & Cheese Twin	2 (3 oz)	290	30	1
Sausage Twin	2 (2.7 oz)	296	30	1
MIX				
Bisquick				
Buttermilk	½ cup	150	0	—
Cheese Garlic	½ cup	160	0	—

FOOD	PORTION	CALS	CHOL	FIBER
Cinnamon Swirl	½ cup	150	0	—
Mix	⅓ cup (1.4 oz)	160	0	—
Reduced Fat	⅓ cup	140	0	tr
Kentucky Kernel				
Biscuit	¼ cup (1 oz)	171	0	1
REFRIGERATED				
buttermilk	1 (1 oz)	98	0	—
1869 Brand				
Buttermilk	1 (1.1 oz)	100	0	0
Hungry Jack				
Butter Tastin' Flaky	1 (1.2 oz)	100	0	0
Cinnamon & Sugar	1 (1.2 oz)	110	0	tr
Flaky	1 (1.2 oz)	100	0	0
Flaky Buttermilk	1 (1.2 oz)	100	0	0
Pillsbury				
Big Country Butter Tastin'	1 (1.2 oz)	100	0	0
Big Country Buttermilk	1 (1.2 oz)	100	0	0
Big Country Southern Style	1 (1.2 oz)	100	0	0
Buttermilk	1 (2.2 oz)	150	0	tr
Country	1 (2.2 oz)	150	0	tr
Grands Blueberry	1 (2.1 oz)	210	0	tr
Grands Butter Tastin'	1 (2.1 oz)	200	0	tr
Grands Buttermilk	1 (2.1 oz)	200	0	tr
Grands Buttermilk Reduced Fat	1 (2.1 oz)	190	0	tr
Grands Extra Rich	1 (2.1 oz)	220	0	tr
Grands Flaky	1 (2.1 oz)	200	0	tr
Grands Golden Corn	1 (1.2 oz)	210	0	tr
Grands HomeStyle	1 (2.1 oz)	210	0	tr
Grands Southern Style	1 (2.1 oz)	200	0	tr
Southern Style Flakey	1 (1.2 oz)	100	0	0
Tender Layer Buttermilk	1 (2.2 oz)	160	0	tr
TAKE-OUT				
buttermilk	1 (2 oz)	212	2	—
plain	1 (35 g)	276	5	—
tea biscuit	1 (3 oz)	210	0	1
w/ egg	1 (4.8 oz)	316	233	—
w/ egg & bacon	1 (5.2 oz)	458	353	1

FOOD	PORTION	CALS	CHOL	FIBER
w/ egg & ham	1 (6.7 oz)	442	300	4
w/ egg & sausage	1 (6.3 oz)	581	302	1
w/ egg & steak	1 (5.2 oz)	410	272	—
w/ egg cheese & bacon	1 (5.1 oz)	477	261	—
w/ ham	1 (4 oz)	386	25	1
w/ sausage	1 (4.4 oz)	485	35	1
w/ steak	1 (4.9 oz)	455	25	—
BISON				
roasted	3 oz	122	70	—
BLACK BEANS				
dried cooked	1 cup	227	0	—
Bean Cuisine				
Pasta & Beans Mediterranean Black Beans & Fusilli	1 serv	210	0	4
Eden				
Organic	½ cup (4.6 oz)	100	0	6
Green Giant				
Black Beans	½ cup (4.5 oz)	50	0	5
Old El Paso				
Black Beans	½ cup (4.6 oz)	100	0	7
Refried	½ cup (4.2 oz)	120	0	6
Progresso				
Black Beans	½ cup (4.6 oz)	110	0	7
BLACKBERRIES				
canned in heavy syrup	½ cup	118	0	—
fresh	½ cup	37	0	3
unsweetened frzn	1 cup	97	0	—
BLACKBERRY JUICE				
Clear Fruit				
Blackberry Rush	8 oz	90	0	—
Everfresh				
Clear Fruit Blackberry Rush	8 oz	90	0	—
Kool-Aid				
Scary Blackberry Ghoul-Aid Drink as prep w/ sugar	1 serv (8 oz)	100	0	0

FOOD	PORTION	CALS	CHOL	FIBER
BLACKEYE PEAS				
CANNED				
w/pork	½ cup	199	17	—
Eden				
Organic	½ cup (4.6 oz)	90	0	4
Green Giant				
Blackeye Peas	½ cup (4.4 oz)	90	0	3
DRIED				
cooked	1 cup	198	0	16
Hurst				
HamBeens California w/ Ham	1 serv	120	0	7
FROZEN				
Birds Eye				
Blackeye Peas	½ cup	110	0	4
BLINTZE				
Empire				
Apple	2 (4.4 oz)	220	<5	5
Blueberry	2 (4.4 oz)	190	10	2
Cheese	2 (4.4 oz)	200	20	3
Cherry	2 (4.4 oz)	200	10	3
Potato	2 (4.4 oz)	190	10	3
Golden				
Apple Raisin	1 (2.25 oz)	80	10	—
Blueberry	1 (2.25 oz)	90	10	—
Cheese	1 (2.1 oz)	80	15	2
Cherry	1 (2.25 oz)	95	5	—
Potato	1 (2.25 oz)	90	5	—
Ratner's				
Cheese	1 (2.1 oz)	90	20	tr
TAKE-OUT				
cheese	1 (2.7 oz)	160	65	tr
BLUEBERRIES				
canned in heavy syrup	1 cup	225	0	—
fresh	1 cup	82	0	—
unsweetened frzn	1 cup	78	0	—
Sonoma				
Dried	¼ cup (1.3 oz)	140	0	5

FOOD	PORTION	CALS	CHOL	FIBER
Tree Of Life				
Organic	1 cup (5 oz)	80	0	2
BLUEBERRY JUICE				
After The Fall				
Maine Coast	1 cup (8 oz)	90	0	0
BLUEFIN				
fillet baked	4.1 oz	186	88	–
BLUEFISH				
fresh baked	3 oz	135	64	–
BOK CHOY (see CABBAGE)				
BORAGE				
fresh chopped	½ cup	9	0	–
fresh chopped cooked	3½ oz	25	0	–
BOTTLED WATER (see WATER)				
BOYSENBERRIES				
in heavy syrup	1 cup	226	0	–
unsweetened frzn	1 cup	66	0	–
BRAINS				
beef pan-fried	3 oz	167	1696	–
beef simmered	3 oz	136	1746	–
lamb braised	3 oz	124	1737	–
lamb fried	3 oz	232	2128	–
pork braised	3 oz	117	2169	0
veal braised	3 oz	115	2635	–
veal fried	3 oz	181	1802	–
Armour				
Pork Brains In Milk Gravy	⅔ cup (5.5 oz)	150	3500	0
BRAN				
corn	1 cup (2.7 oz)	170	0	65
oat	½ cup (1.6 oz)	116	0	7
oat cooked	½ cup (3.8 oz)	44	0	3
rice	½ cup (2.1 oz)	187	0	12
wheat	½ cup (2 oz)	63	0	12

FOOD	PORTION	CALS	CHOL	FIBER
Hodgson Mill				
Oat	¼ cup (1.4 oz)	120	0	6
Mother's				
Oat Bran	½ cup	150	0	6
Quaker				
Oat Bran	½ cup (1.4 oz)	150	0	6
Stone-Buhr				
Oat	⅓ cup (1 oz)	90	0	4
BRAZIL NUTS				
dried unblanched	1 oz	186	0	—
BREAD				
CANNED				
B&M				
Brown Bread	½ in slice (2 oz)	130	0	2
Brown Bread Raisins	½ in slice (2 oz)	130	0	2
FROZEN				
Kineret				
Challah	⅛ loaf (2 oz)	150	15	1
Marie Callender's				
Cornbread & Honey Butter	1 piece + butter	210	15	1
Original Garlic	1 piece	190	<5	2
Parmesan & Romano Garlic	1 piece	200	5	2
New York				
Garlic	1 slice (2 oz)	190	0	1
Garlic Reduced Fat	1 slice (2 oz)	160	0	1
Texas Garlic Toast	1 in slice (1.4 oz)	160	0	1
Pepperidge Farm				
Garlic	1 slice (1.8 oz)	170	30	1
Garlic Sourdough 30% Reduced Fat	1 slice (1.8 oz)	170	5	2
Monterey Jack Jalapeno Cheese	1 slice (2 oz)	145	41	4
Mozzarella Garlic Cheese	1 slice (2 oz)	201	40	1
MIX				
cornbread	1 piece (2 oz)	189	37	1

FOOD	PORTION	CALS	CHOL	FIBER
Aunt Jemima				
Corn Bread Easy Mix	⅓ cup (1.3 oz)	150	0	1
Hodgson Mill				
European Cheese & Herb	¼ cup (1.2 oz)	130	0	tr
Honey Whole Wheat	¼ cup (1.2 oz)	120	0	2
READY-TO-EAT				
baguette whole wheat	2 oz	140	0	1
challah	1 slice (2 oz)	160	0	1
egg	1 slice (1.4 oz)	115	20	—
french	1 slice (1 oz)	78	0	1
french	1 loaf (1 lb)	1270	0	—
gluten	1 slice	47	0	—
italian	1 loaf (1 lb)	1255	0	—
italian	1 slice (1 oz)	81	0	1
navajo fry	1 (10.5 in diam)	527	0	—
navajo fry	1 (5 in diam)	296	0	—
oat bran	1 slice	71	0	1
oat bran reduced calorie	1 slice	46	0	—
oatmeal reduced calorie	1 slice	48	0	—
pita	1 reg (2 oz)	165	0	1
pita	1 sm (1 oz)	78	0	1
pita whole wheat	1 sm (1 oz)	76	0	2
pita whole wheat	1 reg (2 oz)	170	0	5
protein	1 slice	47	0	—
pumpernickel	1 slice	80	0	2
raisin	1 slice	71	0	—
rice bran	1 slice	66	0	—
rye	1 slice	83	0	2
rye reduced calorie	1 slice	47	0	—
seven grain	1 slice	65	0	2
sourdough	1 slice (1 oz)	78	0	1
vienna	1 slice (1 oz)	78	0	1
wheat berry	1 slice	65	0	1
wheat bran	1 slice	89	0	3
white	1 slice	67	0	1
white reduced calorie	1 slice	48	0	2
white toasted	1 slice	67	0	—

FOOD	PORTION	CALS	CHOL	FIBER
white cubed	1 cup	80	0	—
Alvarado St. Bakery				
Barley	1 slice (1.2 oz)	70	0	2
California Style	1 slice (1.2 oz)	60	0	2
French	1 slice (1.2 oz)	80	0	2
Multi-Grain	1 slice (1.2 oz)	60	0	2
Multi-Grain No-Salt	1 slice (1.2 oz)	60	0	2
Oat Berry	1 slice (1.2 oz)	70	0	2
Raisin	1 slice (1.1 oz)	80	0	2
Rye Seed	1 slice (1.2 oz)	60	0	2
Sourdough	1 slice (1.2 oz)	80	0	2
Wheat	1 slice (1.3 oz)	90	0	3
Arnold				
Bran'nola Country Oat	1 slice (1.3 oz)	110	0	3
Country Buttermilk	1 slice (1.3 oz)	110	0	1
Country Wheat	1 slice (1.3 oz)	100	0	1
Country White	1 slice (1.3 oz)	110	0	tr
Natural 100% Whole Wheat	1 slice (1.3 oz)	90	0	3
Raisin Cinnamon	1 slice (1 oz)	80	0	1
August Bros.				
Pumpernickel	1 slice	80	0	1
Rye Onion	1 slice	80	0	1
Rye Thin Unseeded	1 slice	40	0	1
Rye With Seeds	1 slice (1 lb loaf)	80	0	1
Rye	1 slice Without Seeds	80	0	1
Rye N' Pump	1 slice	90	0	1
Bread Du Jour				
French	3 in slice (2 oz)	140	0	1
Cedar's				
Mountain Bread Six Grain	1 piece (2.4 oz)	200	0	4
Damascus				
Mountain Shepard Lahvash	⅓ loaf (2 oz)	135	0	2
Pita	1 (2 oz)	130	0	2
Pita Whole Wheat	1 (2 oz)	160	0	3
Wraps Honey Wheat	½ wrap (2 oz)	130	0	1
Wraps Plain	½ wrap (2 oz)	130	0	1
Wraps Spinach	1 (2 oz)	280	0	2

FOOD	PORTION	CALS	CHOL	FIBER
Wraps Tomato	1 12-inch (4 oz)	240	0	2
Freihofer's				
Country Potato	1 slice (1.3 oz)	100	0	1
Country White	1 slice (1.3 oz)	100	0	tr
Wheat Light	1 slice (1.6 oz)	80	0	4
White Light	2 slices (1.6 oz)	80	0	4
Whole Wheat 100%	1 slice (1.3 oz)	90	0	2
Gold Medal				
100% Whole Wheat	1 slice	70	0	2
Home Pride				
Wheat	1 slice (1 oz)	80	0	1
La Mexicana				
Wraps Chocolate	1 (1.3 oz)	120	0	1
Wraps Southwestern Mild Chili	1 (1.3 oz)	120	0	1
Wraps Spinach	1 (1.3 oz)	120	0	1
Wraps Tomato Basil	1 (1.3 oz)	120	0	1
Mediterranean Magic				
Focaccia	⅛ loaf (1.8 oz)	140	0	tr
Milton's				
Healthy Multi-Grain	1 slice (1.4 oz)	110	0	3
Pepperidge Farm				
Apple Cinammon	1 slice (1 oz)	80	0	1
Deli Swirl Rye & Pump	1 slice (1.1 oz)	80	0	1
Farmhouse Country Wheat	1 slice	110	0	2
Farmhouse Hearty White	1 slice (1.5 oz)	110	<5	tr
Farmhouse Sesame Wheat	1 slice	110	0	2
Farmhouse Sourdough	1 slice (1.5 oz)	110	0	1
Natural Whole Grain Whole Wheat	1 slice (1.2 oz)	90	0	2
Natural Whole Grain Honey Oat	1 slice (1.2 oz)	90	0	2
Sandwich Pocket Wheat	1 (2 oz)	160	0	3
Sandwich Pocket White	1 (2 oz)	150	0	2
Swirl Cinnamon	1 slice (1 oz)	90	0	1
Swirl Raisin Cinnamon	1 slice (1 oz)	80	0	1

FOOD	PORTION	CALS	CHOL	FIBER
Stroehmann				
100% Whole Wheat	1 slice (1.3 oz)	90	0	2
D'Italiano Italian No Seeds	1 slice (1 oz)	80	0	tr
D'Italiano Italian Seeded	1 slice (1 oz)	80	0	tr
Family White	1 slice (0.8 oz)	65	0	0
Homestyle Split Top Wheat	1 slices (0.8 oz)	60	0	tr
Homestyle Split Top White	1 slice (0.8 oz)	65	0	1
Honey Cracked Wheat	1 slice (1.2 oz)	80	0	1
King White	1 slice (0.8 oz)	65	0	0
Potato	1 slice (1.2 oz)	100	0	tr
Ranch White	1 slice (0.8 oz)	65	0	0
Rye	1 slice (1.1 oz)	80	0	tr
Rye w/ Caraway	1 slice (1.1 oz)	80	0	tr
Twelve Grain	1 slice (1.2 oz)	90	0	1
Sunmaid				
Raisin	1 slice	70	0	1
TastyBite				
Nan Kontos Massala	½ loaf (1.4 oz)	120	0	1
Nan Kontos Onion	½ loaf (1.4 oz)	120	0	1
Nan Kontos Roghani	½ loaf (1.4 oz)	125	0	1
Nan Kontos Tandoori	½ loaf (1.4 oz)	120	0	1
Roti Kontos Missy	½ loaf (1.4 oz)	125	0	2
Valley Lahvosh				
Valley Wraps	1 (1 oz)	100	0	1
ZA				
Pit-Za Hearty Multi-Grain	⅛ bread (2 oz)	130	0	2
Pit-Za Salt-Free Garlic Whole Wheat	⅛ bread (2 oz)	150	0	3
REFRIGERATED				
Pillsbury				
Crusty French Loaf	⅕ loaf (2.2 oz)	150	0	tr
Grands Wheat	1 (2.1 oz)	200	0	2
Stefano's				
Stuffed Bread Broccoli & Cheese	½ bread (6 oz)	450	25	7

FOOD	PORTION	CALS	CHOL	FIBER
TAKE-OUT				
chapatis as prep w/ fat	1 bread (1.6 oz)	95	3	3
cornbread	2 in x 2 in (1.4 oz)	107	28	–
cornstick	1 (1.3 oz)	101	30	tr
focaccia	1 piece (2 oz)	130	0	1
focaccia onion	1 piece (4.6 oz)	282	0	2
focaccia rosemary	1 piece (3.5 oz)	251	0	2
focaccia tomato olive	1 piece (4.7 oz)	270	0	2
garlic bread	2 slices (2 oz)	190	0	1
irish soda bread	1 slice (2 oz)	174	11	–
naan	1 bread (3.5 oz)	286	46	2
paratha	1 bread (2.1 oz)	201	27	2
BREAD COATING				
Don's Chuck Wagon				
Chicken Baking Mix	¼ cup (1 oz)	95	0	1
Fish & Chips Mix	¼ cup (1 oz)	100	0	1
Fish Mix	¼ cup (1 oz)	95	0	1
Mushroom Batter Mix	¼ cup (1 oz)	95	0	1
Onion Ring Mix	¼ cup (1 oz)	100	0	1
Seafood Bake & Fry Mix	¼ cup (1 oz)	95	0	1
Luzianne				
Cajun Chicken Coating Mix	2 tbsp (1 oz)	100	0	1
Mrs. Dash				
Crispy Coating	2 tbsp (0.6 oz)	65	0	–
Oven Fry				
Extra Crispy For Chicken	⅛ pkg (0.5 oz)	60	0	0
Extra Crispy For Pork	⅛ pkg (0.5 oz)	60	0	0
Shake 'N Bake				
Buffalo Wings	¹⁄₁₀ pkg (0.4 oz)	40	0	0
Classic Italian Chicken or Pork	⅛ pkg (0.4 oz)	40	0	0
Country Mild Recipe	⅛ pkg (0.3 oz)	35	0	0
Glazes Barbecue Chicken Or Pork	⅛ pkg (0.4 oz)	45	0	0
Glazes Honey Mustard Chicken Or Pork	⅛ pkg (0.4 oz)	45	0	0
Glazes Tangy Honey Chicken Or Pork	⅛ pkg (0.4 oz)	45	0	0

FOOD	PORTION	CALS	CHOL	FIBER
Home Style Flour Recipe For Chicken	⅛ pkg (0.4 oz)	40	0	0
Hot & Spicy Chicken Or Pork	⅛ pkg (0.4 oz)	40	0	0
Original For Chicken	⅛ pkg (0.4 oz)	40	0	0
Original For Fish	¼ pkg (0.7 oz)	80	0	tr
Original For Pork	⅛ pkg (0.4 oz)	45	0	0

BREAD MACHINE MIX

Betty Crocker
FOOD	PORTION	CALS	CHOL	FIBER
Harvest Wheat	¹⁄₁₁ loaf	140	0	2
Home-Style White	¹⁄₁₁ loaf	130	0	0

Fleischmann's
FOOD	PORTION	CALS	CHOL	FIBER
Apple Cinnamon	⅛ loaf	160	0	2
Cinnamon Raisin	⅛ loaf	160	0	2
Country White	⅛ loaf (1.6 oz)	170	0	2
Cranberry Orange	⅛ loaf	150	0	2
Honey Oatmeal	⅛ loaf	160	0	3
Italian Herb	⅛ loaf	160	0	2
Sourdough	⅛ loaf	150	0	2
Stoneground Wheat	⅛ loaf	160	0	3

Sassafras
FOOD	PORTION	CALS	CHOL	FIBER
Apricot Oatmeal	1 slice (1.4 oz)	140	0	2

Wanda's
FOOD	PORTION	CALS	CHOL	FIBER
Dried Tomato Cheddar	¼ cup mix per serv (1.2 oz)	140	0	3
European White	¼ cup mix per serv (1.2 oz)	130	0	1
Oatmeal	¼ cup mix per serv (1.2 oz)	120	0	1
Oatmeal Cinnamon	¼ cup mix per serv (1.2 oz)	120	0	1
Old World Rye	¼ cup mix per serv (1.9 oz)	90	0	3
Onion	¼ cup mix per serv (1.2 oz)	120	0	1
Orange Cinnamon	¼ cup mix per serv (1.3 oz)	130	0	1
Oregano Garlic	¼ cup mix per serv (1.2 oz)	130	0	2

FOOD	PORTION	CALS	CHOL	FIBER
Rosemary Basil	¼ cup mix per serv (1.2 oz)	130	0	1
Rye	¼ cup mix per serv (1.2 oz)	120	0	1
Rye Caraway	¼ cup mix per serv (1.2 oz)	120	0	1
Sourdough	¼ cup mix per serv (1.2 oz)	120	0	1
Sunflower Sesame Poppyseed	¼ cup mix per serv (1.2 oz)	120	0	2
Ten Grain	¼ cup mix per serv (1.4 oz)	140	0	3
Wheat	¼ cup mix per serv (1.2 oz)	130	0	2
White	¼ cup mix per serv (1.2 oz)	130	0	1
Whole Wheat	¼ cup mix per serv (1.3 oz)	130	0	4

BREADCRUMBS

fresh	⅔ cup	76	0	1

Progresso

Garlic & Herb	¼ cup (1 oz)	100	0	1
Italian Style	¼ cup (1 oz)	110	0	1
Parmesan	¼ cup (1 oz)	100	0	1
Plain	¼ cup (1 oz)	110	0	1

BREADFRUIT

fresh	¼ small	99	0	—
seeds cooked	1 oz	48	0	—
seeds raw	1 oz	54	0	—
seeds roasted	1 oz	59	0	—

BREADNUTTREE SEEDS

dried	1 oz	104	0	—

BREADSTICKS

onion poppyseed	1	64	10	—
plain	1 sm	25	0	—
plain	1	41	0	—

Bread Du Jour

Original	1 (1.9 oz)	130	0	1

FOOD	PORTION	CALS	CHOL	FIBER
Sourdough	1 (1.9 oz)	130	0	1
J.J. Cassone				
Garlic	1 (1.6 oz)	150	0	2
New York				
Garlic Soft	1 (1.5 oz)	140	0	1
Pillsbury				
Soft	1 (1.4 oz)	110	0	tr
Soft Garlic & Herb	1 (2.1 oz)	180	0	tr
Stella D'Oro				
Grissini Original Fat Free	3	60	0	—
Grissini Style Fat Free	3 (0.5 oz)	60	0	0
Original	1 (0.4 oz)	45	0	0
Potato 'N Onion	1 (0.4 oz)	45	0	0
Roasted Garlic	1 (0.4 oz)	45	0	tr
Roasted Garlic	1 (0.4 oz)	45	0	0
Sesame	1 (0.4 oz)	50	0	tr
Snack Stix Cracked Pepper	4 (0.5 oz)	70	0	0
Snack Stix Salted	4 (0.5 oz)	70	0	0
Sodium Free	1 (0.4 oz)	45	0	0
Wheat	1 (0.3 oz)	40	0	0

BREAKFAST DRINKS

orange drink powder	3 rounded tsp	93	0	—
orange drink powder as prep w/water	6 oz	86	0	—

BROAD BEANS

canned	1 cup	183	0	—
dried cooked	1 cup	186	0	—
fresh cooked	3½ oz	56	0	—

BROCCOFLOWER

fresh raw	½ cup (1.8 oz)	16	0	—

BROCCOLI
FRESH

chinese broccoli (gai lan) cooked	1 cup (3.1 oz)	19	0	2
chopped cooked	½ cup	22	0	2
raw chopped	½ cup	12	0	1

FOOD	PORTION	CALS	CHOL	FIBER
FROZEN				
chopped cooked	½ cup	25	0	–
spears cooked	10 oz pkg	69	0	4
spears cooked	½ cup	25	0	3
Birds Eye				
Chopped	⅓ cup	25	0	2
Cuts	½ cup	25	0	3
Florets	1 cup	25	0	2
In Cheese Sauce	½ cup	70	5	2
Green Giant				
Butter Sauce	4 oz	50	<5	2
Cheese Sauce	⅔ cup (3.9 oz)	70	<5	2
Chopped	¾ cup (2.8 oz)	25	0	2
Cuts	1 cup (2.9 oz)	25	0	2
Harvest Fresh Cut	⅔ cup (3.2 oz)	25	0	2
Harvest Fresh Spears	3.5 oz	25	0	2
Select Florets	1⅓ cups (2.9 oz)	25	0	2
Select Spears	3 oz	25	0	2
Health Is Wealth				
Broccoli Munchees	2 (1 oz)	60	0	1
Stouffer's				
Au Gratin	1 serv (4 oz)	100	10	2
Tree Of Life				
Cuts	1 cup (3.1 oz)	25	0	2
BROWNIE				
FROZEN				
Greenfield				
Fat Free Homestyle	1 (1.3 oz)	110	0	0
Otis Spunkmeyer				
Blue Yonder w/ Walnuts	1 (2 oz)	230	20	2
Weight Watchers				
Brownie A La Mode	1 (3.14 oz)	190	30	2
Double Fudge Brownie Parfait	1 (5.3 oz)	190	5	2
MIX				
plain	1 (1.2 oz)	139	9	1
plain low calorie	1 (0.8 oz)	84	0	1
Betty Crocker				
Chocolate Chunk as prep	1	180	21	–

FOOD	PORTION	CALS	CHOL	FIBER
Dark Chocolate Fudge as prep	1	170	21	—
Dark Chocolate w/ Syrup as prep	1	170	21	—
Fudge as prep	1	170	21	—
German Chocolate Coconut Pecan Filling as prep	1	200	21	1
Hot Fudge as prep	1	170	21	—
Original as prep	1	180	21	—
Peanut Butter as prep	1	180	21	—
Stir'n Bake w/ Mini Kisses as prep	1 serv	220	0	1
Turtle w/ Caramel & Pecans as prep	1	170	21	—
Walnut as prep	1	180	21	—
Estee				
Brownie Mix as prep	2	100	0	1
No Pudge!				
Cappuccino Fudge	1	100	0	tr
Mint Fudge	½ cup	100	0	tr
Original Fudge	1	100	0	tr
Raspberry Fudge	1	100	0	tr
Sweet Rewards				
Low Fat Fudge as prep	1	130	0	1
Reduced Fat Supreme as prep	1	140	21	—
READY-TO-EAT				
plain	1 sm (1 oz)	115	5	1
plain	1 lg (2 oz)	227	10	1
w/ nuts	1 (1 oz)	100	14	—
Dolly Madison				
Fudge	1 (3 oz)	330	45	1
Entenmann's				
Little Bites	3 (2.2 oz)	290	45	1
Ultimate Fudge	1 (1.6 oz)	220	50	2
Greenfield				
Blondie Fat Free Apple Spice	1 (1.3 oz)	110	0	0

FOOD	PORTION	CALS	CHOL	FIBER
Health Valley				
Bar w/ Fudge Filling	1 bar	110	0	4
Hostess				
Brownie Bites	3 (1.3 oz)	170	30	1
Fudge	1 (3 oz)	330	45	1
Light	1 (1.4 oz)	140	1	1
Lance				
Fudge Nut	1 (2.25 oz)	340	20	2
Little Debbie				
Brownie Lights	1 (2 oz)	190	0	1
Brownie Loaves	1 (2.1 oz)	260	40	1
Fudge	1 pkg (2.1 oz)	270	15	tr
Tastykake				
Fudge Walnut	1 (3 oz)	370	80	1
Tom's				
Fudge Nut	1 pkg (2.5 oz)	300	5	0
REFRIGERATED				
Toll House				
Brownie Dough	1/12 pkg (1.5 oz)	180	15	2
TAKE-OUT				
plain	1 2 in sq (2.1 oz)	243	10	–
BRUSSELS SPROUTS				
FRESH				
cooked	½ cup	30	0	3
cooked	1 sprout	8	0	–
raw	½ cup	19	0	–
raw	1 sprout	8	0	1
FROZEN				
cooked	½ cup	33	0	–
Birds Eye				
Brussels Sprouts	11 sprouts	35	0	3
Green Giant				
Butter Sauce	⅔ cup (3.6 oz)	60	<5	4
BUCKWHEAT				
groats roasted cooked	1 cup (5.9 oz)	647	0	5
groats roasted uncooked	1 cup (5.7 oz)	567	0	17
BUFFALO				
water buffalo roasted	3 oz	111	52	–

FOOD	PORTION	CALS	CHOL	FIBER
BULGUR				
cooked	1 cup (6.3 oz)	151	0	8
uncooked	1 cup (4.9 oz)	479	0	26
Casbah				
Pilaf Mix as prep	1 cup	200	0	4
Salad Mix as prep	⅔ cup	90	0	1
Hodgson Mill				
Bulgur w/ Soygrits	¼ cup (1.4 oz)	120	0	1
BURBOT (FISH)				
fresh baked	3 oz	98	65	—
BURDOCK ROOT				
cooked	1 cup	110	0	—
fresh	1 cup	85	0	—
BUTTER				
clarified butter	3½ oz	876	256	—
ghee cow's milk	1 tbsp	126	39	0
ghee vegetable oil	1 tbsp	126	0	0
stick	1 stick (4 oz)	813	248	—
stick	1 pat (5 g)	36	11	—
whipped	4 oz	542	165	—
whipped	1 pat (4 g)	27	8	—
BREAKSTONE'S				
Salted	1 tbsp (0.5 oz)	100	30	—
Cabot				
Butter	1 tbsp	100	30	0
Corman				
Light	1 tbsp	55	5	0
Hotel Bar				
Stick	1 tbsp (0.5 oz)	100	30	—
Keller's				
European	1 tbsp (0.5 oz)	100	30	0
Land O Lakes				
Salted	1 tbsp (0.5 oz)	100	30	—
Ultra Creamy Salted	1 tbsp (0.5 oz)	110	30	—
Organic Valley				
Butter	1 tbsp (0.5 oz)	100	30	0
Unsalted	1 tbsp (0.5 oz)	110	30	0

FOOD	PORTION	CALS	CHOL	FIBER
BUTTER BEANS				
CANNED				
Green Giant				
Butter Beans	½ cup (4.5 oz)	90	0	4
Van Camp				
Butter Beans	½ cup (4.6 oz)	110	0	7
FROZEN				
Birds Eye				
Speckled	½ cup	100	0	4
BUTTER BLENDS				
stick	1 stick	811	99	—
Brummel & Brown				
Spread Made With Yogurt	1 tbsp (0.5 oz)	50	0	—
BUTTER SUBSTITUTES				
Butter Buds				
Mix	1 tsp (2 g)	5	0	—
Sprinkles	1 tsp (2 g)	5	0	—
Molly McButter				
Cheese	1 tsp	5	0	—
Light Sodium	1 tsp	5	0	—
Natural Butter	1 tsp	5	0	—
Roasted Garlic	1 tsp	5	0	—
Mrs. Bateman's				
Butterlike Baking Butter	1 tbsp (0.5 oz)	36	<5	0
Butterlike Saute Butter	1 tbsp (0.5 oz)	40	5	0
Watkins				
Butter Sprinkles	1 tsp (2 g)	5	0	0
Imitation Butter Flavored Mist	1 tbsp (0.5 oz)	120	0	0
BUTTERBUR				
canned fuki chopped	1 cup	3	0	—
fresh fuki	1 cup	13	0	—
BUTTERFISH				
baked	3 oz	159	71	—
fillet baked	1 oz	47	21	—
BUTTERNUTS				
dried	1 oz	174	0	—

FOOD	PORTION	CALS	CHOL	FIBER
BUTTERSCOTCH (see also CANDY)				
Hershey				
Chips	1 tbsp (0.5 oz)	80	0	–
Nestle				
Morsels	1 tbsp	80	0	0
CABBAGE (see also COLESLAW)				
chinese bok choy shredded cooked	½ cup	10	0	–
chinese pak-choi raw shredded	½ cup	5	0	–
chinese pe-tsai raw shredded	1 cup	12	0	–
chinese pe-tsai shredded cooked	1 cup	16	0	–
danish raw	1 head (2 lbs)	228	0	18
danish raw shredded	½ cup (1.2 oz)	9	0	tr
danish shredded cooked	½ cup (2.6 oz)	17	0	1
green raw	1 head (2 lbs)	228	0	18
green raw shredded	½ cup (1.2 oz)	9	0	tr
green shredded cooked	½ cup (2.6 oz)	17	0	1
napa cooked	1 cup (3.8 oz)	13	0	0
red raw shredded	½ cup	10	0	1
red shredded cooked	½ cup	16	0	–
savoy raw shredded	½ cup	10	0	–
savoy shredded cooked	½ cup	18	0	–
Greenwood				
Sweet & Sour Red	½ cup	100	0	0
TAKE-OUT				
korean kimchee	½ cup	22	0	4
stuffed cabbage	1 (6 oz)	373	95	–
CACTUS				
napoles fresh sliced	½ cup (1.5 oz)	7	0	–
pricklypear fresh	1 cup (5.3 oz)	56	0	4
CAKE (see also CAKE MIX)				
angelfood	1 cake (11.9 oz)	876	0	5

FOOD	PORTION	CALS	CHOL	FIBER
angelfood home recipe	½ cake (1.9 oz)	142	0	1
apple crisp home recipe	1 recipe 6 serv (29.6 oz)	1377	1	–
boston cream pie frzn	⅛ cake (3.2 oz)	232	34	1
carrot w/ cream cheese icing home recipe	1 cake 10 in diam	6175	1183	–
cheesecake	⅙ cake (2.8 oz)	256	44	2
cheesecake	1 cake 9 in diam	3350	2053	–
cheesecake home recipe	½ cake (4.5 oz)	456	155	–
chocolate cupcake creme filled w/ frosting home recipe	1 (1.8 oz)	188	9	–
chocolate w/o frosting home recipe	½ cake (3.3 oz)	340	55	–
chocolate w/o frosting home recipe	2 layers (39.9 oz)	4067	661	–
coffeecake crumb topped cinnamon home recipe	½ cake (2.1 oz)	240	36	2
cream puff shell home recipe	1 (2.3 oz)	239	129	–
crumpet	1 (2.3 oz)	131	0	2
devil's food cupcake w/ chocolate frosting	1	120	19	–
devil's food w/ creme filling	1 (1 oz)	105	15	–
eclair home recipe	1 (3 oz)	262	127	–
fruitcake	1 piece (1.5 oz)	139	2	–
fruitcake dark home recipe	1 cake 7½ in x 2¼ in	5185	640	–
jelly roll lemon filled	1 slice (3 oz)	210	35	tr
pound	1 cake 8½ x 3½ x 3 in	1935	1100	–
pound	⅒ cake (1 oz)	117	66	–
pound fat free	1 cake (12 oz)	961	0	–
pound cake home recipe	1 loaf 8½ in x 3½ in	1935	1100	–

FOOD	PORTION	CALS	CHOL	FIBER
sheet cake w/ white frosting home recipe	1 cake 9 in sq	4020	636	—
sheet cake w/o frosting home recipe	⅑ cake	315	61	—
sheet cake w/o frosting home recipe	1 cake 9 in sq	2830	552	—
shortcake home recipe	1 (2.3 oz)	225	2	—
sour cream pound	¹⁄₁₀ cake (1 oz)	117	17	tr
sponge	¹⁄₁₂ cake (1.3 oz)	110	39	—
sponge home recipe	¹⁄₁₂ cake (2.2 oz)	140	80	—
sponge cake dessert shell	1 (0.8 oz)	75	33	0
sponge w/ creme filling	1 (1.5 oz)	155	7	—
tiramisu	1 cake (4.4 lbs)	5732	2395	3
white w/ coconut frosting home recipe	¹⁄₁₂ cake (3.9 oz)	399	2	—
white w/o frosting home recipe	¹⁄₁₂ cake (2.6 oz)	264	2	—
white w/ white frosting	1 cake 9 in diam	4170	46	—
white w/ white frosting	¹⁄₁₆ cake	260	3	—
yellow w/ chocolate frosting	1 cake 9 diam	3895	609	—
yellow w/ chocolate frosting	⅛ cake (2.2 oz)	242	35	1
yellow w/o frosting home recipe	¹⁄₁₂ cake (2.4 oz)	245	37	—
yellow w/o frosting home recipe	2 layers (28.7 oz)	2947	443	—
Amy's				
Toaster Pops Apple	1	140	0	tr
Toaster Pops Strawberry	1	140	0	tr
Baby Watson				
Cheesecake	1 slice (3 oz)	260	65	tr
Baker Maid				
Creole Royal Pineapple Apricot	1 slice (1.7 oz)	90	5	1
Creole Royal Pineapple Apricot	3 slices (5 oz)	270	20	4

FOOD	PORTION	CALS	CHOL	FIBER
Carousel				
New York Cheese Cake	1 cake (3 oz)	250	95	1
Dolly Madison				
Angel Food	1 slice (2.1 oz)	160	0	1
Apple Crumb	1 (1.6 oz)	160	15	0
Banana Dream Flip	1 (3.5 oz)	390	30	1
Bear Claw	1 (2.75 oz)	270	25	1
Carrot	1 (4 oz)	360	0	1
Chocolate Snack Squares	1 (1.6 oz)	210	10	0
Cinnamon Buttercrumb	1 (1.6 oz)	170	15	0
Cinnamon Buttercrumb Low Fat	1 (1.5 oz)	140	0	0
Cinnamon Stix	1 (1.3 oz)	170	15	0
Creme Cakes	2 (1.9 oz)	210	25	0
Cupcakes Chocolate	1 (2 oz)	210	5	1
Cupcakes Spice	1 (2 oz)	230	20	0
Dunkin' Stix	1 (1.3 oz)	170	15	0
Frosty Angel	1 (3.5 oz)	330	0	1
Holiday Cupcakes	1 (1.9 oz)	180	5	0
Honey Bun	1 (3.7 oz)	440	15	1
Koo Koos	1 (1.8 oz)	200	5	0
Mini Coconut Loaf	1 (3.5 oz)	350	5	1
Mini Pound Cake	1 (3.2 oz)	310	15	1
Raspberry Square	1 (1.8 oz)	190	5	0
Sweet Roll Apple	1 (2.2 oz)	200	5	0
Sweet Roll Cherry	1 (2.2 oz)	210	10	1
Sweet Roll Cinnamon	1 (2.2 oz)	230	10	1
Texas Cinnamon Bun	1 (4.2 oz)	440	25	1
Zingers Devil's Food	2 (2.6 oz)	270	5	1
Zingers Lemon	1 (1.4 oz)	150	5	0
Zingers Raspberry	1 (1.4 oz)	150	5	0
Zingers Yellow	2 (2.5 oz)	280	5	1
Drake's				
Coffee Cake Low Fat	1 (1.1 oz)	110	10	0
Mini Coffee Cakes	4 (1.83 oz)	220	18	1
Yodel's	1 (1 oz)	150	5	–
Dutch Mill				
Dessert Shells Chocolate Covered	1 (0.5 oz)	80	0	0

FOOD	PORTION	CALS	CHOL	FIBER
Entenmann's				
Apple Puffs	1 (3 oz)	270	0	1
Coffee Cake Cheese Filled Crumb	1 serv (1.9 oz)	200	35	tr
Coffee Cake Crumb	1 serv (2 oz)	250	10	1
Cupcakes Light Chocolate Creme Filled	1 (2 oz)	160	0	1
Hot Cross Buns	1 (2.3 oz)	230	20	2
Stollen Fruit	1/8 cake (2 oz)	210	15	1
Fillo Factory				
Apple Turnovers Vegan	5 (5 oz)	270	0	2
Freihofer's				
Angel Food	1/5 cake (2 oz)	150	0	0
Cinnamon Swirl Buns	1 (2.8 oz)	290	30	1
Coffee Cake Cinnamon Pecan	1/8 cake (2 oz)	220	25	1
Crumb	1/8 cake (2 oz)	240	15	1
Homestyle Golden Loaf	1/8 cake (1.8 oz)	200	50	0
Pound	1/5 cake (2.8 oz)	330	65	0
Greenfield				
Blondie Fat Free Chocolate Chip	1 (1.3 oz)	110	0	0
Hostess				
Angel Food	1/8 cake (2 oz)	160	0	1
Chocodiles	1 (1.6 oz)	240	20	1
Chocolicious	1 (1.6 oz)	190	10	1
Coffee Crumb	1 (1.1 oz)	130	10	0
Crumb Cake Light	1 (1 oz)	100	0	0
Cupcakes Chocolate	1 (1.8 oz)	180	5	1
Cupcakes Orange	1 (1.5 oz)	160	10	0
Cupcakes Light Chocolate	1 (1.6 oz)	140	0	1
Ding Dongs	2 (2.7 oz)	360	15	2
Ho Ho's	2 (2 oz)	250	20	1
Honey Bun Glazed	1 (2.7 oz)	320	15	1
Honey Bun Iced	1 (3.4 oz)	410	10	1
Shortcake Dessert Cups	1 (1 oz)	100	15	0
Sno Balls	1 (1.8 oz)	180	5	1
Suzy Q's	1 (2 oz)	230	10	1

FOOD	PORTION	CALS	CHOL	FIBER
Sweet Roll Cherry	1 (2.2 oz)	210	10	1
Sweet Roll Cinnamon	1 (2.2 oz)	230	10	1
Twinkies	1 (1.5 oz)	150	20	0
Twinkies Light	1 (1.5 oz)	130	10	0
Jell-O				
Dessert Delights Cheesecake	1 bar (1.4 oz)	160	5	tr
Dessert Delights Chocolate Fudge Pudding	1 bar (1.4 oz)	150	0	1
Kellogg's				
Pop-Tarts Apple Cinnamon	1 (1.8 oz)	210	0	1
Pop-Tarts Blueberry	1 (1.8 oz)	210	0	1
Pop-Tarts Brown Sugar Cinnamon	1 (1.8 oz)	210	0	1
Pop-Tarts Cherry	1 (1.8 oz)	200	0	1
Pop-Tarts Chocolate Graham	1 (1.8 oz)	210	0	1
Pop-Tarts Frosted Apple Cinnamon	1 (1.8 oz)	190	0	1
Pop-Tarts Frosted Blueberry	1 (1.8 oz)	200	0	1
Pop-Tarts Frosted Brown Sugar Cinnamon	1 (1.8 oz)	210	0	1
Pop-Tarts Frosted Cherry	1 (1.8 oz)	200	0	1
Pop-Tarts Frosted Chocolate Vanilla Creme	1 (1.8 oz)	200	0	1
Pop-Tarts Frosted Chocolate Fudge	1 (1.8 oz)	200	0	1
Pop-Tarts Frosted Grape	1 (1.8 oz)	200	0	1
Pop-Tarts Frosted Raspberry	1 (1.8 oz)	210	0	1
Pop-Tarts Frosted S'mores	1 (1.8 oz)	200	0	1

FOOD	PORTION	CALS	CHOL	FIBER
Pop-Tarts Frosted Strawberry	1 (1.8 oz)	200	0	1
Pop-Tarts Frosted Wild Berry	1 (2 oz)	210	0	1
Pop-Tarts Frosted Wild Watermelon	1 (2 oz)	210	0	1
Pop-Tarts Low Fat Blueberry	1 (1.8 oz)	190	0	1
Pop-Tarts Low Fat Cherry	1 (1.8 oz)	190	0	1
Pop-Tarts Low Fat Frosted Brown Sugar Cinnamon	1 (1.8 oz)	190	0	1
Pop-Tarts Low Fat Frosted Chocolate Fudge	1 (1.8 oz)	190	0	2
Pop-Tarts Low Fat Frosted Strawberry	1 (1.8 oz)	190	0	1
Pop-Tarts Low Fat Strawberry	1 (1.8 oz)	190	0	1
Pop-Tarts Strawberry	1 (1.8 oz)	200	0	1
Lance				
Dunking Sticks	1 (2.75 oz)	180	<5	tr
Fig Cake	½ piece (2.1 oz)	110	0	1
Fig Cake Fat Free	½ piece (2.1 oz)	100	0	1
Honey Bun	1 (3 oz)	330	0	4
Pecan Twirls	1 pkg (2 oz)	220	5	1
Swiss Rolls	1 (2.5 oz)	170	10	tr
Little Debbie				
Angel Cakes Lemon	1 (1.6 oz)	130	0	0
Angel Cakes Raspberry	1 (1.6 oz)	130	0	0
Banana Nut Loaves	1 (1.9 oz)	220	10	tr
Banana Twins	1 (2.2 oz)	250	10	0
Be My Valentine Chocolate	1 (2.2 oz)	280	0	1
Be My Valentine Vanilla	1 (2.2 oz)	290	0	0
Blueberry Loaves	1 (2 oz)	220	0	tr
Chocolate Chip	1 (2.4 oz)	310	0	tr
Christmas Tree Cake	1 pkg (1.5 oz)	190	0	0

FOOD	PORTION	CALS	CHOL	FIBER
Coconut Creme	1 (1.7 oz)	210	0	0
Coffee Cake Apple	1 (2.1 oz)	230	10	0
Cupcake Creme Filled Chocolate	1 (1.6 oz)	180	5	tr
Cupcake Creme Filled Orange	1 (1.7 oz)	210	0	0
Cupcake Creme Filled Strawberry	1 (1.7 oz)	210	0	tr
Devil Cremes	1 (1.6 oz)	190	0	0
Devil Squares	1 (2.2 oz)	270	0	1
Easter Basket Cake Chocolate	1 (2.4 oz)	300	0	tr
Easter Basket Cake Vanilla	1 (2.5 oz)	320	0	0
Fall Party Cake Chocolate	1 (2.4 oz)	290	0	tr
Fall Party Cake Vanilla	1 (2.5 oz)	310	0	0
Fancy Cakes	1 (2.4 oz)	300	0	0
Frosted Fudge	1 (1.5 oz)	200	<5	tr
Golden Cremes	1 (1.5 oz)	150	10	0
Holiday Cake Roll Cherry Creme	1 (2.1 oz)	260	13	tr
Holiday Snack Cake Chocolate	1 (2.4 oz)	300	0	1
Holiday Snack Cake Vanilla	1 (2.5 oz)	320	0	0
Honey Bun	1 (1.8 oz)	220	<5	tr
Pecan Spinwheels	1 (1 oz)	110	0	0
Snack Cake Chocolate	1 (2.5 oz)	310	0	1
Strawberry Shortcake Roll	1 (2.1 oz)	230	15	0
Swiss Rolls	1 (2.1 oz)	270	15	1
Zebra Cakes	1 (2.6 oz)	330	0	0
Marie Callender's				
Cobbler Apple	1 serv (4.25 oz)	370	0	2
Cobbler Berry	1 serv (4.25 oz)	370	<5	1
Cobbler Cherry	1 serv (4.25 oz)	380	5	0
Cobbler Peach	1 serv (4.25 oz)	380	0	0
Nabisco				
Frosted Strawberry	1 (1.7 oz)	190	0	1

FOOD	PORTION	CALS	CHOL	FIBER
Natural Touch				
Toaster Square Blueberry	1 (2.8 oz)	180	0	6
Toaster Squares Date Walnut	1 (2.8 oz)	200	0	8
Pepperidge Farm				
Apple Turnover	1 (3.1 oz)	330	0	6
Blueberry Turnovers	1 (3.1 oz)	340	0	6
Cherry Turnover	1 (3.1 oz)	320	0	6
Large Layer Chocolate Fudge	⅛ cake (2.4 oz)	260	30	1
Large Layer Coconut	⅛ cake (2.4 oz)	260	35	0
Large Layer Vanilla	⅛ cake (2.4 oz)	250	25	0
Mini Turnover Apple	1 (1.4 oz)	140	0	1
Mini Turnover Cherry	1 (1.4 oz)	140	0	1
Mini Turnover Strawberry	1 (1.4 oz)	140	0	0
Peach Turnover	1 (3.1 oz)	340	0	6
Raspberry Turnovers	1 (3.1 oz)	330	0	6
Perugina				
Pannettone Au Beurre	⅛ cake (2.9 oz)	310	110	2
Philadelphia				
Snack Bars Classic Cheesecake	1 (1.5 oz)	200	35	0
Pillsbury				
Apple Turnovers	1 (2 oz)	170	0	tr
Cherry Turnovers	1 (2 oz)	180	0	0
Sara Lee				
Cheesecake 25% Reduced Fat	¼ cake (4.2 oz)	310	70	2
Cheesecake Cherry Cream	¼ cake (4.7 oz)	350	35	2
Cheesecake Chocolate Chip	¼ cake (4.2 oz)	410	65	2
Cheesecake French	⅙ cake (3.9 oz)	350	20	1
Cheesecake French Strawberry	⅙ cake (4.3 oz)	320	20	1
Cheesecake Strawberry Cream	¼ cake (4.7 oz)	330	40	2

FOOD	PORTION	CALS	CHOL	FIBER
Coffee Cake Butter Streusel	⅛ cake (1.9 oz)	220	35	1
Coffee Cake Crumb	⅛ cake (2 oz)	220	15	1
Coffee Cake Pecan	⅙ cake (1.9 oz)	230	25	1
Coffee Cake Raspberry	⅙ cake (1.9 oz)	220	15	1
Coffee Cake Reduced Fat Cheese	⅙ cake (1.9 oz)	180	20	0
Layer Cake Coconut	⅛ cake (2.8 oz)	260	15	1
Layer Cake Double Chocolate	⅛ cake (2.8 oz)	260	10	2
Layer Cake Fudge Golden	⅛ cake (2.8 oz)	260	15	1
Layer Cake German Chocolate	⅛ cake (2.9 oz)	280	15	1
Layer Cake Vanilla	⅛ cake (2.8 oz)	260	15	0
Original Cheesecake	¼ cake (4.2 oz)	350	50	1
Pound Cake All Butter	¼ cake (2.7 oz)	320	85	1
Pound Cake Chocolate Swirl	¼ cake (2.9 oz)	330	75	tr
Pound Cake Family Size	⅙ cake (2.7 oz)	310	75	1
Pound Cake Reduced Fat	¼ cake (2.7 oz)	280	65	tr
Pound Cake Strawberry Swirl	¼ cake (2.9 oz)	290	60	tr
Strawberry Shortcake	⅛ cake (2.5 oz)	180	15	1
Sinbad				
Baklava	1 piece (2 oz)	337	10	2
SnackWell's				
Streusel Squares Apple Cinnamon	1 (1.5 oz)	150	0	tr
Streusel Squares Cherry	1 (1.5 oz)	150	0	tr
Tastykake				
Banana Creamie	1 (1.5 oz)	170	5	0
Bear Claw Apple	1 (3 oz)	280	0	0
Bear Claw Cinnamon	1 (3 oz)	300	0	tr
Big Texas	1 (3 oz)	300	0	tr

FOOD	PORTION	CALS	CHOL	FIBER
Breakfast Bun Chocolate Raisin	1 (3.2 oz)	330	0	1
Bunny Trail Treats	1 (1.3 oz)	150	30	0
Chocolate Creamie	1 (1.5 oz)	180	15	0
Chocolate Krimpies	2 (2.2 oz)	240	45	1
Coffee Roll Glazed	1 (3 oz)	300	0	tr
Coffee Roll Vanilla	1 (3.2 oz)	320	0	tr
Cupcakes	2 (2.1 oz)	200	10	1
Cupcakes Butter Cream Filled Iced	2 (2.2 oz)	240	10	1
Cupcakes Chocolate Cream Filled Iced	2 (2.2 oz)	230	10	1
Cupcakes Low Fat Vanilla Cream Filled	2 (2.2 oz)	190	0	0
Cupid Kake	1 (1.3 oz)	150	30	0
Honey Bun Glazed	1 (3.2 oz)	350	10	0
Honey Bun Iced	1 (3.2 oz)	350	10	0
Junior Chocolate	1 (3.3 oz)	330	80	1
Junior Coconut	1 (3.3 oz)	310	75	0
Junior Koffee Kake	1 (2.5 oz)	270	45	1
Junior Pound Kake	1 (3 oz)	320	100	1
Kandy Kakes Chocolate	3 (2 oz)	250	0	2
Kandy Kakes Coconut	2 (2.7 oz)	330	5	2
Kandy Kakes Peanut Butter	2 (1.3 oz)	190	10	1
Koffee Kake Cream Filled	2 (2 oz)	240	30	0
Koffee Kake Low Fat Apple	2 (2 oz)	170	0	1
Koffee Kake Low Fat Lemon	2 (2 oz)	180	10	0
Koffee Kake Low Fat Raspberry	2 (2 oz)	170	0	1
Koffee Kakes	1 (2 oz)	210	30	tr
Kreepy Kakes	2 (2.2 oz)	240	20	0
Kreme Krimpies	2 (2 oz)	230	55	0
Krimpets Butterscotch Iced	2 (2 oz)	210	60	0
Krimpets Jelly Fillled	2 (2 oz)	190	45	1

FOOD	PORTION	CALS	CHOL	FIBER
Krimpets Strawberry	2 (2 oz)	210	65	0
Kringle Kake	1 (1.3 oz)	150	30	0
Santa Snacks	2 (2.2 oz)	240	20	0
Sparkle Kake	1 (1.3 oz)	150	30	0
Tasty Tweets	2 (2.2 oz)	240	20	0
Tropical Delight Coconut	2 (2 oz)	190	30	0
Tropical Delight Guava	2 (2 oz)	190	15	0
Tropical Delight Papaya	2 (2 oz)	200	20	0
Tropical Delight Pineapple	2 (2 oz)	200	20	0
Vanilla Creamie	1 (1.5 oz)	190	35	0
Witchy Treat	1 (1.3 oz)	150	30	0
Toastettes				
Frosted Blueberry	1 (1.7 oz)	190	0	1
Frosted Brown Sugar Cinnamon	1 (1.7 oz)	190	0	1
Frosted Cherry	1 (1.7 oz)	190	0	1
Frosted Fudge	1 (1.7 oz)	190	0	3
Strawberry	1 (1.7 oz)	190	0	1
Tom's				
Honey Bun	1 pkg (3 oz)	360	10	2
Honey Bun Jelly Filled	1 pkg (4 oz)	490	0	2
Marble Pound	1 pkg (2.5 oz)	300	50	1
Texas Cinnamon Roll	1 pkg (4 oz)	360	0	0
Tortuga				
Cayman Island Rum Cake	1 piece (2 oz)	194	0	0
Weight Watchers				
Chocolate Raspberry Royale	1 (3.5 oz)	190	20	2
Chocolate Eclair	1 (2.1 oz)	150	30	1
Danish Coffee Cake Apple Cinnamon	1 piece (1.9 oz)	160	0	1
Danish Coffee Cake Cheese	1 piece (1.9 oz)	160	5	1
Danish Coffee Cake Raspberry	1 piece (1.9 oz)	160	0	1
Double Fudge	1 piece (2.75 oz)	190	25	2

FOOD	PORTION	CALS	CHOL	FIBER
French Style Cheesecake	1 piece (3.9 oz)	170	15	2
New York Style Cheesecake	1 piece (2.5 oz)	150	15	1
Strawberry Parfait Royale	1 (5.24 oz)	180	10	0
Triple Chocolate Eclair	1 (2.14 oz)	160	30	1
Well-Bred Loaf				
Banana Bread	1 slice (3.5 oz)	330	60	tr
Banana Nut	1 slice (4.3 oz)	440	85	2
Blueberry	1 slice (4.3 oz)	440	110	1
Carrot	1 slice (4.3 oz)	480	125	2
Carrot Traditional	1 slice (4.3 oz)	440	40	2
Chocolate Chip	1 slice (4.3 oz)	490	105	2
Cinnamon Walnut	1 slice (4.3 oz)	480	110	1
Coconut Rum	1 slice (4.3 oz)	490	95	tr
Cranberry	1 slice (4.3 oz)	460	100	1
Marble	1 slice (4.3 oz)	530	115	1
Pound All Butter	1 slice (4.3 oz)	470	115	tr
Pound Mandarin Orange	1 slice (4 oz)	460	70	tr
Raisin	1 slice (4.3 oz)	460	105	2
TAKE-OUT				
angelfood	1/12 cake (1 oz)	73	0	1
apple crisp	1/2 cup (5 oz)	230	0	–
baklava	1 oz	126	23	1
basbousa namoura	1 piece (1 oz)	60	0	2
boston cream pie	1/6 cake (3.3 oz)	293	43	1
carrot w/ cream cheese icing	1/12 cake (3.9 oz)	484	60	–
cheesecake w/ cherry topping	1/12 cake (5 oz)	359	106	–
coffeecake crumb topped cinnamon	1/8 cake (2.2 oz)	263	20	2
cream puff w/ custard filling	1 (4.6 oz)	336	174	–
eclair w/ chocolate icing & custard filling	1	205	35	–
french apple tart	1 (3.5 oz)	302	60	2
fruitcake	1/36 cake (2.9 oz)	302	24	3

FOOD	PORTION	CALS	CHOL	FIBER
gingerbread	⅑ cake (2.6 oz)	264	24	2
panettone	⅟₁₂ cake (2.9 oz)	300	90	2
petit fours	2 (0.9 oz)	120	0	0
pineapple upside down	⅑ cake (4 oz)	367	25	—
pound fat free	1 oz	80	0	—
pound cake	1 slice (1 oz)	120	32	—
sacher torte	1 slice (2.2 oz)	240	50	4
sheet cake w/ white frosting	⅑ cake	445	70	—
tiramisu	1 piece (5.1 oz)	409	171	tr

CAKE ICING

FOOD	PORTION	CALS	CHOL	FIBER
chocolate as prep w/ butter	⅟₁₂ box (1.5 oz)	161	10	—
chocolate as prep w/ butter	1 box (13.7 oz)	1908	121	—
chocolate as prep w/ butter home recipe	1 recipe (21.1 oz)	2409	176	—
chocolate as prep w/ butter home recipe	⅟₁₂ recipe (1.8 oz)	200	15	—
chocolate as prep w/ margarine	⅟₁₂ box (1.5 oz)	161	0	—
chocolate as prep w/ margarine	1 box (13.7 oz)	1909	0	—
chocolate as prep w/ margarine home recipe	1 recipe (21.1 oz)	2411	5	—
chocolate as prep w/ margarine home recipe	⅟₁₂ recipe (1.8 oz)	200	0	—
chocolate ready-to-use	⅟₁₂ pkg (1.3 oz)	151	0	—
chocolate ready-to-use	1 pkg (16 oz)	1834	0	—
coconut ready-to-use	⅟₁₂ pkg (1.3 oz)	157	0	—
coconut ready-to-use	1 pkg (16 oz)	1903	0	—
cream cheese ready-to-use	⅟₁₂ pkg (1.3 oz)	157	0	—
cream cheese ready-to-use	1 pkg (16 oz)	1906	0	—
glaze home recipe	1 recipe (11.5 oz)	1173	7	—
glaze home recipe	⅟₁₂ recipe (1 oz)	97	1	—

FOOD	PORTION	CALS	CHOL	FIBER
seven minute home recipe	1 recipe (13.6 oz)	1231	0	–
seven minute home recipe	½₂ recipe (1.1 oz)	102	0	–
vanilla as prep w/ butter	½₂ pkg (1.5 oz)	182	10	–
vanilla as prep w/ butter	1 pkg (14.5 oz)	2188	126	–
vanilla as prep w/ butter home recipe	½₂ recipe (1.7 oz)	165	6	–
vanilla as prep w/ butter home recipe	1 recipe (20.1 oz)	1972	67	–
vanilla as prep w/ margarine	1 pkg (14.5 oz)	2190	0	–
vanilla as prep w/ margarine	½₂ pkg (1.5 oz)	182	0	–
vanilla as prep w/ margarine home recipe	½₂ recipe (1.7 oz)	195	0	–
vanilla as prep w/ margarine home recipe	1 recipe (20.1 oz)	2326	5	–
vanilla ready-to-use	½₂ pkg (1.3 oz)	159	0	–
vanilla ready-to-use	1 pkg (16 oz)	1936	0	–
Betty Crocker				
HomeStyle Mix Coconut Pecan as prep	2 tbsp	160	0	tr
HomeStyle Mix White Fluffy as prep	6 tbsp	100	0	–
Party Frosting Chocolate w/ Stars	2 tbsp (1.2 oz)	140	0	–
Rich & Creamy Butter Cream	2 tbsp (1.3 oz)	140	0	–
Rich & Creamy Cherry	2 tbsp (1.2 oz)	140	0	–
Rich & Creamy Chocolate	2 tbsp (1.2 oz)	130	0	–

FOOD	PORTION	CALS	CHOL	FIBER
Rich & Creamy Cream Cheese	2 tbsp (1.2 oz)	140	0	–
Rich & Creamy Dark Chocolate	2 tbsp (1.3 oz)	130	0	1
Rich & Creamy French Vanilla	2 tbsp (1.2 oz)	140	0	–
Rich & Creamy Milk Chocolate	2 tbsp (1.3 oz)	130	0	–
Rich & Creamy Rainbow Chip	2 tbsp (1.2 oz)	140	0	–
Rich & Creamy Vanilla	2 tbsp (1.2 oz)	140	0	–
Toppers Milk Chocolate	2 tbsp (1.2 oz)	130	0	–
Toppers Vanilla	2 tbsp (1.2 oz)	140	0	–
Duncan Hines				
Chocolate Creamy Homestyle	2 tbsp	130	0	2
Milk Chocolate Creamy Homestyle	2 tbsp	130	0	1
Vanilla Creamy Homestyle	2 tbsp	140	0	1
Estee				
Frosting as prep	⅓ pkg	100	0	0
Sweet Rewards				
Ready-To-Spread Reduced Fat Chocolate	2 tbsp (1.2 oz)	120	0	–
Ready-To-Spread Reduced Fat Vanilla	2 tbsp (1.2 oz)	130	0	–
CAKE MIX				
angelfood	10 in cake (20.9 oz)	1535	0	9
angelfood	½₂ cake (1.8 oz)	129	0	1
chocolate w/o frosting	2 layers (26.8 oz)	2393	425	–
chocolate w/o frosting	½₂ cake (2.3 oz)	198	35	–
chocolate w/o frosting low sodium	⅒ cake (1.3 oz)	116	0	–
coffeecake crumb topped cinnamon	⅛ cake (2 oz)	178	28	2

FOOD	PORTION	CALS	CHOL	FIBER
devil's food w/o frosting	½₂ cake (2.3 oz)	198	35	–
devil's food w/ chocolate frosting	½₆ cake	235	37	–
devil's food w/ chocolate frosting	1 cake 9 in diam	3755	598	–
fudge w/o frosting	½₂ cake (2.3 oz)	198	35	–
german chocolate pudding type w/ coconut nut frosting	½₂ cake (3.9 oz)	404	53	–
gingerbread	⅑ cake (2.4 oz)	207	24	2
gingerbread	1 cake 8 in sq	1575	6	–
lemon w/o frosting no sugar low sodium	½₀ cake (1.3 oz)	118	0	–
marble pudding type w/o frosting	½₂ cake (2.6 oz)	253	53	–
marble pudding type w/o frosting	2 layers (30.6 oz)	3021	638	–
white w/o frosting no sugar low sodium	½₀ cake (1.3 oz)	118	0	–
yellow w/ chocolate frosting	½₆ cake	235	36	–
yellow w/o frosting	2 layers (26.5 oz)	2415	437	–
yellow w/o frosting	½₂ cake (2.2 oz)	202	37	–
yellow w/ chocolate frosting	1 cake 9 in diam	3895	609	–
Aunt Jemima				
Coffee Cake Easy Mix	⅓ cup (1.4 oz)	170	0	1
Betty Crocker				
Angel Food Fat Free	½₂ cake	140	0	–
Angel Food Fat Free Confetti as prep	½₂ cake	150	0	–
Cheesecake Chocolate Chip as prep	⅛ cake	410	99	1
Cheesecake Original as prep	⅛ cake	400	102	–
Cheesecake Strawberry Swirl as prep	⅛ cake	380	96	–
Pineapple Upside Down as prep	⅙ cake	420	36	–

FOOD	PORTION	CALS	CHOL	FIBER
Quick Bread Banana	1/12 cake	170	36	–
Quick Bread Cinnamon Streusel as prep	1/14 cake	180	30	–
Quick Bread Cranberry Orange as prep	1/12 cake	170	36	–
Quick Bread Lemon Poppy Seed as prep	1/12 cake	170	36	–
Stir'n Bake Coffee Cake w/ Cinnamon Streusel as prep	1/6 cake	230	12	–
Stir'n Bake Devils Food w/ Chocolate Frosting as prep	1/6 cake	240	0	1
Stir'n Bake Yellow w/ Chocolate Frosting as prep	1/8 cake	240	9	1
SuperMoist Butter Pecan as prep	1/12 cake	240	54	–
SuperMoist Butter Yellow as prep	1/12 cake	260	75	–
SuperMoist Carrot as prep	1/10 cake	320	63	–
SuperMoist Cherry Chip	1/10 cake	300	63	–
SuperMoist Chocolate Fudge as prep	1/12 cake	270	54	1
SuperMoist Golden Vanilla as prep	1/12 cake	240	54	–
SuperMoist Lemon as prep	1/12 cake	240	54	–
SuperMoist Milk Chocolate as prep	1/12 cake	240	54	1
SuperMoist Pineapple as prep	1/12 cake	250	54	–
SuperMoist Spice as prep	1/12 cake	240	54	–
SuperMoist Strawberry as prep	1/12 cake	250	39	–
SuperMoist White as prep	1/12 cake	230	0	–

FOOD	PORTION	CALS	CHOL	FIBER
SuperMoist White Light as prep	⅒ cake	210	0	–
Bisquick				
Mix	⅓ cup (1.4 oz)	160	0	–
Reduced Fat	⅓ cup (1.4 oz)	140	0	tr
Dromedary				
Date Bread	⅟₁₁ cake (2 oz)	190	0	1
Duncan Hines				
Angel Food as prep	⅟₁₂ pkg (1.3 oz)	140	0	1
Butter Recipe Golden as prep	⅟₁₂ cake	320	80	–
Cupcake Yellow as prep	1	180	6	–
Dark Chocolate Fudge as prep	⅟₁₂ cake	290	55	–
Devil's Food Moist Deluxe as prep	⅟₁₂ cake (1.5 oz)	290	55	1
French Vanilla	⅟₁₂ cake (1.5 oz)	250	55	–
Fudge Marble Moist Deluxe as prep	⅟₁₂ cake (1.5 oz)	250	45	0
Lemon Supreme Moist Deluxe	⅟₁₂ cake (1.5 oz)	250	55	0
White Moist Deluxe as prep	⅟₁₂ cake	190	0	–
Yellow Moist Deluxe as prep	⅟₁₂ cake (1.5 oz)	250	55	–
Yellow Moist Deluxe as prep	⅟₁₂ cake	250	55	–
Estee				
Chocolate as prep	⅓ cake	190	0	1
White as prep	⅓ cake	200	0	tr
Hodgson Mill				
Gingerbread Whole Wheat	¼ cup (1 oz)	110	0	2
Jell-O				
No Bake Cherry Cheesecake as prep	⅛ cake (4.8 oz)	340	5	tr
No Bake Double Layer Chocolate as prep	⅛ cake (4.4 oz)	260	<5	1

FOOD	PORTION	CALS	CHOL	FIBER
No Bake Double Layer Cookies And Creme as prep	⅛ cake (4.5 oz)	390	<5	1
No Bake Double Layer Lemon as prep	⅛ cake (4.4 oz)	260	<5	tr
No Bake Homestyle Cheesecake as prep	⅛ cake (4.6 oz)	360	10	tr
No Bake Peanut Butter Cup as prep	⅛ cake (3.8 oz)	380	<5	1
No Bake Reduced Fat Strawberry Swirl Cheesecake as prep	⅛ cake (4 oz)	250	5	0
No Bake Strawberry Cheesecake as prep	⅛ cake (4.8 oz)	340	5	tr
Real Cheesecake as prep	⅛ cake (4.6 oz)	360	5	1
Sweet Rewards				
Reduced Fat White as prep	¹⁄₁₂ cake	180	0	—
Reduced Fat Yellow as prep	¹⁄₁₂ cake	200	30	—
Wanda's				
Double Chocolate	¼ cup mix per serv (1.4 oz)	170	0	2

CALZONE
TAKE-OUT

FOOD	PORTION	CALS	CHOL	FIBER
cheese	1 (12 oz)	1020	100	8

CANADIAN BACON

FOOD	PORTION	CALS	CHOL	FIBER
grilled	1 pkg (6 oz)	257	81	0
Boar's Head				
Canadian Bacon	2 oz	70	30	0
Hormel				
Sandwich Style	3 slices (2 oz)	70	30	0
Oscar Mayer				
Canandian Bacon	2 slices (1.6 oz)	50	25	0
Yorkshire Farms				
Uncured	3 oz	100	44	—

FOOD	PORTION	CALS	CHOL	FIBER
CANADIAN BACON SUBSTITUTES				
Yves				
Canadian Veggie Bacon	1 serv (2 oz)	80	0	1
CANDY				
butterscotch	1 piece (6 g)	24	1	—
butterscotch	1 oz	112	3	—
candied cherries	1 (4 g)	12	0	—
candied citron	1 oz	89	0	—
candied lemon peel	1 oz	90	0	—
candied orange peel	1 oz	90	0	—
candied pineapple slice	1 slice (2 oz)	179	0	—
candy corn	1 oz	105	0	—
caramels	1 piece (8 g)	31	1	—
caramels	1 pkg (2.5 oz)	271	5	—
caramels chocolate	1 bar (2.3 oz)	231	0	—
caramels chocolate	1 piece (6 g)	22	0	—
crisped rice bar almond	1 bar (1 oz)	130	0	1
crisped rice bar chocolate chip	1 bar (1 oz)	115	0	1
dark chocolate	1 oz	150	0	—
fondant chocolate coated	1 lg (1.2 oz)	128	0	—
fondant chocolate coated	1 sm (0.4 oz)	40	0	—
fondant mint	1 oz	105	0	—
gumdrops	10 sm (0.4 oz)	135	0	—
gumdrops	10 lg (3.8 oz)	420	0	—
hard candy	1 oz	106	0	—
jelly beans	10 sm (0.4 oz)	40	0	—
jelly beans	10 lg (1 oz)	104	0	—
lollipop	1 (6 g)	22	0	—
marzipan	1 oz	128	0	2
milk chocolate	1 bar (1.55 oz)	226	10	—
milk chocolate crisp	1 bar (1.45 oz)	203	8	—
milk chocolate w/ almonds	1 bar (1.45 oz)	215	8	—
peanuts chocolate covered	1 cup (5.2 oz)	773	13	—

FOOD	PORTION	CALS	CHOL	FIBER
peanuts chocolate covered	10 (1.4 oz)	208	4	–
sesame crunch	1 oz	146	0	–
sesame crunch	20 pieces (1.2 oz)	181	0	–
sweet chocolate	1 oz	143	0	–
sweet chocolate	1 bar (1.45 oz)	201	0	–
100 Grand				
Bar	1 bar (1.5 oz)	200	10	tr
3 Musketeers				
Bar	2 fun size (1.2 oz)	140	5	0
Bar	1 (2.1 oz)	260	5	1
5th Avenue				
Snack Size	1 bar (0.58 oz)	80	0	–
Almond Joy				
Snack Size	1 (0.68 oz)	90	0	–
Andes				
Chocolate Covered Mint Patties	1 (0.5 oz)	60	0	0
Baby Ruth				
Bar	1 bar (2.1 oz)	270	0	2
Fun Size	1 bar (1 oz)	130	0	tr
Barricini				
Dark Chocolate Raspberry Creme Shells	1 piece (0.3 oz)	47	0	0
Bittyfinger				
Bars	2	170	0	tr
Body Smarts				
Chocolate Peanut Crunch	2 bars (1.8 oz)	210	<5	2
Breath Savers				
Sugar Free Mint Cinnamon	1 piece (2 g)	10	0	–
Sugar Free Peppermint	1 piece (2 g)	10	0	–
Butterfinger				
BB's	1 pkg (1.7 oz)	230	0	1
Bar	1 (2.1 oz)	280	0	1
Bar	1 (2.1 oz)	270	0	1
Fun Size	1 bar	100	0	0

FOOD	PORTION	CALS	CHOL	FIBER
Cape Cod Provisions				
Cranberry Bog Frogs	3 pieces (1.9 oz)	250	7	tr
Carmello				
Snack Size	1 (0.66 oz)	90	<5	—
Cellas				
Chocolate Covered Cherries Milk Chocolate	2 pieces (1 oz)	110	0	2
Certs				
Breath Mints	1 piece (1.67 g)	6	0	—
Mini Sugar Free	1 piece (0.365 g)	1	0	—
Sugar Free	1 piece (1.67 g)	7	0	—
Charms				
Blow Pop	1 (0.6 oz)	70	0	—
Lollipop Sour	1 (0.6 oz)	70	0	—
Lollipop Sweet	1 (0.6 oz)	70	0	—
Chuckles				
Candy	4 pieces (1.4 oz)	140	0	—
Chunky				
Bar	1 (1.4 oz)	210	5	1
Clorets				
Mints	1 piece (1.67 g)	6	0	—
Cloud Nine				
Australian Orange Peel	½ bar (1.5 oz)	220	0	2
Butter Nut Toffee	½ bar (1.5 oz)	230	5	1
Cool Mint Crisp	½ bar (⅛ oz)	220	5	2
Espresso Bean Crunch	½ bar (1.5 oz)	220	0	2
Malted Milk Crunch	½ bar (1.5 oz)	230	5	1
Milk Chocolate	½ bar (1.5 oz)	230	5	1
Oregan Red Raspberry	½ bar (1.5 oz)	230	0	2
Peanut Butter Brittle	½ bar (1.5 oz)	230	5	1
Sundried Cherry	½ bar (1.5 oz)	230	5	1
Toasted Coconut Crisp	½ bar (1.5 oz)	230	5	2
Vanilla Dark	½ bar (1.5 oz)	230	0	2
Crunch				
Fun Size	4 bars	210	10	tr
Del Monte				
Radical Raizins Cinnamon	1 pkg (0.7 oz)	70	0	0

FOOD	PORTION	CALS	CHOL	FIBER
Radical Raizins Rainbow	1 pkg (0.7 oz)	70	0	0
Dove				
Dark Chocolate	1 bar (1.3 oz)	200	5	2
Dark Chocolate	¼ bar (1.5 oz)	230	5	3
Dark Chocolate Minatures	7 (1.5 oz)	220	5	2
Milk Chocolate	1 bar (1.3 oz)	200	5	1
Milk Chocolate	¼ bar (1.5 oz)	230	10	1
Milk Chocolate Miniatures	7 (1.5 oz)	230	10	1
Truffles	3 (1.2 oz)	200	5	1
Dream				
Caramel & Nougat In Milk Chocolate	1 bar (1 oz)	90	<5	1
Estee				
Caramels Vanilla & Chocolate	5	115	0	0
Dark Chocolate	½ bar (1.4 oz)	200	10	0
Milk Chocolate	½ bar (1.4 oz)	230	20	0
Milk Chocolate w/ Almonds	½ bar (1.4 oz)	230	20	0
Milk Chocolate w/ Crisp Rice	½ bar (1.2 oz)	370	30	0
Milk Chocolate w/ Fruit & Nuts	½ bar (1.4 oz)	220	20	0
Mint Chocolate	½ bar (1.4 oz)	200	10	0
Peanut Brittle	⅓ box (1.3 oz)	160	10	1
Peanut Butter Cups	5	200	<5	1
Sugar Free Assorted Fruit	5	30	0	0
Sugar Free Assorted Mint	5	30	0	0
Sugar Free Butterscotch	2	25	0	0
Sugar Free Fruit Gum Drops	23	80	0	0
Sugar Free Gourmet Jelly Beans	26	70	0	0
Sugar Free Gummy Apple Rings	5	70	0	0

FOOD	PORTION	CALS	CHOL	FIBER
Sugar Free Gummy Bears Assorted Fruit	17	100	0	0
Sugar Free Licorice Gum Drops	11	90	0	0
Sugar Free Peppermint Swirl	3	30	0	0
Sugar Free Sour Citrus Slices	9	60	0	0
Sugar Free Toffee	5	30	0	0
Sugar Free Tropical Fruit	5	30	0	0
Ferrero Rocher				
Candy	2 pieces (0.9 oz)	150	0	0
Godiva				
Almond Butter Dome	3 pieces (1.5 oz)	240	5	0
Bouchee Au Chocolat	1 piece (1.5 oz)	210	5	0
Bouchee Ivory Raspberry	1 pieces (1 oz)	160	5	0
Chocolatier Dark Chocolate w/ Raspberry	1 bar (1.5 oz)	220	3	0
Chocolatier Milk Chocolate	1 bar (1.5 ox)	230	10	0
Gold Ballotin	3 pieces (1.5 oz)	210	5	0
Mochaccino Mousse	2 pieces (1.25 oz)	210	4	0
Truffle Amaretto Di Saronno	2 pieces (1.5 oz)	210	5	0
Truffles Assorted	2 pieces (1.5 oz)	220	10	0
Goetze's				
Cow Tales	1 pkg (1 oz)	110	tr	tr
Goldenberg's				
Peanut Chews	3 pieces (1.3 oz)	180	0	1
Goo Goo Supreme				
With Pecans	1 pkg (1.5 oz)	188	0	4
Goobers				
Peanuts	1 pkg (1.38 oz)	210	5	1
Good & Plenty				
Snacksize	3 boxes (1.5 oz)	140	0	—

FOOD	PORTION	CALS	CHOL	FIBER
Haviland				
Chocolate Covered Thin Mints	6 (1.5 oz)	170	0	1
Hershey				
Amazin'Fruit Gummy Candy	1 snack pkg (0.7 oz)	60	0	—
Bar	1 (0.6 oz)	100	0	—
Candy-Coated Milk Chocolate Eggs	4 pieces	90	<5	—
Cookies 'n' Mint	1 bar (0.6 oz)	90	<5	—
Hugs	1 piece	25	0	—
Hugs w/ Almonds	1 piece	25	0	—
Kisses	1	25	0	—
Kisses w/ Almond	1	25	0	—
Milk Chocolate	1 bar (0.6 oz)	90	<5	—
Milk Chocolate w/ Almonds	1 bar (0.6 oz)	100	<5	—
Miniature Milk Chocolate	1 (0.3 oz)	45	0	—
Nuggets Cookies 'n' Creme	1 (0.35 oz)	50	0	—
Nuggets Cookies 'n' Mint	1 (0.35 oz)	50	0	—
Nuggets Milk Chocolate	1 (0.35 oz)	50	0	—
Nuggets Milk Chocolate w/ Almonds	1 (0.35 oz)	50	0	—
Pot Of Gold Solitaires	5 pieces	90	<5	—
ReeseSticks Snack Size	2 pieces (1.2 oz)	190	0	1
Special Dark Miniature	1 (0.3 oz)	45	0	—
Sweet Escapes Chocolate Toffee Crisp	1 bar (0.66 oz)	80	<5	—
Sweet Escapes Peanut Butter Crispy	1 bar (0.7 oz)	70	0	—
Sweet Escapes Triple Chocolate Wafer	1 bar (0.7 oz)	80	0	—
Tastetations Butterscotch	3 pieces (0.6 oz)	60	<5	—
Tastetations Caramel	3 pieces (0.6 oz)	60	<5	—

FOOD	PORTION	CALS	CHOL	FIBER
Tastetations Chocolate	3 pieces (0.6 oz)	60	<5	–
Tastetations Chocolate Mint	3 pieces (0.6 oz)	60	<5	–
Tastetations Peppermint	3 pieces (0.6 oz)	60	0	–
Jolly Rancher				
Lollipops All Flavors	1 (0.6 oz)	60	0	–
Joyva				
Halvah	1.5 oz	240	0	2
Halvah Chocolate Covered	1 bar (2 oz)	380	0	3
Jells Raspberry	3 pieces (1.6 oz)	200	0	tr
Joys Raspberry	1 (1.6 oz)	200	0	1
Marshmallow Twists Chocolate Covered	2 (1.5 oz)	190	0	0
Rings Orange & Raspberry	3 pieces (1.5 oz)	190	0	tr
Sesame Crunch	3 pieces (0.5)	80	0	0
Sticks Orange	3 pieces (1.6 oz)	200	0	tr
Twists Vanilla & Cherry	2 pieces (1.5 oz)	190	0	0
Juicefuls				
Candy	3 pieces (0.5 oz)	60	0	–
Junior Mints				
Snack Size	1 pkg (0.7 oz)	75	0	0
Just Born				
Hot Tamales	1 pkg (2.1 oz)	220	0	–
Mike and Ike Berry Fruits	1 pkg (2.1 oz)	220	0	–
Mike and Ike Cherry & Bubble Gum	1 pkg (2.1 oz)	220	0	–
Mike and Ike Chewy Grape	1 pkg (2.1 oz)	220	0	–
Mike and Ike Lemon Watermelon	1 pkg (2.1 oz)	220	0	–
Mike and Ike Original	1 pkg (1.2 oz)	220	0	–
Mike and Ike Strawberry & Banana	1 pkg (2.1 oz)	220	0	–
Mike and Ike Tropical Fruits	1 pkg (2.1 oz)	220	0	–
Super Hot Tamales	1 pkg (2.1 oz)	220	0	–

FOOD	PORTION	CALS	CHOL	FIBER
Teenee Beanee Assorted Fruits	36 pieces (1.4 oz)	150	0	–
Teenee Beanee Berry Berry	36 pieces (1.4 oz)	150	0	–
Teenee Beanee Tropical Mix	36 pieces (1.4 oz)	150	0	–
Kit Kat				
Bar	1 (0.56 oz)	80	0	–
Krackel				
Bar	1 (0.6 oz)	90	<5	–
Miniature	1 (0.3 oz)	45	0	–
Lance				
Chocolaty Peanut Bar	1 (2 oz)	290	0	2
Cinnamon Chews	1 pkg (1.06 oz)	120	0	0
Fruit Chews	1 pkg (1.06 oz)	120	0	0
Gum Ball Pops	1 (0.45 oz)	45	0	tr
K-Nuts	4 pieces (1.5 oz)	240	5	0
Mint Chews	1 pkg (1.06 oz)	120	0	0
Peanut Bar	1 (1.75 oz)	270	0	2
Pop-A-Lance	1 piece (0.42 oz)	45	0	0
Popcorn'n'Carmel	1 bar (0.75 oz)	90	0	0
Starlight Mints	3 pieces (1 oz)	60	0	0
Strawberry Chews	1 pkg (1.06 oz)	120	0	0
Suckers	3 pieces (0.5 oz)	50	0	0
Whistle Pop	1 (0.67 oz)	70	0	tr
Lifesavers				
Big Tablet Candy Cane	4 pieces (0.5 oz)	60	0	–
Cards 'N Candy	4 pieces (0.4 oz)	40	0	–
Christmas Tin	4 pieces (0.5 oz)	60	0	–
Egg-Sortment	1 roll (0.4 oz)	40	0	–
Gummi Bunnies	3 pkg (1.6 oz)	140	0	–
Gummi Savers Five Flavor	1 roll (1.5 oz)	130	0	–
Gummi Savers Five Flavor	1 pkg (1.8 oz)	160	0	–
Gummi Savers Mixed Berry	1 roll (1.5 oz)	130	0	–
Gummi Savers Mixed Berry	1 pkg (1.8 oz)	160	0	–

FOOD	PORTION	CALS	CHOL	FIBER
Gummi Savers Tangy Fruits	1 roll (1.5 oz)	130	0	—
Gummi Savers Tangy Fruits	1 pkg (1.8 oz)	160	0	—
Gummi Savers Variety	2 pkg (1.3 oz)	120	0	—
Gummi Savers Wacky Frootz	1 roll (1.5 oz)	130	0	—
Gummi Savers Wacky Frootz	1 pkg (1.8 oz)	160	0	—
Gummi Shapes Barnum's Animals	1 pkg (0.8 oz)	70	0	—
Holes Five Flavor	20 pieces (5 g)	20	0	—
Holes Island Fruit	20 pieces (5 g)	20	0	—
Holes Sour 'N Sweet	16 pieces (5 g)	20	0	—
Holes Sunshine Fruits	20 pieces (0.2 oz)	20	0	—
Holes Super Tart	20 pieces (5 g)	20	0	—
Holes Wild Fruits	20 pieces (5 g)	20	<5	—
Lollipops Candy Cane	1 (0.4 oz)	40	0	—
Lollipops Christmas	1 (0.4 oz)	40	0	—
Lollipops Easter	1 (0.4 oz)	40	0	—
Lollipops Fruit Flavors	1 (0.4 oz)	45	0	0
Lollipops Swirled Flavors	1 (0.4 oz)	40	0	—
Lollipops Valentine	1 (0.4 oz)	40	0	—
Roll Butter Rum	2 pieces (5 g)	20	0	—
Roll Candy Cane	4 pieces (0.4 oz)	40	0	—
Roll Cryst-O-Mint	2 pieces (5 g)	20	0	—
Roll Five Flavor	2 pieces (5 g)	20	0	—
Roll Fruits On Fire	2 pieces (5 g)	20	0	—
Roll Pep-O-Mint	3 pieces (5 g)	20	0	—
Roll Spear-O-Mint	3 pieces (5 g)	20	0	—
Roll Sunshine Fruits	2 pieces (5 g)	20	0	—
Roll Tangy Fruit Swirl	2 pieces (5 g)	20	0	—
Roll Tangy Fruit Watermelon	1 pieces (5 g)	20	0	—
Roll Tangy Fruits	2 pieces (5 g)	20	0	—
Roll Tropical Fruits	2 pieces (5 g)	20	0	—
Roll Wild Cherry	1 pieces (5 g)	20	0	—
Roll Wild Flavors	2 pieces (5 g)	20	0	—
Roll Wild Sour Berries	2 pieces (5 g)	20	0	—

FOOD	PORTION	CALS	CHOL	FIBER
Roll Wint-O-Green	3 pieces (5 g)	20	0	—
Sack'it Butter Rum	4 pieces (0.5 oz)	60	0	—
Sack'it Five Flavor	4 pieces (0.5 oz)	60	0	—
Sack'it Holiday Tin	4 pieces (0.5 oz)	60	0	—
Sack'it Pep-O-Mint	4 pieces (0.5 oz)	60	0	—
Sack'it Tangy Fruits	4 pieces (0.5 oz)	60	0	—
Sack'it Wild Cherry	4 pieces (0.5 oz)	60	0	—
Sack'it Wint-O-Green	4 pieces (0.5 oz)	60	0	—
Sugar Free Iced Mint	1 pieces (2 g)	10	0	—
Sugar Free Vanilla Mint	1 pieces (2 g)	10	0	—
Valentine Book	2 pieces (5 g)	20	0	—
Lindt				
Truffles Milk Chocolate	3 pieces (1.3 oz)	210	5	tr
M&M's				
Almond	1.5 oz	220	5	2
Almond	1 pkg (1.3 oz)	200	5	2
Mint	1 pkg (1.7 oz)	230	10	1
Mint	1.5 oz	200	5	1
Peanut	½ bag king size (1.6 oz)	240	5	2
Peanut	1.5 oz	220	5	2
Peanut	1 pkg (1.7 oz)	250	5	2
Peanut	1 fun size (0.7 oz)	110	5	1
Peanut Butter	1 pkg (1.6 oz)	240	5	2
Peanut Butter	1.5 oz	220	5	2
Peanut Butter	1 fun size (0.7 oz)	110	0	1
Plain	1 pkg fun size (0.7 oz)	100	5	0
Plain	½ pkg king size (1.6 oz)	220	5	1
Plain	1 pkg (1.7 oz)	230	6	1
Plain	1.5 oz	200	5	1
Mars				
Almond Bar	2 fun size (1.3 oz)	190	5	1
Almond Bar	1 bar (1.8 oz)	240	5	1
Milk Duds				
Snack Size	4 boxes (1.3 oz)	160	0	0
Milky Way				
Bar	2 fun size (1.4 oz)	180	5	0
Bar	⅓ king size (1.2 oz)	160	5	0

FOOD	PORTION	CALS	CHOL	FIBER
Bar	1 (2.1 oz)	280	5	1
Dark	1 bar (1.8 oz)	220	5	1
Dark	1 fun size (0.7 oz)	90	0	0
Miniature	5 (1.5 oz)	190	5	0
Mounds				
Bar	1 (0.68 oz)	90	0	—
Mr. Goodbar				
Miniature	1 (0.3 oz)	45	0	—
Necco				
Bridge Mix	¼ cup (1.5 oz)	180	5	tr
Chocolate Covered Raisins	30 pieces (1.5 oz)	170	0	1
Malted Milk Balls	11 pieces (1.5 oz)	180	0	tr
Mint	1 piece	12	0	—
SkyBar	1 bar (1.5 oz)	190	5	0
Nestle				
Buncha Crunch	1 pkg (1.4 oz)	90	10	tr
Crunch	1 bar (1.55 oz)	230	10	tr
Crunch Disk	1 (1.2 oz)	180	5	tr
Crunchkins	5 pieces	190	5	tr
Jingles Milk Chocolate Butterfinger	5 pieces	180	<5	tr
Jingles Milk Chocolate Crunch	7 pieces	220	10	tr
Jingles White Crunch	7 pieces	230	10	0
Milk Chocolate	1 bar (1.45 oz)	220	10	tr
Nesteggs Milk Chocolate Butterfinger	5 pieces	210	5	tr
Nesteggs Milk Chocolate Crunch	5 pieces	190	5	tr
Nesteggs White Crunch	7 pieces	230	10	0
Pearson's Egg Nog	2 pieces	60	0	0
Treasures Butterfinger	3 pieces	180	5	tr
Treasures Crunch	4 pieces (1.4 oz)	210	10	tr
Treasures Peanut Butter	4 pieces	250	5	1
Turtles	2 pieces (1.2 oz)	160	<5	tr
Turtles Bite Size	1 piece (0.4 oz)	50	1	tr
White Crunch	1 bar (1.4 oz)	220	10	0

FOOD	PORTION	CALS	CHOL	FIBER
Newman's Own				
Organic Peanut Butter Cups Dark Chocolate	3 pieces (1.2 oz)	180	0	tr
Organic Peanut Butter Cups Milk Chocolate	3 pieces (1.2 oz)	180	0	tr
Organic Peppermint Cups	3 pieces (1.2 oz)	180	0	tr
Organics Espresso Sweet Dark Chocolate	1 bar (1.2 oz)	190	0	0
Nibs				
Cherry	1 pkg (0.49 oz)	45	0	—
Licorice	1 pkg (0.49 oz)	40	0	—
Nips				
Butter Rum	2 pieces	60	0	0
Caramel	2 pieces	60	0	0
Chocolate	2 pieces	60	0	0
Chocolate Parfait	2 pieces	60	0	0
Coffee	2 pieces	50	0	0
Vanilla Almond Cafe	2 pieces	50	0	0
Oh Henry!				
Bar	1 (1.8 oz)	120	<5	0
Palmer				
Milk Chocolate Lollipop	1 (0.9 oz)	130	4	2
Pearson's				
Irish Cream Parfait	2 pieces	60	0	0
Mint Patties	5 (1.3 oz)	150	0	tr
Pez				
Candy	1 roll (0.3 oz)	35	0	—
Candy Sugar Free	1 roll (0.3 oz)	30	0	—
Planters				
Original Peanut Bar	1 pkg (1.6 oz)	230	0	2
Raisinets				
Candy	1 pkg (1.58 oz)	200	<5	1
Fun Size	3 pkg (1.7 oz)	200	5	2
Reese's				
Eggs	1 (0.6 oz)	90	0	—
FastBreak	1 bar (2 oz)	270	<5	2
Nutrageous	1 (0.6 oz)	90	0	—
Peanut Butter Cups	1 (0.28 oz)	40	0	—

FOOD	PORTION	CALS	CHOL	FIBER
Pieces	25 (0.7 oz)	100	0	–
ReeseSticks Peanut Butter	2 pieces (1.2 oz)	190	0	1
Riesen				
Candy	5 pieces (1.4 oz)	180	<5	3
Rokeach				
Cotton Candy	2 cups (1 oz)	110	0	0
Rolo				
Caramels In Milk Chocolate	3 pieces (0.64 oz)	90	<5	–
Russell Stover				
Assorted Creams	3 pieces (1.4 oz)	180	<5	0
Looney Tunes Peanut Butter Nougat w/ Peanuts in Milk Chocolate	1 snack size (0.7 oz)	90	<5	tr
Peanut Butter & Grape Jelly	1 piece (0.8 oz)	100	<5	tr
Peanut Butter & Red Raspberry Cups	2 (1.2 oz)	140	<5	tr
Pecan Delights	1 pkg (1.8 oz)	250	10	2
Pecan Roll	1 (1.75 oz)	260	<5	2
S'mores	3 (1.4 oz)	210	<5	tr
Sugar Free Peanut Butter Cups	4 pieces (1.3 oz)	200	0	2
Sugar Free Pecans & Caramel	2 pieces (1.2 oz)	170	0	0
Simply Lite				
Sugar Free Lil'l Bits Chocolatey	36 pieces (1.4 oz)	130	0	1
Sugar Free Lil'l Bits Peanut Buttery	36 pieces (1.4 oz)	140	0	1
Sugar Free Patteez	5 pieces (1.3 oz)	110	0	1
Skittles				
Original	2 pkg fun size (1.6 oz)	180	0	0
Original	1 pkg (2.8 oz)	250	0	0
Original	½ king size (1.3 oz)	150	0	0
Original	1.5 oz	170	0	0
Tropical	1.5 oz	170	0	0
Tropical	1 bag (2.2 oz)	250	0	0

FOOD	PORTION	CALS	CHOL	FIBER
Tropical	2 bags fun size (1.4 oz)	160	0	0
Wild Berry	1.5 oz	170	0	0
Wild Berry	1 bag (2.2 oz)	250	0	0
Wild Berry	2 bags fun size (1.4 oz)	160	0	0
Smucker's				
Fruit Fillers Strawberry	1 pkg (0.9 oz)	80	0	–
Jelly Beans	1 pkg (0.7 oz)	70	0	0
Snickers				
Bar	1 bar (2.1 oz)	280	10	1
Bar	2 bars fun size (1.4 oz)	190	5	1
Bar	⅓ king size (1.2 oz)	170	5	1
Cruncher	3 fun size (1.4 oz)	230	5	1
Miniatures	4 (1.3 oz)	170	5	1
Munch Bar	1 (1.4 oz)	230	10	2
Peanut Butter	1 bar (2 oz)	310	5	1
Sno Caps				
Candies	1 pkg (2.3 oz)	300	0	3
Speakeasy				
Organic Mints All Flavors	4 pieces (2 g)	10	0	–
Starburst				
California Fruits	1 stick (2.1 oz)	240	2	0
California Fruits	8 pieces (1.4 oz)	160	0	0
Original Fruits	⅓ king size (1.2 oz)	140	0	0
Original Fruits	1 stick (2.1 oz)	240	0	0
Original Fruits	8 pieces (1.4 oz)	160	0	0
Strawberry Fruits	8 pieces (1.4 oz)	160	0	0
Strawberry Fruits	1 stick (2.1 oz)	240	0	0
Tropical Fruits	1 stick (2.1 oz)	240	0	0
Tropical Fruits	8 pieces (1.4 oz)	160	0	0
Steel's				
Salt Water Taffy Assorted	3 pieces (1 oz)	90	0	0
Swedish Fish				
Original	19 pieces (1.4 oz)	160	0	0
Sweet'N Low				
Sugar Free Butter Toffee	4 pieces (0.5 oz)	30	<5	–
Sugar Free Butterscotch	1 piece	7	0	–
Sugar Free Cinnamon	1 piece	7	0	–

FOOD	PORTION	CALS	CHOL	FIBER
Sugar Free Fancy Fruit	1 piece	7	0	—
Sugar Free Fruit Flavors	1 piece	7	0	—
Sugar Free Hard Candy Coffee	4 pieces (0.5 oz)	30	0	—
Sugar Free Peppermint	1 piece	7	0	—
Sugar Free Watermelon	1 piece	7	0	—
Sugar Free Wild Cherry	1 piece	7	0	—
Symphony				
Bar	1 (0.6 oz)	100	<5	—
W/ Almonds & Chocolate Chips	1 bar (0.6 oz)	90	<5	—
Tobler				
Orange Dark Chocolate	5 pieces (1.5 oz)	240	<5	3
Toblerone				
Milk Chocolate w/ Honey & Almond Nougat	⅓ bar (1.76 oz)	170	10	tr
Tom's				
Cherry Sours	1 pkg (2.25 oz)	210	0	0
Jelly Beans	1 pkg (2.25 oz)	230	0	0
Tootsie				
Pop	1	60	0	—
Tropical Source				
Butterscotch Dream	4 pieces (0.5 oz)	60	0	0
Chocolate Dairy Free California Raisin & Currant	½ bar (1.5 oz)	230	0	1
Chocolate Dairy Free Hazelnut Espresso Crunch	½ bar (1.5 oz)	250	0	1
Chocolate Dairy Free Maple Almond Granola	½ bar (1.5 oz)	230	0	1
Chocolate Dairy Free Mint Candy Crunch	½ bar (1.5 oz)	220	0	1
Chocolate Dairy Free Red Raspberry Crush	½ bar (1.5 oz)	230	0	1
Chocolate Dairy Free Sundried Jungle Banana	½ bar (1.5 oz)	230	0	2

FOOD	PORTION	CALS	CHOL	FIBER
Chocolate Dairy Free Toasted Almond	½ bar (1.5 oz)	250	0	1
Chocolate Dairy Free Wild Rice Crisp	½ bar (1.5 oz)	230	0	1
Cool Peppermint	4 pieces (0.5 oz)	60	0	0
Lollipops All Flavors	1	24	0	0
Mango Papaya	4 pieces (0.5 oz)	60	0	0
Twix				
Caramel	1 pkg (2 oz)	280	5	0
Caramel	1 fun size (0.5 oz)	80	0	0
Caramel	1 (1 oz)	140	0	0
Caramel	1 king size (0.8 oz)	120	0	1
Peanut Butter	1 (0.9 oz)	130	0	1
Twizzlers				
Cherry	1 pieces	35	0	—
Chocolate	1 piece	30	0	—
Licorice	1 piece	35	0	—
Pull'n'Peel Cherry	1 piece (1 oz)	90	0	—
Strawberry	1 piece	35	0	—
Velamints				
Cocoamint	1 piece (1.7 g)	5	0	—
Peppermint	1 piece (1.7 g)	5	0	—
Spearmint	1 piece (1.7 g)	5	0	—
Wintergreen	1 piece (1.7 g)	5	0	—
Very Special				
Chocolate Bottles Liquor Filled	3 pieces (1 oz)	150	0	2
Werther's				
Original	3 pieces (0.5 oz)	60	<5	0
Whatchamacallit				
Bar	1 (0.58 oz)	80	0	—
Whitman's				
Assorted	3 pieces (1.4 oz)	190	5	0
Dark Chocolate	3 pieces (1.4 oz)	200	<5	1
Little Ambassadors	7 pieces (1.4 oz)	190	5	1
Pecan Delight	1 bar (2 oz)	310	10	2
Pecan Roll	1 bar (2 oz)	300	5	1
Sampler	3 pieces (1.4 oz)	200	5	1
Snoopy Treats Caramel Peanuts Milk Chocolate	1 snack size (1.4 oz)	80	5	tr

FOOD	PORTION	CALS	CHOL	FIBER
Whoppers				
Malted Milk Balls	1 pkg (0.7 oz)	100	0	0
York				
Chocolate Covered Peppermint Bites	15 pieces (1 oz)	150	0	tr
Peppermint Patty	1 (0.49 oz)	50	0	—
CANTALOUPE				
dried	3.5 pieces (1.4 oz)	140	0	1
fresh cubed	1 cup	57	0	1
fresh half	½	94	0	2
Chiquita				
Wedge	¼ med (4.7 oz)	50	0	1
CAPERS				
Reese				
Capers	1 tsp (5 g)	0	0	—
CARAWAY				
seed	1 tsp	7	0	—
CARDAMOM				
ground	1 tsp	6	0	—
CARDOON				
fresh cooked	3½ oz	22	0	—
fresh shredded	½ cup	36	0	—
CARIBOU				
roasted	3 oz	142	93	—
CARISSA				
fresh	1	12	0	—
CAROB				
carob mix	3 tsp	45	0	—
carob mix as prep w/ whole milk	9 oz	195	33	—
flour	1 tbsp	14	0	—
flour	1 cup	185	0	—
Sunspire				
Carob Chips Unsweetened	13 pieces (0.5 oz)	70	0	0
Carob Chips Vegan	13 pieces (0.5 oz)	70	0	0

FOOD	PORTION	CALS	CHOL	FIBER
CARP				
fresh	3 oz	108	56	—
fresh cooked	3 oz	138	72	—
fresh cooked	1 fillet (6 oz)	276	143	—
roe raw	1 oz	37	103	—
roe salted in olive oil	2 tbsp (1 oz)	40	100	0
CARROT JUICE				
canned	6 oz	73	0	—
CARROTS				
CANNED				
slices	½ cup	17	0	1
slices low sodium	½ cup	17	0	1
Del Monte				
Sliced	½ cup (4.3 oz)	35	0	3
Green Giant				
Sliced	½ cup (4.2 oz)	25	0	2
LeSueur				
Baby Whole	½ cup (4.2 oz)	35	0	3
S&W				
Julienne	½ cup (4.3 oz)	30	0	2
Sliced	½ cup (4.3 oz)	30	0	2
Whole Small	½ cup (4.3 oz)	30	0	2
FRESH				
baby raw	1 (½ oz)	6	0	—
raw	1 (2.5 oz)	31	0	2
raw shredded	½ cup	24	0	2
slices cooked	½ cup	35	0	—
Dole				
Shredded	1 cup (3 oz)	40	0	2
FROZEN				
slices cooked	½ cup	26	0	—
Birds Eye				
Baby Whole	½ cup	40	0	2
Sliced	½ cup	35	0	3
Green Giant				
Harvest Fresh Baby	⅔ cup (3 oz)	20	0	2
Select Baby Cut	¾ cup (2.8 oz)	30	0	3

FOOD	PORTION	CALS	CHOL	FIBER
CASABA				
cubed	1 cup	45	0	—
fresh	⅒	43	0	—
CASHEWS				
cashew butter w/o salt	1 tbsp	94	0	—
dry roasted salted	1 oz	163	0	—
dry roasted w/ salt	18 nuts (1 oz)	160	0	1
oil roasted	1 oz	163	0	—
oil roasted salted	1 oz	163	0	—
Frito Lay				
Salted	1 oz	180	0	1
Lance				
Cashews	1 pkg (1⅛ oz)	200	0	3
Maranatha				
Cashew Butter	2 tbsp	190	0	2
Tamari Cashews	¼ cup	160	0	1
Planters				
Fancy Oil Roasted	1 oz	170	0	1
Fancy Oil Roasted	1 pkg (2 oz)	340	0	3
Halves Lightly Salted Oil Roasted	1 oz	160	0	2
Halves Oil Roasted	1 oz	170	0	2
Honey Roasted	1 oz	150	0	1
Honey Roasted	1 pkg (2 oz)	310	0	3
Munch'N Go Honey Roasted	1 pkg (2 oz)	310	0	3
Munch'N Go Singles Oil Roasted	1 pkg (2 oz)	330	0	3
Oil Roasted	1 pkg (1 oz)	160	0	1
Oil Roasted	1 pkg (1.5 oz)	250	0	2
CASSAVA				
fresh	3½ oz	120	0	—
CATFISH				
channel breaded & fried	3 oz	194	69	—
channel raw	3 oz	99	49	—

FOOD	PORTION	CALS	CHOL	FIBER
CAULIFLOWER				
FRESH				
cooked	½ cup (2.2 oz)	14	0	1
flowerets cooked	3 (2 oz)	12	0	1
flowerets raw	3 (2 oz)	14	0	1
green cooked	1½ cup (3.2 oz)	29	0	3
green raw	1 head 7 in diam (18 oz)	158	0	16
green raw	1 cup (2.2 oz)	20	0	2
green raw floweret	1 (0.9 oz)	8	0	1
raw	½ cup (1.8 oz)	13	0	1
FROZEN				
cooked	½ cup	17	0	–
Birds Eye				
Cauliflower	½ cup	20	0	2
Green Giant				
Cheese Sauce	½ cup (3.5 oz)	60	<5	2
Florets	1 cup (2.8 oz)	25	0	2
CAVIAR				
black	1 tbsp	40	94	–
red	1 tbsp	40	94	–
CELERIAC				
fresh cooked	3½ oz	25	0	–
raw	½ cup	31	0	–
CELERY				
diced cooked	½ cup	13	0	–
fresh	1 stalk (1.3 oz)	6	0	1
raw diced	½ cup	10	0	1
seed	1 tsp	8	0	–
CELTUCE				
raw	3½ oz	22	0	–
CEREAL				
bran flakes	¾ cup (1 oz)	90	0	–
corn flakes	1¼ cup (1 oz)	110	0	–
corn flakes low sodium	1 cup (0.9 oz)	100	0	tr
corn grits white regular & quick as prep w/ water & salt	¾ cup (6.4 oz)	109	0	tr

FOOD	PORTION	CALS	CHOL	FIBER
corn grits white regular or quick as prep	¾ cup (6.4 oz)	109	0	tr
corn grits yellow regular & quick as prep w/ water & salt	¾ cup (6.4 oz)	109	0	tr
corn grits yellow regular & quick not prep	1 cup (5.5 oz)	579	0	3
crispy rice	1 cup (1 oz)	111	0	tr
crispy rice low sodium	1 cup (0.9 oz)	105	0	tr
farina as prep w/ water	¾ cup (6.1 oz)	88	0	2
farina not prep	1 tbsp (0.4 oz)	40	0	tr
granola	½ cup (2.1 oz)	285	0	6
oatmeal instant w/ cinnamon & spice as prep w/ water	1 pkg (5.6 oz)	177	0	3
oatmeal instant w/ raisins & spice as prep w/ water	1 cup (5.5 oz)	161	0	2
oatmeal instant w/ bran & raisins as prep w/ water	1 pkg (6.8 oz)	158	0	6
oatmeal instant as prep w/ water	1 cup (8.2 oz)	138	0	4
oatmeal regular & quick as prep w/ water	¾ cup (6.1 oz)	149	0	3
oatmeal regular & quick not prep	⅓ cup (0.9 oz)	104	0	3
oatmeal instant cooked w/o salt	1 cup	145	0	–
oatmeal quick cooked w/o salt	1 cup	145	0	–
oatmeal regular cooked w/o salt	1 cup	145	0	–
puffed rice	1 cup (0.5 oz)	56	0	tr
puffed wheat	1 cup (0.4 oz)	44	0	1
shredded mini wheats	1 cup (1.1 oz)	107	0	3

FOOD	PORTION	CALS	CHOL	FIBER
shredded wheat rectangular	1 biscuit (0.8 oz)	85	0	2
shredded wheat round	2 biscuits (1.3 oz)	136	0	4
sugar-coated corn flakes	¾ cup (1 oz)	110	0	–
whole wheat hot natural as prep w/ water	¾ cup (6.4 oz)	113	0	3
Albers				
Hominy Quick Grits uncooked	¼ cup	140	0	1
Back To Nature				
Hi-Protein	⅔ cup	140	0	3
Muesli	½ cup	160	0	4
Puff Wheat	½ cup	160	0	4
Ultra Flax	¾ cup	150	0	3
Barbara's Bakery				
Apple Cinnamon O's	¾ cup	110	0	2
Bite Size Shredded Oats	1¼ cups (2 oz)	220	0	6
Cinnamon Puffins	1¼ cup (2 oz)	100	0	6
Cocoa Crunch Stars	1 cup (1 oz)	110	0	1
Frosted Corn Flakes	1 cup (1 oz)	110	0	4
Fruit Juice Sweetened Breakfast O's	1 cup (1 oz)	120	0	3
Fruit Juice Sweetened Brown Rice Crisps	1 cup (1 oz)	120	0	1
Fruit Juice Sweetened Corn Flakes	1 cup (1 oz)	110	0	2
GrainShop	⅔ cup (1 oz)	90	0	8
Honey Crunch Stars	1 cup (1 oz)	110	0	2
Honey Nut Toasted O's	¾ cup	120	0	2
Organic Fruity Punch	1 cup (1 oz)	110	0	0
Organic Soy Essence	¾ cup (1 oz)	100	0	5
Puffins	¾ cup (0.9 oz)	90	0	5
Shredded Spoonfuls	¾ cup (1.1 oz)	110	0	4
Shredded Wheat	2 biscuits (1.4 oz)	140	0	5
General Mills				
Basic 4	1 cup (1.9 oz)	200	0	3
Boo Berry	1 cup (1 oz)	120	0	–

FOOD	PORTION	CALS	CHOL	FIBER
Cheerios	1 cup (1 oz)	110	0	3
Cheerios Apple Cinnamon	¾ cup (1 oz)	120	0	1
Cheerios Frosted	1 cup (1 oz)	120	0	1
Cheerios Honey Nut	1 cup (1 oz)	120	0	2
Cheerios Multi Grain	1 cup (1 oz)	110	0	3
Cheerios Team	1 cup (1 oz)	120	0	1
Chex Corn	1 cup (1 oz)	110	0	0
Chex Honey Nut	¾ cup	120	0	–
Chex Morning Mix Cinnamon	1 pkg (1.1 oz)	130	0	1
Chex Morning Mix Fruit & Nut	1 pkg (1.1 oz)	180	0	1
Chex Morning Mix Honey Nut	1 pkg (1.1 oz)	130	0	1
Chex Multi-Bran	1 cup (2 oz)	200	0	8
Chex Rice	1¼ cup (1.1 oz)	120	0	0
Cinnamon Grahams	¾ cup (1 oz)	120	0	1
Cinnamon Toast Crunch	¾ cup (1 oz)	130	1	1
Cocoa Puffs	1 cup (1 oz)	120	0	–
Cookie Crisp	1 cup (1 oz)	120	0	0
Count Chocula	1 cup (1 oz)	120	0	0
Country Corn Flakes	1 cup (1 oz)	120	0	–
Fiber One	½ cup (1 oz)	60	0	14
Franken Berry	1 cup (1 oz)	120	0	–
French Toast Crunch	¾ cup (1 oz)	120	0	0
Gold Medal Raisin Bran	1½ cups (1.9 oz)	170	0	6
Golden Grahams	¾ cup (1 oz)	120	0	1
Harmony	1¼ cups (1.9 oz)	200	0	2
Honey Nut Clusters	1 cup (1.9 oz)	210	0	3
Kaboom	1¼ cup (1 oz)	120	0	1
Kix	1⅓ cup (1 oz)	120	0	1
Kix Berry Berry	¾ cup (1 oz)	120	0	0
Lucky Charms	1 cup (1 oz)	120	0	1
Nature Valley Low Fat Fruit Granola	⅔ cup (1.9 oz)	210	0	3
Newquick	¾ cup (1 oz)	120	0	–
Oatmeal Crisp Almond	1 cup (1.9 oz)	220	0	4

FOOD	PORTION	CALS	CHOL	FIBER
Oatmeal Crisp Apple Cinnamon	1 cup (1.9 oz)	210	0	4
Oatmeal Crisp Raisin	1 cup (1.9 oz)	210	0	4
Para Su Familia Cinnamon Stars	1 cup (1 oz)	120	0	—
Para Su Familia Fruitis	1 cup (1 oz)	120	0	—
Para Su Familia Raisin Bran	1¼ cups (2 oz)	170	0	6
Raisin Nut Bran	¾ cup (1.9 oz)	200	0	4
Reese's Puffs	¾ cup	130	0	0
Snack'N Dash Cinnamon Toast Crunch	1 pkg (1.2 oz)	140	0	1
Snack'N Dash Honey Nut Cheerios	1 pkg (1 oz)	110	0	2
Snack'N Dash Lucky Charms	1 pkg (1 oz)	110	0	1
Sunrise Organic	¾ cup (1 oz)	110	0	1
Total Brown Sugar & Oat	¾ cup (1 oz)	110	0	1
Total Corn Flakes	1⅓ cup (1 oz)	110	0	—
Total Raisin Bran	1 cup (1.9 oz)	170	0	5
Total Whole Grain	¾ cup (1 oz)	110	0	3
Trix	1 cup (1 oz)	120	0	1
Wheat Hearts	¼ cup (1.3 oz)	130	0	2
Wheaties	1 cup (1 oz)	110	0	3
Wheaties Energy Crunch	1 cup (1.9 oz)	210	0	4
Wheaties Frosted	¾ cup (1 oz)	110	0	—
Wheaties Raisin Bran	1 cup (1.9 oz)	180	0	5
Hansen's				
Orange & Chocolate	½ cup	230	0	4
Strawberry & Yogurt	½ cup	230	0	6
Toasted Nut Crunch	½ cup	230	0	7
Tropical Cluster	½ cup	210	0	6
Health Valley				
10 Bran O's Apple Cinnamon	¾ cup	100	0	3

FOOD	PORTION	CALS	CHOL	FIBER
Bran w/ Apples & Cinnamon	¾ cup	160	0	7
Golden Flax	½ cup	190	0	6
Granola 98% Fat Free Date Almond	⅔ cup	180	0	6
Healthy Crunches & Flakes Almond	¾ cup	130	0	4
Healthy Crunches & Flakes Apple Cinnamon	¾ cup	130	0	4
Healthy Crunches & Flakes Honey Crunch	¾ cup	130	0	4
Hot Cereal Cups Amazing Apple!	1 pkg	220	0	4
Hot Cereal Cups Banana Gone Nuts	1 pkg	240	0	4
Hot Cereal Cups Maple Madness!	1 pkg	240	0	4
Hot Cereal Cups Terrific 10 Grain!	1 pkg	220	0	5
Oat Bran O'S	¾ cup	100	0	3
Organic Amaranth Flakes	¾ cup	100	0	4
Organic Blue Corn Bran Flakes	¾ cup	100	0	4
Organic Bran w/ Raisin	¾ cup	160	0	6
Organic Fiber 7 Flakes	¾ cup	100	0	4
Organic Healthy Fiber Flakes	¾ cup	100	0	4
Organic Oat Bran Flakes	¾ cup	100	0	4
Organic Oat Bran Flakes w/ Raisins	¾ cup	110	0	4
Puffed Honey Sweetened Corn	1 cup	110	0	2
Puffed Honey Sweetened Crisp Brown Rice	1 cup	110	0	2
Raisin Bran Flakes	1¼ cup	190	0	5

FOOD	PORTION	CALS	CHOL	FIBER
Real Oat Bran	½ cup	200	0	5
Healthy Choice				
Almond Crunch With Raisins	1 cup (2 oz)	210	0	5
Golden Multi-Grain Flakes	¾ cup (1.1 oz)	110	0	3
Toasted Brown Sugar Squares	1 cup (2 oz)	190	0	5
Hodgson Mill				
Cracked Wheat	¼ cup (1.4 oz)	110	0	8
Multi Grain w/ Flaxseed & Soy	⅓ cup (1.4 oz)	160	0	6
Kashi				
Breakfast Pilaf as prep	½ cup (4.9 oz)	170	0	6
Go Apple Spice	½ cup (4.9 oz)	270	0	6
Go Banana Almond	½ cup (4.9 oz)	280	0	6
Go Berry Tart	½ cup (4.9 oz)	260	0	6
Go Blueberry Bliss	½ cup (4.9 oz)	260	0	6
Go Cherry Vanilla	½ cup (4.9 oz)	260	0	6
Go Just Peachy	½ cup (4.9 oz)	260	0	6
GoLean	¾ cup (1.4 oz)	120	0	10
Good Friends	¾ cup (1 oz)	90	0	8
Honey Puffed	1 cup (1 oz)	120	0	2
Medley	½ cup (1 oz)	100	0	2
Pillows Apple	¾ cup (1.9 oz)	200	0	2
Pillows Chocolate	¾ cup (1.9 oz)	200	0	2
Pillows Strawberry Crisp	¾ cup (1.9 oz)	200	0	2
Puffed	1 cup (0.9 oz)	70	0	2
Kellogg's				
All-Bran	½ cup (1.1 oz)	80	0	10
All-Bran Bran Buds	⅓ cup (1 oz)	80	0	13
All-Bran Extra Fiber	½ cup (0.9 oz)	50	0	13
Apple Jacks	1 cup (1.2 oz)	120	0	1
Cocoa Frosted Flakes	¾ cup (1.1 oz)	120	0	0
Cocoa Krispies	¾ cup (1.1 oz)	120	0	0
Complete Oat Bran Flakes	¾ cup (1 oz)	110	0	4

FOOD	PORTION	CALS	CHOL	FIBER
Complete Wheat Bran Flakes	¾ cup (1 oz)	90	0	5
Corn Flakes	1 cup (1 oz)	100	0	1
Corn Pops K-Sentials	1 oz	100	0	0
Cracklin' Oat Bran	¾ cup (1.7 oz)	190	0	6
Crispix	1 cup (1 oz)	110	0	1
Froot Loops K-Sentials	1 oz	100	0	0
Frosted Flakes	¾ cup (1.1 oz)	120	0	1
Granola Low Fat	½ cup (1.7 oz)	190	0	3
Honey Crunch Corn Flakes	¾ cup (1.1 oz)	120	0	1
Just Right Crunchy Nuggets	1 cup (2 oz)	210	0	3
Just Right Fruit & Nut	1 cup (2.1 oz)	220	0	3
Low Fat With Raisins	⅔ cup (2.1 oz)	220	0	3
Mini-Wheat Frosted	1 cup (1.8 oz)	180	0	5
Mini-Wheat Strawberry Squares	¾ cup (1.8 oz)	170	0	5
Mini-Wheats Apple Cinnamon Squares	¾ cup (1.9 oz)	180	0	5
Mini-Wheats Blueberry Squares	¾ cup (1.9 oz)	180	0	5
Mini-Wheats Frosted Bite Size	24 pieces (2.1 oz)	200	0	6
Mini-Wheats Raisin Squares	¾ cup (1.9 oz)	180	0	5
Mueslix Apple & Almond Crunch	¾ cups (1.9 oz)	200	0	5
Mueslix Raisin & Almond	⅔ cup (1.9 oz)	200	0	4
Nutri-Grain Almond Raisin	1¼ cup (1.7 oz)	180	0	4
Nutri-Grain Golden Wheat	¾ cup (1 oz)	100	0	4
Product 19	1 cup (1 oz)	100	0	1
Raisin Bran	1 cup (2.1 oz)	200	0	8
Rice Krispies	1¼ cup (1.2 oz)	120	0	0
Rice Krispies Razzle Dazzle	¾ cup (1 oz)	110	0	0
Rice Krispies Treats	¾ cup (1 oz)	120	0	0

FOOD	PORTION	CALS	CHOL	FIBER
Smacks	¾ cup (1 oz)	100	0	1
Smart Start	1 cup (1.8 oz)	180	0	2
Special K	1 cup (1.1 oz)	110	0	1
Kolln				
Crispy Oats	1 cup (1.8 oz)	190	0	2
Oat Bran Crunch	⅔ cup (2.1 oz)	220	0	9
Oat Muesli Fruit	¾ cup (2 oz)	200	0	4
Lundberg				
Purely Organic Hot'n Creamy Rice	⅓ cup	190	0	3
McCann's				
Irish Oatmeal	1 oz	110	0	3
Irish Oatmeal Instant Apples & Cinnamon	1 pkg (1 oz)	130	0	2
Irish Oatmeal Instant Maple & Brown Sugar	1 pkg (1 oz)	160	0	3
Irish Oatmeal Instant Regular	1 pkg (1 oz)	100	0	3
Morning Traditions				
Banana Nut Crunch	1 cup (2 oz)	250	0	4
Blueberry Morning	1¼ cup (1.9 oz)	220	0	2
Cranberry Almond Crunch	1 cup (1.9 oz)	220	0	3
Great Grains Crunchy Pecan	⅔ cup (1.9 oz)	220	0	4
Great Grains Raisins Dates & Pecans	⅔ cup (1.9 oz)	210	0	4
Mother's				
Oatmeal Instant	½ cup (1.4 oz)	150	0	4
Whole Wheat Natural	½ cup (1.4 oz)	130	0	4
Mueslix				
Crispy Blend	⅔ cup (1.9 oz)	200	0	4
Nabisco				
100% Bran	⅓ cup (1 oz)	80	0	8
Frosted Shredded Wheat Bite Size	1 cup (1.8 oz)	190	0	5
Honey Nut Shredded Wheat Bite Size	1 cup (1.8 oz)	200	0	4
Original Shredded Wheat	2 biscuits (1.6 oz)	160	0	5

FOOD	PORTION	CALS	CHOL	FIBER
Original Shredded Wheat 'N Bran	1¼ cup (2.1 oz)	200	0	8
Original Shredded Wheat Spoon Size	1 cup (1.7 oz)	170	0	5
Nutri-Grain				
Almond Raisin	1¼ cup (2 oz)	200	0	4
Golden Wheat	¾ cup (1.1 oz)	100	0	4
Post				
Alpha-Bits	1 cup (1 oz)	130	0	1
Alpha-Bits Marshmallow	1 cup (1 oz)	120	0	0
Bran Flakes	¾ cup (1 oz)	100	0	5
Cocoa Pebbles	¾ cup (1 oz)	120	0	0
Fruit & Fibre Dates Raisins & Walnuts	1 cup (1.9 oz)	210	0	5
Fruit & Fibre Peaches Raisins & Almonds	1 cup (1.9 oz)	210	0	5
Fruity Pebbles	¾ cup (1 oz)	110	0	0
Golden Crisp	¾ cup (1 oz)	110	0	0
Grape-Nuts	¾ cup (1 oz)	100	0	3
Grape-Nuts Flakes	¾ cup (1 oz)	100	0	3
Honey Bunches Of Oats	¾ cup (1 oz)	120	0	1
Honey Bunches Of Oats With Almonds	¾ cup (1.1 oz)	130	0	1
Honeycomb	1⅓ cups (1 oz)	110	0	tr
Post Toasties	1 cup (1 oz)	100	0	1
Raisin Bran	1 cup (2 oz)	190	0	8
Selects Blueberry Morning	¾ cup (1.3 oz)	140	0	2
Waffle Crisp	1 cup (1 oz)	130	0	0
Pritikin				
Apple Raisin Spice	1 pkg (1.6 oz)	170	0	—
Multigrain	1 pkg	160	0	—
Quaker				
Instant Grits Original	1 pkg (1 oz)	100	0	1
Multigrain	½ cup (1.4 oz)	130	0	5
Oatmeal Instant	1 pkg (1 oz)	100	0	3
Oatmeal Instant Apples & Cinnamon	1 pkg (1.2 oz)	130	0	3

FOOD	PORTION	CALS	CHOL	FIBER
Oatmeal Instant Bananas & Cream	1 pkg (1.2 oz)	130	0	2
Oatmeal Instant Blueberries & Cream	1 pkg (1.2 oz)	130	0	2
Oatmeal Instant Cinnamon & Spice	1 pkg (1.6 oz)	170	0	3
Oatmeal Instant Kid's Choice Chocolate Chip Cookie	1 pkg (1.5 oz)	160	0	3
Oatmeal Instant Kid's Choice Cookie'n Cream	1 pkg (1.5 oz)	160	0	2
Oatmeal Instant Kid's Choice Fruity Marshmallow	1 pkg (1.4 oz)	150	0	3
Oatmeal Instant Kid's Choice Oatmeal Raisin Cookie	1 pkg (1.5 oz)	160	0	2
Oatmeal Instant Kid's Choice Radical Raspberry	1 pkg (1.4 oz)	150	0	3
Oatmeal Instant Kid's Choice S'mores	1 pkg (1.5 oz)	160	0	2
Oatmeal Instant Kid's Choice Strawberries'n Stuff	1 pkg (1.4 oz)	150	0	3
Oatmeal Instant Kid's Choice Twisted Strawberry Banana	1 pkg (1.4 oz)	150	0	3
Oatmeal Instant Maple & Brown Sugar	1 pkg (1.5 oz)	160	0	3
Oatmeal Instant Peaches & Cream	1 pkg (1.2 oz)	140	0	2
Oatmeal Instant Raisin & Spice	1 pkg (1.5 oz)	150	0	3
Oatmeal Instant Raisin Date & Walnut	1 pkg (1.3 oz)	140	0	3

FOOD	PORTION	CALS	CHOL	FIBER
Oatmeal Instant Strawberries & Cream	1 pkg (1.2 oz)	140	0	2
Oatmeal Nutrition for Women Golden Brown Sugar	1 pkg (1.6 oz)	170	0	3
Oatmeal Quick'n Hearty Microwave	1 pkg (1 oz)	110	0	2
Oatmeal Quick'n Hearty Microwave Apple Spice	1 pkg (1.6 oz)	170	0	3
Oatmeal Quick'n Hearty Microwave Brown Sugar Cinnamon	1 pkg (1.5 oz)	150	0	3
Oatmeal Quick'n Hearty Microwave Cinnamon Double Raisin	1 pkg (1.6 oz)	170	0	3
Oatmeal Quick'n Hearty Microwave Honey Bran	1 pkg (1.4 oz)	150	0	3
Oats Old Fashion	½ cup (1.4 oz)	150	0	4
Oats Quick	½ cup (1.4 oz)	150	0	4
Oats Steel Cut	½ cup (1.4 oz)	150	0	4
Whole Wheat Hot Natural	½ cup (1.4 oz)	130	0	4
Stone-Buhr				
4 Grain	⅓ cup (1.6 oz)	140	0	5
7 Grain	⅓ cup (1.6 oz)	140	0	7
Bran Flakes	¼ cup (0.6 oz)	64	0	2
Cracked Wheat	¼ cup (2.4 oz)	210	0	6
Granola Hot Apple	⅓ cup (1.6 oz)	153	0	5
Manna Golden	6 tsp (1.6 oz)	160	0	1
Rolled Oats Old Fashion	6 tsp (1.6 oz)	150	0	5
Scotch Oats	¼ cup (1.6 oz)	150	0	4
Sunbelt				
Berry Basic	½ cup (1.9 oz)	220	0	5
Granola Banana Nut	½ cup (1.9 oz)	250	0	4

FOOD	PORTION	CALS	CHOL	FIBER
Granola Cinnamon Raisins	½ cup (1.9 oz)	200	0	4
Granola Fruit & Nut	½ cup (1.9 oz)	240	0	3
Muesli 5 Whole Grains	½ cup (1.9 oz)	210	0	3
Uncle Roy's				
Granola Cashew Raisin	½ cup (1.6 oz)	180	0	3
Granola Fruit & Nut	½ cup (1.6 oz)	175	0	3
Granola Maple Date Nut	½ cup (1.6 oz)	180	0	3
Granola Nut Butter & Almonds	½ cup (1.6 oz)	195	0	3
Granola Fat Free Apple Cinnamon	½ cup (1.6 oz)	175	0	3
Granola Fat Free Wild Cherry	½ cup (1.6 oz)	175	0	3
Granola Low Fat Berries Jubilee	½ cup (1.6 oz)	175	0	3
Granola Low Fat Crispy	½ cup (1.4 oz)	160	0	3
Granola Low Fat Luscious Raspberry	½ cup (1.6 oz)	175	0	3
Granola Low Fat True Blueberry	½ cup (1.6 oz)	175	0	3
Granola Organic Golden Honey	½ cup (1.6 oz)	190	0	3
Granola Organic Maple Nut'N Rice	½ cup (1.4 oz)	170	0	3
Granola Organic Maple Raisin	½ cup (1.6 oz)	190	0	3
Muesli Swiss Style	½ cup (1.6 oz)	170	0	3
Uncle Sam				
Cereal	1 cup (1.9 oz)	190	0	10
Wheatena				
Cereal	⅓ cup (1.4 oz)	150	0	5

CEREAL BARS *(see also* ENERGY BARS*)*

FOOD	PORTION	CALS	CHOL	FIBER
granola	1 (1 oz)	134	0	2
Barbara's Bakery				
Nature's Choice Apple Cinnamon	1 bar (1.3 oz)	120	0	2

FOOD	PORTION	CALS	CHOL	FIBER
Nature's Choice Blueberry	1 bar (⅓ oz)	120	0	2
Nature's Choice Cherry	1 bar (1.3 oz)	120	0	2
Nature's Choice Granola Carob Chip	1 bar (0.7 oz)	80	0	2
Nature's Choice Granola Cinnamon & Raisin	1 bar (0.7 oz)	80	0	3
Nature's Choice Granola Oats 'N Honey	1 bar (0.7 oz)	80	0	2
Nature's Choice Granola Peanut Butter	1 bar (0.7 oz)	80	0	2
Nature's Choice Raspberry	1 bar (1.3 oz)	120	0	2
Nature's Choice Strawberry	1 bar (1.3 oz)	120	0	2
Nature's Choice Triple Berry	1 bar (1.3 oz)	120	0	2
Cap'n Crunch				
Bar	1 (0.8 oz)	90	0	—
Berries Bar	1 (0.8 oz)	90	0	—
Dolly Madison				
Apple	1 (1.3 oz)	120	0	1
Blueberry	1 (1.3 oz)	120	0	1
Raspberry	1 (1.3 oz)	120	0	1
Strawberry	1 (1.3 oz)	120	0	1
Entenmann's				
Apple Cinnamon	1 (1.3 oz)	140	0	tr
Blueberry	1 (1.3 oz)	140	0	tr
Oatmeal Apple Cinnamon	1 (1.3 oz)	140	0	1
Oatmeal Apple Raisin	1 (1.3 oz)	140	0	1
Raspberry	1 (1.3 oz)	140	0	1
Strawberry	1 (1.3 oz)	140	0	tr
Estee				
Rice Crunchie Chocolate	1 (0.7 oz)	50	0	tr

FOOD	PORTION	CALS	CHOL	FIBER
Rice Crunchie Chocolate Chip	1 (0.7 oz)	50	0	0
Rice Crunchie Peanut Butter	1 (0.7 oz)	60	0	0
Rice Crunchie Vanilla	1 (0.7 oz)	60	0	0
General Mills				
Milk 'N Cereal Bars Chex	1 bar (1.6 oz)	160	0	–
Milk 'N Cereal Bars Cinnamon Toast Crunch	1 bar (1.6 oz)	180	0	1
Glenny's				
Chocolate Crunch Creamy Low Fat	1 bar (1.75 oz)	190	0	4
Chocolate Crunch Roasted Peanut	1 bar (1.75 oz)	200	0	6
Chocolate Crunch Toasted Almond	1 bar (1.75 oz)	200	0	6
Health Valley				
98% Fat Free Raisin Cinnamon	⅔ cup	180	0	6
98% Fat Free Tropical	⅔ cup	180	0	6
Blueberry	1	140	0	3
Breakfast Bakes Apple Cinnamon	1 bar	110	0	3
Breakfast Bakes California Strawberry	1 bar	110	0	3
Breakfast Bakes Mountain Blueberry	1 bar	110	0	3
Breakfast Bakes Red Raspberry	1 bar	110	0	3
Chocolate Chip	1	140	0	3
Crisp Rice Bars Apple Cinnamon	1	110	0	1
Crisp Rice Bars Orange Date	1	110	0	1
Crisp Rice Bars Tropical Fruit	1	110	0	1
Date Almond	1	140	0	3

FOOD	PORTION	CALS	CHOL	FIBER
Fiber 7 Flakes w/ Strawberry	1 bar	110	0	3
O's Almond	¾ cup	120	0	3
O's Apple Cinnamon	¾ cup	120	0	3
O's Honey Crunch	¾ cup	120	0	3
Oat Bran Flakes w/ Blueberry	1 bar	110	0	3
Raisin	1	140	0	3
Raisin Bran Flakes w/ Apple Raisin	1 bar	110	0	3
Raspberry	1	140	0	3
Strawberry	1	140	0	3
Hershey's				
Crisy Rice Snacks Peanut Butter	1 bar (0.5 oz)	60	0	tr
Hostess				
Apple	1 (1.3 oz)	120	0	1
Banana Nut	1 (1.3 oz)	120	0	2
Blueberry	1 (1.3 oz)	120	0	1
Raspberry	1 (1.3 oz)	120	0	1
Strawberry	1 (1.3 oz)	120	0	1
Kellogg's				
Nutri-Grain Apple Cinnamon	1 (1.3 oz)	140	0	1
Nutri-Grain Peach	1 (1.3 oz)	140	0	1
Nutri-Grain Raspberry	1 (1.3 oz)	140	0	1
Nutri-Grain Strawberry	1 (1.3 oz)	140	0	1
Nutri-Grain Twists Low Fat Apple Cinnamon	1 (1.3 oz)	140	0	1
Nutri-Grain Twists Low Fat Banana Strawberry	1 (1.3 oz)	140	0	1
Nutri-Grain Twists Low Fat Strawberry Blueberry	1 (1.3 oz)	140	0	1
Kudos				
Chocolate Coated Chocolate Chip	1	120	0	1
Chocolate Coated Peanut Butter	1	90	0	1

FOOD	PORTION	CALS	CHOL	FIBER
Low Fat Blueberry	1 (0.7 oz)	90	0	1
Snickers With	1	100	0	0
M&M's	1	90	0	1
Little Debbie				
Raspberry	1 (1.3 oz)	130	0	tr
S'mores Granola Treats	1 (1 oz)	130	0	1
Strawberry	1 (1.3 oz)	130	0	tr
Nabisco				
Nutter Butter Granola Bar	1 (1 oz)	120	0	tr
Oreo Granola Bar	1 (1 oz)	120	0	1
Nature Valley				
Low Fat Chewy Orchard Blend	1 bar (1 oz)	110	0	1
Nutri-Grain				
Blueberry	1 (1.3 oz)	140	0	1
Cherry	1 (1.3 oz)	140	0	1
Fruit-full Squares Apple	1 (1.7 oz)	180	0	1
Fruit-full Squares Banana	1 (1.7 oz)	190	0	1
Fruit-full Squares Cinnamon Raisin	1 (1.7 oz)	180	0	1
Minis Strawberry	1 pkg (1.5 oz)	160	0	
Mixed Berry	1 (1.3 oz)	140	0	1
Quaker				
Chewy Chocolate Chip	1 (1 oz)	120	0	1
Chewy Cookies 'n Cream	1 (1 oz)	110	0	1
Chewy Peanut Butter Chocolate Chunk	1 (1 oz)	120	0	1
Chewy Graham Slam Chocolate Chip	1 (1 oz)	110	0	1
Chewy Graham Slam Peanut Butter	1 (1 oz)	110	0	1
Chewy Low Fat Chocolate Chunk	1 (1 oz)	110	0	1

FOOD	PORTION	CALS	CHOL	FIBER
Chewy Low Fat Oatmeal Raisin	1 (1 oz)	110	0	1
Chewy Low Fat S'mores	1 (1 oz)	110	0	1
Fruit & Oatmeal Apple Cinnamon	1 (1.3 oz)	130	0	1
Fruit & Oatmeal Bites Apple Crisp	1 pkg	140	0	1
Fruit & Oatmeal Bites Strawberry	1 pkg	140	0	1
Fruit & Oatmeal Bites Very Berry	1 pkg	140	0	1
Fruit & Oatmeal Low Fat Cherry Cobbler	1 (1.3 oz)	140	0	1
Fruit & Oatmeal Low Fat Strawberry	1 (1.3 oz)	140	0	1
Fruit & Oatmeal Low Fat Strawberry Banana	1 (1.3 oz)	130	0	tr
Fruit & Oatmeal Low Fat Strawberry Cheesecake	1 (1.3 oz)	130	0	tr
Rice Krispies				
Treats	1 (0.8 oz)	90	0	0
Treats Peanut Butter Chocolate	1 (0.8 oz)	110	0	0
Treats Cocoa	1 (0.8 oz)	100	0	0
SnackWell's				
Country Fruit Medley	1 (1.3 oz)	130	0	tr
Fat Free Apple Cinnamon	1 (1.3 oz)	120	0	1
Fat Free Blueberry	1 (1.3 oz)	120	0	1
Fat Free Strawberry	1 (1.3 oz)	120	0	1
Hearty Fruit'n Grain Crisp Autumn Apple	1 (1.3 oz)	130	0	1
Hearty Fruit'n Grain Mixed Berry	1 (1.3 oz)	120	0	1
Hearty Fruit'n Grain Orchard Cherry	1 (1.3 oz)	130	0	1

FOOD	PORTION	CALS	CHOL	FIBER
Sunbelt				
Apple	1 (1.3 oz)	130	0	tr
Blueberry	1 (1.3 oz)	130	0	tr
Chewy Granola Almond	1 (1 oz)	130	0	1
Chewy Granola Apple Cinnamon	1 (1.2 oz)	140	0	2
Chewy Granola Chocolate Chip	1 (1.2 oz)	160	0	2
Chewy Granola Oatmeal Raisin	1 (1.2 oz)	130	0	1
Chewy Granola Oats & Honey	1 (1 oz)	120	0	1
Granola Fudge Dipped Chocolate Chip	1 (1.5 oz)	200	0	2
Granola Fudge Dipped Macaroon	1 (1.4 oz)	190	0	1
Weight Watchers				
Apple Cinnamon	1 (1 oz)	100	0	2
Blueberry	1 (1 oz)	100	0	1
Raspberry	1 (1 oz)	100	0	2

CHAMPAGNE

FOOD	PORTION	CALS	CHOL	FIBER
sekt german champagne	3.5 fl oz	84	0	–
Andre				
Blush	4 fl oz	88	0	–
Brut	4 fl oz	84	0	–
Cold Duck	4 fl oz	100	0	–
Extra Dry	4 fl oz	92	0	–
Ballatore				
Spumante	4 fl oz	92	0	–
Eden Roc				
Brut	4 fl oz	92	0	–
Brut Rosé	4 fl oz	99	0	–
Extra Dry	4 fl oz	84	0	–
Tott's				
Blanc de Noir	4 fl oz	88	0	–
Brut	4 fl oz	80	0	–
Extra Dry	4 fl oz	84	0	–

FOOD	PORTION	CALS	CHOL	FIBER

CHAYOTE
FOOD	PORTION	CALS	CHOL	FIBER
fresh cooked	1 cup	38	0	—
raw	1 (7 oz)	49	0	—
raw cut up	1 cup	32	0	—

CHEESE (see also CHEESE DISHES, CHEESE SUBSTITUTES, COTTAGE CHEESE, CREAM CHEESE, NEUFCHATEL)
FOOD	PORTION	CALS	CHOL	FIBER
american	1 oz	93	18	—
american cheese food	1 pkg (8 oz)	745	145	—
american cheese spread	1 jar (5 oz)	412	78	—
american cold pack	1 pkg (8 oz)	752	144	—
american cheese spread	1 oz	82	16	—
beaufort	1 oz	115	34	0
blue	1 oz	100	21	—
blue crumbled	1 cup (4.7 oz)	477	102	—
brick	1 oz	105	27	—
brie	1 oz	95	28	—
cacio di roma sheep's milk cheese	1 oz	130	30	—
camembert	1 oz	85	20	—
camembert	1 wedge (1⅓ oz)	114	27	—
cantal	1 oz	105	26	0
chabichou	1 oz	95	23	0
chaource	1 oz	83	20	0
cheddar	1 oz	114	30	—
cheddar low fat	1 oz	49	6	—
cheddar low sodium	1 oz	113	28	—
cheddar shredded	1 cup	455	119	—
cheshire	1 oz	110	29	—
colby	1 oz	112	27	—
colby low fat	1 oz	49	6	—
colby low sodium	1 oz	113	28	—
comte	1 oz	114	34	0
coulommiers	1 oz	88	23	0
crottin	1 oz	105	23	0
edam	1 oz	101	25	—
emmentaler	1 oz	115	26	—
feta	1 oz	75	25	—
fontina	1 oz	110	33	—

FOOD	PORTION	CALS	CHOL	FIBER
goat fresh	1 oz	23	5	0
goat hard	1 oz	128	30	—
goat semisoft	1 oz	103	22	—
goat soft	1 oz	76	13	—
gouda	1 oz	101	32	—
gruyere	1 oz	117	31	—
limburger	1 oz	93	26	—
maroilles	1 oz	97	26	0
morbier	1 oz	99	23	0
mozzarella	1 lb	1276	356	—
mozzarella	1 oz	80	22	—
mozzarella fresh	1 oz	80	20	0
mozzarella low moisture	1 oz	90	25	—
mozzarella part skim	1 oz	72	16	—
muenster	1 oz	104	27	—
parmesan grated	1 oz	129	22	—
parmesan grated	1 tbsp (5 g)	23	4	—
parmesan hard	1 oz	111	19	—
picodon	1 oz	99	23	0
pimento	1 oz	106	27	—
pont l'eveque	1 oz	86	20	0
port du salut	1 oz	100	35	—
provolone	1 oz	100	20	—
pyrenees	1 oz	101	26	0
quark 20% fat	1 oz	33	5	—
quark 40% fat	1 oz	48	11	—
quark made w/ skim milk	1 oz	22	tr	—
queso anego	1 oz	106	30	—
queso asadero	1 oz	101	30	—
queso chichuahua	1 oz	106	30	—
queso manchego	1 oz	107	27	0
raclette	1 oz	102	26	0
reblochon	1 oz	88	23	0
ricotta part skim	½ cup (4.4 oz)	171	38	—
ricotta part skim	1 cup (8.6 oz)	340	76	—
ricotta whole milk	1 cup (8.6 oz)	428	124	—
ricotta whole milk	½ cup (4.4 oz)	216	63	—
romano	1 oz	110	29	—

FOOD	PORTION	CALS	CHOL	FIBER
roquefort	1 oz	105	26	—
rouy	1 oz	95	23	0
saint marcellin	1 oz	94	23	0
saint nectaire	1 oz	97	23	0
saint paulin	1 oz	85	20	0
sainte maure	1 oz	99	23	0
selles sur cher	1 oz	93	20	0
swiss	1 oz	107	26	—
swiss cheese food	1 pkg (8 oz)	734	186	—
swiss processed	1 oz	95	24	—
tilsit	1 oz	96	29	—
tome	1 oz	92	23	0
triple creme	1 oz	113	34	0
vacherin	1 oz	92	23	0
yogurt cheese, nonfat	1 oz	20	7	—
yogurt cheese	1 oz	80	15	0
Alouette				
Garlic & Herbs	2 tbsp (0.8 oz)	70	30	0
Alpine Lace				
American Jalapeno Peppers	1 slice (1 oz)	80	20	0
American Less Fat Less Sodium White	1 slice (1 oz)	50	20	0
American Less Fat Less Sodium Yellow	1 slice (1 oz)	80	20	0
Cheddar Reduced Fat	1 slice (1 oz)	70	15	0
Colby Reduced Fat	1 slice (1 oz)	80	15	0
Fat Free Parmesan	2 tsp (5 g)	10	0	0
Feta Reduced Fat	1 oz	50	10	0
Feta Reduced Fat Sun Dried Tomato & Basil	1 oz	50	10	0
Goat Reduced Fat	1 oz	40	5	0
Mozzarella Reduced Fat	1 oz	70	10	0
Muenster Reduced Sodium	1 slice (1 oz)	100	25	0
Provolone Smoked Reduced Fat	1 slice (1 oz)	70	15	0
Swiss Reduced Fat	1 slice (1 oz)	90	20	0

FOOD	PORTION	CALS	CHOL	FIBER
Boar's Head				
American	1 oz	100	25	0
Baby Swiss	1 oz	110	25	0
Canadian Cheddar	1 oz	110	35	0
Double Glouster Yellow	1 oz	110	35	0
Havarti	1 oz	110	35	0
Havarti w/ Dill	1 oz	110	35	0
Havarti w/ Jalapeno	1 oz	110	35	0
Lacey Swiss	1 oz	90	15	0
Longhorn Colby	1 oz	110	30	0
Monterey Jack	1 oz	100	25	0
Monterey Jack w/ Jalapeno	1 oz	100	25	0
Mozzarella	1 oz	90	25	0
Muenster	1 oz	100	25	0
Muenster Low Sodium	1 oz	100	20	0
Provolone Picante Sharp	1 oz	100	25	0
Swiss	1 oz	110	20	0
Swiss No Salt Added	1 oz	110	25	0
Breakstone's				
Ricotta	¼ cup (2.2 oz)	110	25	0
Cabot				
Cheddar	1 oz	110	30	0
Cheddar Five Peppercorn	1 oz	110	30	0
Cheddar Mediterranean	1 oz	110	30	0
Cheddar Sundried Tomato Basil	1 oz	110	30	0
Cheddar Toasted Onion & Chive	1 oz	110	30	0
Cheddar Light 50% Reduced Fat	1 oz	70	15	0
Cheddar Light 50% Reduced Fat Jalapeno	1 oz	70	15	0
Cheddar Light 50% Reduced Fat Tomato Basil	1 oz	70	15	0

FOOD	PORTION	CALS	CHOL	FIBER
Cheddar Light 75% Reduced Fat	1 oz	60	10	0
Dehydrated Cheddar Powder	2 tsp (5 g)	25	5	0
Monterey Jack	1 oz	110	30	0
Cedar Grove				
Marble Colby	1 oz	110	30	0
Organic Tomato Basil Cheddar	1 oz	110	30	0
Cheez Whiz				
Light	2 tbsp (1.2 oz)	80	15	0
Churney				
Diet Snack Cheddar Flavored	1 oz	70	10	–
Diet Snack Port Wine Flavored	1 oz	70	10	–
Feta	1 oz	80	20	0
Cracker Barrel				
Baby Swiss	1 oz	110	25	0
Cheddar Extra Sharp	1 oz	120	30	0
Cheddar Marbled Sharp	1 oz	110	30	0
Cheddar New York Aged	1 oz	120	30	0
Cheddar Sharp	1 oz	120	30	0
Cheddar Vermont Sharp	1 oz	110	30	0
Reduced Fat Cheddar Extra Sharp	1 oz	90	20	0
Reduced Fat Cheddar Sharp	1 oz	90	20	0
Reduced Fat Cheddar Vermont Sharp	1 oz	90	20	0
Whipped Spreadable Cream Cheese & Extra Sharp Cheddar	2 tbsp (0.9 oz)	80	20	0
Whipped Spreadable Cream Cheese & Sharp Cheddar	2 tbsp (0.9 oz)	80	20	0

FOOD	PORTION	CALS	CHOL	FIBER
Whipped Spreadable Cream Cheese & Sharp Cheddar w/ Herbs	2 tbsp (0.9 oz)	80	20	0
Di Giorno				
Parmesan Grated	2 tsp (5 g)	25	5	0
Parmesan Shredded	2 tsp (5 g)	20	<5	0
Parmesan Shredded	2 tsp (5 g)	20	5	0
Romano Grated	2 tsp (5 g)	25	5	0
Romano Shredded	2 tsp (5 g)	20	5	0
Easy Cheese				
Spread American	2 tbsp (1.2 oz)	100	25	0
Spread Cheddar	2 tbsp (1.2 oz)	100	25	0
Spread Cheddar'n Bacon	2 tbsp (1.2 oz)	100	25	0
Spread Nacho	2 tbsp (1.2 oz)	100	25	0
Spread Sharp Cheddar	2 tbsp (1.2 oz)	100	25	0
Father Time				
Cheddar Extra-Sharp Premium	1 oz	110	30	0
Formagg				
Formaggio D'Oro	1 oz	70	15	0
Friendship				
Farmer	2 tbsp (1 oz)	50	10	0
Farmer No Salt Added	2 tbsp (1 oz)	50	10	0
Hoop	2 tbsp (1 oz)	20	0	0
Handi-Snacks				
Cheez'n Breadsticks	1 pkg (1.1 oz)	120	15	0
Cheez'n Crackers	1 pkg (1.1 oz)	110	15	0
Cheez'n Pretzels	1 pkg (1 oz)	100	15	tr
Mozzarella String Cheese	1 piece (1 oz)	80	20	0
Nacho Stix'n Cheez	1 pkg (1.1 oz)	110	15	0
Healthy Choice				
American Singles White	1 slice (0.7 oz)	30	<5	—
American Singles Yellow	1 slice (0.7 oz)	30	<5	—
Cheddar Fancy Shreds	¼ cup (1 oz)	45	<5	—
Cheddar Shreds	¼ cup (1 oz)	45	<5	—

FOOD	PORTION	CALS	CHOL	FIBER
Loaf	1 in cube (1 oz)	35	<5	–
Mexican Shreds	¼ cup (1 oz)	45	<5	–
Mozzarella	1 oz	45	<5	–
Mozzarella Fancy Shreds	¼ cup (1 oz)	45	<5	–
Mozzarella Shreds	¼ cup (1 oz)	45	<5	–
Mozzarella String Cheese	1 stick (1 oz)	45	<5	–
Pizza Fancy Shreds	¼ cup (1 oz)	45	<5	–
Pizza String	1 stick (1 oz)	45	<5	–
Heluva Good Cheese				
American	1 slice (0.7)	45	15	0
Cheddar Curds Snack	1 oz	113	28	0
Cheddar Extra-Sharp	1 oz	110	30	0
Cheddar Mild	1 oz	110	30	0
Cheddar Mild Reduced Fat	1 oz	80	15	0
Cheddar Mild White	1 oz	110	30	0
Cheddar Sharp	1 oz	110	30	0
Cheddar Sharp White	1 oz	110	30	0
Cheddar Shredded	¼ cup (1 oz)	110	30	0
Cheddar Very Low Sodium	1 oz	110	25	0
Cheddar White Extra-Sharp	1 oz	110	30	0
Cheddar White Very Low Sodium	1 oz	110	25	0
Cheddar White Shredded	¼ cup (1 oz)	110	30	0
Colby	1 oz	117	30	0
Colby-Jack	1 oz	110	30	0
Cold Pack Cheddar Sharp	2 tbsp (1 oz)	90	20	0
Cold Pack Cheddar Sharp With Bacon	2 tbsp (1 oz)	90	20	0
Cold Pack Cheddar Sharp with Horseradish	2 tbsp (1 oz)	90	20	0
Cold Pack Cheddar Sharp With Jalapenos	2 tbsp (1 oz)	90	20	0

FOOD	PORTION	CALS	CHOL	FIBER
Cold Pack Cheddar Sharp With Port Wine	2 tbsp (1 oz)	90	20	0
Monterey Jack	1 oz	100	25	0
Monterey Jack Shredded	¼ cup (1 oz)	100	30	0
Monterey Jack With Jalapenos	1 oz	100	25	0
Mozzarella Part Skim Low Moisture Shredded	¼ cup (1 oz)	80	15	0
Mozzarella Whole Milk	1 oz	80	20	0
Muenster	1 oz	100	25	0
Swiss	1 oz	112	28	0
Washed Curd Cheese	1 oz	110	30	0
Hoffman				
American Yellow	1 oz	110	25	0
Hot Pepper	1 oz	90	20	0
Super Sharp	1 oz	110	25	0
Hollow Road Farms				
Sheep's Milk	1 oz	45	15	—
Kraft				
Cheddar Extra Sharp	1 oz	120	30	0
Cheddar Medium	1 oz	110	30	0
Cheddar Mild	1 oz	110	30	0
Cheddar Sharp	1 oz	120	30	0
Cheddary Melts Medium Cheddar	1 oz	110	30	0
Cheddary Melts Mild Cheddar	1 oz	110	30	0
Cheddary Melts Shreds Medium Cheddar	¼ cup (1.1 oz)	120	30	0
Cheddary Melts Shreds Mild Cheddar	¼ cup (1.1 oz)	120	30	0
Cheese Food w/ Garlic	1 oz	90	20	0
Cheese Food w/ Jalapeno Peppers	1 oz	90	20	0
Colby	1 oz	110	30	0
Colby Monterey Jack	1 oz	110	30	0
Deluxe American	1 oz	100	25	0
Deluxe American White	1 oz	100	25	0

FOOD	PORTION	CALS	CHOL	FIBER
Deluxe Singles American	1 (1 oz)	110	30	0
Deluxe Singles American	1 (0.7 oz)	70	15	0
Deluxe Singles Pimento	1 (1 oz)	100	25	0
Deluxe Singles Swiss	1 (1 oz)	90	25	0
Deluxe Singles Swiss	1 slice (0.7 oz)	70	20	0
Free Grated	2 tsp (5 g)	15	0	0
Free Shredded Cheddar	¼ cup (0.9 oz)	40	<5	0
Free Shredded Mozzarella	¼ cup (1 oz)	45	<5	tr
Grated Parm Plus! Garlic Herb	2 tsp (5 g)	15	0	0
Grated Parm Plus! Zesty Red Pepper	2 tsp (5 g)	15	0	0
Grated Parmesan	2 tsp (5 g)	20	5	0
Grated Romano	2 tsp (5 g)	20	<5	0
Marbled Cheddar Mild	1 oz	110	30	0
Marbled Cheddar & Monterey Jack	1 oz	110	30	0
Marbled Cheddar & Whole Milk Mozzarella	1 oz	100	25	0
Marbled Colby Monterey Jack	1 oz	110	30	0
Monterey Jack	1 oz	110	30	0
Monterey Jack w/ Jalapeno Peppers	1 oz	110	30	0
Mozzarella Part Skim Low Moisture	1 oz	80	15	0
Mozzarella String Cheese Low Moisture Part Skim	1 piece (1 oz)	80	20	0
Pizza Shredded Four Cheese	¼ cup (0.9 oz)	90	20	0
Pizza Shredded Mozzarella & Cheddar	⅓ cup (1.1 oz)	120	30	0

FOOD	PORTION	CALS	CHOL	FIBER
Pizza Shredded Mozzarella & Provolone w/ Smoke Flavor	¼ cup (0.9 oz)	90	20	0
Reduced Fat Cheddar Mild	1 oz	90	20	0
Reduced Fat Cheddar Sharp	1 oz	90	20	0
Reduced Fat Colby	1 oz	80	20	0
Reduced Fat Monterey Jack	1 oz	80	20	0
Shredded Cheddar Medium	¼ cup (0.9 oz)	100	30	0
Shredded Cheddar Mild	¼ cup (0.9 oz)	100	30	0
Shredded Cheddar Sharp	1 oz (0.9 oz)	110	25	0
Shredded Cheddar & Monterey Jack	¼ cup (0.9 oz)	100	25	0
Shredded Colby & Monterey Jack	¼ cup (0.9 oz)	100	25	0
Shredded Hearty Italian	⅓ cup (1.1 oz)	100	25	0
Shredded Italian Style Classic Garlic	⅓ cup (1.1 oz)	100	25	tr
Shredded Italian Style Mozzarelle & Parmesan	⅓ cup (1.1 oz)	100	25	0
Shredded Lower Fat Cheddar Mild	¼ cup (0.9 oz)	80	20	0
Shredded Lower Fat Cheddar Sharp	¼ cup (0.9 oz)	80	20	0
Shredded Lower Fat Colby & Monterey Jack	¼ cup (0.9 oz)	80	15	0
Shredded Lower Fat Mozzarella	⅓ cup (1.1 oz)	80	15	0
Shredded Lower Fat Pizza Cheese	⅓ cup (1.1 oz)	90	20	0

FOOD	PORTION	CALS	CHOL	FIBER
Shredded Mexican Style Cheddar & Monterey Jack	⅓ cup (1.1 oz)	120	30	0
Shredded Mexican Style Cheddar & Monterey Jack w/ Jalapeno Peppers	⅓ cup (1.1 oz)	120	30	0
Shredded Mexican Style Four Cheese	⅓ cup (1.1 oz)	120	30	0
Shredded Mexican Style Taco Cheese	⅓ cup (1.1 oz)	120	30	0
Shredded Monterey Jack	¼ cup (0.9 oz)	100	25	0
Shredded Parmesan	2 tsp (5 g)	20	2	0
Shredded Part Skim Mozzarella	¼ cup (1.1 oz)	90	20	0
Shredded Swiss	¼ cup (0.9 oz)	100	25	0
Shredded Whole Milk Mozzarella	¼ cup (1.1 oz)	100	25	0
Shredded Finely Cheddar Mild	¼ cup (1.1 oz)	120	30	0
Shredded Finely Cheddar Sharp	¼ cup (1.1 oz)	120	30	0
Shredded Finely Colby & Monterey Jack	¼ cup (1 oz)	110	30	0
Shredded Finely Lower Fat Cheddar Mild	⅓ cup (1.1 oz)	100	20	0
Shredded Finely Lower Fat Cheddar Sharp	⅓ cup (1.1 oz)	100	20	0
Shredded Finely Part Skim Mozzarella	¼ cup (1.1 oz)	90	20	0
Shredded Finely Swiss	¼ cup (0.9 oz)	110	25	0
Singles American	1 (1.2 oz)	110	25	0
Singles American	1 (0.7 oz)	60	15	0
Singles American	1 (0.6 oz)	60	15	0
Singles Mild Mexican	1 (0.7 oz)	70	15	0
Singles Monterey	1 slice (0.7 oz)	70	15	0
Singles Pimento	1 (0.7 oz)	60	15	0
Singles Reduced Fat American	1 (0.7 oz)	50	10	0

FOOD	PORTION	CALS	CHOL	FIBER
Singles Reduced Fat American White	1 (0.7 oz)	50	10	0
Singles Sharp	1 slice (0.7 oz)	70	20	0
Singles Swiss	1 slice (0.7 oz)	70	15	0
Singles Nonfat American	1 (0.7 oz)	30	<5	0
Singles Nonfat American White	1 (0.7 oz)	30	<5	0
Singles Nonfat Sharp Cheddar	1 (0.7 oz)	35	<5	0
Singles Nonfat Swiss	1 slice (0.7 oz)	30	<5	0
Slices Cheddar Mild	1 (1 oz)	110	30	0
Slices Colby	1 (1.6 oz)	180	45	0
Slices Part Skim Mozzarella	1 (1.6 oz)	130	25	0
Slices Part Skim Mozzarella	1 (1.5 oz)	120	25	0
Slices Provolone Smoke Flavor	1 (1.5 oz)	150	35	0
SlicesSwiss	1 (1.5 oz)	170	45	0
Slices Swiss	1 (1.3 oz)	150	40	0
Slices Swiss	1 (0.8 oz)	90	25	0
Slices Swiss	1 (1.6 oz)	180	45	0
Slices Swiss Aged	1 (1.5 oz)	170	45	0
Slices Deli-Thin Part Skim Mozzarella	1 (1 oz)	80	15	0
Slices Deli-Thin Swiss	1 (0.8 oz)	90	25	0
Slices Deli-Thin Swiss Aged	1 (0.8 oz)	90	25	0
Slices Reduced Fat Swiss	1 (1.3 oz)	130	25	0
Spread Bacon	2 tbsp (1.1 oz)	90	25	0
Spread Olive & Pimento	2 tbsp (1.1 oz)	70	20	0
Spread Pimento	2 tbsp (1.1 oz)	80	20	0
Spread Pineapple	2 tbsp (1.1 oz)	70	15	0
Spread Roka Brand Blue	2 tbsp (1.1 oz)	90	25	0
Swiss	1 oz	110	30	0
Land O Lakes				
American	1 slice (0.7 oz)	80	20	0

FOOD	PORTION	CALS	CHOL	FIBER
American Jalapeno	1 slice (0.6 oz)	70	15	0
American Light	1 oz	70	20	0
American Reduced Salt	1 oz	110	30	0
American Sharp	2 slices (1 oz)	100	30	0
American & Swiss	1 slice (0.6 oz)	70	15	0
Baby Swiss	1 oz	110	25	0
Chedarella	1 oz	100	25	0
Cheddar	1 oz	100	30	0
Cheddar Extra Sharp	1 oz	110	30	0
Cheddar Sharp	1 oz	110	30	0
Cheese Spread Golden Velvet	1 oz	80	20	0
Colby	1 oz	110	30	0
Jalapeno Light	1 oz	70	15	0
Monterey Jack	1 oz	110	30	0
Monterey Jack Hot Pepper	1 oz	110	30	0
Mozzarella	1 oz	80	15	0
Muenster	1 oz	100	25	0
Parmesan Grated	1 tbsp	35	10	0
Provolone	1 oz	100	20	0
Swiss	1 oz	110	25	0
Swiss Light	1 oz	80	15	0
Laughing Cow				
Assorted Wedge	1 (1 oz)	70	20	0
Babybel	1 oz	90	10	0
Babybel Mini	1 (0.7 oz)	70	15	0
Bonbel	1 oz	100	25	0
Bonbel Mini	1 (0.7 oz)	70	15	0
Cheesebits	6 pieces (1 oz)	70	20	0
Gouda Mini	1 (0.7 oz)	80	20	0
Original Wedge	1 (1 oz)	70	20	0
Wedge Light	1 (1 oz)	50	10	0
Lifetime				
Cheddar Fat Free	1 oz	40	<5	0
Cheddar Fat Free Lactose Free	1 oz	40	<5	0
Garden Vegetable Fat Free	1 oz	40	<5	0

FOOD	PORTION	CALS	CHOL	FIBER
Jalapeno Jack Fat Free	1 oz	40	<5	0
Jalapeno Jack Fat Free Lactose Free	1 oz	40	<5	0
Mild Mexican Fat Free	1 oz	40	<5	0
Monterey Jack Fat Free	1 oz	40	<5	0
Mozzarella Fat Free	1 oz	40	<5	0
Mozzarella Fat Free Lactose Free	1 oz	40	<5	0
Onions & Chives Fat Free	1 oz	40	<5	0
Sharp Cheddar Fat Free	1 oz	40	<5	0
Smoked Cheddar Fat Free	1 oz	40	<5	0
Swiss Fat Free	1 oz	40	<5	0
Light N'Lively				
Singles American	1 (0.7 oz)	45	10	0
MayBud				
Edam	1 oz	100	25	0
Gouda	1 oz	100	25	0
Gouda Round	1 oz	100	25	0
Northfield				
Naturally Slender	1 oz	90	10	—
Old English				
American Sharp	1 slice (1 oz)	100	30	0
Organic Valley				
Aged Swiss Unpasteurized	1 oz	100	25	0
Cheddar Reduced Fat Low Sodium	1 oz	90	15	0
Cheddar Sharp & Mild	1 oz	110	25	0
Cheddar Sharp & Mild Unpasteurized	1 oz	110	25	0
Colby	1 oz	110	28	0
Colby Unpasteurized	1 oz	110	28	0
Farmer Reduced Fat	1 oz	90	15	0
Feta	1 oz	90	20	0
Monterey Jack	1 oz	100	20	0
Monterey Jack Reduced Fat	1 oz	80	15	0

FOOD	PORTION	CALS	CHOL	FIBER
Mozzarella Part Skim	1 oz	80	16	0
Muenster	1 oz	100	25	0
Pepper Jack	1 oz	110	20	0
Provolone	1 oz	100	20	0
String Part Skim	1 oz	80	16	0
Wisconsin Raw Milk Cheese	1 oz	100	20	0
Polly-O				
Mozzarella Free	1 oz	35	<5	—
Mozzarella Lite	1 oz	60	10	—
Mozzarella Part Skim	1 oz	70	15	—
Mozzarella Part Skim Shredded	¼ cup	80	15	—
Mozzarella Shredded Free	¼ cup	45	<5	—
Mozzarella Shredded Lite	¼ cup	60	15	—
Mozzarella Whole Milk	1 oz	80	20	—
Mozzarella Whole Milk Shredded	¼ cup	90	20	—
Ricotta Free	¼ cup	50	<5	—
Ricotta Lite	¼ cup	70	10	—
Ricotta Part Skim	¼ cup	90	20	—
Ricotta Whole Milk	¼ cup	110	25	—
String	1 oz	80	15	—
String Lite	1 piece (1 oz)	60	10	0
President				
Feta Fat Free	1 oz	30	0	0
Price's				
Cheese & Bacon Spread	2 tbsp (1.1 oz)	90	15	0
Jalapeno Nacho Dip Hot	2 tbsp (1.1 oz)	80	15	0
Jalapeno Nacho Dip Mild	2 tbsp (1.1 oz)	80	15	0
Pimento Cheese Spread	2 tbsp (1.1 oz)	80	15	0
Pimento Cheese Spread Light	2 tbsp (1.1 oz)	60	10	0
Vegetable Garden	2 tbsp (1.1 oz)	70	15	0

FOOD	PORTION	CALS	CHOL	FIBER
Rondele				
Light Soft Spreadable Garlic & Herb	2 tbsp (0.9 oz)	60	10	0
Soft Spreadable Garlic & Herbs	2 tbsp (1 oz)	100	25	0
Sargento				
Blue Crumbled	¼ cup (1 oz)	100	20	0
Cheddar	1 slice (1 oz)	110	30	0
Cheddar Shredded	¼ cup (1 oz)	110	30	0
Cheese For Nachos & Tacos Shredded	¼ cup (1 oz)	110	25	0
Cheese For Pizza Shredded	¼ cup (1 oz)	90	20	0
Cheese For Tacos Shredded	¼ cup (1 oz)	110	25	0
Colby	1 slice (1 oz)	110	30	0
Colby-Jack Shredded	¼ cup (1 oz)	110	25	0
Jarlsberg	1 slice (1.2 oz)	120	20	0
Monterey Jack	1 slice (1 oz)	100	30	0
Monterey Jack Shredded	¼ cup (1 oz)	100	30	0
MooTown Snackers Cheddar	1 piece (0.8 oz)	100	25	0
MooTown Snackers Cheddar Mild Light	1 piece (0.8 oz)	60	10	0
MooTown Snackers Cheese & Pretzels	1 pkg (0.9 oz)	90	10	0
MooTown Snackers Colby-Jack	1 piece (0.8 oz)	90	20	0
MooTown Snackers Pizza Cheese & Sticks	1 pkg (1 oz)	100	10	0
MooTown Snackers String	1 piece (0.8 oz)	70	15	0
MooTown Snackers String Light	1 piece (0.8 oz)	60	10	0
Mozzarella	1 slice (1.5 oz)	130	25	0
Mozzarella Shredded	¼ cup (1 oz)	80	15	0
Muenster	1 slice (1 oz)	100	25	0
Parmesan Grated	1 tbsp (5 g)	25	<5	0
Parmesan Shredded	¼ cup (1 oz)	110	25	0

FOOD	PORTION	CALS	CHOL	FIBER
Parmesan & Romano Shredded	¼ cup (1 oz)	110	25	0
Parmesan & Romano Grated	1 tbsp (5 g)	25	<5	0
Pizza Double Cheese Shredded	¼ cup (1 oz)	90	20	0
Preferred Light Cheddar Mild Shredded	¼ cup (1 oz)	70	10	0
Preferred Light Cheese For Tacos Shredded	¼ cup (1 oz)	70	15	0
Preferred Light Mozzarella	1 slice (1.5 oz)	90	15	0
Preferred Light Mozzarella Shredded	¼ cup (1 oz)	70	10	0
Preferred Light Swiss	1 slice (1 oz)	80	15	0
Provolone	1 slice (1 oz)	100	25	0
Recipe Blend 4 Cheese Mexican Shredded	¼ cup (1 oz)	110	25	0
Recipe Blend 6 Cheese Italian Shredded	¼ cup (1 oz)	90	20	0
Ricotta Light	¼ cup (2.2 oz)	60	15	0
Ricotta Old Fashioned	¼ cup (2.2 oz)	90	25	0
Ricotta Part-Skim	¼ cup (2.2 oz)	80	20	0
Swiss	1 slice (0.7 oz)	80	20	0
Swiss Shredded	¼ cup (1 oz)	110	30	0
Swiss Wafer Thin	2 slices (1 oz)	110	25	0
Smart Beat				
American Fat Free	1 slice (0.6 oz)	25	0	—
Lactose Free Fat Free	1 slice (0.6 oz)	25	0	—
Mellow Cheddar Fat Free	1 slice (0.6 oz)	25	0	—
Sharp Cheddar Fat Free	1 slice (0.6 oz)	25	0	—
Sorrento				
Mozzarella Part Skim Jalapeno	1 oz	80	15	0
Treasure Cave				
Blue Crumbled	1 oz	110	25	0
Feta Crumbled	1 oz	80	20	0

FOOD	PORTION	CALS	CHOL	FIBER
Tree Of Life				
Cheddar 33% Reduced Fat Organic Milk	1 oz	90	15	–
Colby	1 oz	110	30	–
Colby Organic Milk	1 oz	120	30	–
Farmer Part-Skim Organic Milk	1 oz	90	15	–
Jalapeno Organic Milk	1 oz	110	20	–
Monterey Jack 35% Reduced Fat Organic Milk	1 oz	80	15	–
Monterey Jack Organic Milk	1 oz	100	20	–
Mozzarella Organic Milk	1 oz	80	16	–
Muenster Organic Milk	1 oz	100	25	–
Provolone	1 oz	100	20	–
Velveeta				
Light	1 oz	60	10	0
Shredded	¼ cup (1.3 oz)	130	30	0
Shredded Mild Mexican w/ Jalapeno Pepper	¼ cup (1.3 oz)	120	30	0
Spread	1 oz	90	25	0
Spread Hot Mexican	1 oz	90	20	0
Spread Mild Mexican	1 oz	90	25	0
Weight Watchers				
Cheddar Mild Yellow	1 oz	80	15	0
Cheddar Sharp Yellow	1 oz	80	15	0
Fat Free Grated Italian Topping	1 tbsp	20	0	0
Fat Free Reduced Sodium Yellow	2 slices (0.75 oz)	30	0	0
Fat Free Sharp Cheddar	2 slices (0.75 oz)	30	0	0
Fat Free Swiss	2 slices (0.75 oz)	30	0	0
Fat Free White	2 slices (0.75 oz)	30	0	0
Fat Free Yellow	2 slices (0.75 oz)	30	0	0
Wholesome Valley				
Organic American Reduced Fat	1 slice (0.7 oz)	50	10	0

FOOD	PORTION	CALS	CHOL	FIBER
WisPride				
Chunk	1 oz	110	20	0
Garlic & Herb Cup	2 tbsp (1.1 oz)	100	20	0
Hickory Smoked Cup	2 tbsp (1.1 oz)	100	20	0
Port Wine Ball	2 tbsp (1.1 oz)	100	20	0
Port Wine Cup	2 tbsp (1.1 oz)	100	20	0
Port Wine Light Cup	2 tbsp (1.1 oz)	80	10	0
Sharp Ball	2 tbsp (1.1 oz)	100	20	0
Sharp Cheddar Ball	2 tbsp (1.1 oz)	100	20	0
Sharp Cup	2 tbsp (1.1 oz)	100	20	0
Sharp Light Cup	2 tbsp (1.1 oz)	80	10	0
Swiss Ball	2 tbsp (1.1 oz)	110	20	0
CHEESE DISHES				
FROZEN				
Banquet				
Mozzarella Nuggets	6	260	40	1
Health Is Wealth				
Mozzarella Sticks	2 (1.3 oz)	120	15	0
Stouffer's				
Welsh Rarebit	½ cup (2.5 oz)	120	20	0
TAKE-OUT				
fondue	½ cup (3.8 oz)	247	49	—
souffle	1 serv (7 oz)	504	370	1
CHEESE SUBSTITUTES				
mozzarella	1 oz	70	0	—
Formagg				
American White	1 slice (0.66 oz)	60	0	0
American Yellow	1 slice (0.66 oz)	60	0	0
Caesar's Italian Garden American	1 oz	60	0	0
Cheddar	1 slice (0.66 oz)	60	0	0
Cheddar Shredded	1 oz	60	0	0
Classic American	1 oz	60	0	0
Macaroni And Cheese Sauce	⅔ cup (5 oz)	190	0	0
Mozzarella Shredded	1 oz	60	0	0
Old World Mozzarella	1 oz	60	0	0
Parmesan Grated	2 tsp (5 g)	15	0	tr
Swiss	1 oz	60	0	0

FOOD	PORTION	CALS	CHOL	FIBER
Swiss White	1 slice (0.66 oz)	60	0	0
Vintage Provolone	1 oz	60	0	0
Zesty Jalapeno American	1 oz	60	0	0
Georgio's				
Imitation Cheddar Shredded	¼ cup (1 oz)	90	0	0
Imitation Mozzarella Shredded	¼ cup (1 oz)	90	0	0
Sargento				
Cheddar Shredded	¼ cup (1 oz)	90	0	0
Mozzarella Shredded	¼ cup (1 oz)	80	0	0
Yves				
Good Slice American	1 slice (0.7 oz)	35	0	0
Good Slice Cheddar	1 slice (0.7 oz)	35	0	1
Good Slice Jalapeno Jack	1 slice (0.7 oz)	35	0	0
Good Slice Mozzarella	1 slice (0.7 oz)	30	0	0
Good Slice Swiss	1 slice (0.7 oz)	35	0	0
CHERIMOYA				
fresh	1	515	0	—
CHERRIES				
CANNED				
sour in heavy syrup	½ cup	232	0	—
sour in light syrup	½ cup	189	0	—
sour water packed	1 cup	87	0	—
sweet in heavy syrup	½ cup	107	0	—
sweet in light syrup	½ cup	85	0	—
sweet juice pack	½ cup	68	0	—
sweet water pack	½ cup	57	0	—
Del Monte				
Dark Pitted In Heavy Syrup	½ cup (4.2 oz)	100	0	1
Sweet Dark Whole Unpitted In Heavy Syrup	½ cup (4.2 oz)	120	0	tr
DRIED				
Sonoma				
Pitted	¼ cup (1.4 oz)	140	0	2

FOOD	PORTION	CALS	CHOL	FIBER
FRESH				
sour	1 cup	51	0	–
sweet	10	49	0	–
Chiquita				
Cherries	21	90	0	9
FROZEN				
sour unsweetened	1 cup	72	0	–
sweet sweetened	1 cup	232	0	–
CHERRY JUICE				
After The Fall				
Black Cherry	1 can (12 oz)	170	0	0
Capri Sun				
Wild Cherry Drink	1 pkg (7 oz)	100	0	0
Eden				
Montmorency Juice	8 oz	140	0	0
Juicy Juice				
Drink	1 box (4.23 oz)	70	0	0
Drink	1 box (8.5 oz)	140	0	0
Kool-Aid				
Black Cherry Drink as prep w/ sugar	1 serv (8 oz)	100	0	0
Bursts Cherry Drink	1 (7 oz)	100	0	0
Splash Drink	1 serv (8 oz)	110	0	0
Sugar Free Drink Mix as prep	1 serv (8 oz)	5	0	0
Mott's				
Cherry	1 box (8 oz)	120	0	–
Ocean Spray				
Black Cherry Blast	8 oz	140	0	0
Veryfine				
Juice-Ups	8 fl oz	130	0	0
CHERVIL				
seed	1 tsp	1	0	–
CHESTNUTS				
chinese cooked	1 oz	44	0	–
chinese dried	1 oz	103	0	–
chinese raw	1 oz	64	0	–
chinese roasted	1 oz	68	0	–

FOOD	PORTION	CALS	CHOL	FIBER
cooked	1 oz	37	0	–
creme de marrons	1 oz	73	0	1
dried peeled	1 oz	105	0	–
japanese cooked	1 oz	16	0	–
japanese dried	1 oz	102	0	–
japanese raw	1 oz	44	0	–
japanese roasted	1 oz	57	0	–
raw peeled	1 oz	56	0	–
roasted	2 to 3 (1 oz)	70	0	–
roasted	1 cup	350	0	–
CHEWING GUM				
bubble gum	1 block (8 g)	27	0	–
stick	1 (3 g)	10	0	–
Aquafresh				
Peppermint	2 pieces	5	0	–
Arm & Hammer				
Dental Care Spearmint or Peppermint	2 pieces (2.5 g)	5	0	–
Bazooka				
Fruit Chunk	1 piece (6 g)	25	0	–
Fruit Soft	1 piece (6 g)	25	0	–
Gum	1 piece (4 g)	15	0	–
Gum	1 piece (6 g)	25	0	–
Beech-Nut				
Peppermint	1 stick (3 g)	10	0	0
Spearmint	1 stick (3 g)	10	0	0
Big Red				
Stick	1	10	0	–
Brock				
Bubble Gum	1 piece (0.2 oz)	20	0	–
Bubble Yum				
Bananaberry Split	1 piece (0.3 oz)	25	0	–
Cotton Candy	1 piece (0.3 oz)	25	0	–
Grape	1 piece (0.3 oz)	25	0	–
Luscious Lime	1 piece (0.3 oz)	25	0	–
Regular	1 piece (0.3 oz)	25	0	0
Sour Apple	1 piece (0.3 oz)	25	0	1
Sour Cherry	1 piece (0.3 oz)	25	0	0
Variety Pack	1 piece (0.3 oz)	25	0	0

FOOD	PORTION	CALS	CHOL	FIBER
Watermelon	1 piece (0.3 oz)	25	0	0
Wild Strawberry	1 piece (0.3 oz)	25	0	0
Bubblicious				
Gum	1 piece (7.9 g)	25	0	–
Care*Free				
Sugarless Wild Cherry	1 stick (3 g)	10	0	–
Chiclets				
Original	1 piece (1.59 g)	6	0	–
Tiny Size	8 pieces (0.13 g)	tr	0	–
Clorets				
Clorets	1 piece (1.59 g)	6	0	–
Dentyne				
Cinn-A-Burst	1 piece (3.2 g)	9	0	–
Gum	1 piece (1.88 g)	6	0	–
Ice Peppermint	2 pieces (3 g)	5	0	–
Sugar Free	1 piece (1.88 g)	5	0	–
Doublemint				
Chewing Gum	1 piece	10	0	–
Eclipse				
Spearmint	2 pieces	5	0	–
Extra Sugar Free				
Cinnamon	1 piece	8	0	–
Spearmint & Peppermint	1 stick	8	0	–
Winter Fresh	1 piece	8	0	–
Freedent				
Spearmint Peppermint & Cinnamon	1 stick	10	0	–
Freshen-Up				
Gum	1 piece (4.2 g)	13	0	–
Fruit Stripe				
Bubble Gum Jumbo Pack	1 stick (3 g)	10	0	0
Variety Pack Chewing & Bubble Gum	1 stick (3 g)	10	0	0
Hubba Bubba				
Bubble Gum Cola	1 piece	23	0	–
Bubble Gum Sugarfree Grape	1 piece	13	0	–

FOOD	PORTION	CALS	CHOL	FIBER
Bubble Gum Sugarfree Original	1 piece	14	0	–
Original	1 piece	23	0	–
Strawberry Grape Raspberry	1 piece	23	0	–
Juicy Fruit				
Stick	1	10	0	–
Lance				
Big Red Cinnamon	1 piece (3 g)	10	0	0
Double Bubble	1 piece (7 g)	25	0	0
Double Mint	1 piece (3 g)	10	0	0
Rain-Blo				
Bubble Gum Balls	1 piece (2 g)	5	0	–
Speakeasy				
Natural Rainforest All Flavors	2 pieces	10	0	–
Trident				
Gum	1 piece (1.88 g)	5	0	–
Soft Bubble Gum	1 piece (3.3 g)	9	0	–
Winterfresh				
Stick	1 stick (3 g)	10	0	–
Wrigley's				
Spearmint	1 stick	10	0	–

CHIA SEEDS

FOOD	PORTION	CALS	CHOL	FIBER
dried	1 oz	134	0	–

CHICKEN (see also CHICKEN DISHES, CHICKEN SUBSTITUTES, DINNER, HOT DOGS)
FRESH

FOOD	PORTION	CALS	CHOL	FIBER
broiler/fryer back w/ skin batter dipped & fried	½ back (2.5 oz)	238	63	–
broiler/fryer back w/ skin floured & fried	1.5 oz	146	39	–
broiler/fryer back w/ skin roasted	1 oz	96	28	–
broiler/fryer back w/ skin stewed	½ back (2.1 oz)	158	48	–
broiler/fryer back w/o skin fried	½ back (2 oz)	167	54	–

FOOD	PORTION	CALS	CHOL	FIBER
broiler/fryer breast w/ skin batter dipped & fried	½ breast (4.9 oz)	364	119	—
broiler/fryer breast w/ skin batter dipped & fried	2.9 oz	218	72	—
broiler/fryer breast w/ skin roasted	½ breast (3.4 oz)	193	83	—
broiler/fryer breast w/ skin roasted	2 oz	115	49	—
broiler/fryer breast w/ skin stewed	½ breast (3.9 oz)	202	83	—
broiler/fryer breast w/o skin fried	½ breast (3 oz)	161	78	—
broiler/fryer breast w/o skin roasted	½ breast (3 oz)	142	73	—
broiler/fryer breast w/o skin stewed	2 oz	86	44	—
broiler/fryer drumstick w/ skin batter dipped & fried	1 (2.6 oz)	193	62	—
broiler/fryer drumstick w/ skin floured & fried	1 (1.7 oz)	120	44	—
broiler/fryer drumstick w/ skin roasted	1 (1.8 oz)	112	48	—
broiler/fryer drumstick w/ skin stewed	1 (2 oz)	116	48	—
broiler/fryer drumstick w/o skin fried	1 (1.5 oz)	82	40	—
broiler/fryer drumstick w/o skin roasted	1 (1.5 oz)	76	41	—
broiler/fryer drumstick w/o skin stewed	1 (1.6 oz)	78	40	—
broiler/fryer leg w/ skin batter dipped & fried	1 (5.5 oz)	431	142	—
broiler/fryer leg w/ skin floured & fried	1 (3.9 oz)	285	105	—

FOOD	PORTION	CALS	CHOL	FIBER
broiler/fryer leg w/ skin roasted	1 (4 oz)	265	105	–
broiler/fryer leg w/ skin stewed	1 (4.4 oz)	275	105	–
broiler/fryer leg w/o skin fried	1 (3.3 oz)	195	93	–
broiler/fryer leg w/o skin roasted	1 (3.3 oz)	182	89	–
broiler/fryer leg w/o skin stewed	1 (3.5 oz)	187	90	–
broiler/fryer neck w/ skin stewed	1 (1.3 oz)	94	27	–
broiler/fryer skin batter dipped & fried	from ½ chicken (6.7 oz)	748	140	–
broiler/fryer skin batter dipped & fried	4 oz	449	84	–
broiler/fryer skin floured & fried	from ½ chicken (2 oz)	281	41	–
broiler/fryer skin floured & fried	1 oz	166	24	–
broiler/fryer skin roasted	from ½ chicken (2 oz)	254	46	–
broiler/fryer skin stewed	from ½ chicken (2.5 oz)	261	45	–
broiler/fryer thigh w/ skin batter dipped & fried	1 (3 oz)	238	80	–
broiler/fryer thigh w/ skin floured & fried	1 (2.2 oz)	162	60	–
broiler/fryer thigh w/ skin roasted	1 (2.2 oz)	153	58	–
broiler/fryer thigh w/ skin stewed	1 (2.4 oz)	158	57	–
broiler/fryer thigh w/o skin fried	1 (1.8 oz)	113	53	–
broiler/fryer thigh w/o skin roasted	1 (1.8 oz)	109	49	–
broiler/fryer thigh w/o skin stewed	1 (1.9 oz)	107	49	–

FOOD	PORTION	CALS	CHOL	FIBER
broiler/fryer w/ skin floured & fried	½ chicken (11 oz)	844	283	—
broiler/fryer w/ skin fried	½ chicken (16.4 oz)	1347	404	—
broiler/fryer w/ skin roasted	½ chicken (10.5 oz)	715	263	—
broiler/fryer w/ skin stewed	½ chicken (11.7 oz)	730	262	—
broiler/fryer w/ skin neck & giblets roasted	1 chicken (1.5 lbs)	1598	730	—
broiler/fryer w/ skin neck & giblets stewed	1 chicken (1.6 lbs)	1625	726	—
broiler/fryer w/o skin roasted	1 cup (5 oz)	266	125	—
broiler/fryer wing w/ skin batter dipped & fried	1 (1.7 oz)	159	39	—
broiler/fryer wing w/ skin floured & fried	1 (1.1 oz)	103	26	—
broiler/fryer wing w/ skin roasted	1 (1.2 oz)	99	29	—
broiler/fryer wing w/ skin stewed	1 (1.4 oz)	100	28	—
capon w/ skin neck & giblets roasted	1 chicken (3.1 lbs)	3211	1458	—
cornish hen w/ skin roasted	1 hen (8 oz)	595	299	—
cornish hen w/o skin & bone roasted	1 hen (3.8 oz)	144	113	—
cornish hen w/o skin & bone roasted	½ hen (2 oz)	72	57	—
cornish hen w/skin roasted	½ hen (4 oz)	296	149	—
roaster w/ skin neck & giblets roasted	1 chicken (2.4 lbs)	2363	1003	—
roaster w/ skin roasted	½ chicken (1.1 lbs)	1071	365	—
roaster w/o skin roasted	1 cup (5 oz)	469	160	—
stewing w/ skin neck & giblets stewed	1 chicken (1.3 lbs)	1636	603	—

FOOD	PORTION	CALS	CHOL	FIBER
stewing w/ skin stewed	½ chicken (9.2 oz)	744	205	—
stewing w/ skin stewed	6.2 oz	507	140	—
Perdue				
Boneless Skinless Breasts Cooked	3 oz	110	70	—
Boneless Breast Roasted Garlic Herb	1 piece (3 oz)	90	50	—
Breaded Breast Strips Barbecue	3 oz	120	30	—
Breaded Breast Strips Hot & Spicy	3 oz	110	30	—
Breaded Breast Strips Original	3 oz	120	35	—
Burger Cooked	1 (3 oz)	160	110	—
Chicken Breast Seasoned Italian Cooked	1 piece (3 oz)	90	50	—
Chicken Breast Seasoned Lemon Pepper Cooked	1 piece (3 oz)	90	50	—
Chicken Breast Seasoned Teriyaki Cooked	1 piece (3 oz)	90	50	—
Ground Cooked	3 oz	170	125	—
Ground Breast Cooked	3 oz	80	55	—
Honey Rotisserie Dark Meat	3 oz	200	80	—
Honey Rotisserie White Meat	3 oz	140	70	—
Oven Stuffer Dark Meat Roasted	3 oz	210	100	—
Oven Stuffer Drumstick Roasted	1 (3.6 oz)	190	120	—
Oven Stuffer White Meat Roasted	3 oz	170	80	—
Oven Stuffer Wingette Roasted	3 (3.4 oz)	220	120	—
Seasoned Roasting Chicken Toasted Garlic Dark Meat	3 oz	190	100	—

FOOD	PORTION	CALS	CHOL	FIBER
Seasoned Roasting Chicken Toasted Garlic White Meat	3 oz	160	75	—
Seasoned Strips Parmesan Garlic cooked	3 oz	100	55	—
Seasoned Strips Savory Classic cooked	3 oz	90	55	—
Seasoned Strips Spicy Fiesta cooked	3 oz	140	75	—
Split Breast Cooked	1 piece (6.8 oz)	370	180	—
Thin Sliced Breast Rosemary Garlic Thyme	1 piece (3 oz)	90	60	—
Thin Sliced Breast Tomato Herb	1 piece (3 oz)	90	60	—
Whole Dark Meat cooked	3 oz	150	110	—
Whole White Meat Cooked	3 oz	170	85	0
Wings Roasted	2 (3.2 oz)	210	115	—
Tyson				
Broth Marinated Breast Filet	1 (4.7 oz)	140	70	0
Broth Marinated Drums	2 (4 oz)	140	90	0
Broth Marinated Thighs	1 (4.9 oz)	380	110	0
Broth Marinated Wings	4 pieces (4.2 oz)	240	95	0
Chicken Broccoli & Cheese	1 piece (5.9 oz)	320	50	3
Chicken Stuffed w/ Wild Rice & Mushroom	1 piece (5.9 oz)	300	50	1
Cordon Bleu	1 piece (5.9 oz)	350	55	3
Cornish Hen	1 serv (4 oz)	180	130	0
Kiev	1 piece (5.9 oz)	460	115	2

FOOD	PORTION	CALS	CHOL	FIBER
Wampler				
Breast Tenders	4 oz	130	70	–
FROZEN				
Banquet				
Breast Nuggets	7	280	40	1
Breast Patties Grilled Honey BBQ	1	110	40	0
Breast Patties Grilled Honey Mustard	1	120	25	0
Breast Tenders Our Original	3	250	40	tr
Breast Tenders Southern	3 pieces	260	40	1
Country Fried	1 serv (3 oz)	270	65	1
Fat Free Baked Breast Patties	1	100	20	1
Fried Our Original	1 serv (3 oz)	280	65	1
Honey BBQ Skinless Fried	1 serv (3 oz)	230	55	1
Hot 'n Spicy Fried	1 serv (3 oz)	260	65	1
Nuggets Our Original	6	270	35	1
Nuggets Southern Fried	5	270	35	2
Patties Our Orignal	1	190	30	1
Patties Southern Fried	1	190	25	tr
Skinless Fried	1 serv (3 oz)	220	65	2
Smokehouse Big Wings	2	200	70	0
Southern Fried	1 serv (3 oz)	280	65	1
Wings Firehouse Big	2	190	70	0
Wings Honey BBQ	4	380	70	1
Wings Hot & Spicy	4 pieces	280	90	tr
Country Skillet				
Bites	5	270	20	1
Breast Tenders	3	240	25	1
Chunks	5	270	20	1
Fried	3 oz	270	65	1
Nuggets	10	280	25	1
Patties	1	190	20	1

FOOD	PORTION	CALS	CHOL	FIBER
Southern Fried Chunks	5	270	20	1
Southern Fried Patties	1	190	20	1
Empire				
Nuggets	5 (3 oz)	180	15	1
Stix	4 (3.1 oz)	180	25	2
Health Is Wealth				
Nuggets	4 (3 oz)	150	40	0
Patties	1 (3 oz)	150	40	0
Tenders	3 (3 oz)	130	35	0
Kid Cuisine				
Dino Mite Nuggets	4 pieces	300	40	1
Radical Racin' Nuggets w/ Cheese	4 pieces	300	35	tr
Sensible Chef				
Fried Breast	1 (3 oz)	200	55	2
Weaver				
Breast Strips	3 pieces (3.3 oz)	210	35	2
Breast Tenders	5 pieces (3 oz)	220	35	1
Croquettes	1 serv (3.5 oz)	290	45	2
Dutch Frye Nuggets	5 pieces (3.3 oz)	280	45	2
Honey Battered Tenders	5 pieces (2.9 oz)	230	35	1
Hot Wings Buffalo Style	3 pieces (2.7 oz)	190	95	0
Mini Drums Crispy	5 pieces (3.3 oz)	250	40	1
Nuggets	4 pieces (2.7 oz)	210	35	1
Patties	1 (2.6 oz)	180	30	1
Rondelet	1 (2.6 oz)	170	20	1
Rondelet Dutch Frye	1 (2.6 oz)	230	35	1
Rondelet Italian	1 (2.6 oz)	210	20	1
READY-TO-EAT				
chicken roll light meat	2 oz	90	28	–
chicken roll light meat	1 pkg (6 oz)	271	85	–
poultry salad sandwich spread	1 oz	238	9	–
poultry salad sandwich spread	1 tbsp (13 g)	109	4	–

FOOD	PORTION	CALS	CHOL	FIBER
Banquet				
Fat Free Baked Breast Tenders	3	120	30	2
Boar's Head				
Breast Hickory Smoked	2 oz	60	30	0
Breast Oven Roasted	2 oz	50	30	0
Breast Bar B Q Sauce Basted	2 oz	60	30	0
Butterball				
Crispy Baked Breasts Italian Style Herb	1 piece (0.5 oz)	190	55	1
Crispy Baked Breasts Lemon Pepper	1 piece (0.5 oz)	200	50	tr
Crispy Baked Breasts Original	1 piece (0.5 oz)	180	45	1
Crispy Baked Breasts Parmesan	1 piece (0.5 oz)	200	55	tr
Crispy Baked Breasts Southwestern	1 piece (0.5 oz)	170	35	2
Tenders Baked Breast	3 pieces	170	35	1
Tenders Hickory Smoked Grilled	4 pieces + sauce	160	50	1
Tenders Oriental Grilled	4 pieces + sauce	160	45	1
Carl Buddig				
Chicken Sliced	1 pkg (2.5 oz)	110	40	—
Lean Slices Honey Smoked Breast	1 pkg (2.5 oz)	70	30	—
Lean Slices Roasted Breast	1 pkg (2.5 oz)	60	30	—
Chicken By George				
Cajun	1 breast (4 oz)	130	60	0
Caribbean Grill	1 breast (4 oz)	150	60	0
Garlic & Herb	1 breast (4 oz)	120	60	0
Italian Bleu Cheese	1 breast (4 oz)	130	60	0
Lemon Herb	1 breast (4 oz)	120	60	0
Lemon Oregano	1 breast (4 oz)	130	50	0
Mesquite Barbecue	1 breast (4 oz)	130	60	0
Mustard Dill	1 breast (4 oz)	140	60	0
Roasted	1 breast (4 oz)	110	55	0

FOOD	PORTION	CALS	CHOL	FIBER
Teriyaki	1 breast (4 oz)	130	55	0
Tomato Herb With Basil	1 breast (4 oz)	140	60	0
Empire				
Barbarcue Whole	5 oz	280	110	0
Battered & Breaded Cutlets	1 (3.3 oz)	200	25	2
Battered & Breaded Fried Breasts	3 oz	170	45	tr
Battered & Breaded Nuggets	5 (3 oz)	200	30	1
Bologna	3 slices (1.8 oz)	200	40	0
Fried Drum & Thigh	3 oz	240	80	2
Falls				
BBQ	3 oz	150	75	–
Healthy Choice				
Deli-Thin Oven Roasted Breast	6 slices (2 oz)	45	25	0
Deli-Thin Smoked Breast	6 slices (2 oz)	60	30	0
Fresh-Trak Oven Roasted Breast	1 slice (1 oz)	30	15	0
Oven Roasted Breast	1 slice (1 oz)	25	15	0
Smoked Breast	1 slice (1 oz)	35	15	0
Hebrew National				
Deli Thin Oven Roasted	1.8 oz	45	20	–
Louis Rich				
Carving Board Classic Baked	2 slices (1.6 oz)	45	25	0
Carving Board Grilled	2 slices (1.6 oz)	45	25	0
Deli-Thin Oven Roasted Breast	4 slices (1.8 oz)	50	25	0
Oven Roasted Deluxe Breast	1 slice (1 oz)	30	15	0
Mr. Turkey				
Deli Cuts Hardwood Smoked	3 slices	30	13	–
Deli Cuts Oven Roasted	3 slices	25	15	–
Oscar Mayer				
Free Oven Roasted Breast	4 slices (1.8 oz)	45	25	0

FOOD	PORTION	CALS	CHOL	FIBER
Lunchables Chicken/ Monterey Jack	1 pkg (4.5 oz)	350	75	1
Lunchables Deluxe Chicken/Turkey	1 pkg (5.1 oz)	380	70	1
Lunchables Dessert Chocolate Pudding/ Chicken/Jack	1 pkg (6.2 oz)	370	55	0
Perdue				
Breast Cutlets Homestyle	1 (2.9 oz)	110	35	–
Breast Cutlets Italian Style	1 (2.9 oz)	120	40	–
Breast Filets In Barbecue Sauce	1 piece + 3 tbsp sauce (5.9 oz)	200	70	–
Breast Strips In Garlic & Herb Sauce	1 serv (5 oz)	100	50	2
Breast Strips In Marinara Sauce	1 serv (5 oz)	120	50	–
Breast Strips In Teriyaki Sauce	1 serv (5 oz)	190	50	–
Carved Breast Honey Roasted	½ cup (2.5 oz)	100	45	–
Carved Breast Original Roasted	½ cup (2.5 oz)	90	50	–
Cutlets Cooked	1 (3.5 oz)	220	55	–
Nuggets	5 (3.4 oz)	210	50	–
Nuggets Chicken & Cheese	5 (3.4 oz)	230	55	–
Short Cuts Entrees In Teriyaki Sauce	5 oz	190	50	–
Short Cuts Italian	½ cup (2.5 oz)	100	60	–
Short Cuts Lemon Pepper	½ cup (2.5 oz)	100	60	–
Short Cuts Southwestern	½ cup (2.5 oz)	100	60	–
Shady Brook				
Slow Roasted Breast	2 oz	60	30	–
Tyson				
Breaded Breast Chunks	6 pieces (2.9 oz)	230	20	1
Breaded Breast Fillet	2 pieces (2.8 oz)	180	25	1

FOOD	PORTION	CALS	CHOL	FIBER
Breaded Breast Pattie	1 (2.6 oz)	190	25	1
Breaded Breast Tenders	5 pieces (3 oz)	220	35	1
Breaded Chicken Chunks	6 pieces (3 oz)	220	40	0
Chick'n Quick Chick'n Cheddar	1 patty (2.6 oz)	220	40	0
Chicken Bits Southern Fried	6 pieces (2.9 oz)	260	40	1
Chicken Strips	1 serv (3 oz)	90	45	0
Chicken Strips Southwestern	1 serv (3 oz)	110	40	0
Country Fried Chicken Fritter	5 pieces (2.9 oz)	260	40	1
Drumsticks Hot BBQ Style	2 (3.5 oz)	160	100	1
Glazed Grilled Breast Pattie	1 (2.7 oz)	120	40	0
Grilled Chicken Pattie	1 (2.9 oz)	170	55	0
Nuggets Breaded White Meat	6 pieces (2.9 oz)	250	35	1
Patties Southern Fried	1 (2.9 oz)	260	40	1
Roasted Drumsticks	3 (5.6 oz)	320	230	0
Roasted Drumsticks w/o Skin	2 (3.3 oz)	140	120	0
Roasted Half Chicken	1 serv (3 oz)	160	75	0
Roasted Whole Chicken	1 serv (3 oz)	160	75	0
Roasted Breast Boneless w/o Skin	1 (3.7 oz)	130	70	0
Roasted Breast Half w/o Skin	1 (4.3 oz)	150	80	0
Roasted Half Breast w/ Skin	1 (5.1 oz)	260	110	0
Roasted Half Chicken w/o Skin	1 serv (3 oz)	120	75	0
Roasted Tabasco Wings	3 (3 oz)	190	100	1
Roasted Thigh w/ Skin	1 (3.6 oz)	270	120	0
Roasted Thighs w/o Skin	1 (2.9 oz)	150	95	0

FOOD	PORTION	CALS	CHOL	FIBER
Roll White Meat	2 oz	90	25	0
Southern Fried Breaded Breast Pattie	1 (2.6 oz)	180	30	0
Southern Fried Breast Fillets	2 pieces (3.4 oz)	210	30	1
Southern Fried Chunks	6 pieces (2.9 oz)	260	40	1
Tenders Breaded Honey Battered	5 pieces (2.9 oz)	230	35	1
Tenders Breaded Pattie	3 pieces (3.2 oz)	100	0	1
Thick'n Crispy Pattie	1 (2.6 oz)	200	40	1
Wings BBQ	3 pieces (3.2 oz)	200	110	0
Wings Hot N'Spicy	4 (3.2 oz)	210	100	0
Wings Teriyaki	4 pieces (3.4 oz)	190	120	2
Wings Of Fire	4 pieces (3.4 oz)	220	110	0
TAKE-OUT				
oven roasted breast of chicken	2 oz	60	25	–

CHICKEN DISHES
CANNED
Bumble Bee

Chicken Salad	1 pkg (3.5 oz)	230	25	0
Dinty Moore				
Noodles & Chicken	1 can (7.5 oz)	180	30	1
Stew	1 cup (8.5 oz)	220	40	2
FROZEN				
Jimmy Dean				
Grilled Breast Sandwich	1 (5.5 oz)	330	70	1
White Castle				
Grilled Chicken Sandwich	2 (4 oz)	250	20	5
Grilled Chicken Sandwich w/ Sauce	2 (4.8 oz)	290	20	5
MIX				
Chicken Skillet Helper				
Stir-Fried Chicken as prep	1 cup	270	105	1

FOOD	PORTION	CALS	CHOL	FIBER
Hamburger Helper				
Reduced Sodium Cheddar Spirals Chicken Recipe as prep	1 cup	240	40	0
Reduced Sodium Italian Herb Chicken Recipe as prep	1 cup	200	35	2
Reduced Sodium Southwestern Beef Chicken Recipe as prep	1 cup	220	35	2
Tyson				
Mandarin Wrap Kit	1½ wraps (14.6 oz)	630	50	5
READY-TO-EAT				
salad low fat	⅓ cup	90	20	—
Shady Brook				
Chicken Breast w/ Rice Pilaf	1 serv (12 oz)	350	120	—
Teriyaki Breast	1 serv (12 oz)	490	15	—
Wampler				
Cacciatore	1 cup	260	90	—
Fajitas	1 cup	210	70	—
Salad	⅓ cup	200	30	—
Salad Lite	⅓ cup	130	25	—
Smokey Barbecue Chicken	1 cup	430	140	—
Sweet-n-Sour	1 cup	250	55	—
SHELF-STABLE				
Dinty Moore				
Microwave Cup Chicken & Dumpling	1 pkg (7.5 oz)	200	35	1
Microwave Cup Stew	1 pkg (7.5 oz)	180	30	2
Lunch Bucket				
Chicken Fiesta	1 pkg (7.5 oz)	160	5	5
Dumplings'n Chicken	1 pkg (7.5 oz)	140	10	1
TastyBite				
Chicken Moglai	1 pkg (9.5 oz)	300	45	3

FOOD	PORTION	CALS	CHOL	FIBER
TAKE-OUT				
boneless breaded & fried w/ barbecue sauce	6 pieces (4.6 oz)	330	61	—
boneless breaded & fried w/ honey	6 pieces 4 oz)	339	61	—
boneless breaded & fried w/ mustard sauce	6 pieces (4.6 oz)	323	62	—
boneless breaded & fried w/ sweet & sour sauce	6 pieces (4.6 oz)	346	61	—
breast & wing breaded & fried	2 pieces (5.7 oz)	494	149	—
chicken & dumplings	¾ cup	256	109	tr
chicken & noodles	1 cup	365	103	—
chicken a la king	1 cup	470	221	—
chicken cacciatore	¾ cup	394	99	2
chicken paprikash	1½ cups	296	90	—
drumstick breaded & fried	2 pieces (5.2 oz)	430	165	—
groundnut stew hkatenkwan	1 serv (15.7 oz)	576	116	4
jamaican jerk wings	4 wings (9.9 oz)	709	172	tr
sancocho de pollo dominican chicken stew	1 serv	702	195	1
thigh breaded & fried	2 pieces (5.2 oz)	430	165	—
CHICKEN SUBSTITUTES				
Health Is Wealth				
Buffalo Wings	3 pieces (2.2 oz)	100	0	3
Chicken-Free Nuggets	3 pieces (2.25 oz)	90	0	2
Chicken-Free Patties	1 (3 oz)	120	0	2
Loma Linda				
Chicken Supreme Mix not prep	⅓ cup (0.9 oz)	90	0	4
Chik Nuggets	5 pieces (3 oz)	240	0	5
Fried Chik'n w/Gravy	2 pieces (2.8 oz)	160	0	2

FOOD	PORTION	CALS	CHOL	FIBER
Morningstar Farms				
Chik Nuggets	4 pieces (3 oz)	160	0	5
Chik Patties	1 (2.5 oz)	150	0	2
Meatless Buffalo Wings	5 pieces (3 oz)	200	0	3
Quorn				
Cutlets	1 (3.5 oz)	200	0	4
Nuggets	3–4 pieces (3 oz)	180	0	3
Patties	1 patty (2.6 oz)	160	0	3
Tenders	1 cup (3 oz)	90	0	3
Soy Is Us				
Chicken Not!	½ cup (1.75 oz)	140	0	9
Worthington				
Chic-Ketts	2 slices (1.9 oz)	120	0	2
Chicken Sliced or Roll	2 slices (2 oz)	80	0	tr
Chicken Sliced	2 slices (2 oz)	80	0	tr
ChikStiks	1 (1.6 oz)	110	0	2
CrispyChik Patties	1 (2.5 oz)	150	0	2
Cutlets	1 slice (2.1 oz)	70	0	2
Diced Chik	¼ cup (1.9 oz)	40	0	1
FriChik	2 pieces (3.2 oz)	120	0	1
FriChik Low Fat	2 pieces (3 oz)	80	0	1
Golden Croquettes	4 pieces (3 oz)	210	0	6
Yves				
Veggie Chicken Burgers	1 (3 oz)	120	0	3

CHICKPEAS
CANNED
chickpeas	1 cup	285	0	—
Green Giant				
Garbanzo	½ cup (4.4 oz)	110	0	5
Old El Paso				
Garbanzo	½ cup (4.6 oz)	120	0	7
Progresso				
Chick Peas	½ cup (4.6 oz)	120	0	5
Garbanzo	½ cup (4.4 oz)	110	0	5
DRIED				
cooked	1 cup	269	0	—

CHICORY
greens raw chopped	½ cup	21	0	—
root raw	1 (2.1 oz)	44	0	—

FOOD	PORTION	CALS	CHOL	FIBER
roots raw cut up	½ cup (1.6 oz)	33	0	—
witloof head raw	1 (1.9 oz)	9	0	—
witloof raw	½ cup (1.6 oz)	8	0	—

CHILI

FOOD	PORTION	CALS	CHOL	FIBER
chili w/ beans	1 cup	286	43	—
dried ancho	1 tsp	3	0	tr
dried casabel	1 tsp	3	0	tr
dried guajillo	1 tsp	3	0	tr
dried mulato	1 tsp	3	0	tr
dried pasilla	1 tsp	3	0	tr
dried smoked chipotle	1 tsp	3	0	tr
powder	1 tsp	8	0	—
Amy's				
Chili & Cornbread	1 pkg (10.5 oz)	320	10	8
Organic Black Bean	1 cup	200	0	15
Organic Medium	1 cup	190	0	7
Organic Medium w/ Vegetables	1 cup	190	0	8
Armour				
Chili No Beans	1 cup (8.7 oz)	390	70	0
Chili W/ Beans Western Style	1 cup (8.8 oz)	370	60	9
Chili w/ Beans	1 cup (8.9 oz)	370	50	10
Chili w/ Beans Hot	1 cup (8.9 oz)	370	50	10
Vienna Sausage & Chili	1 cup (8.7 oz)	410	80	15
Carroll Shelby's				
Original Texas Chili Kit	2 tbsp	60	0	0
Chef Boyardee				
Chili Mac	½ can (7 oz)	260	30	3
Del Monte				
Sauce	1 tbsp (0.6 oz)	20	0	0
Gebhardt				
Chili Powder	¼ tsp (0.3 g)	1	0	tr
Chili Quik Seasoning	1 tbsp (0.3 oz)	43	0	2
Plain	1 cup (9.4 oz)	232	0	3
With Beans	1 cup (9.4 oz)	322	29	15
Health Valley				
Burrito	1 cup	160	0	12
Enchilada	1 cup	160	0	12

FOOD	PORTION	CALS	CHOL	FIBER
Fajita	1 cup	80	0	7
In A Cup Black Bean Mild	¾ cup	120	0	6
In A Cup Texas Style Spicy	¾ cup	120	0	6
Vegetarian Lentil Mild	1 cup	160	0	12
Vegetarian Lentil No Salt	1 cup	80	0	6
Vegetarian Mild	1 cup	160	0	12
Vegetarian Mild No Salt	1 cup	160	0	12
Vegetarian Spicy	1 cup	160	0	12
Vegetarian Spicy No Salt	1 cup	160	0	12
Vegetarian w/ 3 Beans Mild	1 cup	160	0	12
Vegetarian w/ Black Beans Mild	1 cup	160	0	12
Vegetarian w/ Black Beans Spicy	1 cup	160	0	12
Healthy Choice				
Bowls Chili & Cornbread	1 meal (9.5 oz)	350	35	8
Hormel				
Chunky w/ Beans	1 cup (8.7 oz)	270	35	7
Hot No Beans	1 cup (8.3 oz)	210	35	3
Hot With Beans	1 cup (8.7 oz)	270	35	7
Microcup Meals Chili Mac	1 cup (7.5 oz)	200	25	2
Microcup Meals Hot With Beans	1 cup (7.3 oz)	220	30	6
Microcup Meals No Beans	1 cup (7.3 oz)	190	30	2
Microcup Meals With Beans	1 cup (7.3 oz)	220	30	6
No Beans	1 cup (8.3 oz)	210	35	3
Turkey No Beans	1 cup (8.3 oz)	190	75	3
Turkey w/ Beans	1 cup (8.7 oz)	210	35	5
Vegetarian	1 cup (8.7 oz)	200	0	7
With Beans	1 cup (8.7 oz)	270	35	7

FOOD	PORTION	CALS	CHOL	FIBER
Hunt's				
Chili Beans	½ cup (4.5 oz)	87	0	6
Chili Sauce	2 tbsp (1.2 oz)	35	0	1
Hurst				
HamBeens Chili Beans	1 serv	130	0	10
Instant India				
Chili Ginger Paste	2 tbsp (1 oz)	90	0	0
Just Rite				
With Beans	1 cup (9 oz)	379	35	13
Lean Cuisine				
Everyday Favorites Three Bean Chili w/ Rice	1 pkg (10 oz)	250	10	9
Luigino's				
Chili-Mac	1 pkg (8 oz)	230	25	3
Lunch Bucket				
Chili With Beans	1 pkg (7.5 oz)	260	25	8
Manwich				
Homestyle Fixins	½ cup (4.6 oz)	84	0	6
Marie Callender's				
Chili & Cornbread	1 meal (16 oz)	560	60	7
McCormick				
Original Chili Seasoning	1⅓ tbsp (9 g)	30	0	2
Natural Choice				
Organic Vegan Three Bean	½ cup (4.6 oz)	140	0	7
Natural Touch				
Vegetarian	1 cup (8.1 oz)	170	0	11
Nature's Entree				
Texas Chili	1 pkg (12 oz)	320	15	11
Nile Spice				
Chili'n Beans Original	1 pkg	150	0	6
Chili'n Beans Spicy	1 pkg	150	0	6
Old El Paso				
Chili Seasoning Mix	1 tbsp (0.3 oz)	25	0	1
Chili With Beans	1 cup (8 oz)	200	30	6
Open Range				
Plain	1 cup (8.8 oz)	353	48	6
With Beans	1 cup (9 oz)	281	26	10

FOOD	PORTION	CALS	CHOL	FIBER
Soy7				
Chili Mix as prep	1 cup	150	0	7
Stouffer's				
With Beans	1 pkg (8.75 oz)	270	35	8
Tabatchnick				
Vegetarian	7.5 oz	210	0	10
Ultimate				
No Beans Hot	1 cup (8.7 oz)	420	85	5
Turkey w/ Beans	1 cup (8.7 oz)	260	50	9
W/ Beans	1 cup (8.7 oz)	320	50	9
W/ Beans Hot	1 cup (8.7 oz)	320	50	9
Van Camp				
Beanee Weenee Chilee	1 cup (7.7 oz)	240	35	9
Chili With Beans	1 cup (8.9 oz)	350	45	7
Mexican Style Chili Beans	½ cup (4.6 oz)	110	0	8
Wampler				
Turkey	1 cup	250	75	–
Watkins				
Powder	¼ tsp (0.5 g)	0	0	0
Seasoning	1¼ tsp (4 g)	15	0	0
Wick Fowler's				
2 Alarm Chili Kit	3 tbsp	60	0	0
False Alarm Chili Kit	2 tbsp	50	0	0
Worthington				
Chili	1 cup (8.1 oz)	290	0	9
Low Fat	1 cup (8.1 oz)	170	0	11
Yves				
Veggie Chili	1 pkg (10.5 oz)	230	0	14
TAKE-OUT				
con carne w/ beans	8.9 oz	254	133	–

CHILI PEPPER (see PEPPERS)

CHINESE FOOD (see ASIAN FOOD)

CHINESE PRESERVING MELON

cooked	½ cup	11	0	–

CHIPS

barbecue	1 oz	139	0	–

FOOD	PORTION	CALS	CHOL	FIBER
barbecue	1 bag (7 oz)	971	0	—
corn	1 bag (7 oz)	1067	0	9
corn	1 oz	153	0	1
corn barbecue	1 oz	148	0	1
corn barbecue	1 bag (7 oz)	1036	0	10
corn cones	1 oz	145	0	—
corn onion	1 oz	142	0	—
potato	1 bag (8 oz)	1217	0	—
potato	1 oz	152	0	—
potato light	1 oz	134	0	—
potato light	1 bag (6 oz)	801	0	—
potato sour cream & onion	1 oz	150	2	—
potato sour cream & onion	1 bag (7 oz)	1051	14	—
potato sticks	½ cup (0.6 oz)	94	0	1
potato sticks	1 oz	148	0	1
potato sticks	1 pkg (1 oz)	148	0	—
taro	1 oz	141	0	—
taro	10 (0.8 oz)	115	0	—
tortilla	1 oz	142	0	2
tortilla	1 bag (7.5 oz)	1067	0	14
tortilla nacho	1 oz	141	0	2
tortilla nacho	1 bag (8 oz)	1131	0	12
tortilla nacho light	1 oz	126	0	—
tortilla nacho light	1 bag (6 oz)	757	0	—
tortilla ranch	1 oz	139	0	—
tortilla ranch	1 bag (7 oz)	969	1	—
Barbara's Bakery				
Potato	1¼ cup (1 oz)	150	0	1
Potato No Salt Added	1¼ cups (1 oz)	150	0	1
Potato Ripple	1¼ cup (1 oz)	150	0	1
Potato Yogurt & Green Onion	1¼ cup (1 oz)	150	0	1
Tortilla Blue Corn	15 chips (1 oz)	140	0	1
Tortilla Blue Corn No Salt	15 chips (1 oz)	140	0	1
Tortilla Pinta Salsa	15 chips (1 oz)	130	0	2
Barrel O' Fun				
Barbeque	1 oz	145	0	0

FOOD	PORTION	CALS	CHOL	FIBER
Potato	1 oz	150	0	0
Sour Cream & Onion	1 oz	150	0	0
Tortilla Nacho	1 oz	140	0	1
Tortilla White	1 oz	140	0	0
Tostada Yellow	1 oz	140	0	0
Bruno & Luigi's				
Pasta Chips Garlic & Herb	1 oz	117	0	1
Cape Cod				
Potato	19 chips (1 oz)	150	0	1
Potato Golden Russet	1 pkg (0.5 oz)	70	0	tr
Chester's				
Flamin' Hot	1 oz	140	0	tr
Salsa	1 oz	140	0	tr
Doritos				
3D's Cooler Ranch	27 (1 oz)	140	<5	1
3D's Nacho Cheesier	27 (1 oz)	140	<5	1
Cooler Ranch	12 (1 oz)	140	0	1
Flamin' Hot	11 (1 oz)	140	0	1
Nacho Cheesier	11 (1 oz)	140	0	1
Salsa Verde	12 (1 oz)	150	0	1
Smokey Red	12 (1 oz)	150	0	1
Spicy Nacho	12 (1 oz)	140	0	1
Toasted Corn	13 (1 oz)	140	0	1
Wow Nacho Cheesier	1 pkg (0.75 oz)	70	0	1
Durangos				
Tortilla	15 (1 oz)	150	0	2
Eden				
Brown Rice Chips	1 oz	150	0	0
Sea Vegetable Chips	1 oz	140	0	0
Energy Food Factory				
Corn Pops Fat Free	½ oz	50	0	1
Corn Pops Nacho	½ oz	50	0	1
Corn Pops Original	½ oz	50	0	1
Potato Pops Au Gratin	½ oz	60	<5	1
Potato Pops Fat Free	½ oz	50	0	1
Potato Pops Herb & Garlic	½ oz	50	0	1
Potato Pops Mesquite	½ oz	50	0	1
Potato Pops Original	½ oz	50	0	1

FOOD	PORTION	CALS	CHOL	FIBER
Potato Pops Salt N' Vinegar	½ oz	50	0	1
Fritos				
Chili Cheese	31 (1 oz)	160	0	1
Corn Chips BBQ	29 (1 oz)	150	0	1
Corn Chips King Size	12 (1 oz)	150	0	1
Corn Chips Sabrositas Flamin' Hot	30 (1 oz)	150	0	1
Corn Chips Sabrositas Lime'N Chile	28 (1 oz)	150	0	1
Corn Chips Wild N'Mild Ranch	28 (1 oz)	160	0	1
Original	32 (1 oz)	160	0	1
Scoops	11 (1 oz)	160	0	1
Texas Grill Honey BBQ	15 (1 oz)	150	0	1
GeniSoy				
Soy Crisps	1 oz	110	0	2
Soy Crisps Apple Cinnamon Crunch	1 oz	120	0	2
Soy Crisps Creamy Ranch	1 oz	110	0	2
Soy Crisps Deep Sea Salt	1 oz	110	0	2
Soy Crisps Rich Cheddar Cheese	1 oz	110	0	2
Soy Crisps Roasted Garlic & Onion	1 oz	100	0	2
Soy Crisps Zesty Barbeque	1 oz	110	0	2
Guiltless Gourmet				
Tortilla Baked Chili Lime	18 (1 oz)	110	0	2
Tortilla Baked Mucho Nacho	18 (1 oz)	110	0	2
Tortilla Baked Organic Blue Corn	18 (1 oz)	110	0	2
Tortilla Baked Picante Ranch	18 (1 oz)	110	0	2
Tortilla Baked Red Corn	18 (1 oz)	110	0	2

FOOD	PORTION	CALS	CHOL	FIBER
Tortilla Baked Spicy Black Bean	18 (1 oz)	110	0	2
Tortilla Baked Sweet White Corn	18 (1 oz)	110	0	2
Tortilla Baked Yellow Corn	18 (1 oz)	110	0	2
Tortilla Baked Yellow Corn Unsalted	18 (1 oz)	110	0	2
Herr's				
Potato	1 oz	140	0	1
Tortilla Restaurant Style White Corn	10 chips (1 oz)	140	0	2
Husman's				
Deli Style Tortilla	11 chips	150	0	1
Potato	18 (1 oz)	160	0	1
Potato Sour Cream & Onion	18 (1 oz)	150	0	1
Potato Sweet N'Sassy	18 (1 oz)	155	0	1
Lance				
BBQ	22 (1 oz)	160	0	1
Cajun	15 (1 oz)	150	0	1
Corn Chips	39 (1.25 oz)	200	0	1
Corn Chips Hot BBQ	35 (1.25 oz)	210	0	1
Hot Fries	1 pkg (0.9 oz)	140	0	1
Mesquite BBQ	22 (1 oz)	150	0	1
Potato	23 (1 oz)	160	0	1
Ripple	15 (1 oz)	160	0	1
Salt & Vinegar	22 (1 oz)	160	0	2
Sour Cream & Onion	22 (1 oz)	160	0	1
Tortilla Fiesta Salsa Triangles	16 (1 oz)	140	0	2
Tortilla Nacho Mini Round	46 (1.25 oz)	180	0	2
Tortilla Nacho Triangles	15 (1 oz)	140	0	1
Lay's				
Adobadas	16 (1 oz)	170	0	1
Baked KC Masterpiece BBQ	11 (1 oz)	120	0	2
Baked Original	11 (1 oz)	110	0	2
Baked Roasted Herb	12 (1 oz)	130	0	2

FOOD	PORTION	CALS	CHOL	FIBER
Baked Sour Cream & Onion	12 (1 oz)	120	0	2
Classic	20 (1 oz)	150	0	1
Deli Style Hot N'Tangy BBQ	18 (1 oz)	150	0	1
Deli Style Jalapeno	17 (1 oz)	150	0	1
Deli Style Original	17 (1 oz)	140	0	1
Deli Style Salt & Vinegar	16 (1 oz)	90	0	1
Flamin' Hot	17 pieces (1 oz)	150	0	1
KC Masterpiece BBQ	15 (1 oz)	150	0	1
Onion & Garlic	19 (1 oz)	150	0	1
Salt & Vinegar	17 pieces (1 oz)	150	0	1
Sour Cream & Onion	17 pieces (1 oz)	160	<5	1
Toasted Onion & Cheese	17 pieces (1 oz)	160	0	1
Wavy Au Gratin	13 (1 oz)	150	<5	1
Wavy Original	11 pieces (1 oz)	160	0	1
Wavy Ranch	11 (1 oz)	160	0	1
Wow Mesquite BBQ	20 (1 oz)	75	0	1
Wow Mesquite BBQ	20 (1 oz)	75	0	1
Wow Original	20 (1 oz)	75	0	1
Wow Original	1 pkg (0.75 oz)	55	0	1
Wow Sour Cream & Chive	19 (1 oz)	80	0	1
Wow Sour Cream & Chive	19 (1 oz)	80	0	1
Louise's				
"1g" Mesquite BBQ	1 oz	110	0	2
"1g" Original	1 oz	110	0	2
70% Less Fat Mesquite BBQ	1 oz	110	0	2
70% Less Fat Original	1 oz	110	0	2
95% Fat-Free Tortilla	1 oz	120	0	1
Fat-Free Maui Onion	1 oz	110	0	2
Fat-Free Mesquite BBQ	1 oz	110	0	2
Fat-Free No Salt	1 oz	110	0	2
Fat-Free Original	1 oz	110	0	2
Fat-Free Vinegar & Salt	1 oz	110	0	2

FOOD	PORTION	CALS	CHOL	FIBER
Mr. Phipps				
Tater Crisps Bar-B-Que	21 (1 oz)	130	0	1
Tater Crisps Original	23 (1 oz)	120	0	1
Tater Crisps Sour Cream 'n Onion	22 (1 oz)	130	0	1
Tortilla	28 (1 oz)	130	0	3
Tortilla Nacho	28 (1 oz)	130	0	3
Old Dutch Foods				
Potato	12–15 chips (1 oz)	150	0	1
Potato BBQ	12–15 chips (1 oz)	150	0	1
Potato BBQ Ripple	12–15 chips (1 oz)	150	0	tr
Potato Cajun Ripple	12–15 chips (1 oz)	150	0	1
Potato Cheddar & Sour Cream Ripple	12–15 chips (1 oz)	160	0	1
Potato Cheddar & Sour Cream Ripples	12–15 chips (1 oz)	150	0	1
Potato Dill	12–15 chips (1 oz)	140	0	1
Potato Dutch Crunch	15–20 chips (1 oz)	130	0	2
Potato French Onion Ripple	12–15 chips (1 oz)	150	0	1
Potato Jalapeno & Cheddar Dutch Crunch	15–20 chips (1 oz)	130	0	1
Potato Jalapeno Cheese	12–15 chips (1 oz)	150	0	1
Potato Mesquite BBQ Dutch Crunch	15–20 chips (1 oz)	130	0	2
Potato Onion & Garlic	12–15 chips (1 oz)	140	0	1
Potato Outback Spicy BBQ	12–15 chips (1 oz)	150	0	1
Potato Ripples	12–15 chips (1 oz)	150	0	1
Potato Salt & Vinegar Dutch Crunch	15–20 chips (1 oz)	130	0	1
Potato Sour Cream & Onion	12–15 chips (1 oz)	150	0	1
Tortilla Bite Size White Corn	20 chips (1 oz)	150	0	1
Tortilla Nacho Cheese	15 chips (1 oz)	150	0	1

FOOD	PORTION	CALS	CHOL	FIBER
Tortilla Restaurant Style White	9 chips (1 oz)	140	0	2
Tostados White Corn	11 chips (1 oz)	140	0	2
Tostados Yellow	11 chips (1 oz)	140	0	1
Old El Paso				
Tortilla NACHIPS	9 chips (1 oz)	150	0	2
Tortilla White Corn	11 chips (1 oz)	140	0	1
Pita-Snax				
Cheddar Cheese	34 (1 oz)	110	0	tr
Chili & Lime	34 (1 oz)	120	0	tr
Cinnamon	34 (1 oz)	120	0	tr
Dill Ranch	34 (1 oz)	120	0	tr
Garlic	34 (1 oz)	120	0	tr
Lightly Salted	34 (1 oz)	110	0	tr
Planters				
Corn Chips	34 chips (1 oz)	170	0	2
Corn Chips King Size	17 chips (1 oz)	160	0	2
Corn Chips Snacks To Go	1 pkg (1.5 oz)	240	0	3
Pringles				
BBQ	14 chips (1 oz)	150	0	1
Cheese & Onion	14 chips (1 oz)	160	0	1
Cheez-ums	14 chips (1 oz)	150	0	1
Original	14 chips (1 oz)	160	0	1
Pizzalicious	14 chips (1 oz)	160	0	1
Ranch	14 chips (1 oz)	150	0	1
Salt & Vinegar	14 chips (1 oz)	160	0	1
Sour Cream & Onion	14 chips (1 oz)	160	0	1
Robert's American Gourmet				
Spirulina Spirals	1 oz	120	0	3
Ruffles				
Baked	10 (1 oz)	110	0	2
Baked Cheddar & Sour Cream	9 (1 oz)	120	0	2
Buffalo Style	11 chips (1 oz)	160	0	1
Cheddar & Sour Cream	11 chips (1 oz)	160	0	1
French Onion	11 (1 oz)	150	0	1
MC Masterpiece Mesquite BBQ	11 (1 oz)	150	0	1

FOOD	PORTION	CALS	CHOL	FIBER
Original	12 chips (1 oz)	150	0	1
Ranch	13 (1 oz)	150	0	1
Reduced Fat	16 (1 oz)	130	0	1
The Works	12 (1 oz)	160	0	1
Wow Cheddar & Sour Cream	15 (1 oz)	75	0	1
Wow Cheddar & Sour Cream	15 (1 oz)	75	0	1
Wow Original	17 (1 oz)	75	0	1
Santitas				
100% White Corn	6 (1 oz)	130	0	1
Restaurant Style Chips	7 (1 oz)	130	0	1
Restaurant Style Strips	10 (1 oz)	130	0	1
Skinny				
BBQ	1½ cups	90	0	1
Corn	1½ cups	90	0	1
Nacho Cheese	1½ cups	90	0	1
Sour Cream & Onion	1½ cups	90	0	1
Sticks Garden Veggie	1 oz	140	0	1
Sticks Island Lime Chili	1 oz	140	0	1
Sticks Maui Wowie	1 oz	140	0	1
Sticks Original Spud	1 oz	140	0	1
Snyder's Of Hanover				
BBQ Rib	1 oz	140	0	tr
Barbeque Corn	1.5 oz	230	0	2
Cheddar Bacon	1 oz	150	0	3
Corn Chips	1.5 oz	230	0	2
Grilled Steak & Onion	1 oz	140	0	4
Hot Buffalo	1 oz	150	0	4
Kosher Dill	1 oz	140	0	3
No Salt	1 oz	140	0	3
Potato	1 oz	140	0	3
Ripple	1 oz	140	0	4
Salt & Vinegar	1 oz	140	0	4
Sausage Pizza	1 oz	150	0	4
Sour Cream & Onion	1 oz	150	0	4
Tasty Veggie Potato Chips	1 oz	150	0	4
Tortilla Nacho	1 oz	140	0	1

FOOD	PORTION	CALS	CHOL	FIBER
Tortilla No Salt Yellow Corn	1 oz	140	0	1
Tortilla White Corn	1 oz	140	0	1
Tortilla Yellow Corn	1 oz	140	0	1
Tortilla Yellow Corn mini	1 oz	160	0	1
Soya King				
Soy Mongolian BBQ	23 chips (1 oz)	140	0	3
Soy Original	23 chips (1 oz)	140	0	3
Soy Sour Cream & Onion	23 chips (1 oz)	140	0	3
Soy Taco	23 chips (1 oz)	140	0	3
State Line				
Chips	1 pkg (0.5 oz)	80	0	tr
Sunchips				
French Onion	13 (1 oz)	140	0	2
Harvest Cheddar	13 (1 oz)	140	0	2
Original	14 (1 oz)	140	0	2
Terra Chips				
Sweet Potato	1 oz	140	0	1
Sweet Potato Spiced	1 oz	140	0	3
Taro Spiced	1 oz	130	0	2
Vegetable	1 oz	140	0	3
Torengos				
Chips	13 chips (1 oz)	140	0	1
Tostitos				
Baked Bite Size	20 (1 oz)	110	0	2
Baked Bite Size Salsa & Cream Cheese	16 (1 oz)	120	0	1
Baked Original	13 (1 oz)	110	3	1
Bite Size	15 (1 oz)	140	0	1
Crispy Rounds	13 (1 oz)	150	0	1
Nacho Style	6 (1 oz)	140	0	1
Restaurant Style	7 (1 oz)	140	0	1
Restaurant Style Hint Of Lime	6 (1 oz)	140	0	1
Santa Fe Gold	7 (1 oz)	140	0	1
Wow Original	6 (1 oz)	90	0	1
Tyson				
Tortilla Salted	13 (1 oz)	150	0	2

FOOD	PORTION	CALS	CHOL	FIBER
Tortilla Yellow Corn Salted	13 (1 oz)	150	0	2
Utz				
Baked Crisps	12 (1 oz)	110	0	2
Carolina Barbeque	20 (1 oz)	150	0	1
Cheddar & Sour Cream	20 (1 oz)	160	0	1
Corn Chips	24 (1 oz)	160	0	1
Corn Chips Barbecue	24 (1 oz)	160	0	1
Grandma	20 (1 oz)	140	5	1
Grandma BBQ	20 (1 oz)	140	5	1
Home Style Kettle	20 (1 oz)	140	0	1
Home Style Kettle BBQ	20 (1 oz)	140	0	1
Kettle Classics Crunchy	20 (1 oz)	150	0	1
Kettle Classics Crunchy Mesquite BBQ	20 (1 oz)	150	0	1
No Salt Added	20 (1 oz)	150	0	1
Onion & Garlic	20 (1 oz)	150	0	1
Potato	20 (1 oz)	150	0	1
Reduced Fat BBQ	22 (1 oz)	140	0	1
Reducted Fat Ripple	24 (1 oz)	140	0	1
Ripple	20 (1 oz)	150	0	1
Ripple Sour Cream & Onion	20 (1 oz)	160	0	1
Ripple Barbeque	20 (1 oz)	150	0	1
Salt'N Vinegar	20 (1 oz)	150	0	1
The Crab Chip	20 (1 oz)	150	0	1
Tortilla Black Bean & Salsa	13 (1 oz)	150	0	1
Tortilla Low Fat Baked	10 (1 oz)	120	0	2
Tortilla Nacho	13 (1 oz)	150	0	1
Tortilla Restaurant Style	6 (1 oz)	140	0	1
Tortilla Spicy Nacho	13 (1 oz)	150	0	1
Tortilla White Corn	12 (1 oz)	140	0	1
Wavy	20 chips (1 oz)	150	0	1
Yes! Fat Free	20 (1 oz)	75	0	1
Yes! Fat Free Barbeque	20 (1 oz)	75	0	1
Yes! Fat Free Ripple	20 (1 oz)	75	0	1
Wise				
Dipsy Doodles	1 pkg (1.5 oz)	240	0	1

FOOD	PORTION	CALS	CHOL	FIBER
CHITTERLINGS				
pork cooked	3 oz	258	122	0
CHIVES				
freeze-dried	1 tbsp	1	0	–
fresh chopped	1 tbsp	1	0	–
fresh chopped	1 tsp	0	0	–

CHOCOLATE (see also CANDY, COCOA, ICE CREAM TOPPINGS, MILK DRINKS)

FOOD	PORTION	CALS	CHOL	FIBER
BAKING				
baking	1 oz	145	0	–
grated unsweetened	1 cup (4.6 oz)	690	0	18
liquid unsweetened	1 oz	134	0	–
squares unsweetened	1 square (1 oz)	148	0	4
Baker's				
Bittersweet	½ square (0.5 oz)	70	0	1
German's Sweet	2 squares (0.5 oz)	60	0	tr
Semi-Sweet	½ square (0.5 oz)	70	0	1
Unsweetened	½ square (0.5 oz)	70	0	2
White	½ square (0.5 oz)	80	<5	0
Nestle				
Choco Bake	½ oz	80	0	2
Premier White Bar	½ oz	80	<5	0
Premier White Morsels	1 tbsp	80	0	0
Semi-Sweet Bar	½ oz	70	0	tr
Unsweetened Bar	½ oz	80	0	2
chips				
milk chocolate	1 cup (6 oz)	862	38	–
semisweet	1 cup (6 oz)	804	0	–
semisweet	60 pieces (1 oz)	136	0	–
Baker's				
Real Milk Chocolate	½ oz	70	0	0
Real Semi-Sweet	½ oz	60	0	1
Semi-Sweet	½ oz	70	0	0
Cloud Nine				
Double Dark Chocolate	13 pieces (0.5 oz)	80	5	0
Hershey				
Almond Joy Bits	1 tbsp (0.5 oz)	60	0	–
Chocolate & Peanut Butter Chips	1 tbsp (0.5 oz)	70	0	–
Holiday Baking Bits	1 tbsp (0.5 oz)	70	0	–

FOOD	PORTION	CALS	CHOL	FIBER
Milk Chocolate	1 tbsp (0.5 oz)	80	<5	–
Mini Kisses For Baking	11 pieces (0.5 oz)	80	<5	–
Mint Chocolate	1 tbsp (0.5 oz)	80	0	–
Premier White Milk Chips	1 tbsp (0.5 oz)	80	0	–
Raspberry Chips	1 tbsp (0.5 oz)	80	0	–
Semi-Sweet	1 tbsp (0.5 oz)	80	0	–
Semi-Sweet Mini	1 tbsp (0.5 oz)	80	0	–
Skor English Toffee Baking Bits	1 tbsp (0.5 oz)	70	10	–
M&M's				
Baking Bits Milk Chocolate	0.5 oz	70	5	0
Baking Bits Semi-Sweet	0.5 oz	70	0	1
Nestle				
Crunch Baking Pieces	1½ tbsp	80	0	0
Milk Chocolate Morsels	1 tbsp	70	<5	0
Mint Chocolate Morsels	1 tbsp	70	0	tr
Morsels Semi-Sweet	1 tbsp	70	0	tr
Semi-Sweet Mega Morsels	1 tbsp	70	0	tr
Semi-Sweet Mini Morsels	1 tbsp	70	0	tr
Sunspire				
Chocolate Sundrops	47 pieces (1.4 oz)	190	0	1
Dark Chocolate Grain Sweetened	13 pieces (0.5 oz)	70	0	1
Organic	13 pieces (0.5 oz)	70	0	0
Toll House				
Mint-Chocolate	2 tbsp (1.5 oz)	130	0	1
Semi-Sweet	2 tbsp (1.5 oz)	130	0	1
Tropical Source				
Espresso Roast Dairy Free	13 pieces (1.5 oz)	70	0	1
Semi-Sweet Dairy Free	13 pieces (1.5 oz)	80	5	0
MIX				
powder	2-3 heaping tsp	75	0	–
powder as prep w/ whole milk	9 oz	226	33	–

FOOD	PORTION	CALS	CHOL	FIBER
Quik				
Chocolate Powder	2 tbsp (0.8 oz)	90	0	1
Chocolate Powder No Sugar	2 tbsp (0.4 oz)	40	0	2

CHOCOLATE MILK (see MILK DRINKS)

CHOCOLATE SYRUP

syrup	1 cup	653	0	–
syrup	2 tbsp	82	0	–
syrup as prep w/ whole milk	9 oz	232	33	–
Ah!Laska				
Organic	2 tbsp	85	0	–
Estee				
Chocolate	2 tbsp	15	0	0
Hershey				
Chocolate Fudge	1 tbsp (0.7 oz)	70	<5	–
Chocolate Malt	2 tbsp (1.4 oz)	100	0	–
Lite	2 tbsp (1.2 oz)	50	0	–
Syrup	2 tbsp (1.4 oz)	100	0	–
Marzetti				
Syrup	2 tbsp	40	0	0
Quik				
Chocolate	2 tbsp (1.3 oz)	100	0	tr
Red Wing				
Syrup	2 tbsp (1.4 oz)	110	0	0
Toll House				
Mint Chocolate	2 tbsp (1.5 oz)	130	0	1
Semi-Sweet	2 tbsp (1.5 oz)	130	0	1

CHUTNEY

apple cranberry	1 tbsp	16	0	–
coconut	¼ cup	74	0	2
mango	1 tbsp	54	0	tr
tomato	1 tbsp	32	0	tr
Sonoma				
Dried Tomato	1 tbsp (0.7 g)	35	0	0
Wild Thyme Farms				
Apricot Cranberry Walnut	1 tbsp	15	0	–

FOOD	PORTION	CALS	CHOL	FIBER
Pineapple Peach Lime	1 tbsp	14	0	–
CILANTRO				
fresh	1 tsp (2 g)	tr	0	tr
fresh	1 cup (1.6 oz)	11	0	1
Watkins				
Dried	¼ tsp (0.5 oz)	0	0	0
CINNAMON				
ground	1 tsp	6	0	–
Watkins				
Ground	¼ tsp (0.5 g)	0	0	0
CISCO				
smoked	3 oz	151	27	–
smoked	1 oz	50	9	–
CLAMS				
CANNED				
meat only	1 cup	236	107	–
meat only	3 oz	126	57	–
Bumble Bee				
Baby	2 oz	50	40	0
Progresso				
Creamy Clam Sauce	½ cup (4.2 oz)	110	10	0
Minced	¼ cup (2.1 oz)	25	10	0
Red Clam Sauce	½ cup (4.4 oz)	60	10	1
White Clam Sauce	½ cup (4.4 oz)	150	20	0
FRESH				
cooked	3 oz	126	57	–
cooked	20 sm	133	60	–
raw	20 sm (6.3 oz)	133	60	–
raw	9 lg (6.3 oz)	133	60	–
raw	3 oz	63	29	–
TAKE-OUT				
breaded & fried	20 sm	379	115	–
CLOVES				
ground	1 tsp	7	0	–
COCOA				
hot cocoa	1 cup	218	33	–
powder unsweetened	1 tbsp (5 g)	11	0	2

FOOD	PORTION	CALS	CHOL	FIBER
powder unsweetened	1 cup (3 oz)	197	0	29
Ah!Laska				
Organic	2 tbsp	100	0	5
Organic Bakers Cocoa	1 tbsp	20	0	1
Carnation				
Hot Cocoa 70 Calorie	1 pkg (0.7 oz)	70	0	tr
Hot Cocoa Double Chocolate Meltdown	1 pkg (1.2 oz)	150	0	1
Hot Cocoa Fat Free Raspberry	1 pkg (0.3 oz)	30	0	1
Hot Cocoa Fat Free w/ Marshmallows	1 pkg (0.4 oz)	45	0	tr
Hot Cocoa Lactose Free	1 pkg (1 oz)	120	0	1
Hot Cocoa Marshmallow Blizzard	1 pkg (1.5 oz)	180	<5	tr
Hot Cocoa Milk Chocolate	3 tbsp (1 oz)	110	<5	tr
Hot Cocoa Rich Chocolate	3 tbsp (1 oz)	110	<5	tr
Hot Cocoa Rich Chocolate Fat Free	1 pkg (0.3 oz)	25	0	1
Hot Cocoa Rich Chocolate No Sugar Added	3 tbsp (0.5 oz)	50	<5	tr
Hot Cocoa Rich Chocolate w/ Marshmallows	3 tbsp (1 oz)	110	<5	tr
Hershey				
Cocoa	1 tbsp (5 g)	20	0	–
European Cocoa	1 tbsp (5 g)	20	0	–
Nestle				
Cocoa	1 tbsp	15	0	1
Hot Cocoa Rich Chocolate	1 pkg (1 oz)	110	0	tr
Hot Cocoa Rich w/ Marshmallows	1 pkg (1 oz)	110	0	tr
Swiss Miss				
Hot Cocoa And Cream	1 serv	153	6	1

FOOD	PORTION	CALS	CHOL	FIBER
Hot Cocoa Chocolate Sensation	1 serv	148	tr	1
Hot Cocoa Diet	1 serv	22	tr	1
Hot Cocoa Fat Free	1 serv	52	0	1
Hot Cocoa Fat Free Marshmallow Lovers	1 serv	65	0	1
Hot Cocoa Lite	1 serv	76	0	2
Hot Cocoa Marshmallow Lovers	1 serv	142	2	1
Hot Cocoa Milk Chocolate	1 serv	118	1	1
Hot Cocoa Milk Chocolate No Sugar Added	1 serv	55	1	1
Hot Cocoa Milk Chocolate w/ Marshmallows	1 serv	118	tr	1
Hot Cocoa Rich Chocolate	1 serv	110	1	1
Hot Cocoa White Chocolate	1 serv	109	1	tr
Hot Cocoa w/ Marshmallows No Sugar Added	1 serv	56	1	1
Premiere Hot Cocoa Almond Mocha	1 serv	144	1	1
Premiere Hot Cocoa English Toffee	1 serv	142	1	4
Premiere Hot Cocoa Raspberry Truffle	1 serv	144	1	1
Premiere Hot Cocoa Suisse Truffle	1 serv	142	1	1
Rich Hot Cocoa No Sugar Added	1 serv	54	1	1
Sidewalk Cafe Cappuccino	1 serv	119	1	1
Sidewalk Cafe Cinnamon	1 serv	126	1	1

FOOD	PORTION	CALS	CHOL	FIBER
Sidewalk Cafe French Vanilla	1 serv	121	1	tr
Sidewalk Cafe Mocha	1 serv	120	1	1
Weight Watchers				
Hot Cocoa Mix as prep	1 pkg	70	0	1

COCONUT

FOOD	PORTION	CALS	CHOL	FIBER
coconut water	1 tbsp	3	0	–
coconut water	1 cup	46	0	–
cream canned	1 cup	568	0	–
cream canned	1 tbsp	36	0	–
dried sweetened flaked	7 oz pkg	944	0	–
dried sweetened flaked	1 cup	351	0	–
dried sweetened flaked canned	1 cup	341	0	–
dried sweetened shredded	7 oz pkg	997	0	–
dried sweetened shredded	1 cup	466	0	–
dried toasted	1 oz	168	0	–
dried unsweetened	1 oz	187	0	–
fresh	1 piece (1.5 oz)	159	0	4
fresh shredded	1 cup	283	0	7
milk canned	1 tbsp	30	0	–
milk canned	1 cup	445	0	–
milk frozen	1 tbsp	30	0	–
milk frozen	1 cup	486	0	–
Baker's				
Angel Flake	1 tbsp (0.5 oz)	70	0	1
Angel Flake (canned)	2 tbsp (0.5 oz)	70	0	1
Premium Shred	2 tbsp (0.5 oz)	70	0	1

COD

FOOD	PORTION	CALS	CHOL	FIBER
atlantic canned	1 can (11 oz)	327	171	–
atlantic canned	3 oz	89	47	–
atlantic dried	3 oz	246	129	–
atlantic fresh cooked	1 fillet (6.3 oz)	189	99	–

FOOD	PORTION	CALS	CHOL	FIBER
atlantic fresh cooked	3 oz	89	47	—
atlantic fresh raw	3 oz	70	37	—
pacific fresh baked	3 oz	95	43	—
roe raw	1 oz	37	103	—
Van De Kamp's				
Lightly Breaded Fillets	1 (4 oz)	220	35	0

COFFEE *(see also* COFFEE BEVERAGES, COFFEE SUBSTITUTES*)*

FOOD	PORTION	CALS	CHOL	FIBER
INSTANT				
decaffeinated	1 rounded tsp	4	0	—
decaffeinated as prep	6 oz	4	0	—
regular as prep	6 oz	4	0	—
regular w/ chicory	1 rounded tsp	6	0	—
regular w/ chicory as prep	6 oz	6	0	—
Nescafe				
Decafe	1 tsp (2 g)	0	0	0
Decafe w/ Chicory	1 tsp (2 g)	0	0	0
French Vanilla	1 tsp (2 g)	5	0	0
French Vanilla Decaf	1 tsp (2 g)	5	0	0
Hazelnut	1 tsp (2 g)	5	0	0
Irish Creme	1 tsp (2 g)	5	0	0
Regular	1 tsp (2 g)	0	0	0
With Chicory	1 tsp (2 g)	5	0	0
REGULAR				
brewed	8 oz	2	0	—
Folgers				
Colombian Supreme	1 tbsp	16	0	—
Custom Roast	1 tbsp	16	0	—
Decaffeinated	1 tbsp	17	0	—
French Roast	1 tbsp	16	0	—
Gourmet Supreme	1 tbsp	16	0	—
Instant	1 tsp	8	0	—
Instant Decaffeinated	1 tsp	8	0	—
Singles	1 bag	21	0	—
Singles Decaffeinated	1 bag	21	0	—
Special Roast	1 tbsp	16	0	—
Vacuum Pack	1 tbsp	16	0	—
Maryland Club				
Ground	1 tbsp	16	0	—

FOOD	PORTION	CALS	CHOL	FIBER
Nescafe				
Cafe Mocha	1 can (10 oz)	140	10	1
Caffe Latte	1 can (10 oz)	130	15	1
Caffe Latte Decaffeinated	1 can (10 oz)	130	15	0
Espresso	1 tsp (2 g)	0	0	0
Espresso Cafe Latte	1 pkg (0.6 oz)	70	10	0
Espresso Cafe Mocha	1 pkg (1 oz)	110	10	1
Espresso Cappuccino	1 pkg (0.6 oz)	80	10	0
Espresso Roast	1 can (10 oz)	90	<5	0
French Vanilla	1 can (10 oz)	150	15	2
Hazelnut	1 can (10 oz)	130	15	0
Roasted Ground Decaffeinated as prep	1 cup (6 oz)	0	0	0
Roasted Ground as prep	1 cup (6 oz)	0	0	0
TAKE-OUT				
cafe au lait	1 cup (8 fl oz)	77	17	–
cafe brulot	1 cup (4.8 fl oz)	48	0	–
cappuccino	1 cup (8 fl oz)	77	17	–
coffee con leche	1 cup (8 fl oz)	77	17	–
espresso	1 cup (3 fl oz)	2	0	–
irish coffee	1 serv (9 fl oz)	107	12	–
latte w/ skim milk	13 oz	88	4	0
latte w/ whole milk	13 oz	152	33	0
mocha	1 mug (9.6 fl oz)	202	40	–
COFFEE BEVERAGES				
Arizona				
Iced Latte Supreme	8 oz	110	6	1
Iced Mocha Latte	8 oz	110	5	1
Chock full o'Nuts				
New York Cappuccino French Vanilla	1 pkg (0.9 oz)	90	0	0
New York Cappuccino Hazelnut	1 pkg (0.9 oz)	90	0	0
Coffee House USA				
All Flavors	1 bottle (9.5 oz)	100	15	tr
Gehl's				
Iced Cappuccino	1 can (11 oz)	190	13	0

FOOD	PORTION	CALS	CHOL	FIBER
General Foods				
Cappuccino Coolers French Vanilla as prep w/ 2% milk	1 serv	180	21	0
International Coffee Sugar Free Cafe Vienna as prep	1 serv (8 oz)	30	0	0
International Coffee Sugar Free Fat Free Suisse Mocha as prep	1 serv (8 oz)	25	0	tr
International Coffees Cafe Francais as prep	1 serv (8 oz)	60	0	0
International Coffees Cafe Vienna as prep	1 serv (8 oz)	70	0	tr
International Coffees Decaffeinated French Vanilla Cafe as prep	1 serv (8 oz)	60	0	0
International Coffees Decaffeinated Suisse Mocha as prep	1 serv (8 oz)	60	0	0
International Coffees French Vanilla Cafe as prep	1 serv (8 oz)	60	0	0
International Coffees Hazelnut Belgain Cafe as prep	1 serv (8 oz)	70	0	0
International Coffees Irish Creme Cafe as prep	1 serv (8 oz)	60	0	0
International Coffees Italian Cappuccino as prep	1 serv (8 oz)	60	0	0
International Coffees Kahlua Cafe as prep	1 serv (8 oz)	60	0	0

FOOD	PORTION	CALS	CHOL	FIBER
International Coffees Orange Cappuccino as prep	1 serv (8 oz)	70	0	tr
International Coffees Suisse Mocha as prep	1 serv (8 oz)	60	0	0
International Coffees Viennese Chocolate Cafe as prep	1 serv (8 oz)	50	0	0
International Coffees Sugar Free Fat Free Decaffeinated French Vanilla	1 serv (8 oz)	25	0	0
International Coffees Sugar Free Fat Free Decaffeinated Suisse Mocha	1 serv (8 oz)	25	0	tr
International Coffees Sugar Free Fat Free French Vanilla Cafe as prep	1 serv (8 oz)	25	0	0
Jakada				
Latte Mocha	1 bottle (10.5 oz)	180	10	0
Latte Vanilla	1 bottle (10.5 oz)	180	10	0
Maxwell House				
Cafe Cappuccino Amaretto as prep	1 serv (8 oz)	90	0	0
Cafe Cappuccino Decaffeinated Mocha as prep	1 serv (8 oz)	100	0	0
Cafe Cappuccino Decaffeinated Vanilla as prep	1 serv (8 oz)	90	0	0
Cafe Cappuccino Irish Cream as prep	1 serv (8 oz)	90	0	0
Cafe Cappuccino Mocha as prep	1 serv (8 oz)	100	0	0
Cafe Cappuccino Sugar Free Mocha as prep	1 serv (8 oz)	60	0	tr

FOOD	PORTION	CALS	CHOL	FIBER
Cafe Cappuccino Sugar Free Vanilla as prep	1 serv (8 oz)	60	0	0
Iced Cappuccino as prep w/ 2% milk	1 serv (8 oz)	180	20	tr
Silk				
Coffee Soylatte	1 bottle (11 oz)	220	0	0
Starbucks				
Frappuccino	1 bottle (9.5 fl oz)	190	12	0
COFFEE SUBSTITUTES				
powder	1 tsp	9	0	—
powder as prep	6 oz	9	0	—
powder as prep w/ milk	6 oz	121	25	—
Natural Touch				
Kaffree Roma	1 tsp (2 g)	10	0	0
Roma Cappuccino	3 tbsp (0.4 oz)	50	0	0
Pero				
Instant Grain Beverage	1 tsp (1.5 g)	5	0	—
Postum				
Instant Coffee Flavor as prep	1 serv (8 oz)	10	0	0
Instant as prep	1 serv (8 oz)	10	0	0
COFFEE WHITENERS				
liquid nondairy frzn	1 tbsp (0.5 oz)	20	0	—
powder nondairy	1 tsp	11	0	—
Hood				
Non Dairy	1 tbsp (0.5 oz)	20	0	0
International Delight				
Amaretto	1 tbsp (0.6 fl oz)	45	0	0
Cinnamon Hazelnut	1 tbsp (0.6 fl oz)	45	0	0
Irish Creme	1 tbsp (0.6 fl oz)	45	0	0
No Fat Amaretto	1 tbsp (0.5 fl oz)	30	0	0
No Fat French Vanilla Royale	1 tbsp (0.5 fl oz)	30	0	0
No Fat Hawaiian Macadamia	1 tbsp (0.5 fl oz)	30	0	0
No Fat Irish Creme	1 tbsp (0.5 fl oz)	30	0	0

FOOD	PORTION	CALS	CHOL	FIBER
Suisse Chocolate Mocha	1 tbsp (0.6 fl oz)	45	0	0
Mocha Mix				
Fat-Free	1 tbsp (0.5 fl oz)	10	0	0
Lite	1 tbsp (0.5 fl oz)	10	0	0
Lite	4 fl oz	80	0	0
Original	1 tbsp (0.5 fl oz)	20	0	0
Signature Flavors French Vanilla	1 tbsp (0.5 fl oz)	35	0	–
Signature Flavors Irish Creme	1 tbsp (0.5 fl oz)	35	0	–
Signature Flavors Kahlua	1 tbsp (0.5 fl oz)	35	0	–
Signature Flavors Mauna Loa Macadamia Nut	1 tbsp (0.5 fl oz)	35	0	–
N-Rich				
Coffee Creamer	1 tsp (2 g)	10	0	0
Silk				
Creamer	1 tbsp	15	0	0
Creamer French Vanilla	1 tbsp	20	0	0
Creamer Hazelnut	1 tbsp	15	0	0
COLESLAW				
Fresh Express				
Cole Slaw	1½ cups (3 oz)	25	0	2
TAKE-OUT				
coleslaw w/ dressing	½ cup	42	5	–
vinegar & oil coleslaw	3.5 oz	150	0	–
COLLARDS				
fresh cooked	½ cup	17	0	–
frzn chopped cooked	½ cup	31	0	–
raw chopped	½ cup	6	0	–
Birds Eye				
Chopped Greens frzn	1 cup	30	0	2
COOKIES				
MIX				
chocolate chip	1 (0.56 oz)	79	7	–
oatmeal	1 (0.6 oz)	74	7	tr
oatmeal raisin	1 (0.6 oz)	74	7	tr

FOOD	PORTION	CALS	CHOL	FIBER
Betty Crocker				
Chocolate Peanut Butter as prep	1 bar	180	18	−
Date Bar as prep	1 bar	150	0	1
Oatmeal as prep	2	150	12	1
GoldnBrown				
Fat Free	1 (1.1 oz)	120	0	0
READY-TO-EAT				
animal crackers	1 box (2.4 oz)	299	11	−
australian anzac biscuit	1	98	0	1
chocolate chip	1 box (1.9 oz)	233	12	−
chocolate chip low fat	1 (0.25 oz)	45	0	−
chocolate chip low sugar low sodium	1 (0.24 oz)	31	0	−
chocolate chip soft-type	1 (0.5 oz)	69	0	tr
chocolate wafer	1 (0.2 oz)	26	0	−
cream cheese	1 (1.1 oz)	141	25	tr
gingersnaps	1 (0.24 oz)	29	0	−
graham	1 squares (0.24 oz)	30	0	−
graham chocolate covered	1 (0.49 oz)	68	0	−
graham honey	1 (0.24 oz)	30	0	tr
hermits	1 (1 oz)	117	23	1
jumbles coconut	1 (1 oz)	121	26	1
ladyfingers	1 (0.38 oz)	40	40	−
macaroons	1 (0.8 oz)	97	0	−
madeleines	1 (0.8 oz)	86	46	tr
meringue	1 (0.3 oz)	20	0	0
molasses	1 (0.5 oz)	65	0	−
neapolitan tri-color cookie	1 (0.6 oz)	79	17	tr
oatmeal	1 (0.52 oz)	71	0	tr
oatmeal	1 (0.6 oz)	81	0	1
oatmeal raisin	1 (0.6 oz)	81	0	1
oatmeal raisin low sugar no sodium	1 (0.24 oz)	31	0	−
peanut butter sandwich	1 (0.5 oz)	67	0	−
peanut butter soft-type	1 (0.5 oz)	69	0	tr

FOOD	PORTION	CALS	CHOL	FIBER
pinenut cookies	1 (1.1 oz)	134	0	1
raisin soft-type	1 (0.5 oz)	60	0	–
reginette queen'a biscuit	1 (0.8 oz)	86	tr	tr
shortbread	1 (0.28 oz)	40	2	–
shortbread pecan	1 (0.49 oz)	79	5	tr
spritz	1 (0.4 oz)	42	6	tr
sugar	1 (0.52 oz)	72	8	–
sugar low sugar sodium free	1 (0.24 oz)	30	0	–
sugar wafers w/ creme filling	1 (0.12 oz)	18	0	–
sugar wafers w/ creme filling sugar free sodium free	1 (0.14 oz)	20	0	–
toll house original	1 (0.8 oz)	105	15	tr
vanilla sandwich	1 (0.35 oz)	48	0	tr
zeppole	1 (0.8 oz)	78	24	tr
Alternative Baking				
Vegan Chocolate Chip	1 serv (2.5 oz)	280	0	1
Vegan Expresso Chocolate Chip	1 serv (2 oz)	230	0	1
Vegan Lemon	1 serv (2.25 oz)	250	0	1
Vegan Oatmeal	1 serv (2.25 oz)	250	0	2
Vegan Peanut Butter	1 serv (2.25 oz)	270	0	1
Vegan Pumpkin	1 serv (2 oz)	200	0	1
Vegan Wheat Free Choco Cherry Chunk	1 serv (1.75 oz)	190	0	1
Vegan Wheat Free Hula Nut	1 serv (1.75 oz)	190	0	2
Vegan Wheat Free P-nut Fudge Fusion	1 serv (1.75 oz)	190	0	1
Vegan Wheat Free Snickerdoodle	1 serv (1.75 oz)	170	0	1
Amay's				
Chinese Style Almond	1 (0.5 oz)	80	4	0
Archway				
Alpine Fudge	1 (1.3 oz)	160	<5	tr
Carrot Cake	1 (1 oz)	130	5	0
Chocolate Chip	1 (0.9 oz)	120	5	0

FOOD	PORTION	CALS	CHOL	FIBER
Chocolate Chip Sugar Free	1 (0.8 oz)	110	0	0
Coconut Macaroon	2 (1.4 oz)	180	0	1
Devils Food Chocolate Drop Fat Free	1 (0.7 oz)	60	0	0
Dutch Cocoa	1 (0.9 oz)	100	0	0
Frosty Lemon	1 (0.9 oz)	100	0	0
Fruit & Honey Bar	1 (0.9 oz)	110	5	0
Fruit Bar Fat Free	1 (0.9 oz)	90	0	0
Ginger Snaps	5 (1 oz)	120	0	0
Homestyle Chocolate Chip	3 (1 oz)	130	5	1
Iced Spice	1 (1 oz)	120	0	0
Oatmeal	1 (0.9 oz)	100	5	0
Oatmeal Apple Filled	1 (0.9 oz)	90	<5	0
Oatmeal Pecan	1 (0.9 oz)	110	5	1
Oatmeal Raisin Bran	1 (0.9 oz)	100	0	1
Oatmeal Raspberry Fat Free	1 (1.1 oz)	100	0	1
Oatmeal Sugar Free	1 (0.8 oz)	110	0	0
Oatmeal Raisin	1 (0.9 oz)	100	0	1
Oatmeal Raisin Fat Free	1 (1.1 oz)	100	0	1
Old Dutch Apple	1 (0.9 oz)	110	5	0
Peanut Butter	1 (1 oz)	150	5	0
Peanut Butter Fudge	1 (1.3 oz)	220	<5	1
Peanut Butter Sugar Free	1 (0.8 oz)	110	0	0
Pecan Crunch	3 (1.2 oz)	180	5	0
Raspberry Filled	1 (0.8 oz)	90	5	0
Rocky Road	1 (0.8 oz)	110	10	0
Rocky Road Sugar Free	1 (0.8 oz)	100	0	tr
Shortbread Sugar Free	1 (0.8 oz)	110	0	0
Strawberry Filled	1 (0.8 oz)	90	0	0
Arnott's				
Raspberry Tartlets	2	100	0	tr
BP Gourmet				
Biscotti Fat Free Cinnamon Crunch	6 (1 oz)	110	0	0

FOOD	PORTION	CALS	CHOL	FIBER
Biscotti Fat Free Vanilla Crunch	4 (1 oz)	80	0	0
Chocolate Fudge Chip Sugar Free	5 (1 oz)	100	0	0
Dreams Chocolate	7 (1 oz)	120	0	0
Dreams Fat Free Chocolate Fudge	13 (1 oz)	100	0	0
Dreams Fat Free Vanilla	19 (1 oz)	100	0	0
Tangos Fat Free Chocolate Fudge Chip	4 (1 oz)	100	0	0
Bahlsen				
Afrika	8 (1.1 oz)	170	5	2
Butter Leaves	7 (1 oz)	140	15	tr
Choco Leibniz	2 (1 oz)	140	5	tr
Choco Star Dark Chocolate	3 (1.1 oz)	170	0	1
Choco Star Milk Chocolate	3 (1.1 oz)	180	<5	1
Chocolate Hearts	4 (1 oz)	160	5	1
Delice	6 (1 oz)	140	0	tr
Deloba	4 (0.9 oz)	130	0	tr
Hanover Waffelin	5 (1 oz)	160	0	0
Hit Chocolate Vanilla Filled	2 (1 oz)	140	0	tr
Hit Vanilla Chocolate Filled	2 (1 oz)	140	0	tr
Kipferl	4 (1 oz)	150	5	0
Leibniz	6 (1 oz)	130	10	1
Nuss Dessert	3 (1.1 oz)	180	10	tr
Probiers	6 (1.1 oz)	150	0	tr
Twingo	6 (1.1 oz)	170	0	1
Waffeletten	4 (1 oz)	160	<5	1
Baker's Harvest				
Cinnamon Grahams Low Fat	2 (0.9 oz)	110	0	1
Graham Low Fat	2 (0.9 oz)	110	0	1
Iced Oatmeal	1 (0.6 oz)	70	0	0
Pecan Shortbread	1 (0.5 oz)	80	<5	0

FOOD	PORTION	CALS	CHOL	FIBER
Bakery Wagon				
Cobbler Mixed Fruit Fat Free	1	70	0	1
Cobbler Raspberry Fat Free	1	70	0	1
Ginger Snaps	5	160	0	1
Honey Fruit Bars	1	100	5	1
Iced Molasses Mini	3	130	0	1
Oatmeal Raspberry Filled	1	100	0	1
Oatmeal Soft	1	100	0	1
Oatmeal Walnut Raisin	1	100	0	1
Vanilla Wafers Cholesterol Free	6	130	0	1
Barbara's Bakery				
Apple Cinnamon Bars Fat Free Whole Wheat	1 (0.7 oz)	60	0	2
Chocolate Chip	1 (0.6 oz)	80	5	1
Double Dutch Chocolate	1 (0.6 oz)	80	5	1
Fig Bars Fat Free Wheat Free	1 (0.7 oz)	60	0	1
Fig Bars Fat Free Whole Wheat	1 (0.7 oz)	60	0	2
Nature's Choice Coconut Almond	1 bar (1 oz)	120	0	1
Nature's Choice Expresso Bean	1 bar (1 oz)	120	0	1
Nature's Choice Lemon Yogurt	1 bar (1 oz)	120	0	1
Nature's Choice Roasted Peanut	1 bar (1 oz)	130	0	1
Old Fashioned Oatmeal	1 (0.6 oz)	70	5	1
Raspberry Bars Fat Free Wheat Free Raspberry	1 (0.7 oz)	60	0	1
Snackimals Chocolate Chip	8 (1 oz)	120	0	1

FOOD	PORTION	CALS	CHOL	FIBER
Snackimals Oatmeal Wheat Free	8 (1 oz)	120	0	2
Snackimals Vanilla	8 (1 oz	120	0	1
Traditional Blueberry Low Fat	1 (0.7 oz)	60	0	1
Traditional Fig Low Fat	1 (0.7 oz)	60	0	1
Traditional Shortbread	1 (0.6 oz)	80	10	1
Bed & Breakfast				
Cranberry Orange Oatmeal	1 (0.8 oz)	110	10	1
Enrobed Shortbread	2 (1.4 oz)	190	15	1
Fruit Center Key Lime	2 (1.1 oz)	140	<5	0
Fruit Center Raspberry	2 (1.1 oz)	140	<5	0
Beigel's				
Black & White	1 (1 oz)	100	0	0
Breaktime				
Chocolate Chip	1 (1 oz)	37	0	tr
Coconut	1 (0.3 oz)	35	0	tr
Ginger	1 (0.3 oz)	34	0	—
Oatmeal	1 (0.3 oz)	35	0	tr)
Sprinkles	1 (0.3 oz)	36	0	—
Brent & Sam's				
Chocolate Chip Pecan	2 (0.5 oz)	80	<5	0
Chocolate Chip Raspberry	2 (0.5 oz)	70	<5	0
Chocolate Chips	2 (0.5 oz)	70	<5	0
Key Lime White Chocolate	2 (0.5 oz)	70	<5	0
Oatmeal Raisin Pecan	2 (0.5 oz)	70	<5	1
Toffee Pecan	2 (0.5 oz)	80	5	0
White Chocolate Macadamia	2 (0.5 oz)	80	<5	0
Bud's Best				
Caco Creme	7 (1 oz)	140	0	2
Chocolate Chip	6 (1 oz)	140	0	1
French Vanilla	7 (1 oz)	150	0	2
Oatmeal	6 (1 oz)	130	0	tr

FOOD	PORTION	CALS	CHOL	FIBER
Cadbury				
Fingers	3	85	2	tr
Cafe				
Cinnamony Twists Chocolate Chip	1 (0.5 oz)	40	0	0
Sugar Free California Almond	4 (1 oz)	110	0	0
Twists Cinnamony	1 (0.3 oz)	40	0	0
Carr's				
Ginger Lemon Cremes	2 (1 oz)	140	<5	tr
Chortles				
Cookies	½ pkg. (1 oz)	125	0	1
Cookie Lover's				
Chocolate Chip	1 (0.8 oz)	90	10	0
Creme Supremes	2 (0.9 oz)	120	0	1
Creme Supremes Mint	2 (0.9 oz)	120	0	1
Grahams	2 (1 oz)	100	0	1
Grahams Cinnamon	2 (1 oz)	110	0	1
Peanut Butter	1 (0.8 oz)	100	15	0
Shortbread	1 (0.8 oz)	120	15	0
Dare				
Blueberry Cheesecake	1 (0.6 oz)	90	4	tr
Butter Shortbread	1 (0.5 oz)	63	6	tr
Butter Creme	1 (0.6 oz)	85	2	1
Carrot Cake	1 (0.6 oz)	92	3	tr
Chocolate Chip	1 (0.5 oz)	77	2	tr
Chocolate Fudge	1 (0.7 oz)	97	1	1
Cinnamon Danish	1 (0.4 oz)	47	2	tr
Coconut Creme	1 (0.7 oz)	99	1	tr
French Creme	1 (0.5 oz)	80	1	tr
Harvest From The Rain Forest	1 (0.5 oz)	70	2	tr
Key Lime Creme	1 (0.6 oz)	86	0	tr
Lemon Creme	1 (0.7 oz)	95	1	tr
Maple Leaf Creme	1 (0.6 oz)	83	0	tr
Maple Walnut Fudge	1 (0.7 oz)	99	0	tr
Milk Chocolate Fudge	1 (0.7 oz)	99	1	tr
Oatmeal Raisin	1 (0.4 oz)	59	4	tr
Social Tea	1 (0.2 oz)	26	0	tr

FOOD	PORTION	CALS	CHOL	FIBER
Sun Maid Raisin Oatmeal	1 (0.5 oz)	52	5	tr
De Beukelaer				
Pirouline	8 (1 oz)	130	15	tr
Pirouline Viennese Wafers	1 (1 oz)	150	30	tr
Delarce				
Chocosprits	1 (0.6 oz)	90	9	tr
Marquisettes	3 (0.9 oz)	140	5	1
Roules d'Or	4 (1 oz)	180	0	0
Dunkaroos				
Chocolate Chip Frosting w/ Chocolate	1 pkg (1 oz)	120	0	tr
Cinnamon Graham w/ Vanilla Frosting & Sprinkles	1 pkg (1 oz)	130	0	—
Cookies'n Creme	1 pkg (1 oz)	120	0	—
Dutch Mill				
Chocolate Chip	3 (1.1 oz)	160	0	1
Coconut Macaroons	3 (1 oz)	120	0	0
Oatmeal Raisin	3 (1 oz)	130	0	1
Eddyleon				
Jelly Graham Raspberry	1 (0.9 oz)	134	2	tr
Pudding Cookies	1 (0.9 oz)	134	2	tr
Entenmann's				
Little Bites Chocolate Chip	8 (1.8 oz)	240	10	1
Soft Baked Chocolate Chip	1 (0.7 oz)	100	10	tr
Soft Baked Double Chocolate	1 (0.7 oz)	100	10	tr
Soft Baked Milk Chocolate Chips	1 (0.7 oz)	100	10	tr
Soft Baked Original Chocolate Chip	3 (1 oz)	150	10	tr
Soft Baked White Chocolate Macadamia Nut	1 (0.7 oz)	100	10	tr

FOOD	PORTION	CALS	CHOL	FIBER
Soft Baked Light Chocolately Chip	2 (1 oz)	120	0	tr
Soft Baked Light Oatmeal Raisin	2 (1 oz)	100	0	1
Estee				
Chocolate Chip	4	150	0	tr
Coconut	4	140	0	tr
Fig Bars	2	100	0	3
Fudge	4	150	0	1
Lemon Thins	4	140	0	tr
Oatmeal Raisin	4	130	0	1
Sandwich Chocolate	3	160	0	1
Sandwich Original	3	160	0	1
Sandwich Peanut Butter	3	160	0	1
Sandwich Vanilla	3	160	0	tr
Shortbread	4	130	0	tr
Sugar Free Chocolate Chip	3	110	0	1
Sugar Free Chocolate Walnut	3	110	0	1
Sugar Free Coconut	3	110	0	1
Sugar Free Chocolate Grahams	2	110	0	3
Sugar Free Cinnamon Grahams	2	90	0	2
Sugar Free Old Fashion Grahams	2	90	0	2
Sugar Free Lemon	3	110	0	1
Sugar Free Wafer Banana Split	5	155	0	0
Sugar Free Wafer Chocolate	5	150	0	0
Sugar Free Wafer Chocolate Peanut Butter Caramel	5	150	0	0
Sugar Free Wafer Lemon Creme	5	150	0	0
Sugar Free Wafer Peanut Butter Creme	5	150	0	0

FOOD	PORTION	CALS	CHOL	FIBER
Sugar Free Wafer Vanilla	5	150	0	0
Sugar Free Wafer Vanilla Strawberry	5	150	0	0
Vanilla Thins	4	140	0	tr
Falcone's				
Sorrentini	1 (1 oz)	100	10	2
Famous Amos				
Butter Shortie	1 (0.5 oz)	80	10	tr
Chocolate Chip	4 (1 oz)	140	0	tr
Chocolate Chip & Pecan	4 (1 oz)	140	0	tr
Chocolate Chip Toffee	4 (1 oz)	130	0	0
Chocolate Creme Sandwich	3 (1.2 oz)	140	0	tr
Chunky Chocolate Chip	1 (0.5 oz)	70	0	0
Fat Free Fig Bar	2 (1 oz)	90	0	1
Fat Free Strawberry Fruit Bar	2 (1 oz)	90	0	0
Fig Bar	2 (1.1 oz)	120	0	tr
Oatmeal Chocolate Chip Walnut	4 (1 oz)	140	0	tr
Oatmeal Raisin	4 (1 oz)	130	5	tr
Oatmeal Macaroon Creme Sandwich	3 (1.2 oz)	160	0	1
Peanut Butter Chocolate Chunk	1 (0.5 oz)	80	0	tr
Peanut Butter Creme Sandwich	3 (1.2 oz)	160	0	1
Pecan Shortie	1 (0.5 oz)	80	0	tr
Vanilla Creme Sandwich	3 (1.2 oz)	160	0	0
Freihofer's				
Chocolate Chip	2 (0.9 oz)	120	10	1
Frookie				
Animal Frackers	14 (1 oz)	130	0	1
Chocolate Chip Wheat & Gluten Free	3 (1.1 oz)	140	0	1
Double Chocolate Wheat & Gluten Free	3 (1.1 oz)	130	0	1

FOOD	PORTION	CALS	CHOL	FIBER
Dream Creams Strawberry	4 (1 oz)	140	0	4
Dream Creams Vanilla	4 (1 oz)	140	0	4
Funky Monkeys Chocolate	16 (1 oz)	120	0	1
Funky Monkeys Vanilla	16 (1 oz)	120	0	1
Graham Cinnamon	2 (1 oz)	100	0	1
Graham Honey	2 (1 oz)	110	0	1
Lemon Wafers	8 (1 oz)	110	0	tr
Old Fashioned Ginger Snaps	8 (1 oz)	120	0	tr
Organic Chocolate Chip	3 (1.1 oz)	150	0	1
Organic Chip Double Chocolate	3 (1.1 oz)	140	0	1
Organic Iced Lemon	3 (1.3 oz)	165	0	0
Organic Oatmeal Raisin	3 (1.1 oz)	140	0	1
Peanut Butter Chunk Wheat & Gluten Free	3 (1.1 oz)	140	0	0
Sandwich Chocolate	2 (0.7 oz)	100	0	1
Sandwich Lemon	2 (0.7 oz)	100	0	1
Sandwich Peanut Butter	2 (0.7 oz)	100	0	1
Sandwich Vanilla	2 (0.7 oz)	100	0	1
Shortbread	5 (1 oz)	130	15	tr
Vanilla Wafers	8 (1 oz)	110	0	0
General Henry				
Fruit Bars Apple	1 (0.6 oz)	60	0	tr
Fruit Bars Blueberry	1 (0.6 oz)	60	0	tr
Fruit Bars Fig	1 (0.6 oz)	60	0	tr
Girl Scout				
Apple Cinnamon Reduced Fat	3 (1 oz)	120	0	tr
Do-si-dos	3 (1.2 oz)	170	0	1
Lemon Drops	3 (1.2 oz)	160	0	0
Samoas	2 (1 oz)	160	0	2
Striped Chocolate Chip	3 (1.2 oz)	180	0	tr
Tagalongs	2 (0.9 oz)	150	0	2
Thin Mints	4 (1 oz)	140	0	tr

FOOD	PORTION	CALS	CHOL	FIBER
Trefoils	5 (1.1 oz)	160	0	1
Godiva				
Biscotti Dipped In Milk Chocolate	1 (0.9 oz)	120	20	0
Golden Grahams Treats				
Chocolate Chunk	1 bar (0.8 oz)	90	0	0
Honey Graham	1 bar (0.8 oz)	90	0	0
King Size Chocolate Chunk	1 bar (1.6 oz)	190	0	1
King Size Honey Graham	1 bar (1.6 oz)	180	0	1
Gourmet				
Chocolate Chip	2 (1.1 oz)	160	15	1
Lemon Creme	2 (1.4 oz)	210	0	0
Oatmeal Raisin	2 (0.9 oz)	120	15	1
Peanut Butter Chip	2 (1 oz)	150	10	tr
Raspberry Center	2 (1.1 oz)	140	10	tr
Grandma's				
Chocolate Chip	1 (1.4 oz)	190	0	tr
Fudge Chocolate Chip	1 (1.4 oz)	170	<5	1
Fudge Sandwich	3	180	0	tr
Fudge Vanilla Sandwich	3	120	0	tr
Mini Fudge	9	150	0	1
Mini Peanut Butter	9	150	0	1
Mini Vanilla	9	150	<5	tr
Oatmeal Raisin	1 (1.4 oz)	160	5	1
Old Time Molasses	1 (1.4 oz)	160	<5	tr
Peanut Butter	1 (1.4 oz)	190	5	1
Peanut Butter Chocolate Chip	1 (1.4 oz)	190	<5	1
Peanut Butter Sandwich	5	210	0	1
Rich N'Chewy	1 pkg	270	10	1
Vanilla Sandwich	3	180	0	tr
Vanilla Sandwich	5	210	5	tr
Handi-Snack				
Cookie Jammers Cookies & Fruit Spread	1 pkg (1.3 oz)	130	0	tr

FOOD	PORTION	CALS	CHOL	FIBER
Health Valley				
Apple Spice	3	100	0	3
Apricot Delight	3	100	0	3
Biscotti Amaretto	2	120	0	3
Biscotti Chocolate	2	120	0	3
Biscotti Fruit & Nut	2	120	0	3
Cheesecake Bars Blueberry	1 bar	160	0	3
Cheesecake Bars Raspberry	1 bar	160	0	3
Cheesecake Bars Strawberry	1 bar	160	0	3
Chips Double Chocolate	3	100	0	4
Chips Old Fashioned	3	100	0	4
Chips Original	3	100	0	4
Chocolate Fudge Center	2	70	0	3
Chocolate Sandwich Bar Bavarian Creme	1 bar	150	0	3
Chocolate Sandwich Bars Caramel Creme	1 bar	150	0	3
Chocolate Sandwich Bars Vanilla Creme	1 bar	150	0	3
Date Delight	3	100	0	3
Graham Amaranth	8	100	0	3
Graham Oat Bran	8	100	0	3
Graham Original Amaranth	6	120	0	3
Hawaiian Fruit	3	100	0	3
Jumbo Apple Raisin	1	80	0	3
Jumbo Raisin Raisin	1	80	0	3
Jumbo Raspberry	1	80	0	3
Marshmallow Bars Chocolate Chip	1	90	0	1
Marshmallow Bars Old Fashioned	1	90	0	1

FOOD	PORTION	CALS	CHOL	FIBER
Marshmallow Bars Tropical Fruit	1	90	0	1
Oat Bran Fruit Bars Raisin Cinnamon	1 bar	160	0	2
Raisin Oatmeal	3	100	0	3
Raspberry Fruit Center	1	70	0	2
Tarts Baked Apple Cinnamon	1	150	0	3
Tarts California Strawberry	1	150	0	3
Tarts Chocolate Fudge	1	150	0	3
Tarts Cranberry Apple	1	150	0	3
Tarts Mountain Blueberry	1	150	0	3
Tarts Red Raspberry	1	150	0	3
Tarts Sweet Red Cherry	1	150	0	3
Hellema				
Almond	1 pkg (0.6 oz)	90	0	tr
Hershey				
Cripsy Rice Snacks Peanut Butter	1 (0.6 oz)	70	0	tr
Joseph's				
Almond Sugar Free	2 (0.9 oz)	100	0	0
Chocolate Chip Sugar Free	2 (0.9 oz)	100	0	0
Chocolate Walnut Sugar Free	2 (0.9 oz)	100	0	1
Coconut Sugar Free	2 (0.9 oz)	105	0	0
Lemon Sugar Free	2 (0.9 oz)	95	0	0
Oatmeal Raisin Sugar Free	2 (0.9 oz)	100	0	0
Peanut Butter Sugar Free	2 (0.9 oz)	95	0	1
Pecan Shortbread Sugar Free	2 (0.9 oz)	100	0	0
Keebler				
Animal Crackers Chocolate Chip	7 (1 oz)	130	0	0

FOOD	PORTION	CALS	CHOL	FIBER
Animal Crackers Ernie's	1 box	250	0	1
Animal Crackers Iced	6 (1.1 oz)	150	0	0
Animal Crackers Sprinkled	6 (1.1 oz)	150	0	0
Butter	5 (1.1 oz)	150	10	tr
Chips Deluxe	1 (0.5 oz)	80	0	0
Chips Deluxe Chocolate Lovers	1 (0.6 oz)	90	5	0
Chips Deluxe Coconut	1 (0.5 oz)	80	0	tr
Chips Deluxe Rainbow	1 (0.6 oz)	80	<5	tr
Chips Deluxe Soft 'n Chewy	1 (0.6 oz)	80	5	0
Chips Deluxe w/ Peanut Butter Cup	1 (0.6 oz)	90	0	0
Classic Collection Chocolate Fudge Creme	1 (0.6 oz)	80	0	0
Classic Collection French Vanilla Creme	1 (0.6 oz)	80	0	0
Cookie Stix Butter	5 (1.2 oz)	160	10	1
Cookie Stix Chocolate Chip	4 (0.9 oz)	130	5	tr
Cookie Stix Rainbow	5 (1.2 oz)	150	5	tr
Danish Wedding	4 (0.9 oz)	120	0	tr
Droxies	3 (1.1 oz)	140	0	tr
Droxies Reduced Fat	3 (1.1 oz)	140	0	1
E.L. Fudge Butter w/ Fudge Filling	2 (0.9 oz)	120	<5	tr
E.L. Fudge Fudge w/ Fudge Filling	2 (0.9 oz)	120	0	tr
E.L. Fudge w/ Peanut Butter Filling	2 (0.9 oz)	120	0	tr
Fudge Shoppe Deluxe Grahams	3 (1 oz)	140	0	tr
Fudge Shoppe Double Fudge 'n Caramel	2 (1 oz)	140	0	tr
Fudge Shoppe Fudge Sticks	3 (1 oz)	150	0	tr
Fudge Shoppe Fudge Sticks Peanut Butter	3 (1 oz)	150	0	tr

FOOD	PORTION	CALS	CHOL	FIBER
Fudge Shoppe Fudge Stripes	3 (1.1 oz)	160	0	tr
Fudge Shoppe Fudge Stripes Reduced Fat	3 (1 oz)	140	0	0
Fudge Shoppe Grasshoppers	4 (1 oz)	150	0	tr
Fudge Shoppe S'mores	3 (1.2 oz)	160	0	tr
Ginger Snaps	5 (1.1 oz)	150	0	0
Golden Fruit Cranberry	1 (0.7 oz)	80	0	tr
Golden Fruit Raisin	1 (0.7 oz)	80	0	tr
Graham Cinnamon Crisp	8 (1 oz)	140	0	1
Graham Cinnamon Crisp Low Fat	8 (1 oz)	110	0	1
Graham Honey	8 (1.1 oz)	150	0	1
Graham Honey Low Fat	8 (1.1 oz)	120	0	1
Graham Original	8 (1 oz)	130	0	tr
Lemon Coolers	5 (1 oz)	140	0	tr
Oatmeal Country Style	2 (0.8 oz)	120	0	tr
Sandies Almond Shortbread	1 (0.5 oz)	80	5	0
Sandies Pecan Shortbread	1 (0.5 oz)	80	<5	tr
Sandies Simply Shortbread	1 (0.5 oz)	80	10	0
Snack Size Chips Deluxe	1 pkg (2 oz)	300	5	tr
Snack Size Chips Deluxe Chocolate Lovers	1 pkg (2 oz)	280	20	1
Snack Size Mini Fudge Stripes	1 pkg (2 oz)	280	0	2
Snack Size Rainbow Chips Deluxe	1 pkg (2 oz)	290	5	1
Snack Size Sandies w/ Pecans	1 pkg (2 oz)	300	10	1
Snackin' Grahams Cinnamon	21 (1 oz)	130	0	1

FOOD	PORTION	CALS	CHOL	FIBER
Snackin' Grahams Honey	23 (1 oz)	130	0	tr
Soft Batch Chocolate Chip	1 (0.6 oz)	80	0	tr
Soft Batch Homestyle Chocolate Chunk	1 (0.9 oz)	130	0	1
Soft Batch Homestyle Double Chocolate	1 (0.9 oz)	130	0	1
Soft Batch Homestyle Oatmeal Raisin	1 (0.9 oz)	130	0	tr
Soft Batch Oatmeal Raisin	1 (0.5 oz)	70	0	tr
Sugar Wafers Creme	3 (0.9 oz)	130	0	tr
Sugar Wafers Lemon	3 (0.9 oz)	130	0	0
Sugar Wafers Peanut Butter	4 (1.1 oz)	170	0	1
Vanilla Wafers	8 (1.1 oz)	150	0	tr
Vanilla Wafers Reduced Fat	8 (1.1 oz)	130	0	tr
Vienna Fingers	2 (1 oz)	140	0	tr
Vienna Fingers Lemon	2 (1 oz)	140	0	0
Knott's Berry Farm				
Shortbread Apricot	3 (1 oz)	120	4	0
Shortbread Boysenberry	3 (1 oz)	120	4	0
Shortbread Raspberry	3 (1 oz)	120	4	0
LU				
Chocolatier	3 (1 oz)	150	0	1
Le Bastogne	2 (0.8 oz)	120	0	0
Le Dore	4 (1 oz)	140	<5	0
Le Fondant	4 (1.1 oz)	170	0	1
Le Palmier	4 (1.2 oz)	180	0	tr
Le Petit Beurre	4 (1.2 oz)	150	10	tr
Le Petit Ecolier Dark Chocolate	2 (0.9 oz)	130	<5	1
Le Petit Ecolier Hazelnut Milk Chocolate	2 (0.9 oz)	130	5	0

FOOD	PORTION	CALS	CHOL	FIBER
Le Petit Ecolier Milk Chocolate	2 (0.9 oz)	130	5	tr
Le Raisin Dore	4 (1.2 oz)	160	20	tr
Le Truffe Coconut	4 (1.2 oz)	190	0	1
Le Truffe Praline Chocolates	4 (1.2 oz)	170	0	2
Les Varietes	3 (0.9 oz)	140	5	6
Pim's Orange	2 (0.9 oz)	90	10	tr
Pim's Raspberry	2 (0.9 oz)	90	5	tr
La Choy				
Fortune	4 (1 oz)	112	0	1
Lance				
Apple Bar Fat Free	1 (1.75 oz)	160	0	tr
Apple Oatmeal Bar	1 (1.8 oz)	190	10	1
Big Town Banana	1 pkg (2 oz)	250	0	1
Big Town Chocolate	1 pkg (2 oz)	250	0	1
Big Town Vanilla	1 pkg (2 oz)	250	0	1
Choc-O-Lunch	1 pkg (1.5 oz)	200	0	1
Choc-O-Mint	1 pkg (1¼ oz)			
Coated Graham	1 pkg (1.3 oz)	190	0	1
Fig Bar	1 (1.75 oz)	180	0	2
Fudge Chocolate Chip	1 (2 oz)	130	<5	1
Gourmet Chocolate Chip	1 (2 oz)	130	5	1
Lem-O-Lunch	1 pkg (3.4 oz)	240	0	1
Lemon Nekot	1 pkg (1.5 oz)	210	0	1
Nut-O-Lunch	1 pkg (3.3 oz)	240	0	3
Oatmeal	1 (2 oz)	130	0	1
Oatmeal Creme	1 (2 oz)	240	0	1
Peanut Butter	1 (2 oz)	140	<5	1
Peanut Butter Creme Wafer	1 pkg (1.5 oz)	230	0	2
Van-O-Lunch	1 pkg (1.5 oz)	210	0	0
Larzaroni				
Arancelli	8 (1 oz)	160	8	tr
Calypso	3 (1 oz)	150	0	1
Limonelli	5 (1 oz)	140	5	2
Malaika	5 (1 oz)	158	17	1
Nanette	4 (1.2 oz)	170	<5	tr
Okla	3 (1 oz)	186	6	1

FOOD	PORTION	CALS	CHOL	FIBER
Oskar	10 (1 oz)	150	0	tr
Samba	5 (1 oz)	160	0	2
Velieri	3 (0.9 oz)	120	10	tr
Linden's				
Lemon	1 (1 oz)	120	10	—
Little Debbie				
Apple Flips	1 (1.2 oz)	150	5	tr
Caramel Bars	1 (1.2 oz)	160	0	0
Cherry Cordials	1 (1.3 oz)	170	0	tr
Coconut Rounds	1 (1.2 oz)	150	0	tr
Cookie Wreaths	1 (0.6 oz)	100	0	0
Easter Puffs	1 (1.2 oz)	140	0	0
Fig Bars	1 (1.5 oz)	150	0	1
Fudge Delights	1 (1.1 oz)	110	0	tr
Fudge Rounds	1 (1.2 oz)	140	0	tr
German Chocolate Ring	1 (1 oz)	140	0	1
Ginger	1 (0.7 oz)	90	5	0
Jelly Creme Pies	1 (1.2 oz)	160	0	0
Marshmallow Crispy Bar	1 (1.3 oz)	140	0	0
Marshmallow Supremes	1 (1.1 oz)	130	0	tr
Marshmallow Pie Banana	1 pkg (1.5 oz)	180	0	0
Marshmallow Pie Chocolate	1 (1.4 oz)	160	0	1
Nutty Bar	1 (2 oz)	310	0	1
Oatmeal Raisin	1 (1.3 oz)	160	0	tr
Oatmeal Creme Pie	1 (1.3 oz)	170	0	tr
Oatmeal Delights	1 (1.1 oz)	110	0	tr
Oatmeal Lights	1 (1.3 oz)	130	0	tr
Peanut Butter Bars	1 (1.9 oz)	270	0	1
Peanut Butter & Jelly Oatmeal Pie	1 (1.1 oz)	130	0	tr
Peanut Clusters	1 (1.4 oz)	190	0	tr
Pumpkin Delights	1 (1.2 oz)	150	5	0
Raisin Creme Pie	1 (1.2 oz)	140	0	0
Star Crunch	1 (1.1 oz)	140	0	0
Sugar Free Chocolate Chip	3 (1.1 oz)	140	0	tr

FOOD	PORTION	CALS	CHOL	FIBER
Sugar Free Oatmeal	6 (1.1 oz)	120	0	1
Yo-Yo's	1 (1.2 oz)	130	0	tr
M&M's				
Cookies & Milky Way	1 bar (1.2 oz)	180	0	1
Cookies & Milky Way	1 bar (1.20 oz)	180	0	1
Manischewitz				
Macaroons Chocolate	2 (0.9 oz)	90	0	4
Milk Lunch Brand				
New England Biscuits	4 (1.1 oz)	140	<5	1
MoonPie				
Chocolate	1 (2.75 oz)	330	0	0
Mini Banana	1 (1.2 oz)	152	0	0
Mini Chocolate	1 (1.2 oz)	152	0	0
Mini Vanilla	1 (1.2 oz)	152	0	0
Mother's				
Almond Shortbread	3	180	0	1
Checkerboard Wafers	8	150	0	1
Chocolate Chip	2	160	10	0
Chocolate Chip Angel	3	180	0	1
Chocolate Chip Parade	4	130	0	1
Circus Animals	6	140	0	0
Classic Assortments	2	140	0	1
Cocadas	5	150	5	2
Cookie Parade	4	140	0	2
Dinosaur Grrrahams	2	130	0	2
Double Fudge	2	180	0	2
English Tea	2	180	0	1
Flaky Flix Fudge	2	140	0	2
Flaky Flix Vanilla	2	140	0	1
Gaucho Peanut Butter	2	190	0	2
Iced Oatmeal	2	130	0	1
Iced Raisin	2	180	0	1
MLB Double Header Duplex	3	170	5	1
Macaroon	2	150	0	2
Marias	3	170	5	1
Oatmeal	2	110	0	1
Oatmeal Chocolate Chip	2	120	0	1

FOOD	PORTION	CALS	CHOL	FIBER
Oatmeal Raisin	5	150	5	2
Oatmeal Walnut Chocolate Chip	2	130	0	1
Rainbow Wafers	8	150	0	1
Striped Shortbread	3	170	0	1
Sugar	2	140	0	1
Taffy	2	180	0	2
Triplet Assortment	2	140	0	1
Vanilla Wafers	6	150	4	1
Wallops Boysenberry	1	80	0	1
Wallops Honey Crust Fig	1	80	0	0
Wallops Honey Graham Fig	1	80	0	1
Wallops Mixed Berry	1	80	0	1
Wallops Peach Apricot	1	80	0	1
Wallops Raspberry	1	80	0	1
Wallops Strawberry	1	80	0	1
Walnut Fudge	2	130	0	1
Zoo Pals	14	140	0	1
Mrs. Alison's				
Coconut Bar	2 (1 oz)	130	0	0
Creme Wafers	5 (1.1 oz)	170	0	tr
Duplex Sandwich	3 (1 oz)	130	0	0
Fudge Fingers	3 (1 oz)	160	0	0
Ginger Snaps	4 (1 oz)	130	<2	tr
Jelly Tops	5 (1 oz)	140	0	0
Lemon Creme	3 (1 oz)	130	0	0
Macaroons	2 (1 oz)	140	0	tr
Pecan	2 (1 oz)	140	0	0
Shortbread	5 (1 oz)	120	0	0
Vanilla Sandwich	3 (1 oz)	130	0	0
Murray's				
Sugar Free Double Fudge	3 (1.2 oz)	140	0	3
Sugar Free Ginger Snap	6 (1 oz)	110	0	tr
Sugar Free Peanut Butter	6 (1 oz)	130	0	1

FOOD	PORTION	CALS	CHOL	FIBER
Sugar Free Vanilla Sandwich Creme	3 (1 oz)	120	0	2
Sugar Free Vanilla Wafers	9 (1.1 oz)	120	0	tr
Nabisco				
Barnum's Animal Crackers	10 (1 oz)	130	0	tr
Barnum's Animal Crackers Chocolate	10 (1 oz)	130	0	1
Biscos Sugar Wafers	8 (1 oz)	140	0	0
Cafe Cremes Cappuccino	2 (1.1 oz)	160	0	0
Cafe Cremes Vanilla	2 (1.1 oz)	160	0	0
Cafe Cremes Vanilla Fudge	2 (1.1 oz)	200	0	tr
Cameo	2 (1 oz)	130	0	0
Chips Ahoy!	3 (1.1 oz)	160	0	1
Chips Ahoy! Chewy	3 (1.3 oz)	170	0	tr
Chips Ahoy! Chunky	1 (0.5 oz)	80	5	0
Chips Ahoy! Munch Size	6 (1.1 oz)	160	0	1
Chips Ahoy! Reduced Fat	3 (1.1 oz)	140	0	tr
Family Favorites Iced Oatmeal	1 (0.6 oz)	80	0	0
Family Favorites Oatmeal	1 (0.6 oz)	80	0	0
Family Favorites Vanilla Sandwich	3 (1.2 oz)	170	0	0
Famous Chocolate Wafers	5 (1.1 oz)	140	<5	1
Grahams	4 (1 oz)	120	0	1
Honey Maid Chocolate	8 (1 oz)	120	0	1
Honey Maid Cinnamon Grahams	8 (1 oz)	120	0	tr
Honey Maid Honey Grahams	8 (1 oz)	120	0	1
Honey Maid Low Fat Cinnamon Grahams	8 (1 oz)	110	0	tr

FOOD	PORTION	CALS	CHOL	FIBER
Honey Maid Low Fat Grahams	8 (1 oz)	110	0	tr
Honey Maid Oatmeal Crunch	8 (1 oz)	120	0	1
Lorna Doone	4 (1 oz)	140	5	tr
Mallomars	2 (0.9 oz)	120	0	tr
Marshmallow Twirls	1 (1 oz)	130	0	0
Mystic Mint	1 (0.5 oz)	90	0	0
Newton Fat Free Fig	2 (1 oz)	90	0	1
Newtons Fig	2 (1.1 oz)	110	0	1
Newtons Fat Free Apple	2 (1 oz)	90	0	tr
Newtons Fat Free Cobblers Apple Cinnamon	1 (0.8 oz)	70	0	tr
Newtons Fat Free Cobblers Peach Apricot	1 (0.8 oz)	70	0	0
Newtons Fat Free Cranberry	2 (1 oz)	100	0	tr
Newtons Fat Free Raspberry	2 (1 oz)	100	0	tr
Newtons Fat Free Strawberry	2 (1 oz)	90	0	0
Nilla Wafers	8 (1.1 oz)	140	<5	0
Nilla Wafers Chocolate Reduced Fat	8 (1 oz)	110	0	tr
Nilla Wafers Reduced Fat	8 (1 oz)	120	0	0
Nutter Butter Bites	10 (1 oz)	150	<5	tr
Nutter Butter Chocolate Peanut Butter Sandwich	2 (1 oz)	130	0	1
Nutter Butter Peanut Butter Sandwich	2 (1 oz)	130	<5	tr
Old Fashioned Ginger Snaps	4 (1 oz)	120	0	tr
Oreo	3 (1.2 oz)	160	0	1
Oreo Double Stuff	2 (1 oz)	140	0	tr

FOOD	PORTION	CALS	CHOL	FIBER
Oreo Reduced Fat	3 (1.1 oz)	130	0	1
Oreo Halloween	2 (1 oz)	140	0	tr
Pecanz	1 (0.5 oz)	90	<5	0
Pinwheels Chocolate Marshmallow	1 (1 oz)	130	0	tr
Rugrats Chocolate Frosted	8 (1.1 oz)	150	0	tr
Rugrats Vanilla Frosted	8 (1.1 oz)	150	0	tr
Social Tea	6 (1 oz)	120	5	tr
Sweet Crispers Chocolate	18 (1.1 oz)	130	0	1
Sweet Crispers Chocolate Chip	18 (1.1 oz)	130	0	tr
Teddy Grahams Chocolate	24 (1 oz)	130	0	1
Teddy Grahams Chocolately Chip	24 (1 oz)	130	0	tr
Teddy Grahams Cinnamon	24 (1 oz)	130	0	1
Teddy Grahams Honey	24 (1 oz)	130	0	tr
Nestle				
Flipz Crunchy Graham White Fudge Chocolate	8 (1 oz)	140	0	0
Newman's Own				
Fig Newman's Organic	2 (1.3 oz)	120	0	1
Nonni's				
Biscotti Cioccalati	1 (1 oz)	130	5	1
Biscotti Decadence	1 (1.1 oz)	130	5	1
Biscotti Original	1 (1 oz)	100	25	1
Biscotti Paradiso	1 (1.1 oz)	130	5	0
NutraBalance				
Fibre Oatmeal Raisin	1 (0.7 oz)	80	0	3
Protein Fortified	1 (2 oz)	260	10	2
ReNeph Spice	1 (2 oz)	210	0	0
Old Brussels				
Ginger Crisps	2 (0.9 oz)	140	0	2

FOOD	PORTION	CALS	CHOL	FIBER
Old London				
Coffee Toppers Chocolate Creme	3 (0.5 oz)	70	0	0
Coffee Toppers Vanilla Creme	3 (0.5 oz)	70	0	0
Olde World				
Pizzelle Almond	3 (1 oz)	90	45	0
Pizzelle Anise	3 (1 oz)	90	45	0
Pizzelle Chocolate	3 (1 oz)	100	45	0
Pizzelle Lemon	3 (1 oz)	90	45	0
Pizzelle Vanilla	3 (1 oz)	90	45	0
Otis Spunkmeyer				
Butter Sugar	1 med (1.3 oz)	160	15	tr
Butter Sugar	1 (2 oz)	250	20	1
Carnival	1 med (1.3 oz)	170	10	0
Chocolate Chip	1 bite size (0.75 oz)	100	5	0
Chocolate Chip	1 med (1.3 oz)	170	10	0
Chocolate Chip	1 (2 oz)	250	15	tr
Chocolate Chip Pecan	1 med (1.3 oz)	170	10	tr
Chocolate Chip Walnut	1 med (1.3 oz)	180	10	tr
Chocolate Chip Walnut	1 bite size (0.75 oz)	100	5	0
Chocolate Chip Walnut	1 (2 oz)	270	15	tr
Double Chocolate Chip	1 med (1.3 oz)	180	10	tr
Double Chocolate Chip	1 bite size (0.75 oz)	100	5	1
Oatmeal Raisin	1 med (1.3 oz)	160	10	1
Oatmeal Raisin	1 bite size (0.75 oz)	90	5	tr
Otis Express Chocolate Chunk	1 (2 oz)	280	20	1
Otis Express Double Chocolate Chip	1 (2 oz)	270	15	1
Otis Express Oatmeal Raisin	1 (2 oz)	240	15	2
Otis Express Peanut Butter	1 (2 oz)	270	15	2
Peanut Butter	1 med (1.3 oz)	180	10	1
Pinnacle Checkpoint Chocolate Almond Coconut	1 (2.4 oz)	320	25	2

FOOD	PORTION	CALS	CHOL	FIBER
Pinnacle Mach One Mocha Chocolate Chunk	1 (2.4 oz)	300	20	1
Pinnacle Passport Peanut Butter Chocolate Chunk	1 (2.4 oz)	300	25	1
Pinnacle Ripcord Rocky Road	1 (2.4 oz)	310	15	2
Pinnacle Takeoff Triple Chocolate	1 (2.4 oz)	300	20	tr
Pinnacle Transatlantic Turtle	1 (2.4 oz)	310	20	2
Travel Lite Low Fat Apple Cinnamon	1 (1.3 oz)	130	0	tr
Travel Lite Low Fat Chocolate Chip	1 (1.3 oz)	130	0	tr
Travel Lite Low Fats Ginger Spice	1 (1.3 oz)	130	0	tr
Travel Lite Low Fat Oatmeal Rum Raisin	1 (1.3 oz)	130	0	1
White Chocolate Macadamia Nut	1 med (1.3 oz)	180	10	tr
White Chocolate Macadamia Nut	1 (2 oz)	280	20	tr
Pally				
Butter	5 (1 oz)	140	1	1
Carnival	5 (1 oz)	130	0	1
Cinnamon Biscuit	5 (1 oz)	130	0	0
Mariel Biscuit	6 (1 oz)	150	0	1
Tea Biscuits	5 (1 oz)	150	0	1
Pamela's				
Pecan Shortbread Rice Flour	1 (0.8 oz)	130	20	tr
Parmalat				
Grisbi Lemon	1 (0.6 oz)	90	5	1
Grisbi Lemon	1 (0.6 oz)	90	<5	1
Peek Freans				
Arrowroot	4 (1.2 oz)	150	0	1
Assorted Creme	1 (1 oz)	130	<5	0
Dream Puffs	2 (0.9 oz)	110	0	0

FOOD	PORTION	CALS	CHOL	FIBER
Fruit Creme	2 (0.9 oz)	130	0	0
Ginger Crisp	4 (1.2 oz)	150	0	tr
Nice	4 (1.2 oz)	160	0	1
Petit Beret Creme Caramel	2 (0.8 oz)	110	0	tr
Petit Beret Fudge Truffle	2 (0.8 oz)	110	0	tr
Petit Beurre	4 (1 oz)	130	tr	tr
Rich Tea	4 (1.2 oz)	160	0	tr
Shortcake	2 (0.9 oz)	140	20	0
Traditional Oatmeal	1 (0.7 oz)	90	0	tr
Tropical Cremes Calypso Lime	2 (0.9 oz)	130	0	0
Pepperidge Farm				
Biscotti Almond	1 (0.7 oz)	90	5	0
Biscotti Chocolate Hazelnut	1 (0.7 oz)	90	15	2
Biscotti Cranberry Pistachio	1 (0.7 oz)	90	5	0
Bordeaux	4	130	10	tr
Brussels	3	150	5	1
Chantilly Raspberry	2 (1 oz)	120	0	tr
Chessman	3	120	20	tr
Chocoate Chunk Soft Baked Double Chocolate	1 (0.9 oz)	130	0	1
Chocolate Chunk Chesapeake	1 (0.7 oz)	140	10	0
Chocolate Chunk Minis Nantauket	1 pkg (1.75 oz)	260	10	0
Chocolate Chunk Minis Sausalito	4 (1 oz)	160	10	0
Chocolate Chunk Montauk	1 (0.9 oz)	130	10	0
Chocolate Chunk Nantucket	1 (0.9 oz)	140	10	0
Chocolate Chunk Sausalito	1 (0.7 oz)	140	10	0
Chocolate Chunk Soft Baked	1	130	10	0

FOOD	PORTION	CALS	CHOL	FIBER
Chocolate Chunk Soft Baked Milk Chocolate Macademia	1	130	10	0
Chocolate Chunk Soft Baked Reduced Fat	1	110	15	tr
Chocolate Chunk Soft Baked White Chocolate Pecan	1	120	5	1
Chocolate Chunk Tahoe	1 (0.9 oz)	130	10	0
Fruitful Strawberry Cup	3	140	10	tr
Geneva	3	160	0	1
Ginger Man	4 (1 oz)	130	10	tr
Goldfish Grahams Cinnamon	1 pkg (1.75 oz)	240	5	2
Lemon Nut Crunch	3	170	15	2
Lido	1	90	<5	0
Milano Endless Chocolate	3	180	<5	1
Milano Milk Chocolate	3	170	10	tr
Milano Double Chocolate	2 (0.7 oz)	140	10	tr
Milano Mint	2	130	<5	1
Pirouettes Chocolate Laced	5 (1.1 oz)	180	5	tr
Pirouettes Traditional	5 (1.2 oz)	170	5	0
Shortbread	2	140	10	tr
Soft Baked Oatmeal Raisin	1 (0.9 oz)	130	10	0
Soft Baked Reduced Fat Oatmeal Raisin	1 (0.9 oz)	100	10	tr
Spritzers Cool Key Lime	6 (1.1 oz)	140	<5	0
Spritzers Ripe Red Raspberry	5 (1.1 oz)	140	<5	0
Spritzers Zesty Lemon	5 (1.1 oz)	140	<5	0
Verona Strawberry	3 (1.1 oz)	140	10	tr

FOOD	PORTION	CALS	CHOL	FIBER
Ralston				
Cinnamon Grahams Low Fat	2 (0.9 oz)	110	0	1
Real Torino				
Lady Fingers	3 (1 oz)	110	5	0
Reko				
Pizzelle Maple	5 (1 oz)	150	15	0
Pizzelle Vanilla	1 (6 g)	30	3	0
Royal				
Apple Bars	1 (1.1 oz)	100	0	1
Apple Cake	1 (1.1 oz)	110	0	1
Brownie Rounds	1 (1.1 oz)	130	0	0
Chocolate Chip	1 (1.1 oz)	140	0	1
Devilfood	1 (1 oz)	110	0	0
Fig Bars	1 (1.1 oz)	100	0	1
Oatmeal	1 (1.1 oz)	130	0	1
Raisin	1 (1 oz)	110	0	0
Strawberry Bars	1 (1.1 oz)	100	0	1
Salerno				
Mini Butter	25 (1 oz)	180	15	tr
Mini Dinosaur Chocolate Graham	16 (1.1 oz)	140	0	1
Scotter Pie	1 (1.2 oz)	140	0	0
Santa Fe Farms				
Chocolate Chocolate Chip Fat Free	2 (1 oz)	60	0	3
Chocolate Mint Fat Free	2 (1 oz)	60	0	3
Ginger Fat Free	2 (1 oz)	70	0	2
Sargento				
MooTown Snackers Honey Graham Sticks & Vanilla Creme w/ Sprinkles	1 pkg (1 oz)	140	0	0
MooTown Snackers Vanilla Sticks & Chocolate Fudge Creme	1 pkg (1 oz)	130	0	tr
Savion				
Chocolate Biscuits	5 (1 oz)	120	0	0
Tea Biscuits	5 (1 oz)	120	0	0

FOOD	PORTION	CALS	CHOL	FIBER
Tea Biscuits Vanilla	5 (1 oz)	120	0	0
Scotto's				
Biscotti Fat Free French Vanilla	4 (1 oz)	80	0	0
Season				
Hamantashen Poppy	1 (1 oz)	150	7	1
Hamantashen Apricot	1 (1 oz)	150	7	1
Simple Pleasures				
Almond	1 (0.3 oz)	37	0	tr
Cinnamon Snaps	1 (0.2 oz)	31	0	tr
Digestive	1 (0.3 oz)	46	0	tr
Encore Tea Cookie	1 (0.2 oz)	29	0	tr
Lemon Social Tea	1 (0.2 oz)	29	0	tr
Oatmeal	1 (0.5 oz)	74	0	1
Spice Snaps	1 (0.3 oz)	34	0	tr
Sugar	1 (0.4 oz)	45	3	tr
SnackWell's				
Bite Size Chocolate Chip	13 (1 oz)	130	0	tr
Bite Size Double Chocolate Chip	13 (1 oz)	130	0	1
Bite Size Peanut Butter	13 (1 oz)	120	0	tr
Caramel Delights	1 (0.6 oz)	70	0	0
Chocolate Sandwich	2 (0.8 oz)	110	0	tr
Creme Sandwich	2 (0.9 oz)	105	0	tr
Fat Free Devil's Food	1 (0.5 oz)	50	0	0
Golden Devil's Food	1 (0.5 oz)	50	0	0
Mint Creme	2 (0.9 oz)	110	0	tr
Oatmeal Raisin	2 (0.9 oz)	110	<5	tr
Stella D'Oro				
Almond Toast Mandel	2 (1 oz)	110	30	1
Angel Wings	2 (0.9 oz)	140	<5	tr
Angelica	1 (0.8 oz)	100	15	0
Anginetti	4 (1.1 oz)	140	40	tr
Anisette Sponge	2 (0.9 oz)	90	40	tr
Anisette Toast	3 (1.2 oz)	130	35	tr
Biscotti Almond	1 (0.8 oz)	100	10	tr
Biscotti Chocolate Almond	1 (0.8 oz)	90	10	1

FOOD	PORTION	CALS	CHOL	FIBER
Biscotti Chocolate Chunk	1 (0.8 oz)	90	10	0
Biscotti Hazelnut	1 (0.8 oz)	100	10	0
Biscottini Cashews	1 (0.7 oz)	110	5	0
Breakfast Treats	1 (0.8 oz)	100	10	tr
Breakfast Treats Chocolate	1 (0.8 oz)	100	10	tr
Breakfast Treats Viennese Cinnamon	1 (0.8 oz)	100	10	0
Chinese Dessert Cookies	1 (1.2 oz)	170	5	tr
Chocolate Castelets	2 (1 oz)	130	<5	1
Egg Jumbo	2 (0.8 oz)	90	30	tr
Fruit Slices Fat Free	1 (0.6 oz)	50	0	tr
Holiday Rings & Stars	1	47	0	–
Holiday Trinkets	1	40	tr	–
Hostess Assortment	1	40	tr	–
Kichel Low Sodium	21 (1 oz)	150	80	0
Lady Stella Assortment	3 (1 oz)	130	5	0
Margherite Chocolate	2 (1.1 oz)	140	10	1
Margherite Vanilla	2 (1.1 oz)	140	15	tr
Peach Apricot Pastry Sodium Free	1	80	<5	–
Prune Pastry Dietetic	1	90	<5	–
Roman Egg Biscuits	1 (1.2 oz)	140	20	1
Sesame Regina	3 (1.1 oz)	150	10	1
Spice Drops	1	40	tr	–
Swiss Fudge	2 (0.9 oz)	130	5	0
Stieffenhofer				
Choco Minis	4 (1 oz)	160	15	1
Snaky	3 (1 oz)	160	0	0
Streit's				
Wafers	3 (1 oz)	160	0	1
Suissette				
Swiss Chocolate Hearts	4 (1 oz)	170	5	–
Swiss Delight	4 (1 oz)	160	5	–
Swiss Praline	4 (1 oz)	150	15	1
Sunshine				
All American Butter	5 (1.1 oz)	140	<5	tr

FOOD	PORTION	CALS	CHOL	FIBER
All American Lemon Coolers	5 (1 oz)	140	0	tr
All American Mini Chip-A-Roos	5 (1.1 oz)	160	0	1
Animal Crackers	14 (1.1 oz)	140	0	tr
Ginger Snaps	7 (1 oz)	130	0	tr
Golden Fruit Cranberry	1 (0.7 oz)	80	0	tr
Golden Fruit Raisin	1 (0.7 oz)	80	0	tr
Hydrox	3 (1.1 oz)	150	0	1
Hydrox Reduced Fat	3 (1.1 oz)	140	0	1
Oatmeal Country Style	2 (0.8 oz)	120	0	tr
Sugar Wafers Peanut Butter Creme	4 (1.1 oz)	170	0	1
Sugar Wafers Vanilla Creme	3 (0.9 oz)	130	0	tr
Vanilla Wafers	7 (1.1 oz)	150	3	tr
Vienna Fingers	2 (1 oz)	140	0	tr
Vienna Fingers Lemon	2 (1 oz)	140	0	0
Vienna Fingers Reduced Fat	2 (1 oz)	130	0	tr
Sweet'N Low				
Sugar Free Amaretto Biscotti	4 (1 oz)	120	10	tr
Sugar Free Chocolate Chip	4 (1 oz)	135	10	tr
Sugar Free Cinnamon Graham	7 (1 oz)	120	15	tr
Sugar Free Morning Crunch Bars	2 (1 oz)	120	10	tr
Sugar Free Vanilla Wafers	7 (1 oz)	120	15	tr
Sweetzels				
Chocolate Chip	7 (1 oz)	160	5	0
Ginger Snaps	4 (1.2 oz)	140	0	tr
Vanilla Wafers	7 (1.1 oz)	137	0	0
Tastykake				
Chocolate Chip	1 (1.4 oz)	180	10	1
Chocolate Chip Bar	1 (2 oz)	270	10	tr
Chocolate Fudge Iced	1 (1.4 oz)	170	55	1

FOOD	PORTION	CALS	CHOL	FIBER
Fudge Bar	1 (2 oz)	250	5	1
Lemon Bar	1 (2 oz)	260	5	1
Oatmeal Raisin Bar	1 (2 oz)	260	15	2
Oatmeal Raisin Boxed	3 (0.4 oz)	130	5	tr
Oatmeal Raisin Iced	1 (1.4 oz)	170	25	1
Strawberry Bar	1 (2 oz)	260	5	1
Sugar Boxed	3 (0.4 oz)	120	10	0
The Source				
Barry's Raspberry Palmiers	1 (0.7 oz)	80	0	0
Tom's				
Animal Crackers	½ pkg (1 oz)	120	0	tr
Big Cookie Chocolate Chip	1 pkg (2.75 oz)	340	0	1
Big Cookie Peanut Butter Chocolate Chip	1 pkg (2 oz)	280	0	1
Chocolate Chip	1 pkg (2 oz)	280	0	1
Confetti Chip	1 pkg (2 oz)	300	0	tr
Fat Free Apple Bar	1 pkg (1.75 oz)	160	0	1
Fat Free Fig Bar	1 pkg (1.75 oz)	160	0	2
Vanilla Wafers	½ pkg (1 oz)	130	0	tr
Tree Of Life				
Fat Free Almond Butter	1 (0.8 oz)	60	0	1
Fat Free Carrot Cake	1 (0.8 oz)	60	0	1
Fat Free Devil's Food Chocolate	1 (0.8 oz)	70	0	1
Fat Free Oatmeal Raisin	1 (0.8 oz)	70	0	1
Fruit Bars Fat Free Fig	1 (0.8 oz)	70	0	2
Fruit Bars Fat Free Peach Apricot	1 (0.8 oz)	70	0	1
Fruit Bars Fat Free Wildberry	1 (0.8 oz)	70	0	2
Monster Carob Chip	1 (4.7 oz)	700	10	5
Monster Granola	1 (4.7 oz)	700	10	5
Monster Macaroon	1 (4.7 oz)	750	10	5
Monster Peanut Butter	1 (4.7 oz)	700	20	5

FOOD	PORTION	CALS	CHOL	FIBER
Monster Fat Free Carrot Cake	1 cookie (3.8 oz)	240	0	4
Monster Fat Free Devil's Food Chocolate	1 cookie (3.8 oz)	320	0	8
Monster Fat Free Gingerbread	1 cookie (3.8 oz)	320	0	8
Monster Fat Free Maple Pecan	1 cookie (3.8 oz)	360	0	8
Oatmeal	1 (0.8 oz)	100	15	0
Sandwich Royal Vanilla	2 (0.9 oz)	120	0	1
Wheat Free Carob	1 (0.8 oz)	100	0	6
Wheat Free Maple Walnut	1 (0.8 oz)	100	0	6
Wheat Free Oatmeal	1 (0.8 oz)	90	0	1
Wheat Free Peanut Butter	1 (0.8 oz)	109	0	1
Twix				
Bars Chocolate Caramel	1 (0.9 oz)	140	0	0
Voortman				
Almonette	2 (1 oz)	150	0	tr
Chocolate Chip	1 (0.7 oz)	100	0	0
Chocolate Wafers Sugar Free	3 (1 oz)	160	0	0
Coconut Delight	1 (0.6 oz)	90	0	0
Peanut Delight	1 (0.9 oz)	130	<5	tr
Strawberry Wafers Sugar Free	3 (1 oz)	160	0	0
Sugar	1 (0.6 oz)	80	0	0
Turnovers Blueberry	1 (0.9 oz)	100	<5	0
Turnovers Cherry	1 (0.9 oz)	100	<5	0
Turnovers Strawberry	1 (0.9 oz)	100	<5	0
Vanilla Wafers Sugar Free	3 (1 oz)	160	0	0
Windmill	1 (0.7 oz)	90	0	0
Walkers				
Shortbread Triangles	2 (0.7 oz)	100	15	0
Weight Watchers				
Apple Raisin Bar	1 (0.75 oz)	70	0	2
Chocolate Chip	2 (1.06 oz)	140	0	1

FOOD	PORTION	CALS	CHOL	FIBER
Chocolate Sandwich	2 (1.06)	140	0	1
Fruit Filled Fig	1 (0.7 oz)	70	0	0
Fruit Filled Raspberry	1 (0.7 oz)	70	0	0
Oatmeal Raisin	2 (1.06 oz)	120	0	1
Vanilla Sandwich	2 (1.06 oz)	140	0	1
White Eagle Bakery				
Chruscik	2 (1 oz)	140	45	0
REFRIGERATED				
chocolate chip	1 (0.42 oz)	59	3	—
chocolate chip unbaked	1 oz	126	7	—
oatmeal	1 (0.4 oz)	56	3	—
oatmeal raisin	1 (0.4 oz)	56	3	—
peanut butter	1 (0.4 oz)	60	4	—
peanut butter dough	1 oz	130	8	—
sugar	1 (0.42 oz)	58	4	—
sugar dough	1 oz	124	8	—
Pillsbury				
Bunny	2	130	<5	0
Chocolate Chip	1 (1 oz)	130	<5	tr
Chocolate Chip Reduced Fat	1 (1 oz)	110	<5	tr
Chocolate Chip w/ Walnuts	1 (1 oz)	140	<5	tr
Chocolate Chunk	1 (1 oz)	130	<5	tr
Christmas Tree	2	130	<5	0
Double Chocolate	1 (1 oz)	130	<5	tr
Flag	2	130	<5	0
Frosty	2	130	<5	0
M&M's	1 (1 oz)	130	<5	tr
Oatmeal Chocolate Chip	1 (1 oz)	120	<5	tr
One Step Pan Chocolate Chip	⅛ pan (1 oz)	130	<5	tr
One Step Pan M&M's	⅛ pan (1 oz)	130	<5	tr
Peanut Butter	1 (1 oz)	120	<5	tr
Pumpkin	2	130	<5	0
Reeses	1 (1 oz)	130	<5	tr
Shamrock	2	130	<5	0
Sugar	2	130	<5	0
Sugar Holiday Red & Green	2	130	<5	0

FOOD	PORTION	CALS	CHOL	FIBER
Valentine	2	130	<5	0
White Chocolate Chunk	1 (1 oz)	130	<5	0
TAKE-OUT				
biscotti with nuts chocolate dipped	1 (1.3 oz)	117	18	1
black & white	1 lg (3 oz)	302	58	1
finikia	1 (1.2 oz)	171	27	1
koulourakia butter cookie twist	1 (0.9 oz)	113	32	tr

CORIANDER

FOOD	PORTION	CALS	CHOL	FIBER
leaf dried	1 tsp	2	0	—
leaf fresh	¼ cup	1	0	—
seed	1 tsp	5	0	—
Instant India				
Tomato Coriander Paste	2 tbsp (1 oz)	90	0	0

CORN

FOOD	PORTION	CALS	CHOL	FIBER
CANNED				
cream style	½ cup	93	0	—
w/ red & green peppers	½ cup	86	0	—
white	½ cup	66	0	—
yellow	½ cup	66	0	1
Del Monte				
Cream Style Golden	½ cup (4.4 oz)	90	0	2
Cream Style Goldens No Salt Added	½ cup (4.4 oz)	60	0	2
Cream Style White	½ cup (4.4 oz)	100	0	2
Fiesta	½ cup (4.4 oz)	50	0	2
Gold & White Supersweet	½ cup (4.4 oz)	80	0	2
Whole Kernel Golden	½ cup (4.4 oz)	90	0	3
Whole Kernel Golden Supersweet No Salt Added	½ cup (4.4 oz)	60	0	3
Whole Kernel Golden Supersweet No Salt Added	½ cup (4.4 oz)	70	0	3

FOOD	PORTION	CALS	CHOL	FIBER
Whole Kernel Golden Supersweet No Sugar	½ cup (4.4 oz)	60	0	3
Whole Kernel Golden Supersweet Vacuum Packed	½ cup (3.7 oz)	70	0	3
Whole Kernel White Sweet	½ cup (4.4 oz)	60	0	3
Green Giant				
Cream Style	½ cup (4.5 oz)	100	0	1
Mexicorn	⅓ cup (2.7 oz)	60	0	2
Niblets	⅓ cup (2.7 oz)	70	0	2
Niblets 50% Less Sodium	⅓ cup (2.7 oz)	60	0	1
Niblets Extra Sweet	⅓ cup (2.6 oz)	50	0	2
Niblets No Added Sugar or Salt	⅓ cup (2.7 oz)	60	0	2
White Shoepeg	⅓ cup	80	0	1
Whole Sweet	½ cup (4.3 oz)	80	0	2
Whole Sweet 50% Less Sodium	½ cup (4.2 oz)	80	0	2
Owatonna				
Cream Style	½ cup	100	0	—
Whole Kernel In Brine	½ cup	90	0	—
Whole Kernel Vacuum Pack	½ cup	100	0	—
S&W				
Cream Style	½ cup (4.4 oz)	60	0	2
Whole Kernel	⅓ cup (3 oz)	70	0	2
Veg-All				
Whole Kernel	½ cup	80	0	2
DRIED				
Goya				
Giant White	⅓ cup (1.6 oz)	160	0	4
FRESH				
on-the-cob w/ butter cooked	1 ear	155	6	—
white cooked	½ cup	89	0	—
white raw	½ cup	66	0	—
yellow cooked	1 ear (2.7 oz)	83	0	—

FOOD	PORTION	CALS	CHOL	FIBER
yellow cooked	½ cup	89	0	—
yellow raw	1 ear (3 oz)	77	0	—
yellow raw	½ cup	66	0	—
FROZEN				
cooked	½ cup	67	0	—
on-the-cob cooked	1 ear (2.2 oz)	59	0	—
Birds Eye				
Cob Big Ear	1 ear	120	0	3
Cut	⅓ cup	70	0	2
Gold & White Blend	½ cup (3.5 oz)	60	0	2
Green Giant				
Butter Sauce Niblets	⅔ cup (4.3 oz)	130	<5	3
Butter Sauce Shoepeg White	¾ cup (4 oz)	120	<5	3
Cream Corn	½ cup (4.1 oz)	110	0	2
Extra Sweet Niblets	⅔ cup (3.1 oz)	70	0	2
Harvest Fresh Niblets	⅔ cup (3.4 oz)	80	0	3
Harvest Fresh Shoepeg White	½ cup (2.6 oz)	70	0	2
Niblets	⅔ cup (2.9 oz)	80	0	2
On The Cob Extra Sweet	1 ear (4.4 oz)	120	0	3
On The Cob Nibblers	1 ear (2.1 oz)	70	0	1
On The Cob Niblets	1 ear (5 oz)	160	0	3
Select Extra Sweet White	⅔ cup (2.9 oz)	50	0	3
Select Shoepeg White	¾ cup (3.2 oz)	100	0	3
Ore Ida				
Cob Corn	1 ear (6.1 oz)	180	0	4
Cob Corn Mini-Gold	1 ear (3.1 oz)	90	0	2
Stouffer's				
Souffle	½ cup (6 oz)	170	65	1
Tree Of Life				
Corn	⅔ cup (3.2 oz)	80	0	1
TAKE-OUT				
fritters	1 (1 oz)	62	12	1
scalloped	½ cup	258	47	—

CORN CHIPS (see CHIPS)

FOOD	PORTION	CALS	CHOL	FIBER

CORNISH HEN (see CHICKEN)

CORNMEAL

FOOD	PORTION	CALS	CHOL	FIBER
corn grits cooked	1 cup	146	0	–
corn grits uncooked	1 cup	579	0	–
white	1 cup (4.8 oz)	505	0	10
whole grain	1 cup (4.3 oz)	442	0	9
yellow	1 cup (4.8 oz)	505	0	10
yellow self-rising	1 cup (4.3 oz)	407	0	8
Albers				
White	3 tbsp	110	0	tr
Yellow	3 tbsp	110	0	tr
FROZEN				
McKenzie's				
Hush Puppies	1 serv (1.9 oz)	190	0	2
MIX				
Hodgson Mill				
Cornbread Mix Jalapeno Mexican	¼ cup (1 oz)	100	0	1
Yellow Organic	¼ cup (1 oz)	100	0	3
Yellow Self Rising	¼ cup (1 oz)	90	0	3
Kentucky Kernal				
Sweet Cornbread Mix	¼ cup (1 oz)	120	0	0
Stone-Buhr				
Yellow Corn Meal	¼ cup (1 oz)	100	0	1
TAKE-OUT				
hush puppies	1 (0.75 oz)	74	10	1

CORNSTARCH

FOOD	PORTION	CALS	CHOL	FIBER
cornstarch	1 cup (4.5 oz)	488	0	1
Armour				
Cream Cornstarch	1 tbsp (0.4 oz)	40	0	0

COTTAGE CHEESE

FOOD	PORTION	CALS	CHOL	FIBER
creamed	4 oz	117	17	–
creamed	1 cup (7.4 oz)	217	31	–
creamed w/ fruit	4 oz	140	13	–
dry curd	1 cup (5.1 oz)	123	10	–
dry curd	4 oz	96	8	–
lowfat 1%	1 cup (7.9 oz)	164	10	–
lowfat 1%	4 oz	82	5	–

FOOD	PORTION	CALS	CHOL	FIBER
lowfat 2%	1 cup (7.9 oz)	203	19	—
lowfat 2%	4 oz	101	9	—
Axelrod				
Nonfat	½ cup (4.4 oz)	90	10	0
Breakstone's				
2% Fat Large Curd	½ cup (4.2 oz)	90	15	0
2% Fat Small Curd	½ cup (4.2 oz)	90	15	0
4% Fat Large Curd	½ cup (4.2 oz)	120	25	0
4% Fat Small Curd	½ cup (4.2 oz)	120	25	0
Cottage Doubles Peach	1 pkg (5.5 oz)	140	15	tr
Dry Curd	¼ cup (1.9 oz)	45	<5	0
Free	½ cup (4.4 oz)	80	5	0
Snack 2% Fat Small Curd	1 pkg (4 oz)	90	15	0
Snack 4% Fat Small Curd	1 pkg (4 oz)	110	25	0
Snack Free	1 pkg (4 oz)	70	5	0
Friendship				
California Style	½ cup (4 oz)	115	25	0
Lowfat No Salt Added	½ cup (4 oz)	90	10	0
Lowfat Pineapple	½ cup (4 oz)	120	10	0
Lowfat 1%	½ cup (4 oz)	90	10	0
Nonfat	½ cup (4 oz)	80	0	0
Nonfat Plus Peach	½ cup (4 oz)	110	0	0
Pot Style	½ cup (4 oz)	90	15	0
With Pineapple	½ cup (4 oz)	140	15	0
Hood				
1% Fat	½ cup (4 oz)	90	10	0
1% Fat Chive & Onion	½ cup (4 oz)	90	10	0
1% Fat No Salt Added	½ cup (4 oz)	90	10	0
1% Fat Pepper & Herb	½ cup (4 oz)	90	10	0
1% Fat Pineapple Cherry	½ cup (4 oz)	110	10	0
4% Fat	½ cup (4 oz)	120	25	0
4% Fat Chive	½ cup (4 oz)	130	25	0
4% Fat Pineapple	½ cup (4 oz)	130	20	0
Nonfat	½ cup (4 oz)	80	5	0
Nonfat Pineapple	½ cup (4 oz)	110	<5	0

FOOD	PORTION	CALS	CHOL	FIBER
Horizon Organic				
Cottage Cheese	½ cup (3.9 oz)	110	15	0
Knudsen				
1.5% Fat Pineapple Small Curd	½ cup (4.6 oz)	120	10	0
2% Fat Small Curd	½ cup (4.2 oz)	100	15	0
4% Fat Large Curd	½ cup (4.5 oz)	130	30	0
4% Fat Small Curd	½ cup (4.3 oz)	120	25	0
Free	½ cup (4.2 oz)	80	5	0
On The Go! 1.5% Fat Peach	1 pkg (4 oz)	110	10	0
On The Go! 1.5% Fat Pineapple	1 pkg (4 oz)	110	10	0
On The Go! 1.5% Fat Strawberry	1 pkg (4 oz)	110	10	0
On The Go! 1.5% Fat Tropical Fruit	1 pkg (4 oz)	110	10	0
On The Go! 2% Fat	1 pkg (4 oz)	90	15	0
On The Go! Free	1 pkg (4 oz)	70	5	0
Light N'Lively				
1% Fat	½ cup (4 oz)	80	10	0
1% Fat Garden Salad	½ cup (4.2 oz)	80	10	0
1% Fat Peach & Pineapple	½ cup (4.3 oz)	110	10	0
Fat Free	½ cup (4.4 oz)	80	5	0
COTTONSEED				
kernels roasted	1 tbsp	51	0	—
COUGH DROPS				
Halls				
Cough Drops	1 (3.8 g)	15	0	—
Plus	1 (4.7 g)	18	0	—
With Vitamin C	1 (3.8 g)	14	0	—
Lifesavers				
Menthol	2 (0.5 oz)	60	0	—
COUSCOUS				
cooked	1 cup (5.5 oz)	176	0	2
dry	1 cup (6.1 oz)	650	0	9

FOOD	PORTION	CALS	CHOL	FIBER
Casbah				
Almond Chicken Vegetarian	1 pkg (1.5 oz)	160	0	tr
Asparagus Au Gratin Organic	1 pkg (1.5 oz)	150	<5	1
Cheddar Broccoli	1 pkg (1.3 oz)	130	<5	tr
Hearty Harvest Zestful Organic as prep	1 pkg (10 fl oz)	180	0	2
Moroccan Stew	1 pkg (2 oz)	180	0	1
Pilaf as prep	1 cup	200	0	tr
Tomato Parmesan	1 pkg (1.8 oz)	170	<5	2
Kitchen Del Sol				
Spicy Vegetable as prep	½ cup (1.1 oz)	120	0	1
Tomato & Olive	½ cup (1.1 oz)	120	0	1
Melting Pot				
Calypso Cranberry	1 cup	200	0	1
Lentil Curry	1 cup	170	0	1
Lucky Seven	1 cup	190	0	1
Mango Salsa	1 cup	190	0	1
Roasted Garlic	1 cup	170	0	1
Sesame Ginger	1 cup	180	0	0
Sun-Dried Tomatoes	1 cup	190	0	1
Wild Mushroom	1 cup	190	0	1
Near East				
Couscous as prep	1¼ cup	260	0	2
COWPEAS				
catjang dried cooked	1 cup (2.9 oz)	200	0	–
common canned	1 cup	184	0	–
frozen cooked	½ cup	112	0	–
leafy tips chopped cooked	1 cup	12	0	–
leafy tips raw chopped	1 cup	10	0	–
CRAB				
CANNED				
blue	3 oz	84	76	–
blue	1 cup	133	120	–

FOOD	PORTION	CALS	CHOL	FIBER
Bumble Bee				
Fancy Lump Meat	½ can (1.9 oz)	40	50	0
Fancy White Meat	½ can (1.9 oz)	28	43	0
FRESH				
alaska king cooked	1 leg (4.7 oz)	129	72	–
alaska king cooked	3 oz	82	45	–
alaska king raw	3 oz	71	35	–
alaska king raw	1 leg (6 oz)	144	72	–
blue cooked	3 oz	87	85	–
blue cooked	1 cup	138	135	–
blue raw	1 crab (7 oz)	18	16	–
blue raw	3 oz	74	66	–
dungeness raw	3 oz	73	50	–
dungeness raw	1 crab (5.7 oz)	140	97	–
queen steamed	3 oz	98	60	–
TAKE-OUT				
baked	1 (3.8 oz)	160	184	–
cake	1 (2 oz)	160	82	–
mousse	¼ cup	364	136	–
soft-shell fried	1 (4.4 oz)	334	45	–
CRACKER CRUMBS				
chocolate wafer cookie crumbs	½ cup (5.9 oz)	728	0	–
cracker meal	1 cup (4 oz)	440	0	–
graham cracker crumbs	½ cup (4.4 oz)	540	0	3
Baker's Harvest				
Graham	⅓ cup (1 oz)	130	0	1
Honey Maid				
Graham Cracker	0.5 oz	70	0	tr
Kellogg's				
Corn Flake Crumbs	2 tbsp (0.4 oz)	40	0	0
Nabisco				
Nilla Cookie Crumbs	2 tbsp (0.5 oz)	70	<5	tr
Oreo				
Cookie Crumbs	2 tbsp (0.5 oz)	80	0	1
Premium				
Fat Free Cracker Crumbs	¼ cup (1 oz)	100	0	1

FOOD	PORTION	CALS	CHOL	FIBER
Ritz				
Cracker Crumbs	⅓ cup (1 oz)	140	0	1
CRACKERS				
cheese	1 (1 in sq) (1 g)	5	0	—
cheese	14 (½ oz)	71	2	—
cheese low sodium	1 (1 in sq) (1 g)	5	0	—
cheese low sodium	14 (½ oz)	71	2	—
cheese w/ peanut butter filling	1 (0.24 oz)	34	0	tr
crispbread rye	1 (0.35 oz)	37	0	2
melba toast plain	1 (5 g)	19	0	tr
melba toast pumpernickel	1 (5 g)	19	0	tr
melba toast rye	1 (5 g)	19	0	tr
melba toast wheat	1 (5 g)	19	0	tr
oyster cracker	1 (1 g)	4	0	tr
rye w/ cheese filling	1 (0.24 oz)	34	1	—
rye wafers plain	1 (0.9 oz)	84	0	—
rye wafers seasoned	1 (0.8 oz)	84	0	—
saltines	1 (3 g)	13	0	tr
saltines low sodium fat free	6 (1 oz)	118	0	—
saltines low sodium fat free	3 (0.5 oz)	59	0	—
saltines low salt	1 (3 g)	13	0	tr
snack cracker	1 (3 g)	15	0	tr
snack cracker low salt	1 (3 g)	15	0	tr
snack cracker w/ cheese filling	1 (7 g)	33	0	—
soup cracker	1 (1 g)	4	0	tr
wheat w/ cheese filling	1 (0.24 oz)	35	1	—
wheat w/ peanut butter filling	1 (0.24 oz)	35	0	—
wheat thins	1 (2 g)	9	0	—
wheat thins	7 (0.5 oz)	67	0	1
wheat thins low salt	7 (0.5 oz)	67	0	1
whole wheat	1 (4 g)	18	0	—
whole wheat low salt	1 (4 g)	18	0	—

FOOD	PORTION	CALS	CHOL	FIBER
Ak-mak				
100% Whole Wheat	5 (1 oz)	116	0	4
Armenian Cracker Bread	1 sheet (1 oz)	100	0	2
Armenian Cracker Bread Whole Wheat	1 sheet (1 oz)	116	0	4
Round Cracker Bread No Seeds	1 (1 oz)	100	0	1
Round Cracker Bread Seeded	1 (1 oz)	100	0	2
Round Cracker Bread Whole Wheat	1 (1 oz)	116	0	4
Austin				
Cracker Sandwich Cheese On Cheese	6 (1.3 oz)	170	0	tr
Cracker Sandwich Cheese Peanut Butter	6 (1.3 oz)	170	0	1
Cracker Sandwich Toasty Peanut Butter	6 (1.3 oz)	170	0	1
Cracker Sandwich Whole Wheat Cheese	6 (1.3 oz)	170	0	tr
Baker's Harvest				
Cheese	23 (1 oz)	150	0	tr
Cheese Reduced Fat	29 (1 oz)	130	0	tr
Snackers Reduced Fat	10 (1.1 oz)	140	0	tr
Wheat Snacks Reduced Fat	16 (1.1 oz)	140	0	1
Woven Wheats	7 (1.1 oz)	140	0	4
Woven Wheats Reduced Fat	8 (1.1 oz)	130	0	4
Barbara's Bakery				
Cheese Bites	26 (1 oz)	120	0	1
Right Lite Rounds Original	5 (0.5 oz)	55	0	0
Rite Lite Rounds Savory Poppy	5 (0.5 oz)	70	0	0
Rite Lite Rounds Tamari Sesame	5 (0.5 oz)	70	0	0
Wheatines All Flavors	1 lg sq (0.5 oz)	50	0	1

FOOD	PORTION	CALS	CHOL	FIBER
Better Cheddars				
Crackers	22 (1 oz)	70	<5	tr
Low Sodium	22 (1 oz)	150	<5	tr
Reduced Fat	24 (1 oz)	140	<5	tr
Blue Diamond				
Nut Thins Almond	16 (1 oz)	130	0	tr
Nut Thins Hazelnut	16 (1 oz)	120	0	1
Nut Thins Pecan	16 (1 oz)	130	0	tr
Burns & Ricker				
Bagel Crisps Garlic	5 (1 oz)	100	0	1
Cheetos				
Bacon Cheddar	1 pkg	190	<5	1
Cheddar Cheese	1 pkg	210	<5	1
Golden Toast	1 pkg	240	5	1
Cheez It				
Big	13 (1 oz)	150	0	tr
Big Reduced Fat	15 (1 oz)	140	0	tr
Heads & Tails	37 (1 oz)	140	0	1
Hot & Spicy	26 (1 oz)	150	0	tr
Low Sodium	27 (1 oz)	160	0	tr
Nacho	28 (1 oz)	150	0	tr
Original	27 (1 oz)	160	0	tr
Party Mix	½ cup (1 oz)	140	0	1
Party Mix Nacho	½ cup (1 oz)	130	0	1
Party Mix Reduced Fat	½ cup (1 oz)	130	0	1
Peanut Butter	1 pkg (1.3 oz)	190	0	1
Reduced Fat	29 (1 oz)	140	0	tr
Snack Mix	½ cup (1 oz)	130	0	2
Snack Mix Big Crunch	¾ cup (1 oz)	110	0	tr
Snack Mix Double Cheese	¾ cup (1 oz)	110	0	tr
White Cheddar	26 (1 oz)	150	<5	tr
Courtney's				
Sun-Dried Tomato Organic	4 (0.5 oz)	60	0	0
Crown Pilot				
Crackers	1 (0.5 oz)	70	0	tr
Dare				
Breton	1 (5 g)	21	0	tr

FOOD	PORTION	CALS	CHOL	FIBER
Breton Garden Vegetable	1 (5 g)	20	0	tr
Breton Light	1 (5 g)	20	0	tr
Breton Reduced Fat & Sodium	3 (0.5 oz)	60	0	tr
Breton Sesame	1 (5 g)	22	0	tr
Breton Minis	20 (0.6 oz)	89	0	tr
Breton Minis Cheddar Cheese	20 (0.6 oz)	87	3	—
Breton Minis Garden Vegetable	20 (0.6 oz)	87	0	1
Cabaret	1 (5 g)	23	0	tr
Vinta	1 (6 g)	30	0	1
Vivant Italian Bruschetta	1 (5 g)	22	0	tr
Doritos				
Jalapeno Cheese	1 pkg	230	<5	1
Nacho Cheddar	1 pkg	240	<5	1
Eden				
Nori Nori Rice	15 (1 oz)	110	0	2
Estee				
Sugar Free Cracked Pepper	18	120	0	1
Sugar Free Golden	10	130	0	1
Sugar Free Wheat	17	100	0	2
Frito Lay				
Cheddar Snacks	1 pkg	200	<5	1
Frookie				
Cheddar	17 (1 oz)	140	0	1
Cracked Pepper	8 (0.7 oz)	70	0	1
Garden Vegetable	13 (1 oz)	130	0	2
Garlic & Herb	8 (0.7 oz)	70	0	1
Pizza	17 (1 oz)	130	0	1
Snack & Party	10 (1 oz)	140	0	1
Water Crackers	8 (0.7 oz)	70	0	1
Wheat & Onion	12 (1 oz)	120	0	2
Wheat & Rye	13 (1 oz)	120	0	3
Gold'n Krackle				
Cheese	½ oz	65	2	0
Cheese & Oregano	½ oz	65	2	0

FOOD	PORTION	CALS	CHOL	FIBER
Hot & Spicy	½ oz	58	0	0
Onion & Garlic	½ oz	58	0	0
Plain	½ oz	58	0	0
Harvest Crisps				
5 Grain	13 (1.1 oz)	130	0	1
Oat	13 (1.1 oz)	140	0	1
Health Valley				
Healthy Pizza Garlic & Herb	6	50	0	2
Healthy Pizza Italiano	6	50	0	2
Healthy Pizza Zesty Cheese	6	50	0	2
Low Fat Mild Jalapeno	6	60	0	2
Low Fat Mild Ranch	6	60	0	2
Low Fat Roasted Garlic	6	60	0	2
Original Oat Bran	6	120	0	3
Original Rice Bran	6	110	0	3
Whole Wheat	5	50	0	2
Whole Wheat Cheese	5	50	0	2
Whole Wheat Herb	5	50	0	2
Whole Wheat No Salt Vegetable	5	50	0	2
Whole Wheat Onion	5	50	0	2
Whole Wheat Vegetable	5	50	0	2
Healthy Choice				
Bread Crisps Garlic Herb	11 (1 oz)	110	0	2
Kashi				
TLC Honey Sesame	15 (1 oz)	130	0	2
TLC Natural Ranch	15 (1 oz)	130	0	2
TLC Original	15 (1 oz)	130	0	2
Kavli				
Crackers	1 piece	40	0	2
Keebler				
Club 33% Reduced Fat	5 (0.6 oz)	70	0	0

FOOD	PORTION	CALS	CHOL	FIBER
Club 50% Reduced Sodium	4 (0.5 oz)	70	0	tr
Club Orignal	4 (0.5 oz)	70	0	tr
Elfin	23 (1 oz)	130	0	tr
Export Soda	3 (0.5 oz)	60	0	tr
Harvest Bakery Multigrain	2 (0.6 oz)	70	0	tr
Munch'ems Cheddar	39 (1 oz)	140	0	1
Munch'ems Cheddar	30 (1 oz)	130	0	tr
Munch'ems Chili Cheese	28 (1.1 oz)	130	0	1
Munch'ems Mexquite BBQ	40 (1 oz)	140	0	1
Munch'ems Ranch	40 (1 oz)	140	0	1
Munch'ems Ranch	33 (1 oz)	130	0	tr
Munch'ems Salsa	28 (1.1 oz)	130	0	1
Munch'ems Seasoned Original	30 (1 oz)	130	0	tr
Munch'ems Sour Cream & Onion	39 (1 oz)	140	0	1
Munch'ems Sour Cream & Onion 55% Reduced Fat	33 (1 oz)	130	0	0
Paks Cheese & Peanut Butter	1 pkg	190	<5	tr
Paks Club & Cheddar	1 pkg	190	10	tr
Paks Toast & Peanut Butter	1 pkg	190	0	1
Paks Wheat & Cheddar	1 pkg (1.3 oz)	180	5	0
Toasteds Buttercrisp	5 (0.6 oz)	80	0	0
Toasteds Buttercrisp	9 (1 oz)	140	<5	tr
Toasteds Onion	9 (1 oz)	140	0	tr
Toasteds Sesame	5 (0.6 oz)	80	0	tr
Toasteds Sesame	9 (1 oz)	140	0	tr
Toasteds Sesame Reduced Fat	10 (1 oz)	120	0	2
Toasteds Wheat	5 (0.6 oz)	80	0	tr
Toasteds Wheat	9 (1 oz)	140	0	tr
Toasteds Wheat Reduced Fat	5 (0.5 oz)	60	0	tr

FOOD	PORTION	CALS	CHOL	FIBER
Toasteds Wheat Reduced Fat	10 (1 oz)	120	0	1
Town House	5 (0.6 oz)	80	0	tr
Town House 50% Reduced Sodium	5 (0.6 oz)	80	0	tr
Town House Reduced Fat	6 (0.6 oz)	70	0	tr
Town House Wheat	5 (0.6 oz)	80	0	tr
Wheatables Honey Wheat	12 (1 oz)	140	0	1
Wheatables Original	12 (1 oz)	140	0	1
Wheatables Seven Grain	12 (1 oz)	140	0	1
Zesta Saltine 50% Reduced Sodium	5 (0.5 oz)	60	0	tr
Zesta Saltine Fat Free	5 (0.5 oz)	50	0	0
Zesta Saltine Original	5 (0.5 oz)	60	0	tr
Zesta Saltine Unsalted Top	5 (0.5 oz)	70	0	tr
Zesta Soup & Oyster	42 (0.5 oz)	80	0	tr
Lance				
Bonnie	6 (1⅛ oz)	160	10	0
Captain Wafers w/ Cream Cheese & Chives	1 pkg (1.3 oz)	190	0	0
Cheese-On-Wheat	1 pkg (1.3 oz)	190	<5	2
Cranberry Bar Fat Free	1 (1.75 oz)	160	0	1
Lanchee	1 pkg (1¼ oz)	190	0	1
Malt	1 pkg (1¼ oz)	190	0	1
Nekot	1 pkg (1.5 oz)	210	0	1
Nip-Chee	1 pkg (1.3 oz)	190	<5	1
Peanut Butter Wheat	1 pkg (1.3 oz)	190	0	1
Rye-Chee	1 pkg (1.4 oz)	210	<5	1
Sour Dough w/ Cheddar & Sour Cream	1 pkg (1.6 oz)	240	5	1
Toastchee	1 pkg (1.4 oz)	200	0	1
Toasty	1 pkg (1¼ oz)	190	0	1
Wheat Italian	¾ cup (1.4 oz)	200	0	1
Wheat Pizza	¾ cup (1.4 oz)	200	0	1

FOOD	PORTION	CALS	CHOL	FIBER
Little Debbie				
Cheese Crackers With Peanut Butter	1 (0.9 oz)	140	0	tr
Cheese On Cheese Crackers	1 (0.9 oz)	140	<5	0
Cream Cheese & Chive	1 (0.9 oz)	140	0	0
Toasty Crackers With Peanut Butter	1 (0.9 oz)	140	0	tr
Wheat Crackers With Cheddar Cheese	1 (0.9 oz)	140	<5	0
NABS				
Cheese Peanut Butter Sandwich	6 (1.4 oz)	190	0	1
Peanut Butter Toast Sandwich	6 (1.4 oz)	190	0	1
Nabisco				
Bacon Flavored	15 (1.1 oz)	160	0	tr
Chicken In A Biskit	14 (1 oz)	160	0	tr
Garden Crisps	15 (1 oz)	130	0	1
Oat Thins	18 (1 oz)	140	0	2
Royal Lunch	1 (0.4 oz)	60	0	0
Swiss	15 (1 oz)	140	0	tr
Tid-Bit Cheese	32 (1 oz)	150	0	tr
Vegetable Thins	14 (1.1 oz)	160	0	1
Wheat Thins Original	16 (1 oz)	140	0	2
Wheat Thins Reduced Fat	18 (1 oz)	120	0	2
Zings!	1 pkg (1.8 oz)	240	0	2
Zwieback	1 (8 g)	35	0	0
Nips				
Cheese	29 (1 oz)	150	0	tr
No-No				
Flatbreads Tortilla Corn Low Fat Sugar Free Everything	3 (1 oz)	95	0	1
Oysterettes				
Crackers	19 (0.5 oz)	60	0	tr

FOOD	PORTION	CALS	CHOL	FIBER
Partners				
Walla Walla Sweet Onion Perservative Free	0.5 oz	65	3	tr
Pepperidge Farm				
Butter Thins	4 (0.5 oz)	70	10	0
English Water Biscuits	4 (0.5 oz)	70	0	0
Gaint Goldfish Peanut Butter Sandwich	1 pkg (1.4 oz)	190	<5	1
Goldfish Cheddar	55	140	10	tr
Goldfish Cheddar 30% Less Sodium	60 (1.1 oz)	150	10	tr
Goldfish Cheese Trio	58	140	<5	1
Goldfish Original	55	140	0	tr
Goldfish Parmesan Cheese	60	140	0	1
Goldfish Pizza Flavored	55 (1 oz)	140	0	1
Goldfish Pretzel	43 (1 oz)	120	0	tr
Goldfish Toasted Wheat	41	150	0	2
Hearty Wheat	3 (0.6 oz)	80	0	1
Sesame	3 (0.5 oz)	70	0	2
Snack Mix Fat Free Goldfish	⅔ cup (0.9 oz)	90	0	0
Peter Pan				
Cheese Peanut Butter	1 pkg	210	0	1
Toast Peanut Butter	1 pkg	210	0	tr
Planters				
Cheese Peanut Butter Sandwiches	1 pkg (1.4 oz)	190	0	1
Toast Peanut Butter Sandwiches	1 pkg (1.4 oz)	190	0	1
Premium				
Saltine Bits	34 (1 oz)	150	0	tr
Saltine Fat Free	5 (0.5 oz)	50	0	0
Saltine Low Sodium	5 (0.5 oz)	60	0	tr
Saltine Multigrain	5 (0.5 oz)	60	0	tr
Saltine Original	5 (0.5 oz)	60	0	tr
Saltine Unsalted Tops	5 (0.5 oz)	60	0	tr
Soup & Oyster	23 (0.5 oz)	60	0	tr

FOOD	PORTION	CALS	CHOL	FIBER
Ralston				
Cheese	23 (1 oz)	150	0	tr
Cheese Reduced Fat	29 (1 oz)	130	0	tr
Saltines Fat Free	5 (0.5 oz)	60	0	–
Snackers Reduced Fat	10 (1.1 oz)	140	0	tr
Wheat Snacks Reduced Fat	16 (1.1 oz)	140	0	1
Woven Wheats	7 (1.1 oz)	140	0	4
Woven Wheats Reduced Fat	8 (1.1 oz)	130	0	4
RedOval Farms				
Stoned Wheat Thins Cracked Pepper	4 (0.6 oz)	70	0	tr
Ritz				
Bits	48 (1 oz)	160	0	1
Bits Sandwiches With Peanut Butter	13 (1 oz)	150	0	1
Bits Sandwiches With Real Cheese	14 (1.1 oz)	160	5	1
Crackers	5 (0.5 oz)	80	0	tr
Low Sodium	5 (0.5 oz)	80	0	tr
Sandwiches With Real Cheese	1 pkg (1.4 oz)	210	5	1
Savory Thins				
Toasted Onion & Garlic	15 (1 oz)	110	0	2
Sesmark				
Brown Rice	15 (1 oz)	120	0	tr
Cheese Thins	15 (1 oz)	130	0	tr
Rice Thins Original	15 (1 oz)	130	0	tr
Rice Thins Teriyaki Flavored	13 (1 oz)	130	0	tr
Savory Thins Original	15 (1 oz)	125	0	1
Sesame Thins Cheddar	9 (1 oz)	150	0	3
Sesame Thins Garlic	9 (1 oz)	150	0	3
Sesame Thins Original	9 (1 oz)	150	0	2
Sesame Thins Unsalted	11 (1 oz)	150	0	3
Smucker's				
Snackers Grape	1 pkg (3.3 oz)	410	0	3
Snackers Strawberry	1 pkg (3.3 oz)	410	0	3

FOOD	PORTION	CALS	CHOL	FIBER
SnackWell's				
Cracked Pepper	7 (0.5 oz)	60	0	tr
Fat Free Wheat	5 (0.5 oz)	60	0	1
Reduced Fat Cheese	38 (1 oz)	130	0	1
Reduced Fat Classic Golden	6 (0.5 oz)	60	0	0
Salsa Cheddar	32 (1 oz)	120	0	1
Snorkles				
Cheddar	56 (1 oz)	140	5	1
Sociables				
Crackers	7 (0.5 oz)	80	0	tr
Sunshine				
Hi Ho	4 (0.5 oz)	70	0	tr
Hi Ho Reduced Fat	5 (0.5 oz)	70	0	tr
Krispy	5 (0.5 oz)	60	0	tr
Krispy Fat Free	5 (0.5 oz)	50	0	0
Krispy Mild Cheddar	5 (0.5 oz)	60	0	tr
Krispy Soup & Oyster	17 (0.5 oz)	60	0	tr
Krispy Unsalted Tops	5 (0.5 oz)	60	0	tr
Krispy Whole Wheat	5 (0.5 oz)	60	0	tr
Tree Of Life				
Bite Size Fat Free Cracked Pepper	12 (0.5)	55	0	0
Bite Size Fat Free Garden Vegetable	12 (0.5 oz)	55	0	0
Bite Size Fat Free Garlic & Herb	12 (0.5 oz)	55	0	0
Bite Size Fat Free Toasted Onion	12 (0.5 oz)	55	0	0
Oyster	40 (0.5 oz)	60	0	0
Saltine Cracked Pepper Fat Free	4 (0.5 oz)	60	0	1
Saltine Fat Free	4 (0.5 oz)	50	0	0
Triscuit				
Crackers	7 (1.1 oz)	140	0	4
Deli-Style Rye	7 (1.1 oz)	140	0	4
Garden Herb	6 (1 oz)	130	0	3
Low Sodium	7 (1.1 oz)	150	0	3
Reduced Fat	8 (1.1 oz)	130	0	4
Wheat 'n Bran	7 (1.1 oz)	140	0	4

FOOD	PORTION	CALS	CHOL	FIBER
Twigs				
Sesame & Cheese Sticks	15 (1 oz)	150	0	tr
Uneeda Biscuit				
Unsalted Tops	2 (0.5 oz)	60	0	tr
Venus				
Fat Free Cracked Pepper	11 (0.5 oz)	60	0	0
Fat Free Garden Vegetable	5 (0.5 oz)	60	0	0
Fat Free Garlic & Herb	11 (0.5 oz)	60	0	0
Fat Free Multi-Grain	5 (0.5 oz)	60	0	tr
Fat Free Spicy Chili	10 (0.5 oz)	60	0	tr
Fat Free Toasted Onion	5 (0.5 oz)	60	0	0
Fat Free Toasted Wheat	5 (0.5 oz)	60	0	tr
Fat Free Tomato & Basil	10 (0.5 oz)	60	0	tr
Fat Free Zesty Italian	10 (0.5 oz)	60	0	tr
Garden Vegetable	6 (1 oz)	150	0	1
Honey Wheat	1 oz	140	0	1
Low Fat Cracker Bread	5 (0.5 oz)	60	0	tr
Low Fat Water Crackers	4 (0.5 oz)	60	0	0
Sesame & Flaxseed	1 oz	130	0	1
Soup Original	0.5 oz	60	0	0
Toasted Wheat	6 (1 oz)	150	0	tr
Wine Cheese Caviar Original	0.5 oz	60	0	0
Wine Cheese Caviar Pepper & Poppy	0.5 oz	60	0	0
Wasa				
Crisp	3 (0.5 oz)	50	0	2
Crisp'N Light Sourdough Rye	3 (0.6 oz)	60	0	1
Crisp'N Light Wheat	2 (0.5 oz)	50	0	1
Crispbread Cinnamon Toast	1 (0.6 oz)	60	0	1
Crispbread Fiber Rye	1 (0.4 oz)	30	0	2

FOOD	PORTION	CALS	CHOL	FIBER
Crispbread Gluten & Wheat Free Corn	1 (0.4 oz)	40	0	0
Crispbread Hearty Rye	1 (0.5 oz)	45	0	2
Crispbread Light Rye	1 (0.3 oz)	25	0	1
Crispbread Multi Grain	1 (0.5 oz)	45	0	2
Crispbread Organic Rye	1 (0.3 oz)	25	0	1
Crispbread Sodium Free Rye	1 (0.3 oz)	30	0	2
Crispbread Sourdough Rye	1 (0.4 oz)	35	0	1
Crispbread Toasted Wheat	1 (0.5 oz)	50	0	1
Crispbread Whole Wheat	1 (0.5 oz)	50	0	1
Waverly				
Crackers	5 (0.5 oz)	70	0	0
Wheat Thins				
Low Salt	16 (1 oz)	140	0	2
Multi-Grain	17 (1 oz)	130	0	2
Wheatworth				
Stone Ground	5 (0.5 oz)	80	0	1
Wisecrackers				
Low Fat Poblano Chili & Sweet Onion	4 (0.5 oz)	45	0	tr
Wortz				
Cheese	23 (1 oz)	150	0	tr
Saltines Fat Free	5 (0.5 oz)	60	0	–
Wheat Snacks Reduced Fat	16 (1.1 oz)	140	0	1
Woven Wheats	7 (1.1 oz)	140	0	4
CRANBERRIES				
cranberry sauce sweetened	½ cup	209	0	–
fresh chopped	1 cup	54	0	–
Ocean Spray				
Craisins	⅓ cup (1.4 oz)	130	0	2
Cran*Fruit Cranberry Orange	¼ cup	120	0	1
Cranberry Sauce Jellied	¼ cup	110	0	1

FOOD	PORTION	CALS	CHOL	FIBER
Fresh	2 oz	25	0	0
Whole Berry Sauce	¼ cup	110	0	1
Wild Thyme Farms				
Cranberry Sauce	1 tbsp	19	0	–
CRANBERRY BEANS				
canned	1 cup	216	0	–
dried cooked	1 cup	240	0	–
CRANBERRY JUICE				
cocktail	1 cup	147	0	–
cranberry juice cocktail	6 oz	108	0	–
cranberry juice cocktail low calorie	6 oz	33	0	–
cranberry juice cocktail frzn	12 oz can	821	0	–
cranberry juice cocktail frzn as prep	6 oz	102	0	–
After The Fall				
Cape Cod Cranberry	1 bottle (10 oz)	130	0	–
Cranberry Ginger Ale	1 can (12 oz)	140	0	0
Crystal Light				
Cranberry Breeze Drink	1 serv (8 oz)	5	0	0
Cranberry Breeze Drink Mix as prep	1 serv (8 oz)	5	0	0
Everfresh				
Cranberry Cocktail	1 can (8 oz)	140	0	0
Mott's				
Cocktail	8 fl oz	150	0	–
Nantucket Nectars				
Big Cran	8 oz	140	0	0
Ocean Spray				
Cocktail	8 oz	140	0	0
Cocktail Reduced Calorie	8 oz	50	0	0
Lightstyle Cranberry Juice Cocktail	8 oz	40	0	0
White Cranberry	1 cup (8 oz)	120	0	–
White Cranberry Peach	1 cup (8 oz)	120	0	–

FOOD	PORTION	CALS	CHOL	FIBER
White Cranberry Strawberry	1 cup (8 oz)	120	0	–
Snapple				
Cranberry Royal	10 fl oz	150	0	–
Tropicana				
Twister Ruby Red	1 bottle (10 oz)	160	0	–
Veryfine				
Cocktail	1 bottle (10 oz)	180	0	0
Wellfleet Farms				
Cranberry	8 oz	130	0	0
CRAYFISH				
cooked	3 oz	97	151	–
raw	3 oz	76	118	–
raw	8	24	37	–
CREAM (see also WHIPPED TOPPINGS)				
clotted cream	2 tbsp (1 oz)	164	48	0
creme fraiche	2 tbsp (1 oz)	100	40	0
half & half	1 tbsp (0.5 oz)	20	6	–
half & half	1 cup (8.5 oz)	315	89	–
heavy whipping	1 tbsp (0.5 oz)	52	21	–
heavy whipping whipped	1 cup (4.1 oz)	411	163	–
light coffee	1 cup (8.4 oz)	496	159	–
light coffee	1 tbsp (0.5 oz)	29	10	–
light whipping	1 tbsp (0.5 oz)	44	17	–
light whipping cream whipped	1 cup (4.2 oz)	345	132	–
Farmland				
Half & Half	2 tbsp	40	0	0
Light Cream	2 tbsp	30	0	0
Hood				
Half & Half	2 tbsp (1 oz)	40	15	0
Heavy	1 tbsp (0.5 oz)	50	20	0
Light	1 tbsp (0.5 oz)	30	10	0
Whipping Cream	1 tbsp (0.5 oz)	45	20	0
Land O Lakes				
Fat Free Half & Half	2 tbsp (1 oz)	20	0	0
Half & Half	2 tbsp (1 oz)	40	15	0
Heavy Whipping	1 tbsp (0.5 oz)	50	20	0

FOOD	PORTION	CALS	CHOL	FIBER
Organic Valley				
Half & Half	2 tbsp (1 oz)	40	15	0
Parmalat				
Half & Half	2 tbsp (1 oz)	40	15	0
CREAM CHEESE				
cream cheese	1 oz	99	31	–
cream cheese	1 pkg (3 oz)	297	93	–
Alpine Lace				
Reduced Fat Roasted Garlic & Herbs	1 tsp (1 oz)	60	10	0
Reduced Fat Sundried Tomato & Basil	2 tsp (1 oz)	70	15	0
Boar's Head				
Cream Cheese	2 tbsp (1 oz)	100	30	0
Breakstone's				
Temp-Tee Whipped	2 tbsp (0.8 oz)	80	25	0
Fleur De Lait				
Garlic & Spice	2 tbsp (0.9 oz)	90	30	0
Friendship				
NY Style Reduced Fat	2 tbsp (1 oz)	50	10	0
Galaxy				
Slices	1 slice (1 oz)	50	10	0
Healthy Choice				
Herbs & Garlic	2 tbsp (1 oz)	25	<5	–
Plain	2 tbsp (1 oz)	25	<5	–
Strawberry	2 tbsp (1 oz)	30	<5	–
Heluva Good Cheese				
Cream Cheese	1 tbsp (1 oz)	100	30	0
Horizon Organic				
Spreadable	2 tbsp	100	30	0
Organic Valley				
Cream Cheese	1 oz	100	30	0
Philadelphia				
Free	1 oz	30	<5	0
Regular	1 oz	100	30	0
Soft	2 tbsp (1 oz)	100	30	0
Soft Apple Cinnamon	2 tbsp (1.1 oz)	100	25	0
Soft Cheesecake	2 tbsp (1 oz)	110	25	0
Soft Chives & Onions	2 tbsp (1.1 oz)	110	30	0

FOOD	PORTION	CALS	CHOL	FIBER
Soft Garden Vegetable	2 tbsp (1.1 oz)	110	30	0
Soft Honey Nut	2 tbsp (1.1 oz)	110	30	0
Soft Pineapple	2 tbsp (1.1 oz)	100	25	0
Soft Salmon	3 tbsp (1.1 oz)	100	30	0
Soft Strawberry	2 tbsp (1.1 oz)	100	25	0
Soft Free	2 tbsp (1.2 oz)	30	<5	0
Soft Free Garden Vegetable	2 tbsp (1.2 oz)	30	<5	0
Soft Free Strawberries	2 tbsp (1.2 oz)	45	<5	0
Soft Light	2 tbsp (1.1 oz)	70	15	0
Soft Light Jalapeno	2 tbsp (1.1 oz)	60	15	0
Soft Light Raspberry	2 tbsp (1.1 oz)	70	15	0
Soft Light Roasted Garlic	2 tbsp (1.1 oz)	70	15	0
Whipped	2 tbsp (0.7 oz)	70	25	0
Whipped Chives	2 tbsp (0.7 oz)	70	20	0
Whipped Smoked Salmon	2 tbsp (0.7 oz)	70	20	0
With Chives	1 oz	90	30	0

CREAM CHEESE SUBSTITUTES
Tofutti

FOOD	PORTION	CALS	CHOL	FIBER
Better Than Cream Cheese French Onion	1 oz	80	0	–
Better Than Cream Cheese Herb & Chive	1 oz	80	0	–
Better Than Cream Cheese Plain	1 oz	80	0	–

CREAM OF TARTAR

FOOD	PORTION	CALS	CHOL	FIBER
cream of tartar	1 tsp	8	0	–

CREPES

FOOD	PORTION	CALS	CHOL	FIBER
basic crepe unfilled	1	75	55	–

Frieda's

FOOD	PORTION	CALS	CHOL	FIBER
Ready-To-Use	2	50	5	0

CROAKER

FOOD	PORTION	CALS	CHOL	FIBER
atlantic breaded & fried	3 oz	188	71	–

FOOD	PORTION	CALS	CHOL	FIBER
atlantic raw	3 oz	89	52	–

CROISSANT
Rudy's Farm
Ham & Swiss Sandwich	1 (3.4 oz)	310	25	1

Sara Lee
Broccoli & Cheese	1 (3.7 oz)	280	30	2
French Style	1 (1.5 oz)	170	<5	1
Ham & Swiss	1 (3.7 oz)	300	45	2
Petite	2 (2 oz)	230	<5	1

TAKE-OUT
w/ egg & cheese	1 (4.5 oz)	368	216	–
w/ egg cheese & bacon	1 (4.5 oz)	413	215	–
w/ egg cheese & ham	1 (5.3 oz)	474	213	–
w/ egg cheese & sausage	1 (5.6 oz)	523	216	–

CROUTONS
plain	1 cup (1 oz)	122	0	2

Pepperidge Farm
Garlic	6 (0.2 oz)	30	0	0
Homestyle	6 (0.2 oz)	30	0	0
Sourdough	6 (0.2 oz)	35	0	0

Up Country Naturals
Organic Whole Wheat Garlic & Herb	¼ cup (0.3 oz)	35	0	tr

CUCUMBER
fresh raw	1 (11 oz)	38	0	3
fresh raw sliced	½ cup (1.8 oz)	7	0	1

FRESH
Chiquita
Cucumber	⅛ med (3.5 oz)	15	0	1

JARRED
Rosoff's
Salad	3 slices (1 oz)	12	0	–

Schorr's
Cucumber Garden Salad	3 slices (1 oz)	12	0	–

TAKE-OUT
cucumber salad	3.5 oz	50	0	–

FOOD	PORTION	CALS	CHOL	FIBER
kimchee	½ cup (1.8 oz)	36	0	tr
tzatziki	½ cup (3.4 oz)	72	5	1
CUMIN				
seed	1 tsp	8	0	–
CURRANTS				
black fresh	½ cup	36	0	–
zante dried	½ cup	204	0	–
CUSK				
fillet baked	3 oz	106	50	–
CUSTARD				
MIX				
as prep w/ 2% milk	½ cup (4.7 oz)	148	74	–
as prep w/ 2% milk	1 recipe 4 serv (18.7 oz)	595	297	–
flan as prep w/ 2% milk	½ cup (4.7 oz)	135	9	–
flan as prep w/ 2% milk	1 recipe 4 serv (18.7 oz)	542	57	–
flan as prep w/ whole milk	1 recipe 4 serv (18.7 oz)	600	66	–
flan as prep w/ whole milk	½ cup (4.7 oz)	150	17	–
Betty Crocker				
Flan w/ Caramel Sauce as prep	1 serv	330	24	
Jell-O				
Americana Custard Dessert as prep w/ 2% milk	½ cup (5 oz)	140	10	0
Flan as prep w/ 2% milk	½ cup (5.1 oz)	140	10	0
READY-TO-EAT				
Kozy Shack				
Flan	1 pkg (4 oz)	150	40	0
Swiss Miss				
Egg Custard	1 pkg (4 oz)	153	4	0
TAKE-OUT				
baked	½ cup (5 oz)	148	123	–

FOOD	PORTION	CALS	CHOL	FIBER
flan	½ cup (5.4 oz)	220	140	–
zabaione	½ cup (57.2 g)	135	213	0

CUTTLEFISH
| steamed | 3 oz | 134 | 190 | – |

DANDELION GREENS
| fresh cooked | ½ cup | 17 | 0 | – |
| raw chopped | ½ cup | 13 | 0 | – |

DANISH PASTRY
FROZEN
Morton
| Honey Buns | 1 (2.28 oz) | 270 | 0 | 1 |
| Honey Buns Mini | 1 (1.3 oz) | 160 | 0 | 1 |

READY-TO-EAT
| plain ring | 1 (12 oz) | 1305 | 292 | – |

Dolly Madison
| Danish Rollers | 3 (2.8 oz) | 290 | 0 | 1 |

Tastykake
Cheese	1 (3 oz)	290	20	tr
Lemon	1 (3 oz)	290	20	1
Raspberry	1 (3 oz)	290	20	1

TAKE-OUT
almond	1 (4¼ in) (2.3 oz)	280	30	2
cheese	1 (3.2 oz)	353	20	–
cinnamon	1 (3.1 oz)	349	27	–
cinnamon nut	1 (4¼ in) (2.3 oz)	280	30	2
fruit	1 (3.3 oz)	335	19	–
raisin nut	1 (4¼ in) (2.3 oz)	280	30	2

DATES
deglet noor dried	10	240	0	–
dried chopped	1 cup	489	0	–
dried whole	10	228	0	–
jujube fresh	1 oz	30	0	–

Calavo
| Dried Pitted | 5–6 (1.4 oz) | 120 | 0 | 3 |

California Redi-Date
| Deglet Noor Dried | 5–6 (1.4 oz) | 120 | 0 | 3 |

Dromedary
| Chopped Dried | ¼ cup | 130 | 0 | – |

FOOD	PORTION	CALS	CHOL	FIBER
Sonoma				
Dried	5–6 (1.4 oz)	110	0	5

DEER *(see* VENISON*)*

DELI MEATS/COLD CUTS *(see also* BEEF, CHICKEN, HAM, MEAT SUBSTITUTES, TURKEY*)*

FOOD	PORTION	CALS	CHOL	FIBER
barbecue loaf pork & beef	1 oz	49	11	—
beerwurst beef	1 slice (2¾ in x ⅛ in)	20	4	—
beerwurst beef	1 slice (4 in x in)	75	13	—
beerwurst pork	1 slice (2¾ in x ⅛ in)	14	4	—
beerwurst pork	1 slice (4 in x ⅛ in)	55	13	—
berliner pork & beef	1 oz	65	13	—
blood sausage	1 oz	95	30	—
bologna beef	1 oz	88	16	—
bologna beef & pork	1 oz	89	16	—
bologna pork	1 oz	70	17	—
braunschweiger pork	1 slice (2½ in x ¼ in)	65	28	—
braunschweiger pork	1 oz	102	44	—
corned beef loaf	1 oz	43	13	—
dutch brand loaf pork & beef	1 oz	68	13	—
headcheese pork	1 oz	60	23	—
honey loaf pork & beef	1 oz	36	10	—
honey roll sausage beef	1 oz	42	12	—
lebanon bologna beef	1 oz	60	20	—
liver cheese pork	1 oz	86	49	—
liverwurst pork	1 oz	92	45	—
luncheon meat beef	1 oz	87	18	—
luncheon meat pork & beef	1 oz	100	15	—
luncheon meat pork canned	1 oz	95	18	—
luncheon sausage pork & beef	1 oz	74	18	—
luxury loaf pork	1 oz	40	10	—
mortadella beef & pork	1 oz	88	16	—
mother's loaf pork	1 oz	80	13	—

FOOD	PORTION	CALS	CHOL	FIBER
new england sausage pork & beef	1 oz	46	14	—
olive loaf pork	1 oz	67	11	—
peppered loaf pork & beef	1 oz	42	13	—
pickle & pimiento loaf pork	1 oz	74	10	—
picnic loaf pork & beef	1 oz	66	11	—
salami cooked beef & pork	1 oz	71	18	—
salami hard pork & beef	1 pkg (4 oz)	472	89	—
salami hard pork & beef	1 slice (0.3 oz)	42	8	—
sandwich spread pork & beef	1 tbsp	35	6	—
sandwich spread pork & beef	1 oz	67	11	—
summer sausage thuringer cervelat	1 oz	98	19	—
Boar's Head				
Bologna Beef	2 oz	150	35	0
Bologna Garlic	2 oz	150	35	0
Bologna Lowered Sodium	2 oz	150	30	0
Bologna Pork & Beef	2 oz	150	35	0
Braunschweiger Lite	2 oz	120	50	0
Head Cheese	2 oz	90	65	0
Liverwurst Strassburger	2 oz	170	85	0
Olive Loaf	2 oz	130	20	0
Pastrami	2 oz	90	30	0
Prosciutto	1 oz	60	15	0
Red Pastrami	2 oz	90	30	0
Salami Beef	2 oz	120	25	0
Salami Cooked	2 oz	130	40	0
Salami Genoa	2 oz	180	55	0
Salami Hard	1 oz	110	25	0
Spiced Ham	2 oz	120	30	0

FOOD	PORTION	CALS	CHOL	FIBER
Carl Buddig				
Beef	1 pkg (2.5 oz)	100	50	–
Corned Beef	1 pkg (2.5 oz)	100	50	–
Pastrami	1 pkg (2.5 oz)	100	50	–
Healthy Choice				
Bologna	1 slice (1 oz)	30	15	0
Bologna Beef	1 slice (1 oz)	35	10	0
Deli-Thin Bologna	4 slices (1.8 oz)	60	25	0
Well-Pack Bologna	1 slice (1 oz)	30	15	0
Hebrew National				
Bologna Beef	2 oz	180	40	–
Bologna Beef Reduced Fat	2 oz	130	35	–
Bologna Lean Chub	2 oz	90	25	–
Bologna Midget	2 oz	180	40	–
Deli Pastrami	2 oz	80	30	–
Deli Express Corned Beef	2 oz	80	35	–
Deli Express Tongue Sliced	2 oz	120	50	–
Salami Beef	2 oz	170	40	–
Salami Beef Reduced Fat	2 oz	110	30	–
Salami Sean Chub	2 oz	90	30	–
Salami Midget	2 oz	170	40	–
Hormel				
Liverwurst Spread	4 tbsp (2 oz)	130	70	0
Pepperoni Chunk	1 oz	140	35	0
Pepperoni Sliced	15 slices (1 oz)	140	35	0
Pepperoni Twin	1 oz	140	35	0
Pillow Pack Genoa Salami	2 oz	160	50	0
Pillow Pack Pepperoni	16 slices (1 oz)	140	35	0
Jordan's				
Healthy Trim 95% Fat Free Macaroni & Cheese Loaf	2 slices (1.6 oz)	50	15	0
Healthy Trim 95% Fat Free Olive Loaf	2 slices (1.6 oz)	50	15	0

FOOD	PORTION	CALS	CHOL	FIBER
Healthy Trim 95% Fat Free Pickle & Pepper Loaf	2 slices (1.6 oz)	50	15	0
Healthy Trim 97% Fat Free Corned Beef	2 slices (1.6 oz)	45	30	0
Healthy Trim Low Fat Cooked Salami	3 slices (2 oz)	70	25	0
Healthy Trim Low Fat German Brand Bologna	3 slices (2 oz)	70	25	0
Oscar Mayer				
Bologna	1 slice (1 oz)	90	30	0
Bologna Beef	1 slice (1 oz)	90	20	0
Bologna Garlic	1 slice (1.4 oz)	110	40	0
Bologna Wisconsin Made Ring	2 oz	180	35	0
Braunschweiger Spread	2 oz	190	90	0
Brunschweiger	1 slice (1 oz)	100	40	0
Free Bologna	1 slice (1 oz)	20	5	0
Head Cheese	1 slice (1 oz)	50	25	0
Light Bologna	1 slice (1 oz)	60	15	0
Light Bologna Beef	1 slice (1 oz)	60	15	0
Liver Cheese	1 slice (1.3 oz)	120	80	0
Lunchables Bologna/American	1 pkg (4.5 oz)	450	85	0
Lunchables Deluxe Turkey/Ham	1 pkg (5.1 oz)	360	60	1
Lunchables Dessert Jello/Honey Turkey/Cheddar	1 pkg (5.7 oz)	320	50	tr
Lunchables Fun Pack Bologna/Wild Cherry	1 pkg (11.2 oz)	530	60	tr
Lunchables Fun Pack Ham/Fruit Punch	1 pkg (11.2 oz)	450	50	tr
Lunchables Ham/Swiss	1 pkg (4.5 oz)	320	60	0
Lunchables Pepperoni/American	1 pkg (4.5 oz)	480	95	0

FOOD	PORTION	CALS	CHOL	FIBER
Lunchables Salami/American	1 pkg (4.5 oz)	430	80	0
Luncheon Loaf Spiced	1 slice (1 oz)	70	20	0
New England Brand Sausage	2 slices (1.6 oz)	60	25	0
Old Fashioned Loaf	1 slice (1 oz)	70	15	0
Olive Loaf	1 slice (1 oz)	70	20	0
Pepperoni	15 slices (1 oz)	140	25	0
Pickle And Pimiento Loaf	1 slice (1 oz)	80	20	0
Salami Cotto	1 slice (1 oz)	70	25	0
Salami Cotto Beef	1 slice (1 oz)	60	25	0
Salami For Beer	1 slices (1.6 oz)	110	30	0
Salami Genoa	3 slices (1 oz)	100	25	0
Salami Hard	3 slices (1 oz)	100	25	0
Salami Machaich Brand Beef	2 slices (1.6 oz)	120	30	0
Sandwich Spread	2 oz	130	25	0
Summer Sausage	2 slices (1.6 oz)	140	40	0
Summer Sausage Beef	2 slices (1.6 oz)	140	35	0
Russer				
Bologna	2 oz	180	30	—
Bologna Jalapeno Pepper	2 oz	170	25	—
Bologna Wunderbar German Brand	2 oz	190	20	—
Bologna Beef	2 oz	180	30	—
Bologna Garlic	2 oz	180	30	—
Bologna Italian Brand Sweet Red Pepper	2 oz	180	30	—
Braunschweiger	2 oz	170	90	—
Cooked Salami	2 oz	120	50	—
Dutch Brand	2 oz	130	25	—
Hot Cooked Salami	2 oz	110	45	—
Italian Brand Loaf	2 oz	130	25	—
Jalapeno Loaf With Monterey Jack Cheese	2 oz	160	25	—
Kielbasa Loaf	2 oz	120	35	—
Light Bologna	2 oz	120	30	—

FOOD	PORTION	CALS	CHOL	FIBER
Light Bologna Beef	2 oz	120	30	—
Light Braunschweiger	2 oz	120	60	—
Light Old Fashioned Loaf	2 oz	90	30	—
Light P&P Loaf	2 oz	100	30	—
Light Salami Cooked	2 oz	90	40	—
Olive Loaf	2 oz	160	20	—
P&P Loaf	2 oz	160	25	—
Pepper Loaf	2 oz	90	30	—
Polish Loaf	2 oz	140	25	—
Sara Lee				
Pastrami Beef	2 oz	100	25	1
Peppered Beef	2 oz	70	25	—
Shofar				
Salami Beef	2 oz	160	40	0
Spam				
Less Salt	2 oz	170	40	0
Lite	2 oz	110	45	0
Original	2 oz	170	40	0
Smoked	2 oz	170	40	0
TAKE-OUT				
corned beef	2 oz	70	40	—
corned beef brisket	2 oz	90	35	—
DILL				
seed	1 tsp	6	0	—
sprigs fresh	1 cup	4	0	—
sprigs fresh	5	0	0	—
weed dry	1 tsp	3	0	—
Watkins				
Liquid Spice	1 tbsp (0.5 oz)	120	0	0

DINNER *(see also* ASIAN FOOD, PASTA DISHES, POT PIES, SPANISH FOOD*)*

FOOD	PORTION	CALS	CHOL	FIBER
Amy's				
Country Dinner Vegetable Salisbury Steak	1 pkg (11 oz)	380	15	9
Banquet				
Beef Patty w/ Country Style Vegetables	1 meal (9.5 oz)	310	40	2
Boneless Pork Rib	1 meal (10 oz)	400	45	4

FOOD	PORTION	CALS	CHOL	FIBER
Boneless White Fried Chicken	1 meal (8.25 oz)	540	60	3
Chicken Parmigiana	1 meal (9.5 oz)	320	50	3
Chicken Fingers Meal	1 meal (7.1 oz)	740	70	6
Chicken Fried Beef Steak	1 pkg (10 oz)	420	35	4
Chicken Nuggets Meal	1 meal (6.75 oz)	430	50	4
Extra Helping Boneless Pork Riblet	1 meal (15.25 oz)	720	80	7
Extra Helping Fried Beef Steak	1 meal (16 oz)	820	70	6
Extra Helping Fried Chicken	1 meal (14.7 oz)	910	160	5
Extra Helping Meatloaf	1 meal (16 oz)	610	110	6
Extra Helping Salisbury Steak	1 meal (16.5 oz)	740	130	7
Extra Helping Turkey & Gravy w/ Dressing	1 meal (17 oz)	620	80	10
Extra Helping White Fried Chicken	1 meal (13 oz)	690	70	8
Extra Helping Yankee Pot Roast	1 meal (14.5 oz)	410	50	3
Family Size Brown Gravy & Salisbury Steak	1 serv	240	40	1
Family Size Brown Gravy & Sliced Beef	1 serv	140	40	tr
Family Size Chicken & Broccoli Alfredo	1 serv	270	40	3
Family Size Country Style Chicken & Dumplings	1 serv	290	40	7
Family Size Creamy Broccoli Chicken Cheese & Rice	1 serv	280	45	2
Family Size Hearty Beef Stew	1 cup	170	30	4

FOOD	PORTION	CALS	CHOL	FIBER
Family Size Homestyle Gravy & Sliced Turkey	2 slices	140	40	1
Family Size Mushroom Gravy & Charbroiled Beef Patties	1 patty	250	35	2
Family Size Potato Ham & Broccoli Au Gratin	⅔ cup	210	30	2
Family Size Savory Gravy & Meatloaf	1 slice	120	35	1
Fish Sticks	1 meal (6.6 oz)	290	30	4
Grilled Chicken	1 meal (9.9 oz)	330	50	2
Honey Roast Turkey Breast	1 meal (9 oz)	270	30	4
Meatloaf	1 meal (9.5 oz)	280	60	3
Our Original Fried Chicken	1 meal (9 oz)	470	90	2
Pork Cutlet Meal	1 meal (10.25 oz)	420	35	4
Salisbury Steak	1 meal (9.5 oz)	380	60	4
Sliced Beef	1 meal (9 oz)	270	70	4
Turkey	1 meal (9.25 oz)	270	55	3
Veal Parmagiana	1 meal (8.75 oz)	330	20	2
Western Style Beef Patty	1 meal (9.5 oz)	360	40	3
White Meat Fried Chicken	1 meal (8.75 oz)	460	100	2
Yankee Pot Roast	1 meal (9.4 oz)	230	60	4
Birds Eye				
Easy Recipe Creations Sweet & Sour w/ Pineapple Tidbits	1⅔ cups	200	0	3
Viola! Zesty Garlic Chicken	2 cups (6.2 oz)	260	25	1
Voila! Beef Sirloin Steak And Garlic Potatoes	1 cup	240	25	3
Voila! Chicken Alfredo	1 cup	230	20	2
Voila! Garden Herb Chicken	1 cup	310	40	2

FOOD	PORTION	CALS	CHOL	FIBER
Voila! Grilled Salsa Chicken w/ Rice	1 cup	240	25	3
Voila! Homestyle Turkey w/ Roasted Potatoes	1 cup	200	10	3
Voila! Teriyaki	2 cups (6.4 oz)	240	25	2
Budget Gourmet				
Beef Cantonese	1 meal (9.1 oz)	270	40	–
Beef Stroganoff	1 meal (8.75 oz)	260	50	–
Chicken And Egg Noodles	1 meal (10 oz)	440	90	–
Chicken Au Gratin	1 meal (9.1 oz)	230	40	–
Chicken Breast Parmigiana	1 pkg (11 oz)	270	50	–
Chicken Marsala	1 meal (9 oz)	260	90	–
Chicken With Fettucini	1 meal (10 oz)	400	85	–
Chinese Style Vegetables & Chicken	1 meal (10 oz)	280	10	–
French Recipe Chicken	1 meal (10 oz)	220	40	–
Glazed Turkey	1 meal (9 oz)	260	30	–
Ham & Asparagus Au Gratin	1 meal (8.7 oz)	300	50	–
Italian Style Vegetables & Chicken	1 meal (10.25 oz)	310	30	–
Mandarin Chicken	1 meal (10 oz)	240	40	–
Mesquite Chicken Breast	1 pkg (11 oz)	250	40	–
Orange Glazed Chicken	1 meal (9 oz)	270	25	–
Oriental Beef	1 meal (10 oz)	290	30	–
Oriental Chicken With Vegetables	1 meal (9 oz)	280	20	–
Pepper Steak With Rice	1 meal (10 oz)	300	35	–
Pot Roast Beef	1 meal (10.5 oz)	230	60	–
Roast Chicken With Homestyle Gravy	1 meal (11 oz)	280	35	–
Roast Sirloin Supreme	1 meal (9 oz)	320	85	–
Sirloin Salisbury Steak	1 meal (11 oz)	280	40	–
Sirloin Salisbury Steak	1 meal (9 oz)	220	25	–
Sirloin Cheddar Melt	1 meal (9.4 oz)	380	85	–

FOOD	PORTION	CALS	CHOL	FIBER
Sirloin Of Beef In Herb Sauce	1 meal (9.5 oz)	250	30	–
Sirloin Of Beef In Wine Sauce	1 pkg (11 oz)	280	25	–
Sirloin Tips And Country Vegetables	1 meal (10 oz)	290	40	–
Special Recipe Sirloin Of Beef	1 meal (11 oz)	250	60	–
Stuffed Turkey Breast	1 pkg (11 oz)	250	35	–
Swedish Meatballs With Noodles	1 meal (10 oz)	590	145	–
Sweet And Sour Chicken	1 meal (10 oz)	340	30	–
Teriyaki Beef	1 pkg (10.75 oz)	260	30	–
Teriyaki Chicken Breast	1 meal (11 oz)	300	30	–
Fillo Factory				
Fillo Pie Broccoli & Cheese	¼ pie (4 oz)	350	20	3
Fillo Pie Spinach & Cheese	⅓ pie (4.8 oz)	210	15	2
Green Giant				
Create A Meal Broccoli Stir Fry as prep	1⅓ cups (9.9 oz)	290	60	4
Create A Meal Cheese & Herb Primavera as prep	1¼ cups (10 oz)	330	65	4
Create A Meal Garlic Herb as prep	1¼ cups (10 oz)	340	145	4
Create A Meal Hearty Vegetable Stew as prep	1¼ cups (10 oz)	280	55	3
Create A Meal Lemon Herb as prep	1½ cups (10 oz)	360	65	3
Create A Meal Mushroom & Wine as prep	1¼ cups (10 oz)	390	75	4
Create A Meal Vegetable Almond Stir Fry as prep	1⅓ cups (10 oz)	320	65	6

FOOD	PORTION	CALS	CHOL	FIBER
Healthy Choice				
Beef Pepper Steak Oriental	1 meal (9.5 oz)	260	35	2
Beef Pot Roast	1 meal (11 oz)	300	40	6
Beef Stoganoff	1 meal (11 oz)	320	60	7
Beef Tips Francais	1 meal (9.5 oz)	300	40	4
Beef Tips Portabello	1 meal (11.25 oz)	270	40	7
Bowls Chicken Teriyaki w/ Rice	1 meal (9.5 oz)	270	30	4
Bowls Country Chicken Bake	1 meal (9.5 oz)	230	50	4
Bowls Fiesta Chicken	1 meal (9.5 oz)	220	30	3
Bowls Garlic Lemon Chicken w/ Rice	1 meal (9.5 oz)	300	40	4
Bowls Roasted Potatoes w/ Ham	1 meal (8.5 oz)	210	30	6
Bowls Southwestern Chicken & Pasta	1 meal (9.5 oz)	320	40	6
Bowls Turkey Divan	1 meal (9.5 oz)	250	30	4
Charbroiled Beef Patty	1 meal (11 oz)	310	45	4
Chicken Cantonese	1 meal (10.75)	280	50	2
Chicken Parmigiana	1 meal (11.5 oz)	330	40	3
Chicken & Vegetables Marsala	1 meal (11.5 oz)	240	30	3
Chicken Broccoli Alfredo	1 meal (11.5 oz)	300	50	2
Chicken Dijon	1 meal (11 oz)	270	40	6
Chicken Teriyaki	1 meal (11 oz)	270	45	3
Country Breaded Chicken	1 meal (10.25 oz)	350	45	5
Country Glazed Chicken Breast	1 meal (8.5 oz)	250	30	3
Country Herb Chicken	1 meal (12.15 oz)	320	45	3
Country Inn Roast Turkey	1 meal (10 oz)	250	40	4
Garlic Chicken Milano	1 meal (9.5 oz)	260	35	3
Grilled Chicken Sonoma	1 meal (9 oz)	230	45	3

FOOD	PORTION	CALS	CHOL	FIBER
Grilled Chicken w/ Mashed Potatoes	1 meal (8 oz)	180	45	3
Herb Baked Fish	1 meal (10.9 oz)	340	35	5
Herb Breaded Pork Patty	1 meal (8 oz)	280	30	4
Homestyle Chicken & Pasta	1 meal (9 oz)	270	35	5
Honey Glazed Chicken	1 meal (10 oz)	270	45	4
Honey Mustard Chicken	1 meal (9.5 oz)	290	40	1
Lemon Pepper Fish	1 meal (10.7 oz)	320	30	5
Mandarin Chicken	1 meal (10 oz)	280	35	4
Mesquite Beef w/ Barbecue Sauce	1 meal (11 oz)	320	55	5
Mesquite Chicken Barbecue	1 meal (10.5 oz)	310	55	6
Oriental Style Chicken & Vegetable Stir Fry	1 meal (11.9)	360	25	5
Oven Roasted Beef	1 meal (10.15 oz)	280	50	4
Roast Turkey Breast	1 meal (8.5 oz)	220	25	5
Roasted Chicken	1 meal (11 oz)	230	50	4
Sesame Chicken	1 meal (10.8 oz)	360	20	4
Shrimp & Vegetables	1 meal (11.8 oz)	270	50	6
Sweet & Sour Chicken	1 meal (11 oz)	360	45	5
Traditional Meatloaf	1 meal (12 oz)	330	35	6
Tradtional Breast Of Turkey	1 meal (10.5 oz)	290	45	5
Tradtional Salisbury Steak	1 meal (11.5 oz)	330	50	6
Tuna Casserole	1 meal (8 oz)	240	25	4
Kid Cuisine				
Circus Show Corn Dog	1 meal (8.8 oz)	490	30	5
Cosmic Chicken Nuggets	1 meal (9.1 oz)	500	45	5
Futuristic Fish Sticks	1 meal (8.25 oz)	410	20	4
Game Time Taco Roll Up	1 meal (7.35 oz)	420	25	4

FOOD	PORTION	CALS	CHOL	FIBER
High Flying Fried Chicken	1 meal (10.1 oz)	440	70	3
Parachuting Pork Ribettes	1 meal (7.55 oz)	390	50	3
Lean Cuisine				
Cafe Classics Baked Chicken	1 pkg (8.6 oz)	240	30	3
Cafe Classics Baked Fish	1 pkg (9 oz)	290	40	2
Cafe Classics Beef Peppercorn	1 pkg (8.75 oz)	260	25	4
Cafe Classics Beef Portobello	1 pkg (9 oz)	220	35	2
Cafe Classics Beef Pot Roast	1 pkg (9 oz)	210	30	6
Cafe Classics Chicken Carbonara	1 pkg (9 oz)	280	30	4
Cafe Classics Chicken Cheese Medallions w/ Creamy Sauce	1 pkg (9.37 oz)	300	35	2
Cafe Classics Chicken Mediterranean	1 pkg (10.5 oz)	260	20	4
Cafe Classics Chicken & Vegetables	1 pkg (10.5 oz)	240	30	4
Cafe Classics Chicken In Peanut Sauce	1 pkg (9 oz)	260	30	4
Cafe Classics Chicken In Wine Sauce	1 pkg (8.1 oz)	220	45	2
Cafe Classics Chicken L'Orange	1 pkg (9 oz)	230	40	2
Cafe Classics Chicken Parmesan	1 pkg (10.9 oz)	300	35	5
Cafe Classics Chicken Piccata	1 pkg (9 oz)	300	30	2
Cafe Classics Chicken w/ Basil Cream Sauce	1 pkg (8.5 oz)	260	35	2
Cafe Classics Country Vegetables & Beef	1 pkg (9 oz)	210	25	3

FOOD	PORTION	CALS	CHOL	FIBER
Cafe Classics Fiesta Chicken	1 pkg (9.25 oz)	270	30	3
Cafe Classics Glazed Chicken	1 pkg (8.5 oz)	240	55	0
Cafe Classics Glazed Turkey Tenderloins	1 pkg (9 oz)	260	25	4
Cafe Classics Grilled Chicken	1 pkg (9.4 oz)	250	40	3
Cafe Classics Grilled Chicken Salsa	1 pkg (8.9 oz)	270	45	4
Cafe Classics Herb Roasted Chicken	1 pkg (8 oz)	190	35	4
Cafe Classics Honey Mustard Chicken	1 pkg (8 oz)	270	35	1
Cafe Classics Honey Roasted Chicken	1 pkg (8.5 oz)	270	25	5
Cafe Classics Honey Roasted Pork	1 serv (9.5 oz)	250	45	3
Cafe Classics Meatloaf w/ Whipped Potatoes	1 pkg (9.4 oz)	260	45	4
Cafe Classics Oriental Beef	1 pkg (9.25 oz)	210	25	2
Cafe Classics Oven Roasted Beef	1 pkg (9.25 oz)	260	50	4
Cafe Classics Roasted Turkey Breast	1 pkg (9.75 oz)	270	25	3
Cafe Classics Salisbury Steak	1 pkg (9.5 oz)	280	60	4
Cafe Classics Sirlion Beef Peppercorn	1 pkg (8.75 oz)	220	35	2
Cafe Classics Southern Beef Tips	1 pkg (8.75 oz)	270	35	4
Everday Favorites Vegetable Lasagna	1 pkg (10.5 oz)	260	20	5
Everyday Favorites Chicken Florentine	1 pkg (8 oz)	220	25	3
Everyday Favorites Chicken Chow Mein	1 pkg (9 oz)	240	35	3

FOOD	PORTION	CALS	CHOL	FIBER
Everyday Favorites Homestyle Turkey	1 pkg (9.4 oz)	240	40	3
Everyday Favorites Hunan Beef & Broccoli	1 pkg (8.5 oz)	240	20	2
Everyday Favorites Mandarin Chicken	1 pkg (9 oz)	260	35	2
Everyday Favorites Roasted Chicken	1 pkg (8.1 oz)	260	20	4
Everyday Favorites Stuffed Cabbage	1 pkg (9.5 oz)	210	20	5
Everyday Favorites Swedish Meatballs	1 pkg (9.1 oz)	290	45	4
Hearty Portions Cheese & Spinach Manicotti	1 serv	370	35	8
Hearty Portions Chicken & Barbecue Sauce	1 serv	370	40	6
Hearty Portions Homestyle Beef Stroganoff	1 serv	350	30	9
Hearty Portions Jumbo Rigatoni w/ Meatballs	1 serv	440	35	7
Hearty Portions Oriental Glazed Chicken	1 serv	370	35	4
Hearty Portions Roasted Chicken w/ Mushrooms	1 serv	330	40	4
Skillet Sensations Beef Teriyaki & Rice	1 serv	280	25	5
Skillet Sensations Chicken Primavera	1 serv	320	30	4
Skillet Sensations Chicken Oriental	1 serv	280	15	6
Skillet Sensations Fiesta Beef & Rice	1 serv	300	25	6

FOOD	PORTION	CALS	CHOL	FIBER
Skillet Sensations Garlic Chicken	1 serv	340	20	4
Skillet Sensations Herb Chicken & Roasted Potatoes	1 serv	270	40	5
Skillet Sensations Roasted Turkey	1 serv	220	25	6
Skillet Sensations Savory Beef & Vegetables	1 serv	290	35	9
Skillet Sensations Three Cheese Chicken	1 serv	370	50	3
Luigino's				
Chicken A La King With Noodles	1 pkg (8 oz)	240	60	2
Noodles With Chicken Peas & Carrots	1 cup (6.3 oz)	260	40	2
Noodles With Chicken Peas & Carrots	1 pkg (8 oz)	300	50	2
Sweet & Sour Chicken With Rice	1 pkg (8 oz)	300	20	2
Luzianne				
Cajun Creole Dirty Rice	1 serv	160	0	0
Cajun Creole Etouffee	1 serv	200	0	1
Cajun Creole Gumbo	1 serv	160	0	1
Cajun Creole Jambalaya	1 serv	200	0	1
Marie Callender's				
Beef Stroganoff w/ Noodles	1 meal (13 oz)	600	70	4
Beef Tips In Mushroom Sauce	1 meal (13 oz)	430	50	6
Breaded Chicken Parmigiana	1 meal (16 oz)	860	50	5
Breaded Fish w/ Mac & Cheese	1 meal (12 oz)	550	60	3
Cheesy Rice w/ Chicken & Broccoli	1 meal (12 oz)	390	55	6
Chicken & Dumplings	1 meal (14 oz)	390	130	4
Chicken & Noodles	1 meal (13 oz)	520	80	5

FOOD	PORTION	CALS	CHOL	FIBER
Chicken Cordon Bleu	1 meal (13 oz)	610	75	6
Chicken Fried Beef Steak & Gravy	1 meal (15 oz)	650	50	7
Chicken Teriyaki	1 meal (13 oz)	510	55	2
Country Fried Chicken & Gravy	1 meal (16 oz)	620	75	6
Country Fried Pork Chop	1 meal (15 oz)	540	65	8
Escalloped Noodles & Chicken	1 meal (13 oz)	740	90	5
Glazed Chicken	1 meal (13 oz)	490	90	1
Grilled Southwestern Style Chicken	1 meal (14 oz)	410	80	6
Grilled Chicken & Mashed Potatoes	1 meal (10 oz)	340	90	1
Grilled Chicken Breast & Rice Pilaf	1 meal (11.75 oz)	360	40	4
Grilled Chicken In Mushroom Sauce	1 meal (14 oz)	480	65	7
Grilled Turkey Breast & Rice Pilaf	1 meal (11.75 oz)	310	40	4
Herb Roasted Chicken & Mashed Potatoes	1 meal (14 oz)	580	205	7
Homestyle Turkey & Noodles	1 meal (12 oz)	600	90	5
Honey Roasted Chicken	1 meal (14 oz)	440	140	7
Honey Smoked Ham Steak w/ Macroni & Cheese	1 meal (14 oz)	490	80	5
Meatloaf & Gravy w/ Mashed Potatoes	1 meal (14 oz)	540	95	5
Old Fashioned Beef Pot Roast & Gravy	1 meal (15 oz)	500	110	3
Roast Beef	1 meal (14.5 oz)	390	70	11
Sirloin Salisbury Steak & Gravy	1 meal (14 oz)	550	85	6
Skillet Meal Au Gratin Potatoes	⅔ cup (5 oz)	190	30	2
Skillet Meal Beef Pot Roast	½ pkg	290	60	5

FOOD	PORTION	CALS	CHOL	FIBER
Skillet Meal Beef Stroganoff	½ pkg	310	60	5
Skillet Meal Chicken & Rice w/ Broccoli & Cheese	½ pkg	440	70	8
Skillet Meal Chicken Teriyaki	½ pkg	340	30	5
Skillet Meal Herb Chicken	½ pkg	290	35	5
Skillet Meal Roasted Chicken & Vegetables	½ pkg	260	40	7
Skillet Meal White & Wild Rice In Cheese Sauce	1 cup	300	35	2
Swedish Meatballs	1 meal (12.5 oz)	520	65	3
Sweet & Sour Chicken	1 meal (14 oz)	570	40	7
Turkey w/ Gravy & Dressing	1 meal (14 oz)	500	80	4
Morton				
Breaded Chicken Pattie	1 meal (6.75 oz)	290	35	4
Chicken Nuggets	1 meal (7 oz)	340	30	2
Chili Gravy w/ Beef Enchilada & Tamale	1 meal (10 oz)	270	10	7
Fried Chicken	1 meal (9 oz)	470	90	3
Gravy & Charbroiled Beef Patty	1 meal (9 oz)	310	20	5
Gravy & Salisbury Steak	1 meal (9 oz)	310	30	3
Gravy & Turkey w/ Stuffing	1 meal (9 oz)	240	40	4
Tomato Sauce w/ Meat Loaf	1 meal (9 oz)	250	20	3
Veal Parmagiana w/ Tomato Sauce	1 meal (8.75 oz)	290	25	4
My Own Meal				
Beef Stew	1 pkg (10 oz)	260	55	4

FOOD	PORTION	CALS	CHOL	FIBER
Chicken Mediterranean	1 pkg (10 oz)	270	45	4
Chicken Noodles	1 pkg (10 oz)	270	65	3
Chicken & Black Beans	1 pkg (10 oz)	240	40	6
Old World Stew	1 pkg (10 oz)	310	55	3
Nature's Choice				
Broccoli Parmesan Alfredo	1 pkg (12 oz)	270	10	5
Nature's Entrée				
Hearty Stew	1 pkg (12 oz)	290	10	3
Tuscany White Bean	1 pkg (12 oz)	330	5	4
Patio				
Ranchera	1 pkg (13 oz)	470	35	9
Stouffer's				
Baked Chicken Breast w/ Mashed Potatoes	1 serv (12.2 oz)	330	60	3
Beef Stroganoff	1 pkg (9.75 oz)	390	85	2
Chicken A La King	1 pkg (9.5 oz)	350	40	2
Creamed Chicken	1 pkg (6.5 oz)	260	80	0
Creamed Chipped Beef	½ cup (5.5 oz)	160	40	1
Creamy Chicken & Broccoli	1 pkg (8.9 oz)	320	60	2
Escalloped Chicken & Noodles	1 pkg (10 oz)	430	50	3
Fish w/ Macaroni & Cheese	1 serv (9.5 oz)	460	55	2
Glazed Chicken w/ Rice	1 serv (11.8 oz)	290	45	2
Green Pepper Steak	1 pkg (10.5 oz)	330	35	3
Homestyle Baked Chicken & Gravy & Whipped Potatoes	1 pkg (8.9 oz)	270	75	2
Homestyle Beef Pot Roast & Browned Potatoes	1 pkg (8.9 oz)	250	35	4
Homestyle Fish Filet w/ Macaroni & Cheese	1 pkg (9 oz)	430	70	2

FOOD	PORTION	CALS	CHOL	FIBER
Homestyle Fried Chicken & Whipped Potatoes	1 pkg (7.5 oz)	310	45	5
Homestyle Meatloaf & Whipped Potatoes	1 pkg (9.9 oz)	330	70	3
Homestyle Roast Turkey w/ Gravy Stuffing & Whipped Potatoes	1 pkg (9.6 oz)	320	50	3
Homestyle Salisbury Steak & Gravy & Macaroni & Cheese	1 pkg (9.6 oz)	350	70	2
Meatloaf	1 serv (5.5 oz)	210	60	1
Meatloaf w/ Whipped Potatoes	1 serv (11.5 oz)	380	70	4
Stuffed Pepper	1 pkg (10 oz)	200	20	3
Swedish Meatballs	1 pkg (10.25 oz)	480	60	3
Swanson				
Beef Pot Roast	1 pkg (14 oz)	320	35	4
Chicken Parmigiana w/ Spaghetti	1 pkg (11 oz)	380	25	5
Turkey Breast	1 pkg (11.7 oz)	330	40	4
Tamarind Tree				
Alu Chole	1 pkg (9.2 oz)	350	0	9
Channa Dal Masala	1 pkg (9.2 oz)	340	0	10
Dal Makhini	1 pkg (9.2 oz)	330	5	14
Dhingri Mutter	1 pkg (9.2 oz)	290	0	7
Navratan Korma	1 pkg (9.2 oz)	430	5	7
Palak Paneer	1 pkg (9.2 oz)	380	35	6
Saag Chole	1 pkg (9.2 oz)	370	0	13
Vegetable Jalfrazi	1 pkg (9.2 oz)	310	0	7
Tyson				
BBQ Chicken Potato & Vegetable Medley	1 pkg (14.7 oz)	560	30	9
Beef Stir Fry	1 pkg (14 oz)	430	45	4
Blackened Chicken Spanish Rice & Corn	1 pkg (8.8 oz)	260	30	4
Chicken Primavera	1 pkg (11.3 oz)	350	30	5

FOOD	PORTION	CALS	CHOL	FIBER
Chicken Divan Candied Carrots & Pasta	1 pkg (9.8 oz)	370	50	2
Chicken Francais Sliced Potatoes & Green Beans	1 pkg (8.8 oz)	260	45	6
Chicken Kiev Rice Pilaf & Broccoli Carrots	1 pkg (9.1 oz)	440	85	2
Chicken Marsala Carrots & Red Potatoes	1 pkg (8.8 oz)	180	30	4
Chicken Mesquite Corn & Pea Medley & Au Gratin Potatoes	1 pkg (8.8 oz)	320	25	4
Chicken Picatta	1 pkg (8.8 oz)	190	35	5
Chicken Stir Fry Kit	2¾ cups (14 oz)	430	45	5
Chicken w/ Broccoli & Cheese Carrots & Pasta	1 pkg (8.8 oz)	270	40	3
Chicken w/ Mushroom Sauce Rice Pilaf & Candied Carrots	1 pkg (8.8 oz)	220	30	2
Chicken w/ Tabasco BBQ Sauce	1 pkg (8.8 oz)	260	25	5
Fried Chicken & Gravy w/ Mashed Potatoes & Corn	1 pkg (10.8 oz)	360	30	4
Grilled Chicken Corn O'Brien & Ranch Beans	1 pkg (8.8 oz)	230	30	7
Grilled Italian Chicken Pasta & Vegetable Medley	1 pkg (8.8 oz)	190	30	3
Honey Dijon Chicken Pasta & Pea Medley	1 pkg (11.3 oz)	340	25	6

FOOD	PORTION	CALS	CHOL	FIBER
Roasted Chicken w/ Garlic Sauce Pasta & Vegetable Medley	1 pkg (8.8 oz)	210	25	3
Weight Watchers				
Smart One Grilled Salisbury Steak	1 pkg (8.5 oz)	250	40	3
Smart Ones Chicken Mirabella	1 pkg (9.2 oz)	180	20	4
Smart Ones Fiesta Chicken	1 pkg (8.5 oz)	210	25	5
Smart Ones Honey Mustard Chicken	1 pkg (8.5 oz)	200	30	3
Smart Ones Lemon Herb Chicken Piccata	1 pkg (8.5 oz)	190	25	3
Smart Ones Pepper Steak	1 pkg (10 oz)	240	35	4
Smart Ones Risotto w/ Cheese & Mushrooms	1 pkg (10 oz)	290	20	4
Smart Ones Roast Turkey Medallions & Mushrooms	1 pkg (8.5 oz)	180	20	2
Smart Ones Shrimp Marinara	1 pkg (9 oz)	180	40	4
Smart Ones Stuffed Turkey Breast	1 pkg (10 oz)	260	30	5
Smart Ones Swedish Meatballs	1 pkg (9 oz)	280	30	3
Yves				
Veggie Country Stew	1 pkg (10.5 oz)	170	0	7
DIP				
Breakstone's				
Bacon & Onion	2 tbsp (1.1 oz)	60	20	0
Chesapeake Clam	2 tbsp (1.1 oz)	50	20	0
Free Creamy Salsa	2 tbsp (1.1 oz)	20	<5	0
Free French Onion	2 tbsp (1.1 oz)	25	<5	0
Free Ranch	2 tbsp (1.1 oz)	25	<5	0

FOOD	PORTION	CALS	CHOL	FIBER
French Onion	2 tbsp (1.1 oz)	50	20	0
Toasted Onion	2 tbsp (1.1 oz)	50	20	0
Cheez Whiz				
Medium Cheese & Salsa	2 tbsp (1.2 oz)	100	20	0
Mild Cheese & Salsa	2 tbsp (1.2 oz)	100	20	0
Chi-Chi's				
Fiesta Bean	2 tbsp (0.9 oz)	35	0	1
Fiesta Cheese	2 tbsp (0.9 oz)	40	10	0
Fritos				
Bean	2 tbsp (1.2 oz)	40	0	0
Chili Cheese	1.2 oz	45	<5	0
French Onion	2 tbsp (1.1 oz)	60	15	0
Hot Bean	2 tbsp (1.2 oz)	40	0	1
Jalapeno & Cheddar Cheese	2 tbsp (1.2 oz)	50	5	0
Guiltless Gourmet				
Black Bean Mild	2 tbsp (1 oz)	30	0	1
Black Bean Spicy	2 tbsp (1 oz)	30	0	1
Heluva Good Cheese				
Bacon Horseradish	2 tbsp (1.1 oz)	60	20	0
Clam	2 tbsp (1.1 oz)	50	20	0
French Onion	2 tbsp (1.1 oz)	50	20	0
Homestyle Onion	2 tbsp (1.1 oz)	60	20	0
Light French Onion	2 tbsp (1.1 oz)	35	10	0
Light Jalapeno Cheddar	2 tbsp (1.1 oz)	40	10	0
Ranch	2 tbsp (1.1 oz)	60	20	0
Knudsen				
Free Creamy Salsa	2 tbsp (1.1 oz)	20	<5	0
Free French Onion	2 tbsp (1.1 oz)	25	<5	0
Free Ranch	2 tbsp (1.1 oz)	25	<5	0
Kraft				
Avocado	2 tbsp (1.1 oz)	60	0	0
Bacon & Horseradish	2 tbsp (1.1 oz)	60	0	0
Clam	2 tbsp (1.1 oz)	60	0	0
Free French Onion	2 tbsp (1.1 oz)	25	<5	0
Free Ranch	2 tbsp (1.1 oz)	25	<5	0
Free Salsa	2 tbsp (1.1 oz)	20	<5	0
French Onion	2 tbsp (1.1 oz)	60	0	0
Green Onion	2 tbsp (1.1 oz)	60	0	0
Jalapeno Cheese	2 tbsp (1.1 oz)	60	0	0

FOOD	PORTION	CALS	CHOL	FIBER
Premium Sour Cream	2 tbsp (1.1 oz)	50	20	0
Premium Sour Cream Bacon & Horseradish	2 tbsp (1.1 oz)	60	15	0
Premium Sour Cream Bacon & Onion	2 tbsp (1.1 oz)	60	20	0
Premium Sour Cream Creamy Onion	2 tbsp (1.1 oz)	45	15	0
Premium Sour Cream French Onion	2 tbsp (1.1 oz)	45	15	0
Premium Sour Cream Ranch	2 tbsp (1.1 oz)	50	15	0
Ranch	2 tbsp (1.1 oz)	60	0	0
Louise's				
Fat Free Honey Mustard	1 oz	40	0	0
Fat Free Sour Cream & Onion	1 oz	25	0	0
Fat Free White Cheese Peppercorn	1 oz	25	0	0
Marzetti				
Blue Cheese Veggie	2 tbsp	200	20	0
Lemon Dill Veggie	2 tbsp	140	25	0
Light Ranch Veggie	2 tbsp	60	10	1
Ranch Veggie	2 tbsp	140	25	0
Sour Cream & Onion	2 tbsp	130	25	0
Southwestern Veggie	2 tbsp	130	25	0
Spinach Veggie	2 tbsp	130	20	0
Old El Paso				
Black Bean	2 tbsp (1 oz)	20	0	1
Cheese 'n Salsa Medium	2 tbsp (1 oz)	40	<5	0
Cheese 'n Salsa Mild	2 tbsp (1 oz)	40	<5	0
Chunky Salsa Medium	2 tbsp (1 oz)	15	0	1
Chunky Salsa Mild	2 tbsp (1 oz)	15	0	1
Jalapeno	2 tbsp (1 oz)	30	<5	2
Ruffles				
French Onion	2 tbsp	70	0	1
Ranch	2 tbsp (1.2 oz)	70	0	0

FOOD	PORTION	CALS	CHOL	FIBER
Snyder's Of Hanover				
Microwavable Hot Nacho Cheese	2 tbsp	48	3	0
Microwavable Mild Cheese	2 tbsp	45	5	0
Mustard Pretzel	2 tbsp	60	0	0
Sour Cream & Onion	2 tbsp	60	15	0
Taco Bell				
Fat Free Black Bean	2 tbsp (1.2 oz)	30	0	2
Salsa Con Queso Medium	2 tbsp (1.2 oz)	45	<5	tr
Salsa Con Queso Mild	2 tbsp (1.2 oz)	45	<5	tr
Tyson				
Bleu Cheese For Dipping Wings	2 tbsp (1.4 oz)	140	25	1
Utz				
Fat Free Sour Cream & Onion	2 tbsp (1.1 oz)	30	0	0
Jalapeno & Cheddar	2 tbsp (1 oz)	30	0	0
Low Fat Desert Garden	2 tbsp (1.1 oz)	40	0	0
Low Fat Salsa Con Queso	2 tbsp (1 oz)	40	0	0
Mild Cheddar	2 tbsp (1 oz)	45	5	0
Sour Cream & Onion	2 tbsp (1 oz)	60	15	0
DOCK				
fresh cooked	3½ oz	20	0	–
raw chopped	½ cup	15	0	–
DOLPHINFISH				
fresh baked	3 oz	93	80	–
fresh fillet baked	5.6 oz	174	149	–
DOUGHNUTS				
cake type unsugared	1 (1.6 oz)	198	18	1
creme filled	1 (3 oz)	307	20	–
french cruller glazed	1 (1.4 oz)	169	5	–
honey bun	1 (2.1 oz)	242	4	1
jelly	1 (3 oz)	289	22	–
old fashioned	1 (1.6 oz)	198	18	1

FOOD	PORTION	CALS	CHOL	FIBER
sugared	1 (1.6 oz)	192	14	1
wheat glazed	1 (1.6 oz)	162	9	—
wheat sugared	1 (1.6 oz)	162	9	—
yeast glazed	1 (2.1 oz)	242	4	1
Dolly Madison				
Chocolate Frosted	1 (1.1 oz)	140	5	1
Donut Gems Chocolate	4 (2 oz)	260	10	1
Donut Gems Crunch	3 (2 oz)	220	10	0
Donut Gems Powdered	4 (2 oz)	230	15	0
English Cruller	1 (2 oz)	250	30	1
Glazed Whirl	1 (1.6 oz)	210	25	0
Glazed Yeast	1 (1.5 oz)	190	10	0
Old Fashioned	1 (2.1 oz)	280	20	0
Plain	1 (1.2 oz)	140	10	0
Powdered	1 (1 oz)	120	10	0
Dutch Mill				
Cider	1 (2.1 oz)	240	15	1
Cinnamon	1 (1.8 oz)	210	15	1
Donut Holes Double-Dipped Chocolate	3 (1.4 oz)	220	5	0
Donut Holes Shootin' Stars	3 (1.4 oz)	190	5	0
Double-Dipped Chocolate	1 (2.1 oz)	280	15	1
Glazed	1 (2.1 oz)	250	15	1
Glazed Chocolate	1 (2.4 oz)	270	15	1
Plain	1 (1.8 oz)	210	15	1
Sugared	1 (1.8 oz)	220	15	1
Freihofer's				
Assorted	1 (2 oz)	270	10	0
Hostess				
Blueberry	1 (1.7 oz)	210	10	0
Donettes Crumb	3 (1.5 oz)	170	10	0
Donettes Frosted	3 (1.5 oz)	200	10	0
Donettes Powdered	3 (1.5 oz)	180	10	0
Frosted	1 (1.4 oz)	180	5	0
O's Raspberry Filled	1 (2.2 oz)	230	5	1
Old Fashioned Glazed	1 (2.1 oz)	260	25	1
Plain	1 (1.1 oz)	140	10	0

FOOD	PORTION	CALS	CHOL	FIBER
Powdered	1 (1.3 oz)	150	10	0
Little Debbie				
Donut Sticks	1 (1.6 oz)	210	10	0
Mini Powdered	1 pkg (2.5 oz)	290	10	2
Tastykake				
Mini Plain Glaze	1 pkg (2.5 oz)	260	25	1
Mini Powdered Sugar	1 pkg (2.5 oz)	260	30	tr
Mini Rich Frosted	1 pkg (3 oz)	370	25	3
Tom's				
Chocolate Gem	1 pkg (2.5 oz)	320	10	1
Dunkin' Sticks	1 pkg (2.5 oz)	370	10	tr
Powdered Gems	1 pkg (2.5 oz)	320	10	1
DRINK MIXERS				
whiskey sour mix not prep	1 pkg (0.6 oz)	64	0	—
whiskey sour mix	2 oz	55	0	—
whiskey sour mix as prep	3.6 oz	169	0	—
Bacardi				
Margarita Mix w/o liquor	8 fl oz	100	0	—
Pina Colada	8 fl oz	140	0	—
Rum Runner	8 fl oz	140	0	—
Strawberry Daiquiri w/o liquor	8 fl oz	140	0	—
Canada Dry				
Collins Mixer	8 fl oz	120	0	0
Sour Mixer	8 fl oz	90	0	0
Daily's				
Bloody Mary Original	1 serv (6 oz)	50	0	—
Margarita Strawberry Daiquiri	1 serv (4 oz)	180	0	2
Margarita Green Demon	1 serv (3 oz)	80	0	—
Pina Colada	1 serv (3 oz)	160	0	1
Schweppes				
Collins Mixer	8 fl oz	100	0	0
Tabasco				
Bloody Mary Mix	1 serv (8.4 oz)	56	0	1

FOOD	PORTION	CALS	CHOL	FIBER
Bloody Mary Mix Extra Spicy	1 serv (8.4 oz)	58	0	2

DRUM

FOOD	PORTION	CALS	CHOL	FIBER
freshwater fillet baked	5.4 oz	236	126	—
freshwater baked	3 oz	130	70	—

DUCK

FOOD	PORTION	CALS	CHOL	FIBER
w/ skin roasted	1 cup (4.9 oz)	472	118	0
w/ skin w/ bone leg roasted	3 oz	184	97	—
w/ skin w/o bone breast roasted	3 oz	172	116	—
w/o skin roasted	1 cup (4.9 oz)	281	125	0
w/o skin w/ bone leg braised	1 cup (6.1 oz)	310	183	—
w/o skin breast broiled w/o bone	1 cup (6.1 oz)	244	249	—
wild w/ skin raw	½ duck (9.5 oz)	571	216	—
Grimaud Farms				
Muscovy Duck Confit	1 serv (3 oz)	170	95	—

DUMPLING

FOOD	PORTION	CALS	CHOL	FIBER
Health Is Wealth				
Potstickers Chicken Free	2 (1.6 oz)	80	0	1
Potstickers Pork Free	2 (1.6 oz)	80	0	1
Potstickers Vegetable	2 (1.6 oz)	90	0	5
Steamed Dumpling	2 (1.6 oz)	50	0	1
Pepperidge Farm				
Apple	1 (3 oz)	230	0	1
Peach	1 (3 oz)	320	0	4

DURIAN

FOOD	PORTION	CALS	CHOL	FIBER
fresh	3.5 oz	141	0	—

EEL

FOOD	PORTION	CALS	CHOL	FIBER
fresh cooked	1 fillet (5.6 oz)	375	257	—
fresh cooked	3 oz	200	137	—
raw	3 oz	156	107	—

FOOD	PORTION	CALS	CHOL	FIBER
EGG (see also EGG DISHES, EGG SUBSTITUTES)				
CHICKEN				
fresh	1	75	213	–
frozen	1	75	213	–
frozen	1 cup	363	1033	–
hard cooked	1	77	213	–
hard cooked chopped	1 cup	210	578	–
poached	1	74	212	–
white only	1	17	0	–
white only	1 cup	121	0	–
EggsPlus				
Fresh	1 (1.8 oz)	70	215	0
Horizon Organic				
Medium	1 (1.5 oz)	70	190	–
Organic Valley				
Brown Extra Large	1 (2.2 oz)	90	225	–
Brown Large	1 (2 oz)	80	200	–
Brown Medium	1 (1.8 oz)	70	175	–
OTHER POULTRY				
duck	1 (2.5 oz)	130	619	0
duck 100 year old	1 (1 oz)	49	173	–
duck preserved hard core	1 (1.8 oz)	80	220	0
duck preserved soft core	1 (1.8 oz)	80	220	0
duck salted	1 (1 oz)	54	184	–
quail	1 (9 g)	14	76	–
turkey	1 (2.7 oz)	135	737	–
EGG DISHES				
FROZEN				
Weight Watchers				
Handy Ham & Cheese Omelet	1 (4 oz)	220	30	2
TAKE-OUT				
deviled	2 halves	145	280	–
omelette plain	1 serv (3.5 oz)	172	350	0
salad	½ cup	307	562	–
scrambled plain	2 (3.3 oz)	199	400	0
scrambled w/whole milk & margarine	1 serv	365	774	–

FOOD	PORTION	CALS	CHOL	FIBER
sunny side up	1	91	211	—
EGG ROLLS				
egg roll wrapper fresh	1	83	3	—
Chun King				
Chicken Mini	6	210	15	2
Chicken Restaurant Style	1 (3 oz)	190	20	2
Pork & Shrimp Mini	6	210	15	2
Shrimp Mini	6	190	10	2
Shrimp Restaurant Style	1 (3 oz)	180	15	2
Empire				
Large	1 (3 oz)	190	2	2
Miniature	6 (4.8 oz)	280	0	4
Health Is Wealth				
Broccoli	1 (3 oz)	150	5	2
Oriental Vegetable	1 (3 oz)	160	0	2
Oriental Chicken Free	1 (3 oz)	120	0	2
Pizza	1 (3 oz)	200	0	3
Spinach	1 (3 oz)	180	0	3
Spring Rolls	1 (1.6 oz)	70	0	5
Veggie	1 (3 oz)	130	0	3
La Choy				
Chicken Mini	6	210	15	2
Chicken Restaurant Style	1 (3 oz)	210	15	2
Pork Restaurant Style	1 (3 oz)	220	10	2
Pork & Shrimp Bite Size	12	210	10	2
Pork & Shrimp Mini	6	210	15	2
Shrimp Mini	6	190	10	2
Shrimp Restaurant Style	1 (3 oz)	180	15	2
Sweet & Sour Chicken Restaurant Style	1 (3 oz)	220	15	2
Vegetable w/ Lobster Mini	6	190	5	2
Lo-An				
White Meat Chicken	1 (2.7 oz)	140	10	1

FOOD	PORTION	CALS	CHOL	FIBER
Luigino's				
Chicken	1 pkg (6 oz)	360	25	2
Pork & Shrimp	1 pkg (6 oz)	340	25	3
Shrimp	1 pkg (6 oz)	350	20	4
Sweet & Sour Chicken	1 pkg (6 oz)	400	25	4
Sweet & Sour Pork	1 pkg (6 oz)	360	15	4
Szechwan Vegetable	1 pkg (6 oz)	350	10	3
Worthington				
Vegetarian Egg Rolls	1 (3 oz)	180	0	2
TAKE-OUT				
lobster	1 (4.8 oz)	270	0	6
lumpia vegetable & shrimp	2 (3 oz)	120	10	2
meat & shrimp	1 (4.8 oz)	320	10	4
pork & shrimp	1 (5 oz)	300	15	7
shrimp	1 (3 oz)	170	<5	5
spicy pork	1 (3 oz)	200	5	3
vegetable	1 (3 oz)	170	0	4
EGG SUBSTITUTES				
frozen	¼ cup	96	1	—
frozen	1 cup	384	5	—
liquid	1 cup (8.8 oz)	211	3	—
liquid	1½ oz	40	tr	—
powder	0.35 oz	44	57	—
powder	0.7 oz	88	113	—
Better'n Eggs				
Fat Free Cholesterol Free	¼ cup (2 oz)	30	0	0
Egg Beaters				
Egg Substitute	¼ cup	30	0	0
Omelette Cheese	½ cup	110	5	—
Omelette Vegetable	½ cup	50	0	—
Morningstar Farms				
Breakfast Sandwich Bagel Scramblers Pattie Cheese	1 (5.9 oz)	320	10	4
Breakfast Sandwich English Muffin Scramblers Pattie	1 (5.1 oz)	240	5	5

FOOD	PORTION	CALS	CHOL	FIBER
Breakfast Sandwich English Muffin Scramblers Pattie Cheese	1 (6 oz)	280	10	5
Scramblers	¼ cup (2 oz)	35	0	0
Second Nature				
No Cholesterol	2 fl oz	60	0	—
No Fat	2 fl oz	40	0	—
No Fat With Garden Vegetables	2.5 fl oz	40	0	—
Simply Eggs				
Egg Substitute	1.75 fl oz	35	30	1
EGGNOG				
eggnog	1 cup	342	149	—
eggnog	1 qt	1368	596	—
eggnog flavor mix as prep w/ milk	9 oz	260	33	—
Hood				
Fat Free	4 fl oz	100	<5	0
Golden	4 fl oz	180	65	0
Light	4 fl oz	120	40	0
Select	4 fl oz	210	80	0
Oberweis				
Egg Nog	½ cup	240	40	0
EGGNOG SUBSTITUTES				
Silk				
Nog	½ cup	90	0	0
EGGPLANT				
cubed cooked	1 cup	28	0	3
raw cut up	½ cup (1.4 oz)	11	0	—
slices grilled	4 (7 oz)	38	0	—
whole peeled raw	1 (1 lb)	117	0	—
Progresso				
Caponata	2 tbsp (1 oz)	25	0	2
TastyBite				
Punjab Eggplant	½ pkg (5 oz)	130	0	4
TAKE-OUT				
baba ghannouj	¼ cup	55	0	—

FOOD	PORTION	CALS	CHOL	FIBER
caponata	2 tbsp (1 oz)	30	0	–
iman bayildi eggplant w/ onion & tomato	1 serv (15.6 oz)	345	0	2
indian eggplant runi	1 serv	180	0	1
papoutsakis little shoes	1 serv (15.5 oz)	245	40	1
ELDERBERRIES				
fresh	1 cup	105	0	–
ELDERBERRY JUICE				
elderberry	7 oz	76	0	–
ELK				
roasted	3 oz	124	62	–
EMU				
cooked	3 oz	130	111	–
ENDIVE				
fresh	3.5 oz	9	0	2
raw chopped	½ cup	4	0	–
ENERGY BARS				
AllGoode Organics				
Amazin' Peanut Raisin	1 bar	210	0	3
Banana Nut Nirvana	1 bar	190	0	3
Cashew Almond Passion	1 bar	210	0	3
Chocolate Peanut Pleasure	1 bar	200	5	3
Honey Nut Harvest	1 bar	210	0	3
Nutty Chocolate Apricot	1 bar	200	5	5
Back To Nature				
10th Tee Chocolate Fudge	1 bar	200	0	1
10th Tee Peanut Honey	1 bar	260	0	2
1st Tee Chocolate Peanut	1 bar	290	0	1
1st Tee Oatmeal Raisin	1 bar	280	0	1

FOOD	PORTION	CALS	CHOL	FIBER
Balance				
Oasis Strawberry Cheesecake	1 bar (1.69 oz)	180	0	tr
BeneFit				
Nutrition Bar	1 bar (2 oz)	240	0	tr
Benecol				
Chocolate Crisp	1 bar (1.2 oz)	130	5	2
Chocolate Crisp	1 bar (1.2 oz)	130	5	2
Peanut Crisp	1 bar (1.2 oz)	140	5	1
Better Bar				
Chocolate Coated Caramel Pecan	1 bar (1.8 oz)	180	0	0
Chocolate Coated Peanut	1 bar (1.8 oz)	180	0	0
Yogurt Coated Raspberry	1 bar (1.8 oz)	180	0	0
Breakthru				
Organic Chocolate Fudge	1 bar (2.1 oz)	230	0	3
Organic Cinnamon Crunch	1 bar (2.1 oz)	220	0	3
Organic Honey Graham	1 bar (2.1 oz)	220	0	3
Organic Mocha Fudge	1 bar (2.1 oz)	230	0	3
Carbolite				
Chocolate Peanut Butter Sugar Free	1 bar (1 oz)	144	4	0
Centrum				
Energy Chocolate Nougat	1 (1.98 oz)	220	0	tr
Energy Chocolate Peanut Butter	1 (1.98 oz)	220	0	tr
Clif Bar				
Apricot	1 bar (2.4 oz)	220	0	5
Carrot Cake	1 bar (2.4 oz)	240	0	5
Chocolate Brownie	1 bar (2.4 oz)	240	0	6
Chocolate Almond Fudge	1 bar (2.4 oz)	230	0	5

FOOD	PORTION	CALS	CHOL	FIBER
Chocolate Chip	1 bar (2.4 oz)	240	0	5
Chocolate Chip Peanut Crunch	1 bar (2.4 oz)	240	0	5
Cookies'N Cream	1 bar (2.4 oz)	230	0	5
Cranberry Apple Cherry	1 bar (2.4 oz)	220	0	5
Crunchy Peanut Butter	1 bar (2.4 oz)	240	0	5
GingerSnap	1 bar (2.4 oz)	230	0	6
DrSoy				
Double Chocolate	1 bar (1.76 oz)	180	0	1
Ensure				
All Flavors	1 bar (2.1 oz)	230	<5	1
Extend				
Chocolate Chip Crunch	1 bar (1.4 oz)	160	0	tr
Peanut Butter Crunch	1 bar (1.4 oz)	160	0	0
Fast Fuel Up				
Natural Chocolate Espresso	1 bar (2.3 oz)	300	0	3
Natural Chocolate Crunch	1 bar (2.3 oz)	300	0	3
Organic Chocolate Espresso	1 bar (1.8 oz)	230	0	2
Organic Chocolate Crunch	1 bar (1.8 oz)	230	0	2
Gatorade				
GatorBar	1 bar (1.17 oz)	110	0	1
GeniSoy				
Soy Protein Artic Frost Crispy Chocolate Mint	1 bar (2.2 oz)	230	0	2
Soy Protein Dutch Crunch Sour Apple Crisp	1 bar (2.2 oz)	230	0	1
Soy Protein Fair Trade Arabica Cafe Mocha Fudge	1 bar (2.2 oz)	220	0	1
Soy Protein New York Style Blueberry Cheesecake	1 bar (2.2 oz)	220	0	1

FOOD	PORTION	CALS	CHOL	FIBER
Soy Protein Obsession Fudge Cookies & Cream	1 bar (2.2 oz)	230	0	2
Soy Protein Pure Golden Honey Creamy Peanut Yogurt	1 bar (2.2 oz)	230	0	1
Soy Protein Southern Style Chunky Peanut Butter Fudge	1 bar (2.2 oz)	240	0	1
Soy Protein Ultimate Chocolate Fudge Brownie	1 bar (2.2 oz)	230	0	2
Xtreme Carrot Cake Quake	1 bar (1.6 oz)	190	0	1
Xtreme Peanut Butter Fix	1 bar (1.6 oz)	200	0	2
Xtreme Raspberry Rush	1 bar (1.6 oz)	190	0	2
Xtreme Rocky Roadtrip	1 bar (1.6 oz)	190	0	2
Glucerna				
All Flavors	1 bar (1.3 oz)	140	<5	4
Hansen's				
Chocolate Banana Crunch	1 bar	180	0	2
Chocolate Orchard Crunch	1 bar	170	0	2
Natural Bar Tropical Fruit Crunch	1 bar	170	0	1
Natural Bar Yogurt Strawberry Crunch	1 bar	190	0	1
HeartBar				
Cranberry	1 bar (1.8 oz)	190	0	3
Original	1 bar (1.76 oz)	180	0	3
Jenny Craig				
Meal Bar Chocolate Peanut	1 bar (2 oz)	220	0	1

FOOD	PORTION	CALS	CHOL	FIBER
Meal Bar Lemon Meringue	1 bar (2 oz)	210	0	0
Meal Bar Milk Chocolate	1 bar (2 oz)	210	0	1
Meal Bar Oatmeal Raisin	1 bar (1.97 oz)	210	0	3
Meal Bar Yogurt Peanut	1 bar (2 oz)	220	0	0
Kashi				
GoLean Chocolate Peanut Butter	1 (2.7 oz)	280	0	7
GoLean Honey Vanilla Yogurt	1 (2.7 oz)	280	0	7
GoLean Strawberry Vanilla Yogurt	1 (2.7 oz)	280	0	6
Lean Body For Her				
Chocolate Honey Peanut	1 bar (1.76 oz)	190	0	tr
Luna				
Chai Tea	1 bar (1.7 oz)	180	0	2
Chocolate Pecan Pie	1 bar (1.7 oz)	180	0	2
LemonZest	1 bar (1.7 oz)	180	0	2
Nutz Over Chocolate	1 bar (1.7 oz)	180	0	2
S'Mores	1 bar (1.7 oz)	180	0	2
Sesame Raisin Crunch	1 bar (1.7 oz)	170	0	2
Toasted Nuts 'n Cranberry	1 bar (1.7 oz)	170	0	2
Tropical Crisp	1 bar (1.7 oz)	180	0	2
Met-Rx				
Big 100 Gram Bar Peanut Butter	1 bar (3.5 oz)	340	15	2
Source/One Chocolate Cheesecake	1 bar (2.1 oz)	160	5	tr
NiteBite				
Chocolate Fudge	1 bar (0.9 oz)	100	5	0
Peanut Butter	1 bar (0.9 oz)	100	5	0

FOOD	PORTION	CALS	CHOL	FIBER
Nutiva				
Flaxseed & Raisin Organic	1 bar (1.4 oz)	280	0	6
Hempseed Bar Organic	1 bar (1.4 oz)	210	0	5
Nutribar				
Chocolate Covered Chocolate Fudge	1 bar (2.3 oz)	267	5	2
Odwalla Bar!				
Peanut Crunch	1 bar (2.2 oz)	260	0	3
PermaLean				
Protein Crunch Chocoholic Chocolate	1 bar (1.8 oz)	170	0	tr
Protein Crunch Chocolate Raspberry	1 bar (1.8 oz)	180	10	0
Protein Crunch Stark Raving Peanutz	1 bar (1.8 oz)	180	0	0
PowerBar				
Apple Cinnamon	1 bar (2.3 oz)	230	0	3
Banana	1 bar (2.3 oz)	230	0	3
Chocolate	1 bar (2.3 oz)	230	0	3
Essentials Chocolate	1 bar (1.9 oz)	180	0	3
Harvest Blueberry	1 bar (2.3 oz)	240	0	4
Harvest Strawberry	1 bar (2.3 oz)	240	0	4
Malt-Nut	1 bar (2.3 oz)	230	0	3
Mocha	1 bar (2.3 oz)	230	0	3
Oatmeal Raisin	1 bar (2.3 oz)	230	0	3
Peanut Butter	1 bar (2.3 oz)	230	0	3
Power Gel Strawberry Banana	1 pkg	110	0	–
Vanilla Crisp	1 bar (2.3 oz)	230	0	3
Wild Berry	1 bar (2.3 oz)	230	0	3
Revival				
Marshmallow Krunch	1 bar (2.1 oz)	220	0	tr
Protein Bars Chocolate Temptation	1 bar (2.1 oz)	220	0	tr
Protein Bars Peanut Butter Chocolate Pal	1 bar (2.1 oz)	240	0	1

FOOD	PORTION	CALS	CHOL	FIBER
Protein Bars Peanut Butter Pal	1 bar (2.1 oz)	240	0	tr
Slim-Fast				
Crispy Peanut Caramel	1 bar	120	<5	tr
Dutch Chocolate	1 bar	140	5	2
Meal On-The-Go Apple Cobbler	1 bar	220	<5	2
Meal On-The-Go Chocolate Cookie Dough	1 bar	220	<5	2
Meal On-The-Go Honey Peanut	1 bar	220	<5	2
Meal On-The-Go Milk Chocolate Peanut	1 bar	220	<5	2
Meal On-The-Go Oatmeal Raisin	1 bar	220	<5	2
Meal On-The-Go Rich Chocolate Brownie	1 bar	220	<5	2
Meal On-The-Go Toasted Oat & Spice	1 bar	220	<5	2
Peanut Butter	1 bar	150	5	2
Peanut Butter Crunch	1 bar	130	0	tr
Rich Chewy Caramel	1 bar	120	5	2
Sweet Success				
Chewy Chocolate Brownie	1 bar (1.2 oz)	120	3	3
Think!				
Apple Spice	1 bar (2 oz)	205	62	7
Chocolate Almond Coconut Raisin	1 bar (2 oz)	243	9	2
Chocolate Fruit Harvest	1 bar (2 oz)	217	38	7
ZonePerfect				
Honey Peanut	1 bar (1.8 oz)	200	0	1

FOOD	PORTION	CALS	CHOL	FIBER

ENERGY DRINKS
ARIZONA
Extreme Energy Shot	1 bottle (8.3 oz)	130	0	–

Boost
Chocolate	1 can (8 oz)	240	5	0
Vanilla	8 oz	240	5	0

California Joe
All Natural Protein Drink Mix as prep	1 serv (8 oz)	165	0	0

Calorie Shed
Shake Fat Free No Sugar Caramel Ripple	½ cup (4 fl oz)	70	5	2
Shake Fat Free No Sugar Chocolate	½ cup (4 fl oz)	70	5	2
Shake Fat Free No Sugar Marshmellow Nougat	½ cup (4 fl oz)	70	5	2

Fat Burner
Diet Fruit Punch	8 fl oz	0	0	–

Gatorade
Citrus Cooler	1 cup (8 oz)	50	0	–
Fruit Punch	1 cup (8 oz)	50	0	–
GatorLode	1 can (11.6 fl oz)	280	0	–
GatorPro	1 can (11 fl oz)	360	0	0
Grape	1 cup (8 oz)	50	0	–
Iced Tea Cooler	1 cup (8 oz)	50	0	–
Lemon-Lime	1 cup (8 oz)	50	0	–
Lemonade	1 cup (8 oz)	50	0	–
Orange	1 cup (8 oz)	50	0	–
Tropical Fruit	1 cup (8 oz)	50	0	–

GeniSoy
Soy Protein Shake Chocolate	1 scoop (1.2 oz)	120	0	2
Soy Protein Shake Vanilla	1 scoop (1.2 oz)	130	0	0
Soy Protein Shake Strawberry	1 scoop Banana	130	0	1

Hansen's
Energy Kiwi Strawberry	8 oz	120	0	–

FOOD	PORTION	CALS	CHOL	FIBER
EnergyPeach	8 oz	130	0	—
Energy Punch	8 oz	120	0	—
Healthy Start Carrot Orange Antioxidant Blend	8 oz	130	0	—
Healthy Start Citrus Punch Focus Blend	8 oz	130	0	—
Healthy Start Cranberry Grape Defense Blend	8 oz	110	0	—
Healthy Start Tropical Orange Vitamix Blend	8 oz	110	0	—
Healthy Pleasures				
Chocolate Irish Cream	1 bottle (10.5 oz)	260	6	0
Kashi				
GoLean Shake Man	1 pkg (2.5 oz)	260	0	7
GoLean Shake Woman	1 pkg (2.5 oz)	250	0	7
Nancy Grey's				
Shake Hi-Protein Black Raspberry	1 cup (8 fl oz)	340	65	0
Shake Hi-Protein Chocolate	1 cup (8 fl oz)	340	60	—
Shake Hi-Protein Vanilla	1 cup (8 fl oz)	340	65	—
Nantucket Nectars				
Super Nectars Ginkgo Mango	8 oz	150	0	—
Super Nectars Green Angel	8 oz	140	0	—
Super Nectars Protein Smoothie	8 oz	170	0	—
Super Nectars Red Guarana Tea	8 oz	110	0	—
Super Nectars Vital C	8 oz	130	0	—
NutraShake				
Citrus	1 pkg (4 oz)	200	0	—

FOOD	PORTION	CALS	CHOL	FIBER
Citrus Free	1 serv (4 oz)	200	0	0
Vanilla	1 serv (8 oz)	400	36	—
Vanilla No Added Sugar	1 serv (4 oz)	200	18	—
Piranha				
Phunky Fruit Punch	1 can (8.4 oz)	140	0	0
Pounds Off				
Dark Chocolate Ectasy	1 can (11 oz)	200	0	6
French Vanilla	1 can (11 oz)	220	0	5
Powerade				
Fruit Punch	8 fl oz	70	0	—
Lemon Lime	8 fl oz	70	0	—
Mountain Blast	8 fl oz	70	0	—
Red Bull				
Energy Drink	1 can (8.3 oz)	113	0	—
Slice				
All Sport Diet Lemon Lime	8 fl oz	1	0	—
All Sport Lemon Lime	8 fl oz	72	0	—
All Sport Orange	8 fl oz	74	0	—
All Sport Punch	8 fl oz	81	0	—
Slim-Fast				
Chocolate as prep w/ fat free milk	1 serv	190	9	2
Chocolate Malt as prep w/ fat free milk	1 serv	190	8	2
JumpStart Chocolate as prep w/ fat free milk	1 serv	240	14	5
JumpStart Vanilla as prep w/ fat free milk	1 serv	240	9	5
Strawberry as prep w/ fat free milk	1 serv	190	9	2
Vanilla as prep w/ fat free milk	1 serv	190	9	2
Snapple				
Sport Fruit	1 bottle	80	0	—
Sport Lemon	1 bottle	80	0	—
Sport Lemon Lime	1 bottle	80	0	—

FOOD	PORTION	CALS	CHOL	FIBER
Sport Orange	1 bottle	80	0	—
SoBe				
Adrenaline Rush	1 can (8.3 oz)	140	0	—
Drive	8 oz	120	0	—
Edge	8 fl oz	110	0	—
Elixir 3C Strawberry Carrot	8 fl oz	90	0	—
Jing Essentials	1 bottle (14 oz)	140	0	0
Jing Essentials Citrus Soy Blend	1 bottle (14 oz)	170	0	—
Karma	8 oz	120	0	—
Lean Sugar Free Metabolic Enhancer Diet Green Tea	8 fl oz	5	0	—
Lean Sugar Free Metabolic Enhancer Diet Orange Carrot	8 fl oz	10	0	6
Lizard Lightning Orange Mango	8 fl oz	130	0	—
Qi Essentials Berry Soy Blend	1 bottle (14 oz)	170	0	—
Qi Essentials	1 bottle (14 oz)	140	0	0
Shen Essentials	1 bottle (14 oz)	140	0	0
Shen Essentials Peach Soy Blend	1 bottle (14 oz)	170	0	—
Tsunami Orange Cream	8 fl oz	110	0	—
Sustacal				
Vanilla	8 oz	240	<5	tr
Sweet Success				
Creamy Milk Chocolate	1 can	200	4	3
Creamy Milk Chocolate as prep w/ skim milk	1 serv	180	6	6
The Pumper				
Body Building MilkShake Chocolate	1 serv (13.5 oz)	390	5	5
Body Building Milkshake Banana	1 serv (13.5 oz)	390	10	3

FOOD	PORTION	CALS	CHOL	FIBER
TwinLab				
Hydra Fuel	16 fl oz	132	0	–
Nitro Fuel	16 oz	460	0	–
Ultra Fuel	1 bottle (16 oz)	400	0	–
Ultra Slim-Fast				
Cafe Mocha as prep w/ fat free milk	1 serv	200	9	5
Chocolate Fudge as prep w/ fat free milk	1 serv	200	9	5
Chocolate Malt as prep w/ fat free milk	1 serv	200	9	5
Chocolate Royale as prep w/ fat free milk	1 serv	200	9	5
Fruit Juice Mixable as prep w/ juice	1 serv	200	5	5
Milk Chocolate as prep w/ fat free milk	1 serv	210	8	5
Ready-To-Drink Cappuccino Delight	1 serv	220	5	5
Ready-To-Drink Apple Cranberry Raspberry	1 serv	220	10	5
Ready-To-Drink Chocolate Royale	1 serv	220	5	5
Ready-To-Drink Creamy Milk Chocolate	1 serv	220	5	5
Ready-To-Drink Dark Chocolate Fudge	1 serv	220	5	5
Ready-To-Drink Orange Strawberry Banana	1 serv	220	10	5
Ready-To-Drink Orange Pineapple	1 serv	220	10	5
Ready-To-Drink Strawberries N' Cream	1 serv	220	5	5

FOOD	PORTION	CALS	CHOL	FIBER
Strawberry as prep w/ fat free milk	1 serv	200	9	4
Vanilla as prep w/ fat free milk	1 serv	200	9	5
Vita-J				
Apple Juice	11.5 fl oz	8	0	–
Fruit Punch	11.5 fl oz	8	0	–
Grapefruit Cocktail w/ Raspberry	11.5 fl oz	8	0	–
Orange Juice	11.5 fl oz	8	0	–
ENGLISH MUFFIN				
FROZEN				
Weight Watchers				
Sandwich	1 (4 oz)	210	20	2
READY-TO-EAT				
apple cinnamon	1	138	0	–
crumpets	1 (1.5 oz)	80	0	tr
granola	1	155	0	–
mixed grain	1	155	0	–
plain	1	134	0	–
plain toasted	1	133	0	–
raisin cinnamon	1	138	0	–
sourdough	1	134	0	–
wheat	1	127	0	–
whole wheat	1	134	0	4
Milton's				
Multi-Grain	1 (2 oz)	150	0	3
Pepperidge Farm				
Original	1	130	0	2
Wonder				
Cinnamon Raisin	1 (2.1 oz)	140	0	2
Original	1 (2 oz)	130	0	1
Sourdough	1 (2 oz)	130	0	1
TAKE-OUT				
w/ butter	1 (2.2 oz)	189	13	–
w/ cheese & sausage	1 (4 oz)	393	59	–
w/ egg cheese & canadian bacon	1 (4.8 oz)	289	234	2

FOOD	PORTION	CALS	CHOL	FIBER
w/ egg cheese & sausage	1 (5.8 oz)	487	274	—

EPAZOTE

fresh	1 tbsp (1 g)	tr	0	tr
fresh sprig	1 (2 g)	1	0	tr

EPPAW

raw	½ cup	75	0	—

FALAFEL

Casbah

Mix as prep	5	130	0	2

Near East

Falafel as prep patties	2½	230	0	5

TAKE-OUT

falafel	1 (1.2 oz)	57	0	—

FAT *(see also BUTTER, BUTTER SUBSTITUTES, MARGARINE, OIL)*

beef cooked	1 oz	193	27	—
beef suet	1 oz	242	19	—
beef tallow	1 tbsp (13 g)	115	14	—
chicken	1 cup	1846	174	—
chicken	1 tbsp	115	11	—
cocoa butter	1 tbsp	120	0	—
duck	1 tbsp (13 g)	115	13	0
goose	1 tbsp	115	13	—
lamb new zealand	1 oz	182	25	—
lard	1 tbsp (13 g)	115	12	—
lard	1 cup (205 g)	1849	195	—
pork backfat	1 oz	230	16	0
pork cooked	1 oz	178	26	0
salt pork	1 oz	212	25	—
shortening	1 cup	1812	0	—
shortening	1 tbsp	113	0	—
turkey	1 tbsp	115	13	—

Crisco

Butter Flavor	1 tbsp	110	0	—
Shortening	1 tbsp (0.4 oz)	110	0	—
Sticks	1 tbsp (0.4 oz)	110	0	0
Sticks Butter Flavor	1 tbsp (0.4 oz)	110	0	0

FOOD	PORTION	CALS	CHOL	FIBER
Empire				
Chicken Fat Rendered	1 tbsp (0.5 oz)	120	10	0
FAT SUBSTITUTES				
Smucker's				
Baking Healthy 100% Fat Free	1 tbsp	30	0	0
Soy Is Us				
Fat Not! Organic	3 tbsp	66	0	4
FAVA BEANS				
Progresso				
Fava Beans	½ cup (4.6 oz)	110	0	5
FEIJOA				
fresh	1 (1.75 oz)	25	0	–
puree	1 cup	119	0	–
FENNEL				
fresh bulb	1 (8.2 oz)	72	0	–
fresh sliced	1 cup	27	0	–
seed	1 tsp	7	0	–
FENUGREEK				
seed	1 tsp	12	0	–
FIBER				
Apple Fiber				
Pure	2 tbsp (7 g)	16	0	4
Benefiber				
Supplement	1 pkg (4 g)	20	0	3
Metamucil				
Fiber Wafers Apple Crisp	2	120	0	6
ND Labs				
Pure Apple Fiber	1 tbsp (7 g)	16	0	4
FIDDLEHEAD FERNS				
fresh	3.5 oz	34	0	–
FIGS				
calimyrna	3 (5.4 oz)	120	0	4
canned in heavy syrup	3	75	0	–
canned in light syrup	3	58	0	–

FOOD	PORTION	CALS	CHOL	FIBER
canned water pack	3	42	0	—
dried california	½ cup (3.5 oz)	200	0	17
dried cooked	½ cup	140	0	—
dried whole	10	477	0	17
fresh	1 med	50	0	—
Sonoma				
Dried White Misson	3-4 (1.4 oz)	110	0	5

FIREWEED

leaves chopped	1 cup (0.8 oz)	24	0	2

FISH *(see also individual names, FISH SUBSTITUTES, SUSHI)*

CANNED

Holmes

Finest Kippered Snacks drained	1 can (3.2 oz)	135	60	0
Port Clyde				
Fish Steaks In Louisiana Hot Sauce	1 can (3.75 oz)	150	80	0
Fish Steaks In Mustard Sauce	1 can (3.75 oz)	140	70	0
Fish Steaks In Soybean Oil With Hot Chilies drained	1 can (3.3 oz)	155	80	0
Fish Steaks In Soybean Oil drained	1 can (3.3 oz)	220	115	0

FROZEN

breaded fillet	1 (2 oz)	155	64	—
sticks	1 stick (1 oz)	76	31	—
Gorton's				
Baked Au Gratin	1 piece (4.6 oz)	130	50	—
Baked Broccoli Cheddar	1 piece (4.6 oz)	130	50	—
Baked Primavera	1 piece (4.6 oz)	120	50	—
Batter Dipped Portions	1 piece (2.5 oz)	170	20	—
Crunchy Golden Fillets Breaded	2 (3.8 oz)	250	35	—

FOOD	PORTION	CALS	CHOL	FIBER
Crunchy Golden Sticks	6 (3.8 oz)	250	30	—
Garlic & Herb	2 pieces (3.6 oz)	220	30	—
Garlic Butter Crumb	1 piece (4.6 oz)	170	55	—
Grilled Cajun Blackened	1 piece (3.8 oz)	120	60	—
Grilled Garlic Butter	1 piece (3.8 oz)	120	60	—
Grilled Italian Herb	1 piece (3.8 oz)	130	60	—
Grilled Lemon Butter	1 piece (3.8 oz)	120	60	—
Grilled Lemon Pepper	1 piece (3.8 oz)	120	60	—
Parmesan	2 pieces (3.6 oz)	260	30	—
Ranch	1 piece (3.6 oz)	240	30	—
Southern Fried Country Style	2 pieces (3.6 oz)	230	30	—
Tenders	3.5 pieces (4 oz)	250	30	—
Tenders Extra Crunchy	3.5 pieces (4 oz)	270	30	—
Kineret				
Fish Sticks	5 pieces (4 oz)	280	20	1
Van De Kamp's				
Battered Fish Fillets	1 (2.6 oz)	180	20	0
Battered Fish Nuggets	8 (4 oz)	280	25	0
Battered Fish Portions	2 pieces (5 oz)	350	35	0
Battered Fish Sticks	6 (4 oz)	260	30	0
Breaded Fillets	2 (3.5 oz)	280	35	0
Breaded Fish Portions	3 pieces (4.5 oz)	330	35	0
Breaded Fish Sticks	6 (4 oz)	290	35	0
Breaded Mini Fish Sticks	13 (3.3 oz)	250	30	0
Crisp & Healthy Breaded Fillets	2 (3.5 oz)	150	30	0
Crisp & Healthy Fish Sticks	6 (4 oz)	180	25	0
Fish 'n Fries	1 pkg (6.6 oz)	380	25	2
TAKE-OUT				
jamaican brown fish stew	1 serv	426	84	2
taramasalata	2 tbsp	124	10	—

FISH OIL

cod liver	1 tbsp	123	78	—

FOOD	PORTION	CALS	CHOL	FIBER
herring	1 tbsp	123	104	–
menhaden	1 tbsp	123	71	–
salmon	1 tbsp	123	66	–
sardine	1 tbsp	123	97	–

FISH SUBSTITUTES
Loma Linda
Ocean Platter not prep	⅓ cup (0.9 oz)	90	0	4

Worthington
Fillets	2 (3 oz)	180	0	4
Tuno	½ cup (1.9 oz)	80	0	1

FLAXSEED
Bite Me
Flax Bar	1 bar (1.8 oz)	242	0	12

Stone-Buhr
Flaxseed	1 tsp (1 oz)	150	0	5

FLOUNDER
FRESH
cooked	1 fillet (4.5 oz)	148	86	–
cooked	3 oz	99	58	–

FROZEN
Van De Kamp's
Lightly Breaded Fillets	1 (4 oz)	230	40	0
Natural Fillets	1 (4 oz)	110	45	0

TAKE-OUT
battered & fried	3.2 oz	211	31	–
breaded & fried	3.2 oz	211	31	–

FLOUR
buckwheat whole groat	1 cup (4.2 oz)	402	0	12
corn masa	1 cup (4 oz)	416	0	11
cottonseed lowfat	1 oz	94	0	–
peanut defatted	1 cup	196	0	–
peanut defatted	1 oz	92	0	–
peanut lowfat	1 cup	257	0	–
potato	1 cup (6.3 oz)	628	0	–
rice brown	1 cup (5.5 oz)	574	0	7
rice white	1 cup (5.5 oz)	578	0	4
rye dark	1 cup (4.5 oz)	415	0	29

FOOD	PORTION	CALS	CHOL	FIBER
rye light	1 cup (3.6 oz)	374	0	15
rye medium	1 cup (3.6 oz)	361	0	15
sesame lowfat	1 oz	95	0	—
triticale whole grain	1 cup (4.6 oz)	439	0	19
white all-purpose	1 cup (4.4 oz)	455	0	2
white bread	1 cup (4.8 oz)	495	0	3
white cake unsifted	1 cup (4.8 oz)	496	0	2
white self-rising	1 cup (4.4 oz)	443	0	3
white unbleached	1 cup (4.4 oz)	455	0	3
whole wheat	1 cup (4.2 oz)	407	0	15
All Trump				
Flour	¼ cup (1 oz)	100	0	tr
Aunt Jemima				
Self-Rising	3 tbsp	90	0	1
Betty Crocker				
Softasilk Velvet Cake Flour	¼ cup (1 oz)	100	0	tr
Gold Medal				
All Purpose	¼ cup (1 oz)	100	0	tr
Better For Bread	¼ cup (1 oz)	100	0	tr
Organic All Purpose	¼ cup (1 oz)	100	0	tr
Self Rising	¼ cup (1 oz)	100	0	tr
Unbleached	¼ cup (1 oz)	100	0	tr
Wondra	¼ cup oz)	100	0	tr
Hodgson Mill				
White Unbleached Organic	¼ cup (1 oz)	100	0	3
Whole Wheat Graham Organic	¼ cup (1 oz)	100	0	3
King Arthur				
All Purpose Unbleached	¼ cup (1 oz)	100	0	tr
La Pina				
Flour	¼ cup (1 oz)	100	0	1
Red Band				
All Purpose	¼ cup (1 oz)	100	0	tr
Self-Rising	¼ cup (1 oz)	100	0	tr
Robin Hood				
All Purpose	¼ cup (1 oz)	100	0	tr
Self-Rising	¼ cup (1 oz)	100	0	tr

FOOD	PORTION	CALS	CHOL	FIBER
Unbleached	¼ cup (1 oz)	100	0	tr
Whole Wheat	¼ cup (1 oz)	90	0	3
Stone Ground Mills				
White Unbleached Organic	¼ cup (1.4 oz)	130	0	1
Whole Wheat 100% Stone Ground	3 tbsp (1 oz)	90	0	3

FRENCH BEANS

dried cooked	1 cup	228	0	–

FRENCH FRIES (see POTATOES)

FRENCH TOAST
FROZEN

french toast	1 slice (2 oz)	126	48	2
Aunt Jemima				
Cinnamon Swirl	2 pieces (4.1 oz)	240	90	2
Slices	2 pieces (4.1 oz)	240	80	1
TAKE-OUT				
plain	1 slice	151	75	–
sticks	5 (4.9 oz)	513	75	3
w/ butter	2 slices (4.7 oz)	356	116	–

FROG'S LEGS
TAKE-OUT

as prep w/ seasoned flour & fried	1 (0.8)	70	12	–

FRUCTOSE
Estee

Fructose	1 tsp	15	0	0
Packet	1 pkg	10	0	0

FRUIT DRINKS (see also individual names)
FROZEN

limeade	1 can (6 oz)	408	0	–
Bright & Early				
Fruit Punch	8 fl oz	130	0	–
Five Alive				
Berry Citrus	8 fl oz	120	0	–
Citrus	8 fl oz	120	0	–
Tropical Citrus	8 fl oz	120	0	–

FOOD	PORTION	CALS	CHOL	FIBER
Tree Of Life				
Organic Smoothie Banana Raspberry Strawberry	⅔ cup (5 oz)	90	0	3
Organic Smoothie Mango Strawberry Raspberry	⅔ cup (5 oz)	70	0	4
Organic Smoothie Strawberry Banana	⅔ cup (5 oz)	90	0	3
Organic Smoothie Strawberry Blueberry Banana	⅔ cup (5 oz)	90	0	3
MIX				
Crystal Light				
Fruit Punch as prep	1 serv (8 oz)	5	0	0
Lemon-Lime Drink as prep	1 serv (8 oz)	5	0	0
Passion Fruit Pineapple Drink as prep	1 serv (8 oz)	5	0	0
Pineapple Orange Drink as prep	1 serv (8 oz)	5	0	0
Strawberry Orange Banana as prep	1 serv (8 oz)	5	0	0
Strawberry Kiwi as prep	1 serv (8 oz)	5	0	0
Watermelon Strawberry as prep	1 serv (8 oz)	5	0	0
Kool-Aid				
Cherry as prep	1 serv (8 oz)	60	0	0
Grape Berry Splash Drink as prep	1 serv (8 oz)	70	0	0
Grape Berry Splash Drink as prep w/ sugar	1 serv (8 oz)	100	0	0
Kickin' Kiwi Lime Drink as prep	1 serv (8 oz)	60	0	0
Kickin' Kiwi as prep w/ sugar	1 serv (8 oz)v			

FOOD	PORTION	CALS	CHOL	FIBER
Lemon-Lime Drink as prep w/ sugar	1 serv (8 oz)	100	0	0
Man-O-Mango Berry Drink as prep	1 serv (8 oz)	60	0	0
Man-O-Mango Berry Drink as prep w/ sugar	1 serv (8 oz)	100	0	0
Oh Yeah Orange Pineapple Drink as prep	1 serv (8 oz)	60	0	0
Oh Yeah Orange Pineapple Drink as prep w/ sugar	1 serv (8 oz)	100	0	0
Pina-Pineapple Drink as prep	1 serv (8 oz)	60	0	0
Pina-Pineapple Drink as prep w/ sugar	1 serv (8 oz)	100	0	0
Roarin' Raspberry Cranberry Drink as prep	1 serv (8 oz)	70	0	0
Roarin' Raspberry Cranberry Drink as prep w/ sugar	1 serv (8 oz)	100	0	0
Slammin' Strawberry Kiwi Drink as prep	1 serv (8 oz)	70	0	0
Slammin' Strawberry Kiwi Drink as prep w/ sugar	1 serv (8 oz)	100	0	0
Strawberry Raspberry Drink as prep	1 serv (8 oz)	60	0	0
Strawberry Raspberry Drink as prep w/ sugar	1 serv (8 oz)	100	0	0
Sugar Free Tropical Punch as prep	1 serv (8 oz)	5	0	0
Tropical Punch as prep	1 serv (8 oz)	60	0	0
Tropical Punch as prep w/ sugar	1 serv (8 oz)	100	0	0

FOOD	PORTION	CALS	CHOL	FIBER
Watermelon Cherry Drink as prep	1 serv (8 oz)	60	0	0
Watermelon Cherry Drink as prep w/ sugar	1 serv (8 oz)	100	0	0
Tang				
Orange Pineapple as prep	1 serv (8 oz)	100	0	0
READY-TO-DRINK				
fruit punch	6 fl oz	87	0	—
pineapple & orange drink	8 fl oz	125	0	—
After The Fall				
Amaretto Almond	1 can (12 oz)	170	0	0
American Pie Cherry	1 can (12 oz)	190	0	0
Apple Apricot	1 cup (8 oz)	100	0	0
Apple Raspberry	1 bottle (10 oz)	110	0	—
Apple Strawberry	1 bottle (10 oz)	120	0	—
Banana Casablanca	1 bottle (10 oz)	120	0	—
Berrymeister	1 can (12 oz)	160	0	0
Cranberry Meets Raspberry	1 bottle (10 oz)	120	0	—
Georgia Peach Blend	1 bottle (10 oz)	130	0	—
Mango Montage	1 bottle (10 oz)	140	0	—
Maui Grove	1 bottle (10 oz)	120	0	—
Nantucket Ginger Ale	1 can (12 oz)	140	0	0
Orange Icicle Cream	1 can (12 oz)	170	0	0
Oregon Berry	1 bottle (10 oz)	130	0	—
Passion Of The Islands	1 bottle (10 oz)	125	0	—
Peach Vanilla	1 can (12 oz)	170	0	0
Strawberry Vanilla	1 can (12 oz)	160	0	0
Twist O' Strawberry	1 can (12 oz)	190	0	0
Vanilla Bean Cream	1 can (12 oz)	170	0	0
Apple & Eve				
Apple Cranberry	8 oz	120	0	—
Boku				
White Grape Raspberry	16 fl oz	120	0	—
Capri Sun				
Fruit Punch	1 pkg (7 oz)	100	0	0
Maui Punch	1 pkg (7 oz)	100	0	0

FOOD	PORTION	CALS	CHOL	FIBER
Mountain Cooler	1 pkg (7 oz)	90	0	0
Pacific Cooler	1 pkg (7 oz)	100	0	0
Red Berry	1 pkg (7 oz)	100	0	0
Safari Punch	1 pkg (7 oz)	100	0	0
Strawberry Kiwi Drink	1 pkg (7 oz)	100	0	0
Surfer Cooler Drink	1 pkg (7 oz)	100	0	0
Citrus Squeeze				
California Punch	8 oz	130	0	—
Florida Punch	8 oz	120	0	—
Coco Lopez				
Mango Kiwi	8 fl oz	130	0	—
Crystal Geyser				
Juice Squeeze Citrus Grape	1 bottle (12 fl oz)	145	0	—
Juice Squeeze Orange & Passion Fruit	1 bottle (12 fl oz)	130	0	—
Juice Squeeze Passion Fruit & Mango	1 bottle (12 fl oz)	125	0	—
Juice Squeeze Wild Berry	1 bottle (12 fl oz)	130	0	—
Crystal Light				
Fruit Punch	1 serv (8 oz)	5	0	0
Kiwi Strawberry	1 serv (8 oz)	5	0	0
Orange Strawberry Banana Drink	1 serv (8 oz)	5	0	0
Del Monte				
Peach Raspberry	5.5 fl oz	160	0	3
Pineapple Banana Orange	5.5 fl oz	170	0	1
Strawberry Peach Banana	5.5 fl oz	150	0	1
Dole				
Apple Berry Burst	8 fl oz	120	0	—
Cranberry Apple	8 fl oz	120	0	—
Fruit Fiesta	8 fl oz	140	0	—
Fruit Punch	1 carton (10 oz)	160	0	—
Mountain Cherry	8 fl oz	150	0	—
Orange Peach Mango	8 oz	120	0	—
Orange Strawberry Banana	8 oz	120	0	—

FOOD	PORTION	CALS	CHOL	FIBER
Orchard Peach	8 oz	140	0	–
Pineapple Orange	8 oz	120	0	–
Pineapple Orange Strawberry	8 oz	130	0	–
Tropical Fruit	8 oz	160	0	0
Eden				
Organic Apple Cherry	8 oz Juice	120	0	1
Everfresh				
Cranberry-Apple Drink	1 can (8 oz)	120	0	0
Grape-Strawberry	1 can (8 oz)	120	0	0
Kiwi-Strawberry	1 can (8 oz)	120	0	0
Mandarin Orange Mango Drink	1 can (8 oz)	120	0	0
Orange Banana Strawberry Drink	1 can (8 oz)	120	0	0
Tropical Fruit Punch	1 can (8 oz)	120	0	0
Wild Blackberry Lime Drink	1 can (8 oz)	120	0	0
Five Alive				
Citrus	1 bottle (16 fl oz)	120	0	–
Citrus	1 can (11.5 fl oz)	170	0	–
Citrus Chilled	8 fl oz	120	0	–
Fresh Samantha				
Banana Strawberry	1 cup (8 oz)	130	0	6
Carrot Orange	1 cup (8 oz)	100	0	4
Desperately Seeking C	1 cup (8 oz)	110	0	7
The Big Bang	1 cup (8 oz)	100	0	8
Fruitopia				
Fruit Integration	8 fl oz	110	0	–
Guzzler				
Citrus Punch	8 fl oz	140	0	–
Island Punch	8 fl oz	140	0	0
Hansen's				
Juice Slam Wild Berry	1 box	120	0	–
Smoothie Apricot Nectar	1 can	170	0	–

FOOD	PORTION	CALS	CHOL	FIBER
Smoothie Cranberry Twist	1 can	180	0	—
Smoothie Energy Island Blast	1 can	170	0	—
Smoothie Guava Strawberry	1 can	170	0	—
Smoothie Mango Pineapple	1 can	170	0	—
Smoothie Peach Berry	1 can	170	0	—
Smoothie Pineapple Coconut	1 can	180	0	—
Smoothie Strawberry Banana	1 can	180	0	—
Smoothie Tropical Passion	1 can	170	0	—
Smoothie Whipped Orange	1 can	180	0	—
Smoothie Lite Cranberry Raspberry	1 can	50	0	—
Hood				
Natural Blenders Apple Cranberry Raspberry	1 cup (8 oz)	130	0	—
Natural Blenders Apple Grape Cherry	1 cup (8 oz)	130	0	—
Natural Blenders Apple Peach Pear	1 cup (8 oz)	120	0	—
Natural Blenders Apple Wild Blueberry Strawberry	1 cup (8 oz)	120	0	—
Natural Blenders Pineapple Orange Kiwi	1 cup (8 oz)	120	0	—
Juicy Juice				
Apple Grape	1 box (8.45 oz)	140	0	0
Berry	1 box (8.45 oz)	130	0	0
Punch	1 box (8.45 oz)	140	0	0
Punch	1 box (4.23 oz)	70	0	0
Tropical	1 box (8.45 oz)	140	0	0

FOOD	PORTION	CALS	CHOL	FIBER
Kool-Aid				
Bursts Great Bluedini	1 (7 oz)	100	0	0
Bursts Kickin' Kiwi Lime	1 (7 oz)	100	0	0
Bursts Oh Yeah Orange Pineapple	1 (7 oz)	100	0	0
Bursts Slammin' Strawberry Kiwi	1 (7 oz)	100	0	0
Bursts Tropical Punch	1 (7 oz)	100	0	0
Splash Grape Berry Punch	1 serv (8 oz)	120	0	0
Splash Kiwi Strawberry Drink	1 serv (8 oz)	110	0	0
Splash Tropical Punch	1 serv (8 oz)	120	0	0
Mauna La'i				
Island Guava	8 oz	130	0	0
Paradise Passion	8 oz	130	0	0
Mott's				
Berry	1 box (8 oz)	100	0	—
Fruit Punch	1 box (8 oz)	110	0	—
Fruit Punch	8 fl oz	130	0	—
Nantucket Nectars				
Apple Raspberry	8 oz	140	0	—
California Melonberry	8 oz	110	0	—
Cranberry Apple	8 oz	140	0	—
Fruit Punch	8 oz	130	0	—
Kiwi Berry	8 oz	120	0	—
Orange Passionfruit	8 oz	120	0	—
Orange Mango	8 oz	130	0	0
Peach Orange	8 oz	130	0	1
Pineapple Orange Banana	8 oz	140	0	—
Pineapple Orange Guava	8 oz	120	0	—
Watermelon Strawberry	8 oz	120	0	—
Oberweis				
Fruit Punch	8 oz	120	0	0
Ocean Spray				
Cran*Blueberry	8 oz	160	0	0

FOOD	PORTION	CALS	CHOL	FIBER
Cran*Cherry	8 oz	160	0	0
Cran*Currant	8 oz	140	0	0
Cran*Grape	8 oz	170	0	0
Cran*Mango	8 oz	130	0	0
Cran*Raspberry	8 oz	140	0	0
Cran*Raspberry Reduced Calorie	8 oz	50	0	0
Cran*Strawberry	8 oz	140	0	1
Cran*Tangerine	8 oz	130	0	0
Cranapple	8 oz	160	0	1
Cranapple Reduced Calorie	8 oz	50	0	0
Cranicot	8 oz	160	0	0
Crazy Kiwi Passion	8 oz	130	0	0
Fruit Punch	8 oz	130	0	0
Kiwi Strawberry	8 oz	120	0	0
Lightstyle Cran*Grape	8 oz	40	0	0
Lightstyle Cran*Mango	8 oz	40	0	0
Lightstyle Cran*Raspberry	8 oz	40	0	0
Mandarin Magic	8 oz	120	0	0
Ruby Red & Tangerine Grapefruit	8 oz	130	0	0
Ruby Red & Mango	8 oz	130	0	0
Pek				
Mango Guava Ecstasy	1 bottle (20 fl oz)	110	0	0
Passionate Peach Grapefruit	8 fl oz	110	0	0
Shasta Plus				
Apple-Strawberry	1 can (11.5 oz)	160	0	0
Fruit Punch	1 can (11.5 oz)	160	0	0
Pineapple-Cherry	1 can (11.5 oz)	160	0	0
Sipps				
Fruit Punch	8.45 oz	130	0	—
Snapple				
Cranberry Raspberry	8 fl oz	120	0	—

FOOD	PORTION	CALS	CHOL	FIBER
Diet Cranberry Raspberry	8 fl oz	10	0	—
Diet Kiwi Strawberry	8 fl oz	13	0	—
Fruit Punch	8 fl oz	110	0	—
Kiwi Strawberry	8 fl oz	110	0	—
Snapricot Orange	8 fl oz	120	0	—
Squeezit				
Berry B. Wild	1 bottle (7 oz)	110	0	0
Blue Raspberry	1 bottle (7 oz)	110	0	0
Cherry Cola	1 bottle (7 oz)	110	0	0
Chucklin' Cherry	1 bottle (7 oz)	110	0	0
Green Apple	1 bottle (7 oz)	110	0	0
Grumpy Grape	1 bottle (7 oz)	110	0	0
Lemon Lime	1 bottle (7 oz)	110	0	0
Rockin' Red Puncher	1 bottle (7 oz)	110	0	0
Smarty Arty Orange	1 bottle (7 oz)	110	0	0
Strawberry	1 bottle (7 oz)	110	0	0
Tropical Punch	1 bottle (7 oz)	110	0	0
Watermelon	1 bottle (7 oz)	110	0	0
Tropicana				
Berry Punch	8 fl oz	130	0	—
Citrus Punch	8 fl oz	140	0	—
Fruit Punch	1 container (10 fl oz)	160	0	—
Fruit Punch	8 oz	130	0	—
Orange Pineapple	8 fl oz	110	0	—
Tangerine Orange Juice	8 fl oz	110	0	—
Tropics Orange Strawberry Banana	8 fl oz	110	0	—
Tropics Orange Kiwi Passion	8 fl oz	100	0	—
Tropics Orange Peach Mango	8 fl oz	110	0	—
Tropics Orange Pineapple	8 fl oz	110	0	—
Twister Apple Raspberry Blackberry	1 bottle (10 fl oz)	160	0	—
Twister Citrus Punch	1 bottle (10 oz)	180	0	—

FOOD	PORTION	CALS	CHOL	FIBER
Twister Cranberry Punch	1 bottle (10 oz)	170	0	—
Twister Fruit Punch	1 bottle (10 oz)	170	0	—
Twister Light Orange Strawberry Banana	1 bottle (10 oz)	45	0	—
Twister Orange Cranberry	1 bottle (10 fl oz)	160	0	—
Twister Orange Strawberry Banana	1 bottle (10 oz)	160	0	—
Twister Ruby Red Tangerine	1 bottle (10 oz)	160	0	—
Twister Strawberry Kiwi	1 bottle (10 oz)	160	0	—
V8				
Splash Berry Blend	8 oz	110	0	—
Veryfine				
Apple Cranberry	1 bottle (10 oz)	190	0	0
Apple Quenchers Black Cherry White Grape	8 fl oz	120	0	0
Apple Quenchers Cranberry Tangerine	8 fl oz	120	0	0
Apple Quenchers Peach Kiwi	8 fl oz	130	0	0
Apple Quenchers Peach Plum	8 fl oz	130	0	0
Apple Quenchers Pear Passionfruit	8 fl oz	120	0	0
Apple Quenchers Raspberry Cherry	8 fl oz	120	0	0
Apple Quenchers Raspberry Lime	8 fl oz	120	0	0
Apple Quenchers Strawberry Banana	8 fl oz	120	0	0
Chillers Artic Mango Tangerine	8 fl oz	110	0	tr
Chillers Freezing Fruit Punch	8 fl oz	130	0	0

FOOD	PORTION	CALS	CHOL	FIBER
Chillers Lemon Lime Blizzard	8 fl oz	120	0	0
Chillers Shivering Strawberry Melon	1 can (11.5 oz)	160	0	0
Chillers Tropical Freeze	8 fl oz	120	0	0
Cranberry Raspberry	8 fl oz	160	0	0
Fruit Punch	1 bottle (10 oz)	170	0	0
Juice-Ups Berry	8 fl oz	140	0	0
Juice-Ups Fruit Punch	8 fl oz	140	0	0
Juice-Ups Orange Punch	8 fl oz	140	0	0
Orange Strawberry	8 fl oz	120	0	0
Papaya Punch	1 bottle (10 oz)	160	0	0
Pineapple Orange	1 bottle (10 oz)	160	0	0
Strawberry Banana	1 can (11.5 oz)	160	0	0
Strawberry Banana Punch	1 can (11.5 oz)	190	0	0
Wellfleet Farms				
Cranberry & Georgia Peach	8 oz	140	0	0
Cranberry & Granny Smith Apple	8 oz	130	0	0
Cranberry & Key Lime	8 oz	140	0	0

FRUIT MIXED (see also individual names)
CANNED

FOOD	PORTION	CALS	CHOL	FIBER
fruit cocktail in heavy syrup	½ cup	93	0	–
fruit cocktail juice pack	½ cup	56	0	–
fruit cocktail water pack	½ cup	40	0	–
fruit salad in heavy syrup	½ cup	94	0	–
fruit salad in light syrup	½ cup	73	0	–
fruit salad juice pack	½ cup	62	0	–
fruit salad water pack	½ cup	37	0	–
mixed fruit in heavy syrup	½ cup	92	0	–

FOOD	PORTION	CALS	CHOL	FIBER
tropical fruit salad in heavy syrup	½ cup	110	0	—
Del Monte				
Cherry Mixed Light Syrup	½ cup (4.4 oz)	90	0	1
Chunk Mixed In Heavy Syrup	½ cup (4.5 oz)	100	0	1
Chunky Mixed Fruit Naturals	½ cup (4.4 oz)	60	0	1
Chunky Mixed In Extra Light Syrup	½ cup (4.4 oz)	60	0	1
Citrus Salad	½ cup (4.4 oz)	80	0	0
Fruit Cocktail Fruit Naturals	½ cup (4.4 oz)	60	0	1
Fruit Cocktail In Extra Light Syrup	½ cup (4.4 oz)	60	0	1
Fruit Cocktail In Heavy Syrup	½ cup (4.5 oz)	100	0	1
Fruit Cup Fruit Naturals Mixed	1 pkg (4 oz)	50	0	1
Fruit Cup Mixed In Extra Light Syrup	1 pkg (4 oz)	50	0	1
Fruit Salad In Extra Light Syrup	½ cup (4.5 oz)	70	0	2
Fruit To Go Fruity Combo	1 pkg (4 oz)	70	0	1
Fruit To Go Wild Berry Jumble	1 pkg (4 oz)	80	0	1
Fruitrageous Crazy Cherry Mixed	1 pkg (4 oz)	90	0	1
Orchard Select California Mixed	½ cup (4.5 oz)	80	0	1
Orchard Select Premium Mixed	½ cup (4.4 oz)	80	0	tr
Snack Cups Mixed Fruit In Heavy Syrup	1 serv (4 oz)	80	0	1
SunFresh Ambrosia Salad	½ cup	70	0	1
Tropical Fruit Salad	½ cup (4.3 oz)	60	0	1

FOOD	PORTION	CALS	CHOL	FIBER
Tropical Fruit Salad In Light Syrup	½ cup (4.4 oz)	80	0	1
Very Cherry Mixed Fruit	½ cup (4.4 oz)	90	0	1
Dole				
FruitBowls Tropical Fruit	1 pkg (4 oz)	60	0	2
Tropical Fruit Salad	½ cup (4.3 oz)	80	0	1
Mott's				
Fruitsations Banana	1 pkg (4 oz)	90	0	—
Fruitsations Cherry	1 pkg (4 oz)	70	0	—
Fruitsations Mango Peach	1 pkg (4 oz)	70	0	—
Fruitsations Mixed Berry	1 pkg (4 oz)	90	0	1
Fruitsations Pear	1 pkg (4 oz)	90	0	—
Fruitsations Strawberry	1 pkg (4 oz)	80	0	—
Fruitsations Tropical Fruit	1 pkg (4 oz)	70	0	—
Hearlthy Harvest Peach Medley	1 pkg (3.9 oz)	50	0	1
Ocean Spray				
Cran*Fruit Cranberry Raspberry	¼ cup	120	0	2
Cran*Fruit Cranberry Strawberry	¼ cup	120	0	2
Sunfresh				
Ambrosia Salad	½ cup (4.5 oz)	70	0	1
Mixed Fruit In Light Syrup	½ cup (4.6 oz)	90	0	2
Tropical Salad In Extra Light Syrup	½ cup (4.5 oz)	80	0	0
White House				
Apple Banana Sauce	1 pkg (4 oz)	100	0	1
Apple Mixed Berry Sauce	1 pkg (4 oz)	110	0	1
Apple Peach Sauce	1 pkg (4 oz)	100	0	1
DRIED				
mixed	11 oz pkg	712	0	—

FOOD	PORTION	CALS	CHOL	FIBER
Del Monte				
Mixed	⅓ cup (1.4 oz)	110	0	5
Paradise				
Old English Fruit & Peel Mix	1 tbsp (0.8 oz)	70	0	1
Planters				
Fruit'n Nut Mix	1 oz	140	0	2
Sonoma				
Diced	⅓ cup (1.4 oz)	120	0	3
Mixed Fruit	5-8 pieces (1.4 oz)	120	0	3
Sun-Maid				
Tropical Medley	¼ cup (1.4 oz)	130	0	1
FROZEN				
mixed fruit sweetened	1 cup	245	0	—
Birds Eye				
Mixed Fruit	½ cup	90	0	—
Tree Of Life				
Organic Mixed Berries	¾ cup (5 oz)	60	0	3
FRUIT SNACKS				
fruit leather	1 bar (0.8 oz)	81	0	—
fruit leather pieces	1 oz	97	0	—
fruit leather pieces	1 pkg (0.9 oz)	92	0	—
fruit leather rolls	1 sm (0.5 oz)	49	0	—
fruit leather rolls	1 lg (0.7 oz)	73	0	—
Betty Crocker				
Fruit Gushers All Flavors	1 pkg (0.9 oz)	90	0	0
Fruit String Thing All Flavors	1 pkg (0.7 oz)	80	0	0
Brock				
Beauty & The Beast	1 pkg (0.9 oz)	90	0	—
Cinderella	1 pkg (0.9 oz)	90	0	—
Dinosaurs	1 pkg (0.9 oz)	90	0	—
Ninja Trolls	1 pkg (0.9 oz)	90	0	—
Sharks	1 pkg (0.9 oz)	90	0	—
CoolFruits				
Apple Grape	1 bar (0.5 oz)	51	0	1
Apple Strawberry	1 bar (0.5 oz)	51	0	1
Wild Blueberry	1 bar (0.5 oz)	51	0	1

FOOD	PORTION	CALS	CHOL	FIBER
Del Monte				
Sierra Trail Mix	1 pkg (0.9 oz)	110	0	2
Sierra Trail Mix	¼ cup (1.2 oz)	150	0	3
Sierra Trail Mix	1 pkg (1 oz)	120	0	2
Favorite Brands				
Cherry Fruit Snack	1 pkg (0.9 oz)	80	0	—
Creepy Crawler Fruit Snacks	1 pkg (0.9 oz)	80	0	—
Dinosaur Fruit Snack	1 pkg (0.9 oz)	80	0	—
Grape Fruit Snack	1 pkg (0.9 oz)	80	0	—
Space Alien Fruit Snack	1 pkg (0.9 oz)	80	0	—
Sports Fruit Snacks	1 pkg (0.9 oz)	80	0	—
Strawberry Fruit Snack	1 pkg (0.9 oz)	80	0	—
Teenage Mutant Ninja Turtle Fruit Snacks	1 pkg (0.9 oz)	80	0	—
Troll Fruit Snacks	1 pkg (0.9 oz)	80	0	0
Zoo Animal Fruit Snacks	1 pkg (0.9 oz)	80	0	—
General Mills				
Fruit Snacks All Flavors	1 pkg (0.9 oz)	80	0	0
Health Valley				
Bakes Apple	1 bar	70	0	2
Bakes Date	1 bar	70	0	2
Bakes Raisin	1 bar	70	0	2
Fruit Bars Apple	1	140	0	3
Fruit Bars Apricot	1	140	0	4
Fruit Bars Date	1	140	0	3
Fruit Bars Raisin	1	140	0	3
Seneca				
Apple Chips	12 chips (1 oz)	140	0	2
Sensible Foods				
Crackin' Fruit Cherry Berry	1 pkg (0.6 oz)	51	0	1
Crackin' Fruit Tropical Fruit	1 pkg (0.6 oz)	65	0	1
Sonoma				
Trail Mix	¼ cup (1.4 oz)	160	0	2
Stretch Island				
Fruit Leather Berry Blackberry	2 pieces (1 oz)	90	0	3

FOOD	PORTION	CALS	CHOL	FIBER
Fruit Leather Chunky Cherry	2 pieces (1 oz)	90	0	2
Fruit Leather Great Grape	2 pieces (1 oz)	90	0	2
Fruit Leather Organic Apple	2 pieces (1 oz)	90	0	2
Fruit Leather Organic Grape	2 pieces (1 oz)	90	0	2
Fruit Leather Organic Raspberry	2 pieces (1 oz)	90	0	2
Fruit Leather Rare Raspberry	2 pieces (1 oz)	90	0	2
Fruit Leather Snappy Apple	2 pieces (1 oz)	90	0	3
Fruit Leather Tangy Apricot	2 pieces (1 oz)	90	0	2
Fruit Leather Truly Tropical	2 pieces (1 oz)	90	0	1
Sunbelt				
Fruit Jammers	1 pkg (1 oz)	100	0	0
Sunkist				
100% Fruit Roll All Flavors	1 (0.5 oz)	50	0	1
Weight Watchers				
Apple & Cinnamon	1 pkg (0.5 oz)	50	0	2
Apple Chips	1 pkg (0.75 oz)	70	0	3
Peach & Strawberry	1 pkg (0.5 oz)	50	0	2
GARLIC				
clove	1	4	0	–
fresh chopped	1 tsp	4	0	1
powder	1 tsp	9	0	–
Dorot				
Frozen Crushed Cubes	1 cube (4 g)	5	0	0
Watkins				
Garlic & Chive Seasoning	1 tbsp (7 g)	25	5	0
Garlic Lover's Herb Blend	¼ tsp (0.5 oz)	0	0	0
Liquid Spice	1 tbsp (0.5 oz)	120	0	0

FOOD	PORTION	CALS	CHOL	FIBER
GEFILTE FISH				
sweet	1 piece (1.5 oz)	35	12	–
GELATIN				
MIX				
low calorie	½ cup	8	0	0
mix as prep	½ cup (4.7 oz)	80	0	–
mix not prep	1 pkg (3 oz)	324	0	–
mix w/ fruit	½ cup (3.7 oz)	73	0	–
Jell-O				
1-2-3-Brand Strawberry as prep	⅔ cup (5.2 oz)	130	0	0
Apricot as prep	½ cup (5 oz)	80	0	0
Berry Black as prep	½ cup (5 oz)	80	0	0
Berry Blue as prep	½ cup (5 oz)	80	0	0
Black Cherry as prep	½ cup (5 oz)	80	0	0
Cherry as prep	½ cup (5 oz)	80	0	0
Cranberry Raspberry as prep	½ cup (5 oz)	80	0	0
Cranberry Strawberry as prep	½ cup (5 oz)	80	0	0
Cranberry as prep	½ cup (5 oz)	80	0	0
Grape as prep	½ cup (5 oz)	80	0	0
Lemon as prep	½ cup (5 oz)	80	0	0
Lime as prep	½ cup (5 oz)	80	0	0
Mango as prep	½ cup (5 oz)	80	0	0
Mixed Fruit as prep	½ cup (5 oz)	80	0	tr
Orange as prep	½ cup (5 oz)	80	0	0
Peach as prep	½ cup (5 oz)	80	0	0
Peach Passion Fruit as prep	½ cup (5 oz)	80	0	0
Pineapple as prep	½ cup (5 oz)	80	0	0
Raspberry as prep	½ cup (5 oz)	80	0	0
Sparkling White Grape as prep	½ cup (5 oz)	80	0	0
Strawberry Banana as prep	½ cup (5 oz)	80	0	0
Strawberry Kiwi as prep	½ cup (5 oz)	80	0	0
Strawberry as prep	½ cup (5 oz)	80	0	0

FOOD	PORTION	CALS	CHOL	FIBER
Sugar Free Cherry as prep	½ cup (4.2 oz)	10	0	0
Sugar Free Cranberry as prep	½ cup (4.2 oz)	10	0	0
Sugar Free Lemon	½ cup (4.2 oz)	10	0	0
Sugar Free Lime as prep	½ cup (4.2 oz)	10	0	0
Sugar Free Mixed Fruit as prep	½ cup (4.2 oz)	10	0	0
Sugar Free Orange as prep	½ cup (4.2 oz)	10	0	0
Sugar Free Raspberry as prep	½ cup (4.2 oz)	10	0	0
Sugar Free Strawberry Banana as prep	½ cup (4.2 oz)	10	0	0
Sugar Free Strawberry as prep	½ cup (4.2 oz)	10	0	0
Sugar Free Strawberry Kiwi as prep	½ cup (4.2 oz)	10	0	0
Sugar Free Watermelon as prep	½ cup (4.2 oz)	10	0	0
Watermelon as prep	½ cup (5 oz)	80	0	0
Wild Strawberry as prep	½ cup (5 oz)	80	0	0
READY-TO-EAT				
Handi-Snacks				
Gels Blue Raspberry	1 serv (4 oz)	80	0	0
Gels Cherry	1 serv (4 oz)	80	0	0
Gels Orange	1 serv (3.5 oz)	80	0	0
Gels Strawberry	1 serv (3.5 oz)	80	0	0
Hunt's				
Snack Pack Juicy Gels Mixed Fruit	1 (4 oz)	100	0	0
Snack Pack Gels Cherry	1 serv (3.5 oz)	100	0	0
Snack Pack Gels Raspberry Berry	1 serv (3.5 oz)	100	0	0
Snack Pack Gels Strawberry	1 serv (3.5 oz)	100	0	0

FOOD	PORTION	CALS	CHOL	FIBER
Snack Pack Gels Strawberry Orange	1 serv (3.5 oz)	100	0	0
Jell-O				
Berry Black	1 serv (3.5 oz)	70	0	0
Berry Blue	1 serv (3.5 oz)	70	0	0
Cherry	1 serv (3.5 oz)	70	0	0
Orange	1 serv (3.5 oz)	70	0	0
Orange Strawberry Banana	1 serv (3.5 oz)	70	0	0
Raspberry	1 serv (3.5 oz)	70	0	0
Rhymin' Lymon	1 serv (3.5 oz)	70	0	0
Strawberry	1 serv (3.5 oz)	70	0	0
Strawberry Kiwi	1 serv (3.5 oz)	10	0	0
Sugar Free Orange	1 serv (3.2 oz)	10	0	0
Sugar Free Raspberry	1 serv (3.2 oz)	10	0	0
Sugar Free Strawberry	1 serv (3.2 oz)	10	0	0
Tropical Berry	1 serv (3.5 oz)	10	0	0
Tropical Fruit Punch	1 serv (3.5 oz)	70	0	0
Wild Watermelon	1 serv (3.5 oz)	70	0	0
Kozy Shack				
Gel Treat Cherry	1 pkg (4 oz)	100	0	1
Gel Treat Lemon Lime	1 pkg (4 oz)	100	0	1
Gel Treat Orange	1 pkg (4 oz)	100	0	1
Gel Treat Strawberry	1 pkg (4 oz)	100	0	1
Gel Treat Sugar Free Orange	1 pkg (4 oz)	10	0	1
Gel Treat Sugar Free Strawberry	1 pkg (4 oz)	10	0	1
Swiss Miss				
Gels Berry Strawberry	1 pkg (3.5 oz)	79	0	0
Gels Berry Lemon	1 pkg (3.5 oz)	79	0	0
Gels Raspberry Orange	1 pkg (3.5 oz)	79	0	0
Gels Strawberry Raspberry	1 pkg (3.5 oz)	79	0	0

GIBLETS

FOOD	PORTION	CALS	CHOL	FIBER
capon simmered	1 cup (5 oz)	238	629	–

FOOD	PORTION	CALS	CHOL	FIBER
chicken floured & fried	1 cup (5 oz)	402	647	—
chicken simmered	1 cup (5 oz)	228	570	—
turkey simmered	1 cup (5 oz)	243	606	—

GINGER
ground	1 tsp (1.8 g)	6	0	—
pickled	0.5 oz	5	0	tr
root fresh	¼ cup	17	0	—
root fresh	5 slices	8	0	—
root fresh sliced	¼ cup	17	0	—
Eden				
Pickled w/ Shiso Leaves	1 tbsp	15	0	1

GINKGO NUTS
canned	1 oz	32	0	—
dried	1 oz	99	0	—
raw	1 oz	52	0	—

GIZZARDS
chicken simmered	1 cup (5 oz)	222	281	—
turkey simmered	1 cup (5 oz)	236	336	—
Shady Brook				
Turkey	4 oz	130	180	—

GOAT
roasted	3 oz	122	64	—

GOOSE
w/ skin roasted	½ goose (1.7 lbs)	2362	708	—
w/ skin roasted	6.6 oz	574	172	—
w/o skin roasted	5 oz	340	138	—
w/o skin roasted	½ goose (1.3 lbs)	1406	569	—

GOOSEBERRIES
canned in light syrup	½ cup	93	0	—
fresh	1 cup	67	0	—

GRAPE JUICE
bottled	1 cup	155	0	—
frzn sweetened as prep	1 cup	128	0	—

FOOD	PORTION	CALS	CHOL	FIBER
frzn sweetened not prep	6 oz	386	0	—
grape drink	6 oz	84	0	—
Bright & Early				
Frozen	8 fl oz	140	0	—
Capri Sun				
Drink	1 pkg (7 oz)	100	0	0
Daily				
Drink	8 oz	110	0	
Everfresh				
Juice	1 can (8 oz)	150	0	0
Juicy Juice				
Drink	1 box (4.23 oz)	70	0	—
Drink	1 box (8.45 oz)	140	0	0
Kool-Aid				
Bursts Grape Drink	1 (7 oz)	100	0	0
Drink as prep w/ sugar	1 serv (8 oz)	100	0	0
Drink Mix as prep	1 serv (8 oz)	60	0	0
Sugar Free Drink Mix as prep	1 serv (8 oz)	5	0	0
Mott's				
100% Juice	1 box (8 oz)	130	0	—
Grape Juice	8 fl oz	130	0	—
Nantucket Nectars				
Grapeade	8 oz	130	0	—
Shasta Plus				
Grape Drink	1 can (11.5 oz)	160	0	0
Snapple				
Grapeade	8 fl oz	120	0	—
Veryfine				
100% Juice	1 bottle (10 oz)	200	0	0
Chillers Glacial Grape	1 can (11.5 oz)	160	0	0
Grape Drink	1 bottle (10 oz)	160	0	0
Juice-Ups	8 fl oz	130	0	0
Welch's				
100% White	8 oz	160	0	—
GRAPE LEAVES				
canned	1 (4 g)	3	0	0

FOOD	PORTION	CALS	CHOL	FIBER
fresh raw	1 (3 g)	3	0	tr
Cedar's				
Grape Leaves Stuffed With Rice	6 pieces (4.9 oz)	180	0	8
TAKE-OUT				
dolmas	5 (4.2 oz)	200	0	2
GRAPEFRUIT				
CANNED				
juice pack	½ cup	46	0	—
unsweetened	1 cup	93	0	—
water pack	½ cup	44	0	—
Sunfresh				
Red & White	½ cup (4.4 oz)	45	0	2
FRESH				
pink	½	37	0	1
pink sections	1 cup	69	0	1
red	½	37	0	—
red sections	1 cup	69	0	—
white	½	39	0	1
white sections	1 cup	76	0	1
Ocean Spray				
Fresh	2 oz	50	0	0
GRAPEFRUIT JUICE				
fresh	1 cup	96	0	—
frzn as prep	1 cup	102	0	—
frzn not prep	6 oz	302	0	—
sweetened	1 cup	116	0	—
After The Fall				
Pink	1 bottle (10 oz)	100	0	—
Apple & Eve				
Made In The Shade Ruby Red	8 fl oz	130	0	—
Crystal Geyser				
Juice Squeeze	1 bottle (12 fl oz)	150	0	—
Everfresh				
Juice	1 can (8 oz)	90	0	0
Ruby Red Cocktail	1 can (8 oz)	130	0	0
Fresh Samantha				
Juice	1 cup (8 oz)	90	0	0

FOOD	PORTION	CALS	CHOL	FIBER
Hood				
Select	1 cup (8 oz)	100	0	—
Mott's				
100% Juice	8 fl oz	110	0	—
Nantucket Nectars				
100% Juice	8 oz	100	0	—
100% Ruby Red	8 oz	100	0	—
Ocean Spray				
100% Juice	8 oz	100	0	0
100% Juice Pink	8 oz	110	0	0
Ruby Red Drink	8 oz	130	0	0
Snapple				
Juice	10 fl oz	110	0	—
Pink Grapefruit Cocktail	8 fl oz	120	0	—
Tropicana				
Golden	8 oz	90	0	—
Ruby Red	8 oz	90	0	—
Season's Best	8 oz	90	0	—
Twister Pink	1 bottle (10 oz)	140	0	—
W/ Double Vitamin C	8 fl oz	110	0	—
Veryfine				
100% Juice	1 bottle (10 oz)	110	0	0
Pink	1 bottle (10 oz)	150	0	0
Ruby Red	8 fl oz	120	0	0
GRAPES				
fresh	10	36	0	tr
thompson seedless in heavy syrup	½ cup	94	0	—
thompson seedless water pack	½ cup	48	0	—
Chiquita				
Grapes	1 ½ cups (4.8 oz)	90	0	1
GRAVY				
CANNED				
au jus	1 cup	38	1	—
beef	1 cup	124	7	—
beef	1 can (10 oz)	155	9	—
chicken	1 cup	189	5	—
mushroom	1 cup	120	0	—

FOOD	PORTION	CALS	CHOL	FIBER
turkey	1 cup	122	5	—
Campbell's				
Beef	¼ cup	29	1	tr
Brown	¼ cup	46	tr	1
Chicken	¼ cup	42	3	1
Turkey	¼ cup	29	2	tr
Rudy's Farm				
Sausage Gravy	¼ cup (2 oz)	50	10	0
MIX				
au jus as prep w/ water	1 cup	32	1	—
brown as prep w/ water	1 cup	75	2	—
chicken as prep	1 cup	83	3	—
mushroom as prep	1 cup	70	1	—
onion as prep w/ water	1 cup	77	tr	—
pork as prep	1 cup	76	3	—
turkey as prep	1 cup	87	3	—
Durkee				
Au Jus as prep	¼ cup	5	0	0
Brown as prep	¼ cup	10	0	0
Brown Mushroom as prep	¼ cup	15	0	0
Brown Onion as prep	¼ cup	15	0	0
Chicken as prep	¼ cup	20	0	0
Country as prep	¼ cup	35	0	0
Homestyle as prep	¼ cup	15	0	0
Mushroom as prep	¼ cup	15	0	0
Onion as prep	¼ cup	10	0	0
Pork as prep	¼ cup	10	0	0
Sausage as prep	¼ cup	35	0	0
Swiss Steak as prep	¼ cup	15	0	0
Turkey as prep	¼ cup	20	0	0
French's				
Au Jus as prep	¼ cup	5	0	0
Brown as prep	¼ cup	10	0	0
Chicken as prep	¼ cup	25	0	0
Country as prep	¼ cup	35	0	0
Herb Brown as prep	¼ cup	15	0	0
Homestyle as prep	¼ cup	10	0	0
Mushroom as prep	¼ cup	10	0	0
Onion	¼ cup	15	0	0

FOOD	PORTION	CALS	CHOL	FIBER
Pork as prep	¼ cup	10	0	0
Turkey as prep	¼ cup	20	0	0
Loma Linda				
Gravy Quik Brown	1 tbsp (5 g)	20	0	0
Gravy Quik Chicken	1 tbsp (5 g)	20	0	0
Quik Gravy Country	1 tbsp (5 g)	25	0	0
Quik Gravy Mushroom	1 tbsp (5 g)	15	0	tr
Quik Gravy Onion	1 tbsp (5 g)	20	0	tr
McCormick				
Beef & Herb as prep	¼ cup	30	<5	—

GREAT NORTHERN BEANS
CANNED

FOOD	PORTION	CALS	CHOL	FIBER
great northern	1 cup	300	0	14
Eden				
Organic	½ cup (4.6 oz)	110	0	8
Green Giant				
Great Northern	½ cup (4.4 oz)	100	0	6

DRIED

FOOD	PORTION	CALS	CHOL	FIBER
cooked	1 cup	210	0	—
Hurst				
HamBeens w/ Ham	3 tbsp (1.2 oz)	120	0	11

GREEN BEANS
CANNED

FOOD	PORTION	CALS	CHOL	FIBER
green beans	½ cup	13	0	1
italian	½ cup	13	0	1
italian low sodium	½ cup	13	0	1
low sodium	½ cup	13	0	1
Del Monte				
Cut	½ cup (4.2 oz)	20	0	2
Cut Italian	½ cup (4.2 oz)	30	0	3
Cut No Salt Added	½ cup (4.2 oz)	20	0	2
French Style	½ cup (4.2 oz)	20	0	2
French Style No Salt Added	½ cup (4.2 oz)	20	0	2
French Style Seasoned	½ cup (4.2 oz)	20	0	2
Whole	½ cup (4.2 oz)	20	0	2
Green Giant				
Cut	½ cup (4.2 oz)	20	0	1
Cut 50% Less Sodium	½ cup (4.2 oz)	20	0	1)

FOOD	PORTION	CALS	CHOL	FIBER
French Style	½ cup (4.1 oz)	20	0	1
Kitchen Sliced	½ cup (4.2 oz)	20	0	1
Whole	½ cup (4.1 oz)	25	0	2
Owatonna				
Cut	½ cup	20	0	—
French	½ cup	20	0	—
S&W				
Blue Lake Cut	½ cup (4.2 oz)	20	0	2
French Style	½ cup (4.2 oz)	20	0	2
Whole Small	½ cup (4.2 oz)	20	0	2
Veg-All				
French Style	½ cup	20	0	2
FRESH				
cooked	½ cup	22	0	—
raw	½ cup	17	0	1
FROZEN				
cooked	½ cup	18	0	—
italian cooked	½ cup	18	0	—
Birds Eye				
Cut	½ cup	25	0	2
Italian	½ cup	35	0	3
Green Giant				
Cut	¾ cup (2.8 oz)	25	0	2
Harvest Fresh & Almonds	⅔ cup (2.8 oz)	60	0	2
Harvest Fresh Cut	⅔ cup (2.9 oz)	25	0	2
Stouffer's				
Green Bean Mushroom Casserole	1 serv (4 oz)	130	2	2
Tree Of Life				
Cut	⅔ cup (2.8 oz)	25	0	2
GROUNDCHERRIES				
fresh	½ cup	37	0	—
GROUPER				
cooked	1 fillet (7.1 oz)	238	95	—
cooked	3 oz	100	40	—
raw	3 oz	78	31	—

FOOD	PORTION	CALS	CHOL	FIBER
GUAVA				
fresh	1	45	0	–
guava sauce	½ cup	43	0	–
GUAVA JUICE				
Nantucket Nectars				
Guava	8 oz	130	0	0
Snapple				
Guava Mania	8 fl oz	110	0	–
GUINEA HEN				
w/o skin raw	½ hen (9.3 oz)	292	166	–
HADDOCK				
fresh cooked	3 oz	95	63	–
fresh cooked	1 fillet (5.3 oz)	168	110	–
fresh raw	3 oz	74	49	–
roe raw	1 oz	37	103	–
smoked	3 oz	99	65	–
smoked	1 oz	33	21	–
Van De Kamp's				
Battered Fillets	2 (4 oz)	260	30	0
Breaded Fillets	2 (3.5 oz)	280	25	0
Lightly Breaded Fillets	1 (4 oz)	220	30	0
TAKE-OUT				
breaded & fried	1 piece (3.5 oz)	187	63	tr
HALIBUT				
atlantic & pacific cooked	½ fillet (5.6 oz)	223	65	–
atlantic & pacific cooked	3 oz	119	35	–
atlantic & pacific raw	3 oz	93	27	–
greenland baked	3 oz	203	50	–
Van De Kamp's				
Battered Fillets	3 (4 oz)	300	20	0
HALVA (see SESAME)				
HAM				
canned extra lean roasted	3 oz	116	26	0

FOOD	PORTION	CALS	CHOL	FIBER
center slice country style lean roasted	4 oz	220	80	0
chopped canned	1 oz	68	14	–
ham & cheese loaf	1 oz	73	16	–
ham & cheese spread	1 tbsp	37	9	–
ham salad spread	1 tbsp	32	6	–
minced	1 oz	75	20	–
patty cooked	1 patty (2 oz)	203	43	0
prosciutto	1 oz	55	20	0
sliced extra lean 5% fat	1 oz	37	13	–
sliced regular 11% fat	1 oz	52	16	–
steak boneless extra lean	1 (2 oz)	69	26	0
Alpine Lace				
Boneless Cooked 98% Fat Free	2 slices (2 oz)	60	25	0
Honey Ham 98% Fat Free	2 slices (2 oz)	60	25	0
Smoked Virginia 98% Fat Free	2 slices (2 oz)	60	25	0
Armour				
Chopped Ham canned	2 oz	130	35	0
Deviled Ham Spread	1 pkg (3 oz)	210	60	0
Lean Slices Brown Sugar	1 pkg (2.5 oz)	90	35	–
Star Canned	1 oz	34	11	–
Boar's Head				
Black Forest Smoked	2 oz	60	30	0
Cappy	2 oz	60	15	0
Deluxe	2 oz	60	25	0
Deluxe Lowered Sodium	2 oz	50	20	0
Maple Glazed Honey	2 oz	60	20	0
Pepper	2 oz	60	20	0
Rosemary & Sundried Tomato	2 oz	70	10	0
Sweet Slice Smoked	3 oz	100	30	0
Virgina	2 oz	60	25	0
Virginia Smoked	2 oz	60	25	0
Carl Buddig				
Ham Sliced w/ Natural Juices	1 pkg (2.5 oz)	120	40	–

FOOD	PORTION	CALS	CHOL	FIBER
Honey Ham Sliced w/ Natural Juice	1 pkg (2.5 oz)	120	40	—
Lean Slices Oven Roasted Honey Ham	1 pkg (2.5 oz)	90	35	—
Lean Slices Smoked	1 pkg (2.5 oz)	80	35	—
Healthy Choice				
Baked Cooked	3 slices (2.2 oz)	70	30	0
Cooked	3 slices (2.2 oz)	70	30	0
Deli-Thin Baked Cooked With Natural Juices	6 slices (2 oz)	60	25	0
Deli-Thin Cooked	6 slices (2 oz)	60	30	0
Deli-Thin Honey With Natural Juices	6 slices (2 oz)	60	25	0
Deli-Thin Smoked With Natural Juices	6 slices (2 oz)	60	25	0
Fresh-Trak Cooked	1 slice (1 oz)	30	10	0
Fresh-Trak Honey	1 slice (1 oz)	30	15	0
Honey Boneless	3 oz	100	40	0
Smoked	3 slices (2.2 oz)	70	30	0
Hillshire				
Deli Select Honey Ham	6 slices (2 oz)	60	25	0
Hormel				
Black Label Canned (refrigerated)	3 oz	100	40	0
Black Label Canned (self stable)	3 oz	110	45	0
Cure 81 Half Ham	3 oz	100	45	0
Curemaster	3 oz	80	40	0
Deviled Ham	4 tbsp (2 oz)	150	40	0
Ham & Cheese Patties	1 patty (2 oz)	190	45	0
Ham Patties	1 (2 oz)	180	35	0
Light & Lean 97 Sliced	1 slice (1 oz)	25	15	0
Primissimo Proscuitti	2 oz	120	50	0
Spiral Cure 81	3 oz	150	50	0
Jordan's				
Healthy Trim 97% Fat Free Cooked	1 slice (1 oz)	30	10	0

FOOD	PORTION	CALS	CHOL	FIBER
Healthy Trim 97% Fat Free EZ Serve	1 slice (1 oz)	30	15	0
Healthy Trim 97% Fat Free Virginia	1 slice (1 oz)	30	15	0
Louis Rich				
Carving Board Baked	2 slices (1.6 oz)	50	25	0
Carving Board Honey Glazed Thin	6 slices (2.1 oz)	70	30	0
Carving Board Honey Glazed Traditional	2 slices (1.6 oz)	50	25	0
Carving Board Smoked	1 slice (1.6 oz)	45	20	0
Dinner Slices Baked	1 slice (3.3 oz)	80	40	0
Mr. Turkey				
Deli Cuts Honey Cured	3 slices	35	20	—
Oscar Mayer				
Baked	3 slices (2.2 oz)	70	30	0
Boiled	3 slices (2.2 oz)	60	30	0
Chopped	1 slice (1 oz)	50	15	0
Dinner Slice	3 oz	80	40	0
Dinner Steaks	1 (2 oz)	60	30	0
Free Baked	3 slices (1.6 oz)	35	15	0
Free Honey	3 slices (1.6 oz)	35	15	0
Free Smoked	3 slices (1.6 oz)	35	15	0
Ham & Cheese Loaf	1 slice (1 oz)	70	20	0
Honey	3 slices (2.2 oz)	70	30	0
Lower Sodium	3 slices (2.2 oz)	70	30	0
Lunchables Cookies/Ham/Swiss	1 pkg (4.2 oz)	360	50	tr
Lunchables Dessert Chocolate Pudding/ Ham/American	1 pkg (6.2 oz)	390	55	tr
Lunchables Ham/Cheddar	1 pkg (4.5 oz)	340	75	0
Smoked	3 slices (2.2 oz)	60	30	0
Russer				
Baked	2 oz	70	30	—
Canadian Brand Maple	2 oz	70	30	—
Chopped	2 oz	130	30	—
Cooked Ham	2 oz	60	30	—
Ham & Cheese Loaf	2 oz	120	30	—

FOOD	PORTION	CALS	CHOL	FIBER
Honey & Maple Cured	2 oz	70	30	—
Honey Cured	2 oz	60	30	—
Hot	2 oz	70	30	—
Light Cooked	2 oz	60	30	—
Light Smoked	2 oz	60	30	—
Smoked Virginia	2 oz	70	30	—
Spiced	2 oz	160	30	—
Sara Lee				
Bavarian Brand Baked	2 oz	80	40	—
Bavarian Brand Baked Honey	2 oz	80	40	—
Golden Cure Smoked	2 oz	80	30	—
Honey Ham	2 oz	60	25	—
Honey Roasted	2 oz	90	30	—
Spam				
Spread	4 tbsp (2 oz)	140	40	0
Wampler				
Black Forest	2 oz	60	25	—

HAM DISHES
TAKE-OUT

FOOD	PORTION	CALS	CHOL	FIBER
croquettes	1 (3.1 oz)	217	77	tr
salad	½ cup	287	237	tr

HAM SUBSTITUTES
Yves

FOOD	PORTION	CALS	CHOL	FIBER
Veggie Ham Deli Slices	1 serv (2.2 oz)	80	0	1

HAMBURGER
Jimmy Dean

FOOD	PORTION	CALS	CHOL	FIBER
Burger	1 (2 oz)	220	40	0
Flamed Broiled Cheeseburger	1 (6.3 oz)	540	80	1
Mini Cheeseburger	2 (3 oz)	270	35	1
Kid Cuisine				
Buckaroo Beef Patty Sandwich w/ Cheese	1 meal (8.5 oz)	410	30	4
Rudy's Farm				
Mild Burger	1 (3 oz)	360	65	0
White Castle				
Cheeseburger	2 (3.6 oz)	310	30	6

FOOD	PORTION	CALS	CHOL	FIBER
Hamburger	2 (3.2 oz)	270	20	5
TAKE-OUT				
double patty w/ bun	1 reg	544	99	–
double patty w/ cheese & bun	1 reg	457	110	–
double patty w/ cheese & double bun	1 reg	461	80	–
double patty w/ cheese ketchup mayonnaise onion pickle tomato & bun	1 reg	416	60	–
double patty w/ ketchup mayonnaise onion pickle tomato & bun	1 reg	649	94	–
double patty w/ ketchup cheese mayonnaise mustard pickle tomato & bun	1 lg	706	141	–
double patty w/ ketchup mustard mayonnaise onion pickle tomato & bun	1 lg	540	122	–
double patty w/ ketchup mustard onion pickle & bun	1 reg	576	102	–
single patty w/ bacon ketchup cheese mustard onion pickle & bun	1 lg	609	112	–
single patty w/ bun	1 lg	400	71	–
single patty w/ bun	1 reg	275	36	–
single patty w/ cheese & bun	1 lg	608	96	–
single patty w/ cheese & bun	1 reg	320	50	–
single patty w/ ketchup cheese ham mayonnaise pickle tomato & bun	1 lg	745	122	–

FOOD	PORTION	CALS	CHOL	FIBER
single patty w/ ketchup mustard mayonnaise onion pickle tomato & bun	1 reg	279	26	—
triple patty w/ cheese & bun	1 lg	769	161	—
triple patty w/ ketchup mustard pickle & bun	1 lg	693	142	—

HAMBURGER SUBSTITUTES *(see also MEAT SUBSTITUTES)*
Amy's

All American Burger	1 (2.5 oz)	120	0	3
California Burger	1 (2.5 oz)	130	0	5
Chicago Burger	1 (2.5 oz)	160	5	3
Boca Burgers				
Hint of Garlic	1 patty (2.5 oz)	110	3	4
Vegan Original	1 patty (2.5 oz)	84	0	5
Franklin Farms				
Veggiburger Portabella	1 (3 oz)	120	0	4
GardenVegan				
Fat-Free Patty	1 patty (2.5 oz)	140	0	4
Gardenburger				
Classic Greek	1 (2.5 oz)	120	10	2
Fire Roasted Vegetable	1 (2.5 oz)	120	10	2
Hamburger Style	1 (2.5 oz)	90	0	3
Hamburger Style w/ Cheese	1 (2.5 oz)	110	5	3
Savory Mushroom	1 (2.5 oz)	120	10	4
Green Giant				
Southwestern Style	1 patty (3.2 oz)	140	0	5
Harmony Farms				
Soy Burgers Onion	1 (2.5 oz)	90	0	3
Soy Burgers Garlic	1 (2.5 oz)	110	0	23
Soy Burgers Mushroom	1 (2.5 oz)	110	0	3
Soy Burgers Original	1 (2.5 oz)	110	0	4
Lightlife				
Barbecue Grilles	1 patty (2.7 oz)	120	0	0
Lemon Grilles	1 patty (2.7 oz)	140	0	0
Light Burgers	1 (3 oz)	130	0	2
Tamari Grilles	1 patty (2.7 oz)	120	0	0

FOOD	PORTION	CALS	CHOL	FIBER
Loma Linda				
Patty Mix not prep	⅓ cup (0.9 oz)	90	0	5
Redi-Burger	⅝ in slice (3 oz)	120	0	4
Vege-Burger	¼ cup (1.9 oz)	70	0	2
Morningstar Farms				
Better'n Burger	1 (2.7 oz)	80	0	3
Garden Grille	1 patty (2.5 oz)	120	<5	4
Garden Veggie Patties	1 patty (2.4 oz)	100	0	4
Hard Rock Cafe Veggie Burger	1 (3 oz)	170	0	3
Harvest Burger Italian Style	1 patty (3.2 oz)	140	0	5
Harvest Burger Original	1 (3.2 oz)	140	0	5
Harvest Burger Southwestern	1 (3.2 oz)	140	0	5
Spicy Black Bean Burger	1 (2.7 oz)	110	0	5
Natural Touch				
Garden Veggie Pattie	1 (2.4 oz)	110	0	3
Okara Pattie	1 (2.2 oz)	110	0	3
Original Veggie Burger Kit not prep	¼ pkg (0.8 oz)	80	0	4
Southwestern Veggie Burger Kit not prep	¼ pkg (0.9 oz)	90	0	4
Spicy Black Bean Burger	1 (2.7 oz)	100	0	5
Vegan Burger	1 (2.7 oz)	70	0	3
NewMenu				
VegiBurger	1 patty (3 oz)	110	0	1
Sovex				
Better Than Burger?	½ cup (1.9 oz)	165	0	9
Superburgers				
Vegan Organic Original	1 (3 oz)	98	0	2
Vegan Organic Smoked	1 (3 oz)	98	0	2
Vegan Organic TexMex	1 (3 oz)	110	0	3
V'dora				
Vegetable BurgerLites	1 (3.3 oz)	58	0	0
Veggie Patch				
Burgeriffics	1 (2.5 oz)	110	0	4
Worthington				
Granburger not prep	3 tbsp (0.6 oz)	60	0	2
Prosage Patties	1 (1.3 oz)	80	0	2

FOOD	PORTION	CALS	CHOL	FIBER
Vegetarian Burger	¼ cup (1.9 oz)	60	0	1
Yves				
Black Bean & Mushroom Burgers	1 (3 oz)	100	0	7
Garden Vegetable Patties	1 (3 oz)	90	0	7
Veggie Burger	1 (3 oz)	119	0	4
Zoglo's				
Tender Vegetarian Burgers	1 (2.6 oz)	150	0	2
Vegetable Patties	1 (2.6 oz)	130	0	2
HAZELNUTS				
dried blanched	1 oz	191	0	—
dried unblanched	1 oz	179	0	—
dry roasted unblanched	1 oz	188	0	—
oil roasted unblanched	1 oz	187	0	2
Crumpy				
Chocolate Hazelnut Spread	1 tbsp (0.5 oz)	80	0	0
HEART				
beef simmered	3 oz	148	164	—
chicken simmered	1 cup (5 oz)	268	350	—
lamb braised	3 oz	158	212	—
pork braised	1 cup	215	320	0
pork braised	1	191	285	0
turkey simmered	1 cup (5 oz)	257	327	—
veal braised	3 oz	158	150	—
HEARTS OF PALM				
canned	1 cup (5.1 oz)	41	0	—
canned	1 (1.2 oz)	9	0	—
HEMP				
HempNut				
Shelled Hempseed	1 oz	162	0	2
Nutiva				
Hempseed	1½ tbsp (0.5 oz)	70	0	2

HERBAL TEA *(see* TEA/HERBAL TEA*)*

FOOD	PORTION	CALS	CHOL	FIBER
HERBS/SPICES (see also individual names)				
curry powder	1 tsp	6	0	—
garam masala	1 tsp	8	0	—
poultry seasoning	1 tsp	5	0	—
pumpkin pie spice	1 tsp	6	0	—
Chi-Chi's				
Seasoning Mix	1 tsp (3 g)	10	0	0
Eden				
Furikake Seasoning	½ tsp	5	0	1
Instant India				
Curry Paste Cilantro Garlic	2 tbsp (1 oz)	110	0	0
Curry Paste Ginger Garlic	2 tbsp (1 oz)	90	0	0
Lawry's				
Seasoning Blend Sloppy Joe	1 pkg	126	0	1
Mrs. Dash				
Extra Spicy	⅛ tsp (0.02 oz)	2	0	—
Garlic & Herb	⅛ tsp (0.02 oz)	2	tr	—
Lemon & Herb	⅛ tsp (0.02 oz)	2	0	—
Low Pepper	⅛ tsp (0.02 oz)	2	0	—
Original Blend	⅛ tsp (0.02 oz)	2	0	—
Table Blend	⅛ tsp (0.02 oz)	2	0	—
Watkins				
Apple Bake Seasoning	¼ tsp (0.5 g)	0	0	0
Barbecue Spice	¼ tsp (0.5 g)	0	0	0
Bean Soup Seasoning	¾ tsp (2 g)	5	0	0
Beef Jerky Seasoning	2 tsp (6 g)	15	0	0
Chicken Seasoning	½ tsp (1 g)	0	0	0
Cole Slaw Seasoning	½ tsp (1.5 g)	5	0	0
Egg Sensations	1 tsp (3 g)	10	0	0
Fajita Seasoning	½ tsp (3 g)	10	0	0
Grill Seasoning	¼ tsp (1 g)	0	0	0
Ground Beef Seasoning	⅛ tsp (0.5 g)	0	0	0
Italian Blend	1 tsp (3 g)	1	0	0
Meat Tenderizer	⅛ tsp (0.5 g)	0	0	0
Meatloaf Seasoning	½ tsp (5 g)	15	0	0
Mexican Blend	½ tbsp (4 g)	15	0	0

FOOD	PORTION	CALS	CHOL	FIBER
Omelet & Souffle Seasoning	¾ tsp (2 g)	5	0	0
Oriental Ginger Garlic Liquid Spice Blend	1 tbsp (0.5 oz)	120	0	0
Potato Salad Seasoning	¼ tsp (1 g)	0	0	0
Pumpkin Pie Spice	¼ tsp (0.5 g)	0	0	0
Smokehouse Liquid Blend	1 tbsp (0.5 oz)	120	0	0
Soup & Vegetable Seasoning	¼ tsp (0.5 g)	0	0	0
Spanish Seasoning Blend	¼ tsp (0.5 oz)	0	0	0
HERRING				
atlantic cooked	3 oz	172	65	—
atlantic cooked	1 fillet (5 oz)	290	110	—
atlantic raw	3 oz	134	51	—
pacific baked	3 oz	213	84	—
pacific fillet baked	5.1 oz	360	142	—
roe raw	1 oz	37	103	—
smoked	3.5 oz	210	70	0
TAKE-OUT				
atlantic kippered	1 fillet (1.4 oz)	87	33	—
atlantic pickled	½ oz	39	2	—
fried	1 serv (3.5 oz)	233	69	0
HICKORY NUTS				
dried	1 oz	187	0	—
HOMINY				
CANNED				
white	1 cup (5.6 oz)	482	0	4
Van Camp				
Golden	½ cup (4.3 oz)	80	0	1
White	½ cup (4.3 oz)	80	0	1
HONEY				
honey	1 cup (11.9 oz)	1031	0	—
honey	1 tbsp (0.7 oz)	64	0	—
wild honey	1 tbsp	60	0	—
HONEYDEW				
FRESH				
cubed	1 cup	60	0	—

FOOD	PORTION	CALS	CHOL	FIBER
wedge	1/10	46	0	–
Chiquita				
Wedge	1/10 melon (4.7 oz)	50	0	1

HORSE

roasted	3 oz	149	58	–

HORSERADISH

japanese wasabi	1/4 tsp	1	0	0
wasabi root raw	1 (5.9 oz)	184	0	12
wasabi root raw sliced	1 cup (4.6 oz)	142	0	10
Boar's Head				
Horseradish	1 tsp (5 g)	5	0	0
Eden				
Wasabi Powder	1 tsp	10	0	1
Hebrew National				
White	1 tbsp	7	0	–
Heluva Good Cheese				
Horseradish	1 tsp (5 g)	0	0	–
Kraft				
Cream Style	1 tsp (5 g)	0	0	0
Horseradish Sauce	1 tsp (5 g)	20	<5	0
Prepared	1 tsp (5 g)	0	0	0
Rosoff's				
Red	1 tbsp (0.5 oz)	8	0	–
White	1 tbsp (0.5 oz)	7	0	–
Schorr's				
Red	1 tbsp (0.5 oz)	8	0	–
White	1 tbsp (0.5 oz)	7	0	–

HOT COCOA (see COCOA)

HOT DOG

beef	1 (2 oz)	180	35	–
beef	1 (1.5)	142	27	–
beef & pork	1 (2 oz)	183	29	–
beef & pork	1 (1.5 oz)	144	22	–
chicken	1 (1.5 oz)	116	45	–
pork cheesefurter smokie	1 (1.5 oz)	141	29	–
turkey	1 (1.5 oz)	102	48	–

FOOD	PORTION	CALS	CHOL	FIBER
Applegate Farms				
Chicken Natural Uncured	1 (1.5 oz)	120	40	0
Natural Turkey	1 (1.5 oz)	120	40	0
Armour				
Star Jumbo Beef	1	190	30	—
Boar's Head				
Beef	1 (2 oz)	160	30	0
Beef Lite	1 (1.6 oz)	90	25	0
Pork & Beef	1 (2 oz)	150	25	0
Empire				
Chicken	1 (2 oz)	100	70	0
Turkey	1 (2 oz)	90	35	0
Health Is Wealth				
Uncured Beef	1 (1.5 oz)	80	20	—
Uncured Chicken	1 (1.5 oz)	100	30	—
Healthy Choice				
Beef Low Fat	1 (1.8 oz)	70	15	0
Bunsize	1 (2 oz)	70	20	0
Jumbo	1 (2 oz)	70	20	0
Low Fat Turkey Pork Beef	1 (1.4 oz)	60	10	—
Hebrew National				
Beef	1 (1.7 oz)	150	30	—
Cocktail Beef	6 (1.8 oz)	160	35	—
Dinner Beef	1 (4 oz)	350	75	—
Reduced Fat Beef	1 (1.7 oz)	120	25	—
Hormel				
Fat Free	1 (1.8 oz)	45	15	0
Fat Free Beef	1 (1.8 oz)	45	10	0
Jordan's				
Healthy Trim Low Fat	1 (1.8 oz)	70	25	0
Healthy Trim Low Fat Skinless	1 (1.8 oz)	70	25	0
Kid Cuisine				
Mystical Mini Corn Dogs	4 pieces	230	35	0
Louis Rich				
Bun Length	1 (2 oz)	110	55	0
Cheese	1 (1.6 oz)	90	40	0

FOOD	PORTION	CALS	CHOL	FIBER
Franks	1 (1.6 oz)	80	40	0
Mr. Turkey				
Bun Size	1	130	50	—
Cheese	1	140	50	—
Hot Dog	1	110	40	—
Organic Valley				
All-Natural Beef	1 (1.6 oz)	90	25	—
Oscar Mayer				
Beef	1 (1.6 oz)	140	30	0
Big & Juicy Franks Deli Style	1 (2.7 oz)	230	50	0
Big & Juicy Franks Original	1 (2.7 oz)	240	45	0
Big & Juicy Franks Quarter Pound	1 (4 oz)	350	65	0
Big & Juicy Weiners Hot 'N Spicy	1 (2.7 oz)	220	45	0
Big & Juicy Weiners Smokie Links	1 (2.7 oz)	220	50	0
Big & Juicy Wieners Original	1 (2.7 oz)	240	45	0
Bun-Length Beef	1 (2 oz)	180	35	0
Cheese	1 (1.6 oz)	140	35	0
Fat Free Beef	1 (1.8 oz)	40	15	0
Fat Free Turkey & Beef	1 (1.8 oz)	40	15	0
Jumbo Beef	1 (2 oz)	180	35	0
Light Beef	1 (2 oz)	110	30	0
Wieners	1 (1.6 oz)	150	35	0
Wieners Bun-Length	1 (2 oz)	190	40	0
Wieners Jumbo	1 (2 oz)	180	40	0
Wieners Light	1 (2 oz)	110	35	0
Wieners Little	6 (2 oz)	180	35	0
Russer				
Lil'Salt Deli Franks	1 (2.67 oz)	160	40	—
Shofar				
Kosher Beef	1 (1.8 oz)	150	20	0
Kosher Beef Reduced Fat Reduced Sodium	1 (1.8 oz)	120	25	0
Wampler				
Chicken	1 (2 oz)	120	60	1

FOOD	PORTION	CALS	CHOL	FIBER
TAKE-OUT				
corndog	1	460	79	–
w/ bun chili	1	297	51	–
w/ bun plain	1	242	44	–
HOT DOG SUBSTITUTES				
Lightlife				
Smart Deli Jumbo's	1 link (2.7 oz)	80	0	1
Smart Dogs	1 (1.5 oz)	45	0	0
Tofu Pups	1 (1.4 oz)	60	0	0
Wonder Dogs	1 (1.5 oz)	60	0	0
Loma Linda				
Big Franks	1 (1.8 oz)	110	0	2
Big Franks Low Fat	1 (1.8 oz)	80	0	2
Corn Dogs	1 (2.5 oz)	150	0	3
Morningstar Farms				
America's Original Veggie Dog	1 (2 oz)	80	0	1
Meatfree Corn Dog	1 (2.5 oz)	150	0	3
Meatfree Mini Corn Dog	4 (2.7 oz)	170	0	1
Natural Touch				
Vege Frank	1 (1.6 oz)	100	0	2
NewMenu				
VegiDogs	1 (1.5 oz)	45	0	0
Veggie Patch				
Perfectly Franks	1 (1.7 oz)	70	0	1
Worthington				
Veja Links Low Fat	1 (1.1 oz)	40	0	0
Yves				
Good Dog	1 (1.8 oz)	70	0	1
Tofu Dogs	1 (1.3 oz)	45	0	0
Veggie Dogs	1 (1.6 oz)	60	0	1
Veggie Dogs Chili	1 (1.6 oz)	50	0	2
Veggie Dogs Jumbo	1 (2.7 oz)	100	0	2
Veggie Dogs Jumbo Hot N' Spicy	1 (2.7 oz)	106	0	2
Zoglo's				
Vegetarian Franks	1 (2.6 oz)	125	0	2
HUMMUS				
hummus	1 cup	420	0	–

FOOD	PORTION	CALS	CHOL	FIBER
Athenos				
Roasted Red Pepper	2 tbsp (1.1 oz)	60	0	1
Casbah				
Mix as prep	¼ cup	120	0	1
Cedar's				
No Salt Added Hommus Tahini	2 tbsp (1 oz)	50	0	3
TAKE-OUT				
hummus	⅓ cup	140	0	—

HYACINTH BEANS

FOOD	PORTION	CALS	CHOL	FIBER
dried cooked	1 cup	228	0	—

ICE CREAM AND FROZEN DESSERTS *(see also* ICES AND ICE POPS, PUDDING POPS, SHERBET, YOGURT FROZEN)

FOOD	PORTION	CALS	CHOL	FIBER
chocolate	½ cup (4 fl oz)	143	22	—
dixie cup chocolate	1 (3.5 fl oz)	125	20	—
dixie cup strawberry	1 (3.5 fl oz)	112	17	—
dixie cup vanilla	1 (3.5 fl oz)	116	25	—
freeze dried ice cream chocolate strawberry & vanilla	1 pkg (0.75 oz)	158	1	1
strawberry	½ cup (4 fl oz)	127	19	—
vanilla	½ cup (4 fl oz)	132	29	—
vanilla soft serve	½ cup	111	10	—
3 Musketeers				
Single Chocolate	1 (2 fl oz)	160	20	0
Single Vanilla	1 (2 fl oz)	160	15	0
Snack Chocolate	1 (0.72 fl oz)	60	5	0
Snack Vanilla	1 (0.72 fl oz)	60	5	0
Ben & Jerry's				
Bovinity Divinity	½ cup	290	40	1
Butter Pecan	½ cup	330	65	2
Cherry Garcia	½ cup	260	70	0
Chocolate Chip Cookie Dough	½ cup	300	65	0
Chocolate Fudge Brownie	½ cup	280	45	2
Chubby Hubby	½ cup	350	55	1
Chunky Monkey	½ cup	310	55	3

FOOD	PORTION	CALS	CHOL	FIBER
Coconut Almond Fudge Chip	½ cup	310	40	2
Coffee Heath Bar Crunch	½ cup	310	65	0
Dilbert's World Totally Nuts	½ cup	310	45	tr
Low Fat Blackberry Cobbler	½ cup	180	20	tr
Low Fat Coconut Cream Pie	½ cup	160	15	0
Low Fat Mocha Latte	½ cup	150	10	tr
Low Fat S'mores	½ cup	190	15	1
Mint Chocolate Cookie	½ cup	280	70	1
New York Super Fudge Chunk	½ cup	320	50	4
No Fat Chocolate Comfort	½ cup	150	10	tr
Orange & Cream	½ cup	230	40	0
Peanut Butter Cup	½ cup	380	65	2
Phish Food	½ cup	300	35	3
Phish Stick	1	330	25	2
Pistachio Pistachio	½ cup	240	50	0
Pop Cookie Dough	1	420	55	tr
Pop Totally Nuts	1	370	30	1
Pop Vanilla	1	330	75	tr
Pop Vanilla Heath Bar Crunch	1	330	65	tr
S'mores Bar	1	350	25	1
Smooth White Russian	½ cup (3.8 oz)	240	90	0
Triple Caramel Chunk	½ cup	290	40	0
Vanilla World's Best	½ cup	250	75	0
Vanilla Caramel Fudge	½ cup	300	70	1
Vanilla Heath Bar Crunch	½ cup	310	70	0
Wavy Gravy	½ cup	340	60	9
Better Than Ice Crème				
Soy Vanilla as prep	½ cup	110	0	0
Bon Bons				
Dark Chocolate	5 pieces	190	15	0
Milk Chocolate	5 pieces	200	10	0

FOOD	PORTION	CALS	CHOL	FIBER
Bounty				
Cherry/Dark	1 (0.84 fl oz)	70	5	0
Coconut/Dark	1 (0.84 fl oz)	70	5	0
Coconut/Milk	1 (0.84 fl oz)	70	5	0
Breyers				
Butter Pecan	½ cup (2.4 oz)	180	35	0
Caramel Praline Crunch	½ cup (2.6 oz)	180	30	0
Cherry Vanilla	½ cup (2.4 oz)	150	30	0
Chocolate	½ cup (2.4 oz)	160	30	tr
Chocolate Chip	½ cup (2.4 oz)	170	35	0
Chocolate Chip Cookie Dough	½ cup (2.5 oz)	180	35	0
Chocolate Rainbow	½ cup (2.4 oz)	120	25	0
Coffee	½ cup (2.4 oz)	150	35	0
Cookies N Cream	½ cup (2.4 oz)	170	30	0
Creamsicle	½ cup (2.8 oz)	130	15	0
Double Chocolate Fudge	½ cup (2.6 oz)	150	40	tr
Fat Free Caramel Praline	½ cup (2.5 oz)	120	<5	0
Fat Free Chocolate	½ cup (2.4 oz)	90	0	tr
Fat Free Mint Cookies N Cream	½ cup (2.4 oz)	100	<5	0
Fat Free Strawberry	½ cup (2.4 oz)	90	0	0
Fat Free Take Two Vanilla Strawberry	½ cup (2.4 oz)	80	<5	0
Fat Free Vanilla	½ cup (2.4 oz)	90	0	tr
Fat Free Vanilla Chocolate Strawberry	½ cup (2.4 oz)	90	0	0
Fat Free Vanilla Fudge Twirl	½ cup (2.5 oz)	100	0	tr
French Vanilla	½ cup (2.4 oz)	160	105	0
Fruit Rainbow	½ cup (2.4 oz)	140	30	0
Hershey w/ Almonds	½ cup (2.7 oz)	190	25	tr
Light Butter Pecan	½ cup (2.3 oz)	120	<5	0
Light Caramel Praline Pecan	½ cup (3 oz)	180	15	0
Light French Chocolate	½ cup (2.4 oz)	150	30	tr

FOOD	PORTION	CALS	CHOL	FIBER
Light Mint Chocolate Chip	½ cup (2.4 oz)	140	10	0
Light Vanilla	½ cup (2.4 oz)	130	35	0
Light Vanilla Chocolate Strawberry	½ cup (2.4 oz)	120	10	0
Light Low Fat Brown Marble Fudge	½ cup (2.6 oz)	130	5	tr
Light Low Fat French Vanilla	½ cup (2.3 oz)	110	30	0
Light Low Fat Swiss Almond Fudge	½ cup (2.5 oz)	130	5	tr
Low Fat Butter Pecan	½ cup (2.6 oz)	150	15	0
Low Fat Vanilla	½ cup (2.6 oz)	120	15	0
Low Fat Vanilla Chocolate Strawberry	½ cup (2.6 oz)	120	10	0
Mint Chocolate Chip	½ cup (2.4 oz)	170	35	0
No Sugar Added Fudge Twirl	½ cup (2.6 oz)	100	25	0
No Sugar Added Mint Chocolate Chip	½ cup (2.4 oz)	100	25	0
No Sugar Added Vanilla	½ cup (2.4 oz)	90	25	0
No Sugar Added Vanilla Chocolate Strawberry	½ cup (2.4 oz)	90	25	0
Peach	½ cup (2.4 oz)	130	25	0
Peanut Butter Cup	½ cup (2.7 oz)	210	30	tr
Rocky Road	½ cup (2.5 oz)	180	25	tr
Soft'N Creamy Vanilla	½ cup (2.3 oz)	150	30	0
Soft'N Creamy Vanilla Chocolate Strawberry	½ cup (2.3 oz)	150	30	0
Strawberry	½ cup (2.4 oz)	130	30	0
Take Two Vanilla Chocolate	½ cup (2.5 oz)	160	35	0
Take Two Vanilla Orange Sherbet	½ cup (2.7 oz)	130	20	0
Vanilla	½ cup (2.4 oz)	150	35	0
Vanilla Chocolate Strawberry	½ cup (2.4 oz)	150	30	0
Vanilla Fudge Twirl	½ cup (2.6 oz)	160	35	tr
Viennetta Cappuccino	½ cup (2.4 oz)	190	35	0
Viennetta Chocolate	½ cup (2.4 oz)	190	25	0

FOOD	PORTION	CALS	CHOL	FIBER
Viennetta Vanilla	½ cup (2.4 oz)	190	40	0
Butterfinger				
Bar	1 (2.5 oz)	190	15	0
California Joe				
Soft Serve Chocolate	½ cup (2.5 oz)	72	0	1
Soft Serve Vanilla	½ cup (2.5 oz)	70	0	1
Carnation				
Cup Chocolate	1 (3 oz)	140	25	0
Cup Chocolate Malt	1 (12 oz)	270	20	1
Cup Strawberry	1 (3 oz)	100	20	0
Cup Vanilla	1 (5 oz)	170	35	0
Cup Vanilla	1 (3 oz)	100	20	0
Cup Vanilla Malt	1 (12 oz)	260	20	0
Sundae Cup Strawberry	1 (5 oz)	200	30	0
Sunday Cup Chocolate	1 (5 oz)	210	30	1
Cool Creations				
Cookies & Cream Sandwich	1 (3.5 oz)	240	15	1
Mickey Mouse Bar	1 (2.5 oz)	120	15	0
Mini Sandwich	1 (2.3 oz)	110	10	0
Dippin' Dots				
Dippin' Dots Chocolate	⅝ cup (3 oz)	190	40	0
DoveBar				
Almond	1 (3.67 fl oz)	335	35	0
Bite Size Almond Praline	1 (0.75 fl oz)	80	7	0
Bite Size Cherry Royale	1 (0.75 fl oz)	70	8	0
Bite Size Classic Vanilla	1 (0.75 fl oz)	70	8	0
Bite Size French Vanilla	1 (0.75 fl oz)	70	15	0
Bite Size Mint Supreme	1 (0.75 fl oz)	80	7	0
Caramel Pecan	1 (3.67 fl oz)	350	35	0
Chocolate Milk Chocolate	1 (3.8 fl oz)	340	40	0
Coffee Cashew	1 (3.67 fl oz)	335	35	0

FOOD	PORTION	CALS	CHOL	FIBER
Crunchy Cookie	1 (3.8 fl oz)	340	40	0
Peanut	1 (3.8 fl oz)	380	40	0
Single Vanilla/Dark	1 (2 fl oz)	200	20	0
Vanilla Dark Chocolate	1 (3.8 fl oz)	340	45	0
Vanilla Milk Chocolate	1 (3.8 fl oz)	340	40	0
Drumstick				
Cone Chocolate	1 (4.6 oz)	320	25	2
Cone Chocolate Dipped	1 (4.6 oz)	320	25	1
Cone Vanilla	1 (4.6 oz)	340	20	2
Cone Vanilla Caramel	1 (4.6 oz)	360	25	2
Cone Vanilla Fudge	1 (4.6 oz)	360	20	2
Edy's				
3 Musketeers	½ cup	160	20	–
Dreamery Banana Split	½ cup	240	60	1
Dreamery Black Raspberry Avalanche	½ cup	270	80	1
Dreamery Caramel Toffee Bar Heaven	½ cup	290	75	0
Dreamery Cashew Praline Parfait	½ cup	280	75	0
Dreamery Chocolate Truffle Explosion	½ cup	280	8	1
Dreamery Chocolate Peanut Butter Chunk	½ cup	310	50	2
Dreamery Coney Island Waffle Cone	½ cup	310	70	1
Dreamery Cool Mint	½ cup	300	75	1
Dreamery Deep Dish Apple Pie	½ cup	280	75	0
Dreamery Dulce De Leche	½ cup	270	70	0
Dreamery Grandma's Cookie Dough	½ cup	300	75	0
Dreamery Harvest Peach	½ cup	230	70	0
Dreamery New York Strawberry Cheesecake	½ cup	260	80	0

FOOD	PORTION	CALS	CHOL	FIBER
Dreamery Nothing But Chocolate	½ cup	280	65	1
Dreamery Nuts About Malt	½ cup	290	70	1
Dreamery Raspberry Brownie A La Mode	½ cup	270	75	1
Dreamery Raspberry Brownie A La Mode	½ cup	130	75	1
Dreamery Strawberry Fields	½ cup	220	65	1
Dreamery Tiramisu	½ cup	260	75	0
Dreamery Vanilla	½ cup	260	70	0
Grand Black Cherry Vanilla	½ cup	140	25	—
Grand Blue Ribbon Chocolate Cake	½ cup	180	25	—
Grand Butter Pecan	½ cup	170	25	—
Grand Cherry Chocolate Chip	½ cup	160	25	—
Grand Chocolate	½ cup	150	25	—
GrandChocolate Caramel Swirl	½ cup	170	25	—
Grand Chocolate Chips	½ cup	170	25	—
Grand Chocolate Fudge Mousse	½ cup	160	25	—
Grand Chocolate Fudge Sundae	½ cup	170	20	—
Grand Coffee	½ cup	140	25	—
Grand Cookie Dough	½ cup	180	25	—
Grand Cookies'N Cream	½ cup	160	25	—
Grand Double Fudge Brownie	½ cup	170	30	—
Grand Espresso Chip	½ cup	150	25	—
Grand French Vanilla	½ cup	160	50	—
Grand French Vanilla Fudge Pie	½ cup	160	45	—
Grand Mint Chocolate Chips	½ cup	170	25	—

FOOD	PORTION	CALS	CHOL	FIBER
Grand Neapolitan	½ cup	140	25	–
Grand Nutty Cone Crunch	½ cup	180	25	–
Grand Real Strawberry	½ cup	130	20	–
Grand Rocky Road	½ cup	170	25	–
Grand Spumoni	½ cup	150	25	–
Grand Strawberry Cupcake	½ cup	140	25	–
Grand Tin Roof Sundae	½ cup	170	25	–
Grand Utimate Caramel Cup	½ cup	170	20	–
Grand Vanilla	½ cup	140	25	–
Grand Vanillaberry Bar	½ cup	130	20	–
Grand Light Butter Pecan	½ cup	120	20	–
Grand Light Chocolate Raspberry Escape	½ cup	130	15	–
Grand Light Chocolate Fudge Mousse	½ cup	120	20	–
Grand Light Cookie Dough	½ cup	130	20	–
Grand Light Cookies'N Cream	½ cup	120	15	–
Grand Light Crazy For Caramel	½ cup	120	15	–
Grand Light French Silk	½ cup	130	15	–
Grand Light Mint Chocolate Chips	½ cup	120	20	–
Grand Light Peanut Butter Cups	½ cup	120	20	–
Grand Light Rocky Road	½ cup	120	20	–
Grand Light S'Mores & More	½ cup	130	15	–
Grand Light Strawberry Shortcake	½ cup	110	20	•
Grand Light Vanilla	½ cup	100	20	–
Homemade All Natural Vanilla	½ cup	130	30	–

FOOD	PORTION	CALS	CHOL	FIBER
Homemade Brownies A La Mode	½ cup	150	30	—
Homemade Chocolate Chip Cookie Jar	½ cup	180	25	—
Homemade Chocolate Chip Mousse	½ cup	170	30	—
Homemade Double Chocolate Chunk	½ cup	170	30	—
Homemade Mint Chocolate Chunk	½ cup	170	25	—
Homemade Old Fashioned Butter Pecan	½ cup	160	30	—
Homemade Strawberries & Cream	½ cup	120	25	—
Homemade Vanilla Custard	½ cup	150	55	—
M&M's Almond	½ cup	180	25	—
M&M's Chocolate Brownie Sundae	½ cup	180	25	—
M&M's Mint	½ cup	200	25	—
M&M's Vanilla	½ cup	180	25	—
Milky Way	½ cup	160	25	—
Snickers	½ cup	180	25	—
Snickers Cruncher	½ cup	190	25	—
Twix	½ cup	190	25	—
Twix Peanut Butter	½ cup	190	25	—
Flintstones				
Cool Cream	1 (2.75 oz)	90	5	0
Push-Up Pebbles Treats	1 (2.75 oz)	120	20	0
Friendly's				
Black Raspberry	½ cup	150	30	0
Chocolate Almond Chip	½ cup	170	35	0
Forbidden Chocolate	½ cup	150	30	0
Fudge Nut Brownie	½ cup	200	25	0
Heath English Toffee	½ cup (2.7 oz)	190	30	0
Purely Pistachio	½ cup	160	35	0
Vanilla	½ cup	150	35	0

FOOD	PORTION	CALS	CHOL	FIBER
Vanilla Chocolate Strawberry	½ cup	150	30	tr
Vienna Mocha Chunk	½ cup	180	30	0
Good Humor				
Banana Bob	1 (3 fl oz)	155	5	0
Bar Classic Toasted Almond	1 (3.1 fl oz)	170	10	1
Bar Classic Vanilla	1 (3.1 fl oz)	190	15	0
Bar Classic Almond	1 (3.1 fl oz)	210	15	1
Bar Sidewalk Sundae	1	280	15	2
Bubble O'Bill	1 (3.6 fl oz)	170	15	1
Chip Burrrger	1 (4.7 oz)	320	20	1
Chip Sandwich	1 (4.7 fl oz)	320	20	1
Choco Taco	1 (4.4 fl oz)	320	20	1
Chocolate Eclair Classic	1 (3.1 fl oz)	170	10	1
Classic Candy Center Crunch Vanilla	1	280	15	0
Colonel Crunch Chocolate	1 (3.1 oz)	160	10	1
Colonel Crunch Strawberry	1 (3.1 oz)	170	10	0
Combo Cup	1 (6.2 fl oz)	200	35	1
Cone Olde Nut Sundae	1 (3.9 oz)	230	5	2
Cone Sidewalk Sundae	1 (4.2 oz)	270	10	1
Creamee Burrrger	1 (4.7 oz)	310	20	1
Crunch Classic Candy Center	1 (3.1 fl oz)	260	10	1
Far Frog	1 (3.6 fl oz)	150	20	1
Fun Box Ice Cream Sandwich	1 (3.1 fl oz)	160	10	1
King Cone	1 (5.7 fl oz)	300	25	2
King Cone Classic Vanilla	1 (4.8 oz)	300	20	1
King Cone Strawberry	1 (5.7 oz)	250	25	1
Light Chocolate Chip	½ cup (2.4 oz)	130	10	0

FOOD	PORTION	CALS	CHOL	FIBER
Light Coffee	½ cup (2.4 oz)	110	15	0
Light Cookies N'Cream	½ cup (2.4 oz)	130	10	0
Light Heavenly Hash	½ cup (2.4 oz)	140	10	tr
Light Praline Almond Crunch	½ cup (2.4 oz)	130	15	0
Light Toffee Bar Crunch	½ cup (2.4 oz)	130	15	0
Light Vanilla	½ cup (2.4 oz)	110	15	0
Light Vanilla Chocolate Strawberry	½ cup (2.4 oz)	110	10	0
Light Vanilla Fudge	½ cup (2.6 oz)	120	15	0
Magnum Almond	1 (4.2 fl oz)	270	30	5
Magnum Chocolate	1 (4.2 fl oz)	260	30	2
Number One Bar	1 (4.1 fl oz)	190	15	1
Popsicle Ice Cream Bar	1 (3.1 fl oz)	160	15	1
Popsicle Ice Cream Sandwich	1 (3.6 fl oz)	190	15	1
Sandwich Classic Chip Cookie	1 (4.1 fl oz)	300	18	1
Sandwich Giant Neapolitan	1 (5.2 fl oz)	260	20	1
Sandwich Giant Vanilla	1 (5.2 fl oz)	240	20	1
Sandwich Ice Cream	1	190	15	1
Sandwich Sidewalk Sundae	1 (3.1 oz)	160	10	1
Sandwich Sprinkle	1 (3.1 fl oz)	180	10	1
Strawberry Shortcake Bar Classic	1 (3.1 fl oz)	160	10	1
Sundae Twist Cup	1	160	10	0
Toffee Taco	1 (4.4 fl oz)	300	15	1
WWF Bar	1 (3.7 fl oz)	200	15	1
X-Men Bar	1 (3 fl oz)	150	15	0
Häagen-Dazs				
Bars Chocolate & Almonds	1 (3.7 oz)	380	90	2

FOOD	PORTION	CALS	CHOL	FIBER
Bars Chocolate & Dark Chocolate	1 (3.6 oz)	350	65	2
Bars Chocolate Peanut Butter Swirl	1 (3 oz)	320	60	2
Bars Coffee & Almond Crunch	1 (3.7 oz)	370	90	tr
Bars Cookies & Cream Crunch	1 (3.6 oz)	370	85	tr
Bars Dulce De Leche Caramel	1 (3.7 oz)	370	75	0
Bars Tropical Coconut	1 (3.5 oz)	340	90	0
Bars Vanilla & Almonds	1 (3.7 oz)	380	90	1
Bars Vanilla & Dark Chocolate	1 (3.6 oz)	350	85	1
Bars Vanilla & Milk Chocolate	1 (3.5 oz)	340	90	tr
Butter Pecan	½ cup	310	110	tr
Cappuccino Commotion	½ cup	310	100	1
Cherry Vanilla	½ cup	240	100	0
Chocolate	½ cup	270	115	1
Chocolate Brownie w/ Walnuts	½ cup	290	100	1
Chocolate Chocolate Fudge	½ cup	290	100	tr
Chocolate Chocolate Chip	½ cup	300	105	2
Chocolate Swiss Almond	½ cup	300	100	2
Cinnamon	½ cup	250	110	0
Coffee	½ cup	270	120	0
Coffee Mocha Chip	½ cup	290	110	tr
Cookie Dough Chip	½ cup	310	95	0
Cookies & Cream	½ cup	270	105	0
Creme Caramel Pecan	½ cup	320	95	0
Dulce De Leche Caramel	½ cup	290	100	0
Low Fat Chocolate	½ cup	170	30	tr

FOOD	PORTION	CALS	CHOL	FIBER
Low Fat Coffee Fudge	½ cup	170	25	0
Low Fat Strawberry	½ cup	150	15	0
Low Fat Vanilla	½ cup	170	20	0
Macadamia Brittle	½ cup	300	110	0
Mango	½ cup	250	85	tr
Mint Chip	½ cup	300	105	tr
Pineapple Coconut	½ cup	230	90	0
Pistachio	½ cup	290	110	tr
Rum Raisin	½ cup	270	110	0
Strawberry	½ cup	250	95	tr
Vanilla	½ cup	270	120	0
Vanilla Chocolate Chip	½ cup	310	105	tr
Vanilla Fudge	½ cup	290	100	0
Vanilla Swiss Almond	½ cup	300	105	tr
Healthy Choice				
Butter Pecan Crunch	½ cup	120	5	tr
Cappuccino Chocolate Chunk	½ cup	120	10	1
Cappuccino Mocha Crunch	½ cup	120	5	tr
Cherry Chocolate Chunk	½ cup	110	<5	tr
Chocolate Chocolate Chunk	½ cup	120	5	2
Coconut Cream Pie	½ cup	120	5	1
Cookies 'N Cream	½ cup	120	5	tr
Cookies Creme De Mint	½ cup	130	5	tr
Fudge Brownie	½ cup	120	5	tr
Mint Chocolate Chip	½ cup	120	5	tr
Old Fashioned Blueberry Hill	½ cup	120	<5	1
Old Fashioned Butterscotch Blonde	½ cup	140	10	tr
Old Fashioned Cherry Vanilla	½ cup	120	5	tr
Old Fashioned Strawberry	½ cup	110	0	1
Peanut Butter Cup	½ cup	110	5	tr
Praline & Caramel	½ cup	130	5	tr

FOOD	PORTION	CALS	CHOL	FIBER
Praline Caramel Cluster	½ cup	130	<5	tr
Rocky Road	½ cup	140	5	tr
Turtle Fudge Cake	½ cup	130	<5	2
Vanilla	½ cup	100	5	tr
Vanilla Bean	½ cup	110	5	tr
Wild Raspberry Truffle	½ cup	120	6	tr
Heaven				
Sundae Bars Chocolate Fudge	1 bar	150	7	—
Sundae Bars Vanilla Fudge	1 bar	150	7	—
Vanilla Caramel Nut	1 bar	225	9	—
Vanilla Nut Fudge	1 bar	222	9	—
Hood				
Bar Orange Cream	1 bar (1.8 oz)	90	5	0
Bar Vanilla	1 bar (1.6 oz)	160	15	0
Caramel Butterscotch Blast	½ cup (2.3 oz)	160	25	0
Chocolate	½ cup (2.3 oz)	140	30	0
Chocolate Chip	½ cup (2.3 oz)	160	30	0
Chocolate Eclair	1 bar (1.6 oz)	150	5	0
Christmas Tree	½ cup (2.3 oz)	140	30	0
Coffee	½ cup (2.3 oz)	140	30	0
Cookie Dough Delight	½ cup (2.3 oz)	160	30	0
Cookies N Cream	½ cup (2.3 oz)	160	30	0
Cooler Cups	1 (2.1 oz)	80	<5	0
Crispy Bar	1 (1.9 oz)	180	20	0
Egg Nog	½ cup (2.3 oz)	130	25	0
Fabulous Fudge & Peanut Butter Swirled Fudge Bars	1 bar (2.1 oz)	110	10	0
Fabulous Fudgies Assorted Bars	1 bar (2.1 oz)	100	10	0
Fat Free Chocolate Passion	½ cup (2.5 oz)	100	0	0
Fat Free Classic Harlequin	½ cup (2.5 oz)	100	0	0
Fat Free Double Brownie Sundae	½ cup (2.5 oz)	120	0	0

FOOD	PORTION	CALS	CHOL	FIBER
Fat Free Heavenly Hash	½ cup (2.5 oz)	120	0	0
Fat Free Mississippi Mud Pie	½ cup (2.5 oz)	130	0	0
Fat Free Praline Pecan Delight	½ cup (2.5 oz)	120	0	0
Fat Free Raspberry Blush	½ cup (2.5 oz)	120	0	0
Fat Free Super Strawberry Swirl	½ cup (2.5 oz)	100	0	0
Fat Free Vanilla Fudge Twist	½ cup (2.5 oz)	120	0	0
Fat Free Very Vanilla	½ cup (2.5 oz)	100	0	0
Fudge Bars	1 bar (2.7 oz)	100	0	0
Grasshopper Pie	½ cup (2.3 oz)	160	25	0
Heavenly Hash	½ cup (2.3 oz)	140	20	0
Hendrie's Cherry Chocolate Dips	1 bar (1.3 oz)	120	15	0
Hoodsie Cup Vanilla & Chocolate	1 (1.7 oz)	100	20	0
Light Almond Praline Delight	½ cup (2.4 oz)	110	15	0
Light Brownie Nut Sundae	½ cup (2.4 oz)	140	10	0
Light Caribbean Coffee Royale	½ cup (2.4 oz)	110	15	0
Light Chocolate Almond Chip Sundae	½ cup (2.4 oz)	140	10	0
Light Chocolate Chocolate Chip Cookie Dough	½ cup (2.4 oz)	140	15	0
Light Cookies N Cream	½ cup (2.4 oz)	130	15	0
Light Heath Toffee Chunk Swirl	½ cup (2.4 oz)	140	15	0
Light Heavenly Hash	½ cup (2.4 oz)	130	10	0

FOOD	PORTION	CALS	CHOL	FIBER
Light Maple Sugar Shack	⅓ cup (2.4 oz)	130	10	0
Light Massachusetts Mud Pie	½ cup (2.4 oz)	140	10	0
Light Raspberry Swirl	½ cup (2.4 oz)	120	10	0
Light Strawberry Supreme	½ cup (2.4 oz)	110	15	0
Light Triple Nut Cluster Sundae	½ cup (2.4 oz)	140	10	0
Light Vanilla	½ cup (2.4 oz)	110	15	0
Light Vanilla Chocolate Strawberry	½ cup (2.4 oz)	110	15	0
Low Fat No Sugar Added Caramel Swirl	½ cup (2.4 oz)	120	10	0
Low Fat No Sugar Added Chocolate Supreme	½ cup (2.4 oz)	120	10	0
Low Fat No Sugar Added Mocha Fudge	½ cup (2.4 oz)	110	10	0
Low Fat No Sugar Added Raspberry Swirl	½ cup (2.4 oz)	110	10	0
Low Fat No Sugar Added Vanilla	½ cup (2.4 oz)	100	10	0
Maple Walnut	½ cup (2.3 oz)	160	30	0
Rockets	1 (2 oz)	120	20	1
Sandwich Light	1 (2.2 oz)	160	10	1
Sandwich Vanilla	1 (2.2 oz)	180	20	1
Sports Bar	1 (2.9 oz)	250	25	0
Spumoni	½ cup (2.3 oz)	140	30	0
Strawberry	½ cup (2.3 oz)	130	30	0
Super Sortment Chocolate & Banana Fudge Bar	1 bar (2.1 oz)	100	10	0
Super Sortment Root Beer Float & Orange Cream Bar	1 bar (1.5 oz)	70	10	0
Vanilla	½ cup (2.3 oz)	140	30	0

FOOD	PORTION	CALS	CHOL	FIBER
Vanilla Chocolate Patchwork	½ cup (2.3 oz)	140	30	0
Vanilla Chocolate Strawberry	½ cup (2.3 oz)	140	30	0
Vanilla Fudge	½ cup (2.3 oz)	140	25	0
Klondike				
Almond Bar	1 (5.2 fl oz)	310	25	3
Caramel Crunch	1 (5.2 fl oz)	300	30	tr
Choco Taco Fudge Grande	1 bar (3.2 oz)	310	15	tr
Chocolate Chocolate Bar	1 (5.2 fl oz)	280	20	tr
Coffee Bar	1 (5.2 fl oz)	290	15	0
Dark Chocolate Bar	1 (5.2 fl oz)	290	30	tr
Gold Bar	1 (5.2 fl oz)	340	34	1
Krispy Bar	1 (5.2 fl oz)	300	25	0
Krunch	1 (3.1 fl oz)	200	20	1
Lite Bar	1 (2.3 fl oz)	110	5	1
Lite Bar Caramel	1 (2.4 fl oz)	120	5	1
Movie Bites Chocolate	8 pieces (4.6 oz)	340	25	1
Movie Bites Vanilla	8 pieces (4.6 oz)	320	25	1
Oreo Ice Cream Cookie Sandwich	1 (2.6 oz)	240	15	2
Original	1 (3.3 oz)	290	30	0
Original Bar	1 (5.2 fl oz)	290	15	0
Sandwich Chocolate	1 (5.2 fl oz)	270	20	2
Sandwich Lite	1 (2.9 fl oz)	100	5	1
Mars				
Almond Bar	1 (1.85 fl oz)	210	15	0
Milky Way				
Single Chocolate/Milk	1 (2 fl oz)	210	20	0
Snack Chocolate/Milk	1 (0.72 fl oz)	70	5	0
Snack Vanilla/Dark	1 (0.72 fl oz)	70	5	0
Mocha Mix				
Berry Berry Berry	½ cup	140	0	0
Dutch Chocolate	½ cup (2.3 oz)	140	0	0
Mocha Almond Fudge	½ cup (2.3 oz)	150	0	0

FOOD	PORTION	CALS	CHOL	FIBER
Neapolitan	½ cup (2.3 oz)	140	0	0
Strawberry Swirl	½ cup (2.3 oz)	140	0	0
Vanilla	½ cup (2.3 oz)	140	0	0
Nestle Crunch				
Chocolate	1 bar (3 oz)	200	15	0
Cones	1 (4.6 oz)	300	25	2
Crunch King	1 (4 oz)	270	20	0
Nuggets	8 pieces	310	20	0
Reduced Fat	1 (2.5 oz)	130	5	0
Vanilla	1 bar (3 oz)	200	15	0
NutraShake				
High Calorie High Protein All Flavors	1 serv (4 oz)	200	60	—
Perry's				
No Fat No Sugar Added Caramel	½ cup (2.8 oz)	90	0	1
No Fat No Sugar Added Chocolate	½ cup (2.6 oz)	80	0	2
No Fat No Sugar Added Peach	½ cup (2.9 oz) 90	0	tr	
No Fat No Sugar Added Strawberry	½ cup (2.8 oz)	90	0	tr
No Fat No Sugar Added Vanilla	½ cup (2.6 oz)	80	0	tr
Rice Dream				
Cappuccino	½ cup (3.2 oz)	150	0	1
Carob	½ cup (3.2 oz)	150	0	2
Carob Almong	½ cup (3.2 oz)	170	0	2
Cherry Vanilla	½ cup (3.2 oz)	150	0	1
Cocoa Marble Fudge	½ cup (3.2 oz)	150	0	2
Cookies N' Dream	½ cup (3.2 oz)	170	0	1
Mint Chocolate Chip	½ cup (3.2 oz)	170	0	1
Neapolitan	½ cup (3.2 oz)	150	0	2
Orange Vanilla Swirl	½ cup (3.2 oz)	250	0	1
Strawberry	½ cup (3.2 oz)	140	0	1
Vanilla Swiss Almond	½ cup (3.2 oz)	180	0	1
Rice Dream Supreme				
Cappuccino Almond Fudge	½ cup (3.2 oz)	170	0	2

FOOD	PORTION	CALS	CHOL	FIBER
Cherry Chocolate Chunk	½ cup (3.2 oz)	170	0	1
Chocolate Almond Chunk	½ cup (3.2 oz)	170	0	2
Chocolate Fudge Brownie	½ cup (3.2 oz)	170	0	2
Double Espresso Bean	½ cup (3.2 oz)	160	0	1
Mint Chocolate Cookie	½ cup (3.2 oz)	170	0	1
Peanut Butter Cup	½ cup (3.2 oz)	180	0	2
Pralines N' Dream	½ cup (3.2 oz)	180	0	1
Sealtest				
American Glory	½ cup (2.4 oz)	130	25	0
Butter Pecan	½ cup (2.4 oz)	160	30	0
Candy Cane Crunch	½ cup (2.4 oz)	150	25	0
Chocolate	½ cup (2.4 oz)	140	25	tr
Chocolate Butter Pecan	½ cup (2.4 oz)	150	30	0
Chocolate Chip	½ cup (2.4 oz)	150	30	0
Coconut Chocolate	½ cup (2.4 oz)	160	25	tr
Coffee	½ cup (2.4 oz)	140	30	0
Cupid's Scoops	½ cup (2.5 oz)	140	25	0
French Vanilla	½ cup (2.4 oz)	140	60	0
Fudge Royale	½ cup (2.5 oz)	150	25	0
Heavenly Hash	½ cup (2.4 oz)	150	25	tr
Maple Walnut	½ cup (2.4 oz)	160	30	0
Strawberry	½ cup (2.4 oz)	130	25	0
Triple Chocolate Passion	½ cup (2.5 oz)	160	25	tr
Vanilla	½ cup (2.4 oz)	140	30	0
Vanilla Chocolate Strawberry	½ cup (2.4 oz)	140	25	0
Vanilla With Orange Sherbet	½ cup (2.7 oz)	130	20	0
Silhouette				
The Skinny Cow Low Fat Ice Cream Sandwich Vanilla	1	130	0	2
Snickers				
Single	1 (2 fl oz)	220	15	0
Snack	1 (1 fl oz)	110	5	0

FOOD	PORTION	CALS	CHOL	FIBER
Starbucks				
Biscotti Bliss	½ cup	240	55	—
Caffe Almond Fudge	½ cup	260	55	—
Caffe Almond Roast	1 bar	280	3	—
Dark Roast Expresso Swirl	½ cup	220	55	—
Frappuccino	1 bar (2.8 oz)	110	10	0
Italian Roast Coffee	½ cup	230	65	—
Javachip	½ cup	250	60	—
Low Fat Latte	½ cup	170	10	—
Low Fat Mocha Mambo	½ cup	170	10	—
Vanilla Mochachip	½ cup	270	75	—
Tofutti				
Cuties Chocolate	1 (1.4 oz)	130	0	0
Cuties Vanilla	1 (1.4 oz)	121	0	0
Monkey Bars Peanut Butter	1 bar (2.5 oz)	220	0	tr
Turkey Hill				
Black Cherry	½ cup	140	25	0
Black Raspberry	½ cup	140	30	—
Butter Pecan	½ cup	170	30	0
Chocolate Marshmallow	½ cup	160	30	—
Chocolate Mint Chip	½ cup	180	30	—
Chocolate Peanut Butter Cup	½ cup	180	30	—
Colombian Coffee	½ cup	140	30	—
Cookies 'N Cream	½ cup	160	30	0
Death By Chocolate	½ cup	160	30	—
Dutch Chocolate	½ cup	150	30	—
Egg Nog	½ cup	150	45	—
Fat Free No Sugar Added Caramel Fudge Decadence	½ cup	100	0	—
Fat Free No Sugar Added Cherry Vanilla Fudge	½ cup	90	0	—
Fat Free No Sugar Added Dutch Chocolate	½ cup	90	0	—

FOOD	PORTION	CALS	CHOL	FIBER
Fat Free No Sugar Added Vanilla Bean	½ cup	90	0	—
Fudge Ripple	½ cup	140	30	—
Light Butter Pecan	½ cup	130	15	0
Light Choco Mint Chip	½ cup	140	15	0
Light Tin Lissie Sundae	½ cup	140	10	—
Light Vanilla & Chocolate	½ cup	110	15	0
Light Vanilla Bean	½ cup	110	15	0
Neapolitan	½ cup	150	30	0
Orange Swirl	½ cup	140	20	—
Original Vanilla	½ cup	140	30	—
Peanut Butter Ripple	½ cup	170	30	—
Philadelphia Style Butter Almond	½ cup	180	35	—
Philadelphia Style Chocolate	½ cup	170	35	—
Philadelphia Style Mint Chocolate Chip	½ cup	180	35	—
Philadelphia Style Sweet Cherry Vanilla	½ cup	160	30	—
Philadelphia Style Vanilla Bean	½ cup	170	35	—
Rocky Road	½ cup	170	30	0
Rum Raisin	½ cup	150	30	—
Sandwich Choco Mint Chip	1	200	25	—
Sandwiches Vanilla	1	190	25	—
Strawberries 'N Cream	½ cup	140	25	—
Sundae Cones Rocky Road	1	340	25	—
Sundae Cones Tin Roof Sundae	1	290	25	—
Tin Roof Sundae	½ cup	160	30	0
Vanilla & Chocolate	½ cup	150	30	0

FOOD	PORTION	CALS	CHOL	FIBER
Vanilla Bean	½ cup	140	30	0
Weight Watchers				
Chocolate Chip Cookie Dough Sundae	1 (2.64 oz)	190	5	1
Chocolate Mousse	1 bar	40	5	1
Chocolate Treat	1 bar	100	0	1
English Toffee Crunch	1 bar	110	5	1
Orange Vanilla Treat	1 bar	40	5	0
Vanilla Sandwich	1 bar	150	5	1
TAKE-OUT				
cone vanilla light soft serve	1 (4.6 oz)	164	28	–
gelato chocolate hazelnut	½ cup (5.3 oz)	370	92	2
gelato vanilla	½ cup (3 oz)	211	151	0
sundae caramel	1 (5.4 oz)	303	25	–
sundae hot fudge	1 (5.4 oz)	284	21	–
sundae strawberry	1 (5.4 oz)	269	21	–

ICE CREAM CONES AND CUPS

FOOD	PORTION	CALS	CHOL	FIBER
sugar cone	1	40	0	tr
wafer cone	1	17	0	tr
Comet				
Cups	1 (5 g)	20	0	tr
Sugar Cones	1 (12 g)	50	0	tr
Waffle Cone	1 (17 g)	70	0	1
Dutch Mill				
Chocolate Covered Wafer Cups	1 (0.5 oz)	80	0	0
Frookie				
Chocolate Crunch	1 (0.4 oz)	50	0	tr
Honey Crunch	1 (0.4 oz)	45	0	tr
Keebler				
Chocolatey Cone	1 (0.4 oz)	50	0	0
Fudge Dipped Cup	1 (0.3 oz)	35	0	0
Ice Creme Cup	1 (0.2 oz)	15	0	0
Sugar Cone	1 (0.4 oz)	50	0	0
Waffle Bowl	1 (0.4 oz)	50	0	0
Waffle Cone	1 (0.4 oz)	50	0	0

FOOD	PORTION	CALS	CHOL	FIBER
Oreo				
Chocolate Cones	1 (13 g)	50	0	tr
Teddy Grahams				
Cinnamon Cones	1 (0.5 oz)	60	0	tr
ICE CREAM TOPPINGS				
marshmallow cream	1 oz	88	0	—
marshmallow cream	1 jar (7 oz)	615	0	—
pineapple	2 tbsp (1.5 oz)	106	0	—
pineapple	1 cup (11.5 oz)	861	0	—
strawberry	1 cup (11.5 oz)	863	0	—
strawberry	2 tbsp (1.5 oz)	107	0	—
walnuts in syrup	2 tbsp (1.4 oz)	167	0	—
Ben & Jerry's				
Hot Fudge	(1.3 oz)	140	10	2
Crumpy				
Chocolate Hazelnut Spread	1 tbsp (0.5 oz)	80	0	0
Hershey				
Chocolate Shoppe Double Chocolate	1 tbsp (0.7 oz)	50	0	—
Chocolate Shoppe Apple Pie A La Mode	2 tbsp (1.3 oz)	100	0	—
Chocolate Shoppe Butterscotch Caramel	1 tbsp (0.7 oz)	70	<5	—
Chocolate Shoppe Caramel	2 tbsp (1.3 oz)	100	0	—
Chocolate Shoppe Chocolate Mini	1 tbsp (0.7 oz)	50	0	—
Chocolate Shoppe Double Chocolate	1 tbsp (0.6 oz)	60	0	—
Chocolate Shoppe Hot Fudge	1 tbsp (0.7 oz)	70	<5	—
Chocolate Shoppe Hot Fudge Fat Free	2 tbsp (1.4 oz)	100	0	—
Chocolate Shoppe Sprinkles Milk Chocolate	1 tbsp (0.5 oz)	70	<5	—

FOOD	PORTION	CALS	CHOL	FIBER
Chocolate Shoppe Sprinkles Reeses	1 tbsp (0.5 oz)	70	0	—
Chocolate Shoppe Sprinkles York	1 tbsp (0.6 oz)	80	0	—
Kraft				
Butterscotch	2 tbsp (1.4 oz)	130	<5	0
Caramel	2 tbsp (1.4 oz)	120	0	0
Chocolate	2 tbsp (1.4 oz)	110	0	1
Hot Fudge	2 tbsp (1.4 oz)	140	0	tr
Pineapple	2 tbsp (1.4 oz)	110	0	0
Strawberry	2 tbsp (1.4 oz)	110	0	0
Marzetti				
Caramel Apple	2 tbsp	60	5	0
Caramel Apple Reduced Fat	2 tbsp	30	5	0
Peanut Butter Caramel	2 tbsp	60	0	1
Planters				
Nut	2 tbsp (0.5 oz)	100	0	1
Smucker's				
Plate Scapers Caramel	2 tbsp	100	0	—
ICED TEA				
MIX				
instant artificially sweetened lemon flavored as prep w/ water	8 oz	5	0	—
instant sweetened lemon flavor as prep w/ water	9 oz	87	0	—
instant unsweetened lemon flavor as prep w/ water	8 oz	4	0	—
Crystal Light				
Decaffeinated as prep	1 serv (8 oz)	5	0	0
Iced Tea as prep	1 serv (8 oz)	5	0	0
Peach Tea as prep	1 serv (8 oz)	5	0	0
Raspberry Tea as prep	1 serv (8 oz)	5	0	0

FOOD	PORTION	CALS	CHOL	FIBER
Lipton				
100% Tea Decaffeinated as prep	1 serv	0	0	—
100% Tea Unsweetened as prep	1 serv	0	0	—
100% Tea as prep	1 serv	0	0	—
Calorie Free as prep	1 serv	0	0	—
Decaffeinated Ice Tea Brew as prep	1 serv (8 oz)	0	0	0
Decaffeinated Lemon as prep	1 serv	90	0	—
Diet Decaffeinated Lemon as prep	1 serv	5	0	—
Diet Lemon as prep	1 serv	5	0	—
Diet Peach as prep	1 serv	5	0	—
Diet Raspberry as prep	1 serv	5	0	—
Diet Tea & Lemonade as prep	1 serv	10	0	—
Herbal Iced Collection	1 tea bag	0	0	—
Ice Tea Brew as prep	1 serv (8 oz)	0	0	0
Lemon as prep	1 serv	90	0	—
Lemon as prep	1 pkg (0.5 oz)	50	0	—
Natural Brew 100% Tea Decaffeinated as prep	1 serv	0	0	—
Natural Brew 100% Tea as prep	1 serv	0	0	—
Natural Brew Diet Lemon as prep	1 serv	5	0	—
Natural Brew Diet Peach as prep	1 serv	5	0	—
Natural Brew Diet Tropical as prep	1 serv	5	0	—
Natural Brew Tropical as prep	1 serv	90	0	—
Natural Brew Unsweetened Lemon as prep	1 serv	0	0	—
Peach as prep	1 serv	90	0	—

FOOD	PORTION	CALS	CHOL	FIBER
Rasberry as prep	1 serv	90	0	–
Tea & Lemonade as prep	1 serv	90	0	–
Nestea				
100% Tea	2 tsp (1 g)	0	0	0
100% Tea Decafe	2 tsp (1 g)	0	0	0
Ice Teasers Lemon	1 serv (0.5 oz)	5	0	0
Ice Teasers Orange	1 serv (0.5 oz)	5	0	0
Ice Teasers Wild Cherry	1 serv (0.5 oz)	5	0	0
Lemon	2 tsp (1 g)	5	0	0
Lemon & Sugar	2 tbsp (0.7 oz)	80	0	0
Lemonade Tea	2 tbsp (0.7 oz)	80	0	0
Sugar Free	2 tbsp (0.7 oz)	5	0	0
Sugar Free Decafe	1 tbsp (0.7 oz)	5	0	0
Sun Tea	1 tsp (1 g)	0	0	0
READY-TO-DRINK				
Arizona				
Lemon	1 bottle (16 oz)	180	0	–
Raspberry	8 fl oz	95	0	–
Crystal Light				
Lemon	1 serv (8 oz)	5	0	0
Peach Tea	1 serv (8 oz)	5	0	0
Raspberry Tea	1 serv (8 oz)	5	0	0
Honest Tea				
Gold Rush Herbal Cinnamon	8 fl oz	9	0	–
Lipton				
Carribean Cooler	1 can (12 oz)	130	0	–
Diet Lemon	8 oz	0	0	–
Diet Lemon	1 bottle (16 oz)	10	0	–
Green Tea & Passion Fruit	1 bottle (16 oz)	160	0	–
Lemon	8 oz	80	0	–
Lemon	1 can (12 oz)	120	0	–
Lemon	1 bottle (16 oz)	180	0	–
Natural Lemon	1 box (8 oz)	100	0	–
Peach	8 oz	80	0	–
Peach	1 bottle (16 oz)	220	0	–
Raspberry	8 oz	80	0	–

FOOD	PORTION	CALS	CHOL	FIBER
Raspberry	1 bottle (16 oz)	220	0	–
Raspberry Blast	1 can (12 oz)	130	0	–
Southern Style Extra Sweet No Lemon	1 bottle (16 oz)	240	0	–
Southern Style Lemon	1 bottle (16 oz)	200	0	–
Southern Style Sweetened No Lemon	1 bottle (16 oz)	200	0	–
Sweet	8 oz	80	0	–
Sweetened No Lemon	1 bottle (16 oz)	140	0	–
Sweetened Lemon	8 oz	80	0	–
Tangerine Twist	1 can (12 oz)	120	0	–
Tea & Lemonade	1 bottle (16 oz)	220	0	–
Unsweetened No Lemon	1 bottle (16 oz)	0	0	–
Mad River				
Red Tea w/ Guarana	8 oz	90	0	–
Nantucket Nectars				
Diet	8 oz	5	0	–
Diet Green Tea	8 oz	5	0	–
Half & Half	8 oz	90	0	–
Iced Tea	8 oz	80	0	–
Matt Fee	8 oz	80	0	–
Raspberry	8 oz	90	0	–
Savannah	8 oz	80	0	–
Schweppes				
Ice Tea	8 fl oz	90	0	0
Snapple				
Diet Lemon	8 fl oz	0	0	–
Diet Peach	8 fl oz	0	0	–
Diet Raspberry	8 fl oz	0	0	–
Ginseng Tea	8 fl oz	80	0	–
Green Tea w/ Lemon	8 fl oz	100	0	–
Lemon	8 fl oz	100	0	–
Lemonade Ice Tea	8 fl oz	110	0	–
Orange	8 fl oz	110	0	–
Peach	8 fl oz	100	0	–
Raspberry	8 fl oz	100	0	–
Strawberry	8 fl oz	100	0	–

FOOD	PORTION	CALS	CHOL	FIBER
Turkey Hill				
Blueberry Oolong w/ Vitamins C & E	1 cup	100	0	—
Decaffeinated	1 cup	80	0	—
Decaffeinated Orange	1 cup	10	0	—
Diet	1 cup	0	0	—
Diet Decaffeinated	1 cup	0	0	—
Diet Green Tea w/ Ginseng & Honey	1 cup	5	0	—
Green Tea w/ Ginseng & Honey	1 cup	70	0	—
Lemon	1 cup	100	0	—
Mint Tea w/ Chamomile	1 cup	90	0	—
Oolong w/ Ginkgo Biloba & Ginseng	1 cup	100	0	—
Orange	1 cup	100	0	—
Peach	1 cup	110	0	—
Raspberry Tea	1 cup	110	0	—
Regular	1 cup	90	0	—
ICES AND ICE POPS				
fruit & juice bar	1 (3 fl oz)	75	0	—
gelatin pop	1 (1.5 oz)	31	0	—
ice coconut pineapple	½ cup (4 fl oz)	109	0	—
ice fruit w/ Equal	1 bar (1.7 oz)	12	0	—
ice lime	½ cup (4 fl oz)	75	0	—
ice pop	1 (2 fl oz)	42	0	—
Ben & Jerry's				
Sorbet Devil's Food Chocolate	½ cup	170	0	2
Sorbet Doonesberry	½ cup	140	0	0
Sorbet Lemon Swirl	½ cup	120	0	0
Sorbet Purple Passion Fruit	½ cup	140	0	0
Carnation				
Cup Orange Sherbet	1 (5 oz)	150	5	0
Cup Orange Sherbet	1 (3 oz)	90	5	0

FOOD	PORTION	CALS	CHOL	FIBER
Cold Fusion				
Protein Juice Bar All Flavors	1 bar (3.8 oz)	130	0	0
Cool Creations				
Ice Pop	1 pop (2 oz)	50	0	0
Mickey Mouse Bar	1 (4 oz)	170	15	0
Surprise Pops	1 (2 oz)	60	0	0
CoolFruits				
Fruite Juice Freezer Pops Grape & Cherry	3 pops (3 oz)	70	0	0
Dole				
Fruit'n Juice Coconut	1 bar (4 oz)	210	10	0
Fruit'n Juice Lemonade	1 bar (4 oz)	120	0	0
Fruit'n Juice Lime	1 bar (4 oz)	110	0	0
Fruit'n Juice Peach Passion	1 bar (2.5 oz)	70	0	0
Fruit'n Juice Pineapple Coconut	1 bar (4 oz)	150	0	0
Fruit'n Juice Pineapple Orange Banana	1 bar (2.5 oz)	70	0	0
Fruit'n Juice Pineapple Orange Banana	1 bar (4 oz)	110	0	0
Fruit'n Juice Raspberry	1 bar (2.5 oz)	70	0	0
Fruit'n Juice Strawberry	1 bar (2.5 oz)	70	0	0
Fruit'n Juice Strawberry	1 bar (4 oz)	110	0	0
Grape No Sugar Added	1 bar (1.75 oz)	25	0	0
Raspberry	1 bar (1.75 oz)	45	0	0
Raspberry No Sugar Added	1 bar (1.75 oz)	25	0	0
Strawberry	1 bar (1.75 oz)	45	0	0
Strawberry No Sugar Added	1 bar (1.75 oz)	25	0	0
Edy's				
Fruit Bars Strawberry	1 (3 oz)	80	0	0
Sherbet Berry Rainbow	½ cup	130	5	—
Sherbet Lime	½ cup	130	5	—
Sherbet Orange Cream	½ cup	120	10	—
Sherbet Raspberry	½ cup	130	5	—
Sherbet Starburst Orange & Cherry	½ cup	150	5	—

FOOD	PORTION	CALS	CHOL	FIBER
Sherbet Starburst Strawbery	½ cup	160	5	—
Sherbet Swiss Orange	½ cup	150	5	—
Sherbet Tropical Rainbow	½ cup	130	5	—
Sorbet Coconut	½ cup	140	5	0
Sorbet Lemon	½ cup	140	0	0
Sorbet Mandarin Orange	½ cup	130	0	0
Sorbet Peach	½ cup	130	0	1
Sorbet Raspberry	½ cup	130	0	1
Sorbet Strawberry	½ cup	120	0	0
Whole Fruit Bars Creamy Coconut	1 bar	120	0	—
Whole Fruit Bars Lemonade	1 bar	80	0	—
Whole Fruit Bars Lime	1 bar	80	0	—
Whole Fruit Bars Tangerine	1 bar	80	0	—
Whole Fruit Bars Wild Berry	1 bar	80	0	—
Flintstones				
Push-Up Sherbet Treats	1 (2.75 oz)	100	5	0
Frozfruit				
Banana Cream	1 bar (4 oz)	150	25	1
Cantaloupe	1 bar (4 oz)	60	0	0
Cappuccino Cream	1 bar (3 oz)	140	25	0
Cherry	1 bar (4 oz)	70	0	1
Coconut Cream	1 bar (4 oz)	170	20	2
Kiwi Strawberry	1 bar (4 oz)	90	0	2
Lemon	1 bar (4 oz)	90	0	0
Lemon Iced Tea	1 bar (4 oz)	80	0	0
Lime	1 bar (4 oz)	90	0	0
Orange	1 bar (4 oz)	90	0	0
Pina Colada Cream	1 bar (4 oz)	170	20	1
Pineapple	1 bar (4 oz)	80	0	0
Raspberry	1 bar (4 oz)	80	0	1
Strawberry	1 bar (4 oz)	80	0	1
Strawberry Banana Cream	1 bar (4 oz)	140	20	1

FOOD	PORTION	CALS	CHOL	FIBER
Strawberry Cream	1 bar (4 oz)	130	20	1
Tropical	1 bar (4 oz)	90	0	1
Watermelon	1 bar (4 oz)	50	0	0
Good Humor				
Big Stick Cherry Pineapple	1 (3.6 fl oz)	50	0	0
Big Stick Popsicle	1 (3.6 fl oz)	50	0	—
Calippo Cherry	1 (3.8 fl oz)	100	0	—
Calippo Grape Lemon	1 (3.9 fl oz)	90	0	—
Calippo Orange	1 (3.9 fl oz)	90	0	—
Citrus Bites	1 (1.8 fl oz)	35	0	—
Creamsicle Orange	1 (2.8 fl oz)	110	10	0
Creamsicle Orange	1 (1.8 fl oz)	70	5	0
Creamsicle Orange Raspberry	1 (2.6 fl oz)	100	10	0
Creamsicle Sugar Free	1 (1.8 fl oz)	25	0	—
Fudgsicle Bar	1 (2.8 fl oz)	90	5	1
Fudgsicle Pop	1 (1.8 fl oz)	60	5	0
Fudgsicle Sugar Free	1 (1.8 fl oz)	40	<5	1
Fun Box Fudge Bar	1 (2.3 fl oz)	80	5	0
Fun Box Pops	1 (2 fl oz)	35	0	—
Fun Box Twin Box Cherry	1 (2.6 fl oz)	50	0	—
Fun Box Twin Pop Banana	1 (2.6 fl oz)	50	0	—
Fun Box Twin Pop Blue Raspberry	1 (2.6 fl oz)	50	0	—
Fun Box Twin Pop Cherry Lemon	1 (2.6 fl oz)	50	0	—
Fun Box Twin Pop Orange Cherry Grape	1 (2.6 oz)	50	0	—
Fun Box Twin Pop Root Beer	1 (2.6 fl oz)	50	0	—
Garfield Bar	1 (3.9 fl oz)	90	0	—
Hyperstripe	1 (2.8 fl oz)	80	0	—
Ice Stripe Cherry Orange	1 (1.5 fl oz)	35	0	0
Jumbo Jet Star	1 (4.7 fl oz)	80	0	—
Laser Blazer	1 (2.6 oz)	70	0	—

FOOD	PORTION	CALS	CHOL	FIBER
Popsicle All Natural	1 (1.8 fl oz)	45	0	—
Popsicle Orange Cherry Grape	1 (1.8 fl oz)	45	0	—
Popsicle Rainbow Pops	1 (1.8 fl oz)	45	0	—
Popsicle Rootbeer Banana Lime	1 (1.8 fl oz)	45	0	—
Popsicle Strawberry Raspberry Wildberry	1 (1.8 fl oz)	45	0	—
Popsicle Supersicle Traffic Signal	1	80	0	—
Popsicle Twin Pop Cherry	1 (2.6 fl oz)	70	0	—
Popsicle Twin Pop Orange Cherry Grape Lime	1 (2.6 fl oz)	70	0	—
Snow Cone	1	60	5	—
Snowfruit Coconut Bar	1 (3.75 fl oz)	150	10	1
Snowfruit Orange Bar	1	140	0	tr
Snowfruit Strawberry Bar	1	120	0	tr
Snowfruit Tropical Fruit Bar	1	110	0	—
Sugar Free Pop Orange Cherry Grape	1 (1.8 fl oz)	15	0	—
Supersicle Cherry Banana	1 (4.7 fl oz)	80	0	—
Supersicle Cherry Cola	1 (4.7 fl oz)	80	0	—
Supersicle Double Fudge	1 (4.7 fl oz)	150	10	1
Supersicle Firecracker	1 (4.7 fl oz)	90	0	—
Supersicle Firecracker Jr.	1	72	0	—
Supersicle Sour Tower	1	80	0	—
Swirl Bubble Gum	1 (2.7 fl oz)	55	0	—
Swirl Cherry Banana	1 (2.7 fl oz)	55	0	—
Torpedo Cherry	1 (1.8 fl oz)	35	0	0
Twister Blue Raspberry Cherry Cherry Cola	1 (1.8 fl oz)	45	0	—

FOOD	PORTION	CALS	CHOL	FIBER
Twister Cherry Lemon Orange Lemon	1 (1.8 fl oz)	45	0	—
Vampire's Deadly Secret	1 (2.8 fl oz)	100	0	—
Watermelon Bar	1 (3.6 fl oz)	80	0	—
Häagen-Dazs				
Sorbet Chocolate	½ cup	120	0	2
Sorbet Mango	½ cup	120	0	tr
Sorbet Orange	½ cup	120	0	tr
Sorbet Orchard Peach	½ cup	130	0	tr
Sorbet Raspberry	½ cup	120	0	2
Sorbet Strawberry	½ cup	120	0	1
Sorbet Zesty Lemon	½ cup	120	0	tr
Sorbet Bar Chocolate	1 (2.7 oz)	80	0	1
Sorbet Bars Raspberry & Vanilla Yogurt	1 (2.5 oz)	90	0	tr
Sorbet Bars Strawberry & Vanilla Ice Cream	1 (2.5 oz)	110	35	0
Hood				
Hendrie's Sizzle'N Sour Stix	1 bar (2 oz)	80	5	0
Hoodsie Pop	1 (3.3 oz)	60	0	—
Natural Blenders Pineappple	1 bar (1 oz)	60	0	—
Natural Blenders Raspberry	1 bar (1 oz)	60	0	—
Natural Blenders Strawberry	1 bar (1 oz)	60	0	—
Pop Banana	1 (3.3 oz)	60	0	—
Pop Blue Raspberry	1 (3.3 oz)	60	0	—
Pop Cherry	1 (3.3 oz)	60	0	—
Pop Grape	1 (3.3 oz)	60	0	—
Pop Orange	1 (3.3 oz)	60	0	—
Pop Root Beer	1 (3.3 oz)	60	0	—
Super Sortment Juice Bars	1 bar (1.9 oz)	40	0	—
Lifesavers				
Ice Pops	1 (1.75 oz)	35	0	0
Mr. Freeze				
Assorted	2 bars (3 oz)	45	0	0

FOOD	PORTION	CALS	CHOL	FIBER
Tropical	2 bars (3 oz)	45	0	0
Natural Choice				
Organic Banana	½ cup (3.6 oz)	110	0	tr
Organic Blueberry	½ cup (3.6 oz)	100	0	tr
Organic Kiwi	½ cup (3.6 oz)	110	0	tr
Organic Lemon	½ cup (3.6 oz)	110	0	tr
Organic Mango	½ cup (3.6 oz)	110	0	tr
Organic Strawberry	½ cup (3.6 oz)	110	0	tr
Organic Strawberry Kiwi	½ cup (3.6 oz)	110	0	tr
Silhouette				
Fat Free Fudge Bars	1	90	0	—
Tofutti				
Frutti Apricot Mango	4 fl oz	100	0	—
Frutti Three Berry	4 fl oz	100	0	—
Frutti Vanilla Apple Orchard	4 fl oz	100	0	—
JACKFRUIT				
fresh	3.5 oz	70	0	—
JALAPENO (see PEPPERS)				
JAM/JELLY/PRESERVES				
all flavors jam	1 pkg (0.5 oz)	34	0	tr
all flavors jam	1 tbsp (0.7 oz)	48	0	tr
all flavors jelly	1 tbsp (0.7 oz)	52	0	tr
all flavors jelly	1 pkg (0.5 oz)	38	0	tr
all flavors preserve	1 pkg (0.5 oz)	34	0	tr
all flavors preserve	1 tbsp (0.7 oz)	48	0	tr
apple butter	1 cup (9.9 oz)	519	0	—
apple butter	1 tbsp (0.6 oz)	33	0	—
apple jelly	1 pkg (0.5 oz)	38	0	tr
apple jelly	1 tbsp (0.7 oz)	52	0	tr
apricot jam	0.5 oz	36	0	—
blackberry jam	0.5 oz	34	0	—
cherry jam	0.5 oz	36	0	—
orange jam	0.5 oz	35	0	—
orange marmalade	1 tbsp (0.7 oz)	49	0	—
orange marmalade	1 pkg (0.5 oz)	34	0	—
plum jam	0.5 oz	34	0	—

FOOD	PORTION	CALS	CHOL	FIBER
quince jam	0.5 oz	43	0	–
raspberry jam	0.5 oz	35	0	–
raspberry jelly	0.5 oz	37	0	–
red currant jam	0.5 oz	34	0	–
red currant jelly	0.5 oz	38	0	–
rose hip jam	0.5 oz	36	0	–
strawberry jam	1 tbsp (0.7 oz)	48	0	tr
strawberry jam	1 pkg (0.5 oz)	34	0	tr
strawberry preserve	1 pkg (0.5 oz)	34	0	tr
strawberry preserve	1 tbsp (0.7 oz)	48	0	tr
Eden				
Cherry Butter	1 tbsp	35	0	1
Organic Apple Butter	1 tbsp	20	0	0
Estee				
Fruit Spread Apple Spice	1 tbsp	16	0	0
Fruit Spread Apricot	1 tbsp	16	0	0
Fruit Spread Grape	1 tbsp	16	0	0
Fruit Spread Peach	1 tbsp	16	0	0
Fruit Spread Red Raspberry	1 tbsp	16	0	0
Fruit Spread Strawberry	1 tbsp	16	0	0
Polaner				
All Fruit Peach	1 tbsp	40	0	–
All Fruit Raspberry	1 tbsp	40	0	–
Red Wing				
Apple Jelly	1 tbsp (0.7 oz)	50	0	0
Apple Blackberry Jelly	1 tbsp (0.7 oz)	50	0	0
Apple Cherry Jelly	1 tbsp (0.7 oz)	50	0	0
Apple Currant Jelly	1 tbsp (0.7 oz)	50	0	0
Apple Grape Jelly	1 tbsp (0.7 oz)	50	0	0
Apple Raspberry Jelly	1 tbsp (0.7 oz)	50	0	0
Apple Strawberry Jelly	1 tbsp (0.7 oz)	50	0	0
Black Raspberry Jelly	1 tbsp (0.7 oz)	50	0	0
Blackberry Jelly	1 tbsp (0.7 oz)	50	0	0
Cherry Jelly	1 tbsp (0.7 oz)	50	0	0
Concord Grape Jelly	1 tbsp (0.7 oz)	50	0	0
Crabapple Jelly	1 tbsp (0.7 oz)	50	0	0
Cranberry Jelly	1 tbsp (0.7 oz)	50	0	0
Cranberry Grape Jelly	1 tbsp (0.7 oz)	50	0	0

FOOD	PORTION	CALS	CHOL	FIBER
Currant Jelly	1 tbsp (0.7 oz)	50	0	0
Damson Plum Jelly	1 tbsp (0.7 oz)	50	0	0
Elderberry Jelly	1 tbsp (0.7 oz)	50	0	0
Grape Jelly	1 tbsp (0.7 oz)	50	0	0
Mint Jelly	1 tbsp (0.7 oz)	50	0	0
Mint Apple Jelly	1 tbsp (0.7 oz)	50	0	0
Mixed Fruit Jelly	1 tbsp (0.7 oz)	50	0	0
Red Plum Jelly	1 tbsp (0.7 oz)	50	0	0
Red Raspberry Jelly	1 tbsp (0.7 oz)	50	0	0
Strawberry Jelly	1 tbsp (0.7 oz)	50	0	0
Strawberry Apple Jelly	1 tbsp (0.7 oz)	50	0	0
Sarabeth's				
Spreadable Fruit	1 tbsp	40	0	tr
Strawberry				
Raspberry				
Smucker's				
Concord Grape Jelly	1 tbsp	50	0	—
Peach Preserves	1 tbsp	50	0	—
Simply Fruit	1 tbsp	40	0	—
Red Raspberry				
Tabasco				
Spicy Pepper Jelly	1 tbsp (0.6 oz)	50	0	0
Welch's				
Grape Jam	1 tbsp	50	0	—
White House				
Apple Butter	1 tbsp (0.6 oz)	35	0	—
Wild Thyme Farms				
Fruit Spreads	1 tsp	8	0	—
Blackberry				
Currant Ginger				
Fruit Spreads	1 tsp	7	0	—
Mango Apricot				

JAPANESE FOOD (see ASIAN FOOD, SUSHI)

JAVA PLUM

fresh	1 cup	82	0	—
fresh	3	5	0	—

JELLY (see JAM/JELLY/PRESERVE)

FOOD	PORTION	CALS	CHOL	FIBER
JUTE				
cooked	1 cup	32	0	2
KALE				
chopped cooked	½ cup	21	0	–
frzn chopped cooked	½ cup	20	0	–
raw chopped	½ cup	21	0	–
scotch chopped cooked	½ cup	18	0	–
KETCHUP				
ketchup	1 tbsp	16	0	tr
ketchup	1 pkg (0.2 oz)	6	0	tr
low sodium	1 tbsp	16	0	tr
Del Monte				
Ketchup	1 tbsp (0.5 oz)	15	0	0
Estee				
Ketchup	1 tbsp	15	0	0
Healthy Choice				
Ketchup	1 tbsp (0.5 oz)	9	0	tr
Heinz				
Ketchup	1 tbsp (0.6 oz)	15	0	0
Hunt's				
Ketchup	1 tbsp (0.6 oz)	16	0	0
No Salt Added	1 tbsp (0.6 oz)	16	0	0
McIlhenny				
Spicy	1 tbsp (0.6 oz)	20	0	0
Muir Glen				
Organic	1 tbsp (0.6 oz)	15	0	0
Red Wing				
Extra Fancy	1 tbsp (0.6 oz)	20	0	0
Smucker's				
Tomato	1 tbsp	25	0	–
Tree Of Life				
Ketchup	1 tbsp (0.5 oz)	10	0	–
KIDNEY				
beef simmered	3 oz	122	329	–
lamb braised	3 oz	117	481	–
pork cooked	3 oz	128	408	0
pork cooked	1 cup	211	672	0
veal braised	3 oz	139	672	–

FOOD	PORTION	CALS	CHOL	FIBER
KIDNEY BEANS				
CANNED				
kidney beans	1 cup	208	0	—
red	1 cup	216	0	—
B&M				
Red Baked Beans	½ cup (4.6 oz)	170	<5	6
Friend's				
Red Baked Beans	½ cup (4.6 oz)	160	<5	6
Green Giant				
Dark Red	½ cup (4.5 oz)	110	0	5
Light Red	½ cup (4.5 oz)	110	0	6
Hunt's				
Kidney	½ cup (4.5 oz)	94	0	5
Progresso				
Dark Red	½ cup (4.5 oz)	110	0	6
Red	½ cup (4.6 oz)	110	0	8
S&W				
Dark Red Premium	½ cup (4.6 oz)	100	0	6
Van Camp				
Dark Red	½ cup (4.6 oz)	90	0	6
Light Red	½ cup (4.6 oz)	90	0	6
DRIED				
california red cooked	1 cup	219	0	—
cooked	1 cup	225	0	—
red cooked	1 cup	225	0	—
royal red cooked	1 cup	218	0	—
KIWI JUICE				
After The Fall				
Kiwi Bear	1 cup (8 oz)	100	0	0
KIWIS				
fresh	1 med	46	0	3
Chiquita				
Fresh	2 med (5.2 oz)	100	0	4
Sonoma				
Dried	7-8 pieces (1 oz)	90	0	2
KNISH				
Joshua's				
Coney Island Potato	1 (4.6 oz)	280	0	1

FOOD	PORTION	CALS	CHOL	FIBER
TAKE-OUT				
cheese & blueberry	1 (7 oz)	378	40	–
cheese & cherry	1 (7 oz)	378	40	–
everything	1 (7 oz)	221	0	–
kashe	1 (7 oz)	270	0	–
potato	1 lg (7 oz)	332	72	1
potato	1 med (3.5 oz)	166	36	tr
potato w/ broccoli & cheese	1 (7 oz)	312	24	–
potato w/ spinach & mushroom	1 (7 oz)	214	0	–
KOHLRABI				
raw sliced	½ cup	19	0	–
sliced cooked	½ cup	24	0	–
KUMQUATS				
fresh	1	12	0	–
LAMB				
cubed lean only braised	3 oz	190	92	–
cubed lean only broiled	3 oz	158	77	–
ground broiled	3 oz	240	82	–
leg lean & fat Choice roasted	3 oz	219	79	–
loin chop w/ bone lean & fat Choice broiled	1 chop (2.3 oz)	201	64	–
loin chop w/ bone lean only Choice broiled	1 chop (1.6 oz)	100	44	–
new zealand lean & fat cooked	3 oz	259	93	–
new zealand lean only cooked	3 oz	175	93	–
rib chop lean & fat Choice broiled	3 oz	307	84	–
rib chop lean only Choice broiled	3 oz	200	78	–

FOOD	PORTION	CALS	CHOL	FIBER
shank lean & fat Choice braised	3 oz	206	90	–
shank lean & fat Choice roasted	3 oz	191	77	–
shoulder chop w/ bone lean & fat Choice braised	1 chop (2.5 oz)	244	84	–
shoulder chop w/ bone lean only Choice braised	1 chop (1.9 oz)	152	66	–
sirloin lean & fat Choice roasted	3 oz	248	82	–

LAMB DISHES
TAKE-OUT

FOOD	PORTION	CALS	CHOL	FIBER
curry	¾ cup	345	89	–
stew	¾ cup	124	29	2

LAMBSQUARTERS

FOOD	PORTION	CALS	CHOL	FIBER
chopped cooked	½ cup	29	0	–

LEEKS

FOOD	PORTION	CALS	CHOL	FIBER
chopped cooked	¼ cup	8	0	–
cooked	1 (4.4 oz)	38	0	–
freeze dried	1 tbsp	1	0	–
raw	1 (4.4 oz)	76	0	–
raw chopped	¼ cup	16	0	–

LEMON

FOOD	PORTION	CALS	CHOL	FIBER
fresh	1 med	22	0	–
peel	1 tbsp	0	0	–
wedge	1	5	0	

LEMON EXTRACT
Virginia Dare

FOOD	PORTION	CALS	CHOL	FIBER
Extract	1 tsp	22	0	–

LEMON GRASS

FOOD	PORTION	CALS	CHOL	FIBER
fresh	1 tbsp (5 g)	5	0	0
fresh	1 cup (2.4 oz)	66	0	0

FOOD	PORTION	CALS	CHOL	FIBER
LEMON JUICE				
bottled	1 tbsp	3	0	–
fresh	1 tbsp	4	0	–
frzn	1 tbsp	3	0	–
After The Fall				
Spicy Lemon	1 can (12 oz)	150	0	0
Canarino				
Italian Hot	1 cup	0	0	0
Lemon Beverage	(8 oz)			
Realemon				
Juice	1 tsp (5 ml)	0	0	–
LEMONADE				
FROZEN				
as prep w/ water	1 cup	100	0	–
not prep	1 can (6 oz)	397	0	–
Bright & Early				
Lemonade	8 fl oz	120	0	–
MIX				
powder	9 fl oz	113	0	–
as prep w/ water				
powder w/ equal	1 pitcher (67 oz)	40	0	–
Country Time				
Lem'n Berry Sippers	1 serv (8 oz)	90	0	0
Cranberry Raspberry				
Lemonade as prep				
Lem'n Berry Sippers	1 serv (8 oz)	90	0	0
Raspberry Lemonade				
as prep				
Lem'n Berry Sippers	1 serv (8 oz)	90	0	0
Strawberry Lemonade				
as prep				
Lem'n Berry Sippers	1 serv (8 oz)	90	0	0
Wildberry Lemonade				
as prep				
Lem'n Berry Sippers	1 serv (8 oz)	5	0	0
Sugar Free Strawberry				
Lemonade as prep				
Lemonade as prep	1 serv (8 oz)	70	0	0
Pink as prep	1 serv (8 oz)	70	0	0

FOOD	PORTION	CALS	CHOL	FIBER
Sugar Free Pink as prep	1 serv (8 oz)	5	0	0
Sugar Free as prep	1 serv (8 oz)	5	0	0
Crystal Light				
Lemonade as prep	1 serv (8 oz)	5	0	0
Pink as prep	1 serv (8 oz)	5	0	0
Kool-Aid				
Lemonade as prep	1 serv (8 oz)	70	0	0
Mix as prep w/ sugar	1 serv (8 oz)	100	0	0
Pink as prep w/ sugar	1 serv (8 oz)	100	0	0
Soarin' Strawberry Lemonade as prep	1 serv (8 oz)	70	0	0
Soarin' Strawberry Lemonade as prep w/ sugar	1 serv (8 oz)	100	0	0
Sugar Free Soarin' Strawberry Lemonade as prep	1 serv (8 oz)	5	0	0
Sugar Free Mix as prep	1 serv (8 oz)	5	0	0
READY-TO-DRINK				
After The Fall				
Apple Raspberry	1 bottle (10 oz)	120	0	–
Crystal Geyser				
Juice Squeeze Pink	1 bottle (12 fl oz)	140	0	–
Crystal Light				
Lemonade	1 serv (8 oz)	5	0	0
Pink	1 serv (8 oz)	5	0	0
Diet Rite				
Salt/Sodium Free	8 fl oz	2	0	–
Everfresh				
Lemonade	1 can (8 oz)	120	0	0
Ruby Red	1 can (8 oz)	110	0	0
Fruitopia				
Lemonade	8 fl oz	120	0	–
Hansen's				
Sparkling	8 fl oz	100	0	–
Sparkling Pink	8 fl oz	120	0	–
Nantucket Nectars				
Authentic	8 oz	120	0	–
Pink	8 oz	120	0	–

FOOD	PORTION	CALS	CHOL	FIBER
Nehi				
Lemonade	8 fl oz	130	0	–
Newman's Own				
Lemonade	1 bottle (10 oz)	140	0	0
Roadside Virginia	8 fl oz	110	0	0
Santa Cruz				
Organic	8 oz	100	0	–
Shasta Plus				
Lemonade	1 can (11.5 oz)	160	0	0
Snapple				
Diet Pink	8 fl oz	20	0	–
Lemonade	8 fl oz	120	0	–
Pink	8 fl oz	120	0	–
Strawberry	8 fl oz	110	0	–
Turkey Hill				
Lemonade	1 cup	120	0	–
Raspberry	1 cup	120	0	–
Strawberry Kiwi	1 cup	120	0	–
Veryfine				
Chillers	1 can (11.5 oz)	190	0	0
Chillers Cherry	8 fl oz	120	0	0
Chillers Peach	8 fl oz	120	0	0
Chillers Pink	1 can (11.5 oz)	180	0	0
Chillers Strawberry	1 can (11.5 oz)	170	0	0
LENTILS				
dried cooked	1 cup	231	0	–
Casbah				
Pilaf as prep	1 cup	200	0	2
Natural Touch				
Lentil Rice Loaf	1 in slice (3.2 oz)	170	0	4
Shiloh Farms				
Organic Green not prep	¼ cup (1.6 oz)	150	0	7
TastyBite				
Bengal Lentils	½ pkg (5 oz)	190	0	1
Jodhpur Lentils	½ pkg (5 oz)	190	0	2
Madras Lentils	½ pkg (5 oz)	130	22	5
TAKE-OUT				
indian sambar	1 serv	236	10	9

FOOD	PORTION	CALS	CHOL	FIBER
yemiser selatta eithopian lentil salad	1 serv (3 oz)	115	0	2

LETTUCE *(see also SALAD)*

arugula	½ cup (0.4 oz)	3	0	tr
bibb	1 head (6 oz)	21	0	2
boston	2 leaves	2	0	tr
boston	1 head (6 oz)	21	0	2
cornsalad field salad	1 cup (1.9 oz)	7	0	1
iceberg	1 leaf	3	0	tr
iceberg	1 head (19 oz)	70	0	5
looseleaf shredded	½ cup	5	0	–
romaine shredded	½ cup	4	0	tr
Dole				
Iceberg	1 cup (3 oz)	15	0	1
Romaine	1 ½ cups (3 oz)	15	0	2
Shredded	1 ½ cup (3 oz)	15	0	1
Earthbound Farm				
Romaine Salad Organic	1 ½ cups (2.9 oz)	15	0	1
Western Express				
Hearts Of Romaine	6 leaves (3 oz)	20	0	1

LIMA BEANS
CANNED

large	1 cup	191	0	–
lima beans	½ cup	93	0	–
Del Monte				
Green	½ cup (4.4 oz)	80	0	4
Eden				
Organic Baby	½ cup (4.6 oz)	100	0	4
S&W				
Small Green	½ cup (4.4 oz)	80	0	4
Veg-All				
Baby Green	½ cup	90	0	3
DRIED				
baby cooked	1 cup	229	0	17
cooked	½ cup	104	0	–
large cooked	1 cup	217	0	14

FOOD	PORTION	CALS	CHOL	FIBER
Hurst				
HamBeens Baby Limas w/ Ham	1 serv	120	0	9
HamBeens Large Limas w/ Ham	1 serv	120	0	9
FROZEN				
cooked	½ cup	94	0	–
fordhook cooked	½ cup	85	0	–
Birds Eye				
Baby	½ cup	130	0	6
Fordhook	½ cup	100	0	5
Green Giant				
Butter Sauce	⅔ cup (3.6 oz)	120	<5	6
Harvest Fresh Baby	½ cup (2.7 oz)	80	0	4
LIME				
fresh	1	20	0	–
LIME JUICE				
bottled	1 tbsp	3	0	–
fresh	1 tbsp	4	0	–
After The Fall				
Caribbean Lime	1 can (12 oz)	170	0	0
Key West	1 cup (8 oz)	100	0	0
Realime				
Juice	1 tsp (5 ml)	0	0	–
LINGCOD				
baked	3 oz	93	57	–
fillet baked	5.3 oz	164	101	–
LIQUOR/LIQUEUR *(see also BEER AND ALE, CHAMPAGNE, WINE)*				
anisette	⅔ oz	74	0	0
apricot brandy	⅔ oz	64	0	0
benedictine	⅔ oz	69	0	0
bloody mary	5 oz	116	0	–
bourbon & soda	4 oz	105	0	–
coffee liqueur	1 ½ oz	174	0	–
cognac	1 oz	67	0	0
cosmopolitan	1 (4 oz)	213	0	0
creme de menthe	1 ½ oz	186	0	–
curacao liqueur	⅔ oz	54	0	0

FOOD	PORTION	CALS	CHOL	FIBER
daiquiri	2 oz	111	0	–
gin	1 ½ oz	110	0	–
gin & tonic	7.5 oz	171	0	–
gin ricky	4 oz	150	0	–
long island iced tea	1 serv (7.5 oz)	159	0	0
manhattan	2 oz	128	0	–
martini	2 ½ oz	156	0	–
mint julep	10 oz	210	0	0
old-fashioned	2 ½ oz	127	0	0
pina colada	4 ½ oz	262	0	–
planter's punch	3 ½ oz	175	0	–
rum	1 ½ oz	97	0	–
screwdriver	7 oz	174	0	–
sloe gin fizz	2 ½ oz	132	0	0
tequila sunrise	5 ½ oz	189	0	–
tom collins	7 ½ oz	121	0	–
vodka	1 ½ oz	97	0	–
whiskey	1 ½ oz	105	0	–
whiskey sour	3 oz	123	0	–
LIVER (see also PATE)				
beef braised	3 oz	137	331	–
beef pan-fried	3 oz	184	410	–
chicken stewed	1 cup (5 oz)	219	883	–
duck raw	1 (1.5 oz)	60	227	–
lamb braised	3 oz	187	426	–
lamb fried	3 oz	202	419	–
pork braised	3 oz	140	302	0
turkey simmered	1 cup (5 oz)	237	876	–
veal braised	3 oz	140	477	–
veal fried	3 oz	208	280	–
Shady Brook				
Turkey	4 oz	160	530	
LOBSTER				
northern cooked	1 cup	142	104	–
northern cooked	3 oz	83	61	–
northern raw	3 oz	77	81	–
northern raw	1 lobster (5.3 oz)	136	143	–
spiny steamed	3 oz	122	76	–
spiny steamed	1 (5.7 oz)	233	146	–

FOOD	PORTION	CALS	CHOL	FIBER
Progresso				
Lobster Sauce	½ cup (4.3 oz)	100	5	2
TAKE-OUT				
newburg	1 cup	485	455	—
LOGANBERRIES				
frzn	1 cup	80	0	—
LONGANS				
fresh	1	2	0	—
LOQUATS				
fresh	1	5	0	—
LOTUS				
root raw sliced	10 slices	45	0	—
root sliced cooked	10 slices	59	0	—
seeds dried	1 oz	94	0	—
Eden				
Root	1 serv (0.3 oz)	35	0	2
LOX *(see* SALMON*)*				
LUPINES				
dried cooked	1 cup	197	0	—
LYCHEES				
fresh	1	6	0	—
MACADAMIA NUTS				
dry roasted w/ salt	10-12 nuts (1 oz)	200	0	1
oil roasted	1 oz	204	0	
Hawaiian Host				
Chocolate Covered	1 piece (0.5 oz)	53	2	t
MacFarms of Hawaii				
Chocolate Covered	¼ cup (1.3 oz)	210	5	2
Dry Roasted Salted	¼ cup (1.3 oz)	220	0	3
Kona Coffee Dark Chocolate Covered	¼ cup (1.3 oz)	210	5	2
MACE				
ground	1 tsp	8	0	—

FOOD	PORTION	CALS	CHOL	FIBER
MACKEREL				
CANNED				
jack	1 can (12.7 oz)	563	285	—
jack	1 cup	296	150	—
DRIED				
Eden				
Bonito Flakes	2 tbsp	4	1	0
FRESH				
atlantic cooked	3 oz	223	64	—
atlantic raw	3 oz	174	60	—
jack baked	3 oz	171	51	—
jack fillet baked	6.2 oz	354	106	—
king baked	3 oz	114	58	—
king fillet baked	5.4 oz	207	105	—
pacific baked	3 oz	171	51	—
pacific fillet baked	6.2 oz	354	106	—
spanish cooked	3 oz	134	62	—
spanish cooked	1 fillet (5.1 oz)	230	107	—
spanish raw	3 oz	118	65	—
SMOKED				
atlantic	3.5 oz	296	93	—
MALT				
nonalcoholic	12 fl oz	32	0	—
Bartles & Jaymes				
Malt Cooler Berry	12 fl oz	210	0	—
Malt Cooler Black Cherry	12 fl oz	190	0	—
Malt Cooler Light Berry	12 fl oz	140	0	—
Malt Cooler Mandarin Lemon	12 fl oz	210	0	—
Malt Cooler Margarita	12 fl oz	250	0	—
Malt Cooler Original	12 fl oz	180	0	—
Malt Cooler Peach	12 fl oz	200	0	—
Malt Cooler Pina Colada	12 fl oz	270	0	—
Malt Cooler Planter's Punch	12 fl oz	220	0	—

FOOD	PORTION	CALS	CHOL	FIBER
Malt Cooler Red Sangria	12 fl oz	190	0	—
Malt Cooler Strawberry	12 fl oz	200	0	—
Malt Cooler Strawberry Daiquiri	12 fl oz	220	0	—
Malt Cooler Tropical	12 fl oz	220	0	—
MALTED MILK				
chocolate as prep w/ milk	1 cup	229	34	—
chocolate flavor powder	3 heaping tsp (¾ oz)	79	1	—
natural flavor as prep w/ milk	1 cup	237	37	—
natural flavor powder	3 heaping tsp (¾ oz)	87	4	—
Carnation				
Chocolate	3 tbsp (0.7 oz)	90	0	tr
Original	3 tbsp (0.7 oz)	90	5	tr
MAMMY-APPLE				
fresh	1	431	0	—
MANGO				
fresh	1	135	0	—
Del Monte				
In Extra Light Syrup	½ cup (4.4 oz)	100	0	0
Rainforest Farms				
Slices Dried	6 slices (1.3 oz)	140	0	2
Sonoma				
Pieces Dried	8 pieces (2 oz)	180	0	0
MANGO JUICE				
After The Fall				
Hawaiian Mango	1 can (12 oz)	180	0	0
Mango Ginger	1 can (12 oz)	150	0	0
Fresh Samantha				
Mango Mama	1 cup (8 oz)	120	0	8
Guzzler				
Mango Passion	8 fl oz	140	0	—
Ocean Spray				
Mango Mango	8 oz	130	0	0

FOOD	PORTION	CALS	CHOL	FIBER
Snapple				
Diet Mango Madness	8 fl oz	13	0	–
Mango Madness	8 fl oz	110	0	–
Tang				
Drink Mix as prep	1 serv (8 oz)	100	0	0
MARGARINE				
squeeze	1 tsp	34	0	–
stick corn	1 tsp	34	0	–
stick corn	1 stick (4 oz)	815	0	–
tub corn	1 tsp	34	0	–
tub diet	1 tsp	17	0	–
Benecol				
Single Serve Light	1 pkg (0.3 oz)	30	0	–
Tub Light	1 tbsp (0.5 oz)	45	0	–
Tub Regular	1 tbsp (0.5 oz)	80	0	–
I Can't Believe Its Not Butter				
Spray	5 sprays	0	0	0
Krona				
Stick	1 tbsp	100	15	–
Parkay				
Squeeze	1 tbsp (0.5 oz)	80	0	0
Stick	1 tbsp (0.5 oz)	90	0	0
Stick ⅓ Less Fat	1 tbsp (0.5 oz)	70	0	0
Tub	1 tbsp (0.5 oz)	60	0	0
Tub Light	1 tbsp (0.5 oz)	50	0	0
Tub Soft	1 tbsp (0.5 oz)	100	0	0
Tub Soft Diet	1 tbsp (0.5 oz)	50	0	0
Whipped	1 tbsp (0.3 oz)	70	0	0
Promise				
Spread Soft	1 tbsp	80	0	–
Spread Stick	1 tbsp	90	0	–
Spread Light Soft	1 tbsp	50	0	–
Spread Light Stick	1 tbsp	50	0	–
Ultra Soft	1 tbsp	30	0	–
Ultra Spread Fat Free	1 tbsp	5	0	–
Smart Balance				
No Trans Fat	1 tbsp (0.5 oz)	120	0	–
No Trans Fat Light	1 tbsp (0.5 oz)	45	0	–
No Trans Fat Spread	1 tbsp (0.5 oz)	80	0	–

FOOD	PORTION	CALS	CHOL	FIBER
Smart Beat				
Light Unsalted	1 tbsp (0.5 oz)	25	0	—
Squeeze Fat Free	1 tbsp (0.5 oz)	5	0	—
Super Light Trans Fat Free	1 tbsp (0.5 oz)	20	0	—
Take Control				
Spread	1 tbsp (0.5 oz)	50	<5	0
Weight Watchers				
Light	1 tbsp	45	0	0
Light Sodium Free	1 tbsp	45	0	0

MARINADE *(see SAUCE)*

MARJORAM
dried	1 tsp	2	0	—

MARSHMALLOW
marshmallow	1 reg (0.3 oz)	23	0	—
marshmallow	1 cup (1.6 oz)	146	0	—
Joyva				
Twists Chocolate Covered	2 (1.5 oz)	190	0	0
Just Born				
Peeps	5 (1.5 oz)	160	0	—

MATZO
plain	1 (1 oz)	112	0	1
whole wheat	1 (1 oz)	99	0	3
Goodman's				
Matzo Ball Mix 50% Less Salt	2 tbsp (0.5 oz)	50	0	0
Matzo Ball Mix as prep	2 tbsp (0.5 oz)	60	0	1
Horowitz Margareten				
Egg Milk Chocolate Coated	1 oz	97	8	1
Manischewitz				
Egg Dark Chocolate Coated	½ matzo (1 oz)	97	8	1
Matzo Meal	¼ cup (1 oz)	130	0	1
Streit's				
Dietetic	1 (1 oz)	100	0	1

FOOD	PORTION	CALS	CHOL	FIBER
Lightly Salted	1 (1 oz)	110	0	1
Matzoh Meal	¼ cup (1 oz)	110	0	1
Passover	1 (1 oz)	110	0	1
Unsalted	1 (0.9 oz)	100	0	1
Whole Wheat	1 (1 oz)	110	0	4
MAYONNAISE				
mayonnaise	1 tbsp	99	8	—
mayonnaise	1 cup	1577	130	—
reduced calorie	1 tbsp	34	4	—
reduced calorie	1 cup	556	58	—
sandwich spread	1 tbsp	60	12	—
Blue Plate				
Squeeze	1 tbsp	100	10	0
Hellman's				
Mayonnaise	1 tbsp	100	5	—
Kraft				
Fat Free	1 tbsp (0.6 oz)	10	0	0
Light	1 tbsp (0.5 oz)	50	5	0
Real	1 tbsp (0.5 oz)	100	5	0
Mother's				
Mayonnaise	1 tbsp	100	10	—
Red Wing				
"H" Style	1 tbsp (0.5 oz)	110	10	0
Smart Beat				
Fat Free	1 tbsp	10	0	—
Weight Watchers				
Fat Free	1 tbsp	10	0	0
Light	1 tbsp	25	5	0
Light Low Sodium	1 tbsp	25	5	0
MAYONNAISE TYPE SALAD DRESSING				
mayonnaise type salad dressing	1 cup	916	60	—
mayonnaise type salad dressing	1 tbsp	57	4	—
reduced calorie w/o cholesterol	1 cup	1084	0	—
reduced calorie w/o cholesterol	1 tbsp	68	0	—

FOOD	PORTION	CALS	CHOL	FIBER
Miracle Whip				
Free	1 tbsp (0.5 oz)	15	0	0
Light	1 tbsp (0.5 oz)	35	<5	0
Salad Dressing	1 tbsp (0.6 oz)	70	5	0
Nasoya				
Nayonaise	1 tbsp	35	0	0
Nayonaise Dijon	1 tbsp	30	0	0
Weight Watchers				
Fat Free Whipped Dressing	1 tbsp	15	0	0

MEAT STICKS

FOOD	PORTION	CALS	CHOL	FIBER
jerky beef	1 lg piece (0.7 oz)	67	22	–
jerky beef	1 oz	96	32	–
smoked	1 (0.7 oz)	109	26	–
smoked	1 oz	156	38	–
Big Ones				
BBQ	1 (1 oz)	130	35	0
Hot n'Spicy	1 (1 oz)	130	35	0
Original	1 (1 oz)	130	35	0
Teriyaki	1 (1 oz)	130	35	0
Jack Link's				
Kippered Beefsteak Teriyaki	1 oz	80	25	0
Lance				
Beef & Cheese	1 pkg (1.5 oz)	150	45	0
Beef Jerky	1 piece (0.25 oz)	30	<5	0
Beef Snack	1 piece (0.63 oz)	100	10	0
Hot Sausage	1 piece (0.9 oz)	60	15	0
Lowrey's				
Smokehouse Tender Hickory Smoked	1 pkg (1 oz)	80	25	0
Smokehouse Tender Original	1 pkg (1 oz)	60	25	1
Smokehouse Tender Peppered	1 pkg (1 oz)	60	25	1
Oberto				
Beef Jerky	1 pkg (1.3 oz)	100	25	–

FOOD	PORTION	CALS	CHOL	FIBER
Pemmican				
Original Tender Kippered Beef Steak	1	110	35	0
Peppered Tender Kippered Beef Steak	1	110	35	0
Rough Cut				
Beef Steak Hot	1 pkg (1 oz)	70	25	0
Beef Steak Original	1 pkg (1 oz)	60	25	0
Beef Steak Peppered	1 pkg (1 oz)	60	25	0
Rustlers Roundup				
Beef Jerky	1 serv (5 g)	20	5	tr
Flamin' Hot	1 serv (8 g)	40	10	tr
Smoky Steak	1 serv (0.8 oz)	60	20	0
Spicy	1 serv (0.5 oz)	70	20	tr
Slim Jim				
Spicy	1 (4½ in) (0.3 oz)	50	5	0
Spicy Big	1 (.44 oz)	70	10	0
Spicy Giant	1 (0.97 oz)	150	15	1
Spicy Super	1 (0.64 oz)	100	10	0

MEAT SUBSTITUTES *(see also* BACON SUBSTITUTES, CANADIAN BACON SUBSTITUTES, CHICKEN SUBSTITUTES, HAMBURGER SUBSTITUTES, SAUSAGE SUBSTITUTES, TURKEY SUBSTITUTES*)*

FOOD	PORTION	CALS	CHOL	FIBER
simulated meat product	1 oz	88	0	—
Boca Burgers				
Chef Max's Original	1 patty (2.5 oz)	110	3	4
Frieda's				
SoyTaco	1 oz	50	0	2
Soyrizo	4 tbsp (1.9 oz)	120	0	3
Ken & Robert's				
Veggie Pockets	1 (4.5 oz)	250	0	5
Veggie Pockets Bar B Que	1 (4.5 oz)	290	0	5
Veggie Pockets Broccoli & Cheddar	1 (4.5 oz)	250	0	4
Veggie Pockets Greek	1 (4.5 oz)	250	0	4
Veggie Pockets Indian	1 (4.5 oz)	260	0	5
Veggie Pockets Pizza	1 (4.5 oz)	270	0	4
Veggie Pockets Pot Pie	1 (4.5 oz)	250	0	2

FOOD	PORTION	CALS	CHOL	FIBER
Veggie Pockets Potato & Cheddar	1 (4.5 oz)	260	0	2
Veggie Pockets Santa Fe	1 (4.5 oz)	250	0	5
Veggie Pockets Tex Mex	1 (4.5 oz)	260	0	6
Lightlife				
Foney Baloney	3 slices (1.5 oz)	60	0	0
Gimme Lean Beef	2 oz	70	0	1
Smart Deli Bologna	3 slices (1.5 oz)	50	0	0
Smart Deli Ham	3 slices (1.5 oz)	50	0	0
Smart Deli Peppercorn	3 slices (1.5 oz)	45	0	0
Smart Deli Stickes Soylami	1 oz	40	0	0
Smart Deli Sticks Pepperoni	1 oz	45	0	0
Smart Ground Original	⅓ cup (1.9 oz)	70	0	3
Smart Ground Taco	⅓ cup (2 oz)	60	0	3
Loma Linda				
Dinner Cuts	2 slices (3.2 oz)	90	0	2
Nuteena	⅜ in slice (1.9 oz)	160	0	2
Sandwich Spread	¼ cup (1.9 oz)	80	0	3
Savory Dinner Loaf Mix not prep	⅓ cup (0.9 oz)	90	0	5
Swiss Stake	1 piece (3.2 oz)	120	0	4
Tender Bits	6 pieces (3 oz)	110	0	3
Tender Rounds	6 pieces (2.8 oz)	120	0	3
Vita Burger Chunks not prep	¼ cup (0.7 oz)	70	0	3
Vita Burger Granules	3 tbsp (0.7 oz)	70	0	3
Midland Harvest				
Burger n' Loaf Chili w/o Beans	0.8 oz	90	0	2
Burger n' Loaf Herbs & Spice	3.2 oz	140	0	4
Burger n' Loaf Italian	3.2 oz	140	0	4
Burger n' Loaf Original	3.2 oz	140	0	4

FOOD	PORTION	CALS	CHOL	FIBER
Burger n' Loaf Sloppy Joe w/o Sauce	0.8 oz	80	0	1
Burger n' Loaf Taco	2.7 oz	90	0	1
Morningstar Farms				
Burger Style Recipe Crumbles	⅔ cup (1.9 oz)	80	0	2
Ground Meatless	½ cup (1.9 oz)	60	0	2
Harvest Burger Recipe Crumbles	½ cup (2 oz)	70	0	3
Quarter Prime	1 patty (3.4 oz)	140	0	3
Natural Touch				
Dinner Entree	1 patty (3 oz)	220	0	2
Loaf Mix not prep	4 tbsp (1 oz)	100	0	7
Stroganoff Mix not prep	4 tbsp (0.8 oz)	90	10	3
Taco Mix not prep	3 tbsp (0.6 oz)	60	0	3
Vegan Burger Crumbles	½ cup (1.9 oz)	60	0	2
Quorn				
Grounds	⅔ cup (3 oz)	80	0	4
Soy Is Us				
Beef Not!	½ cup (1.75 oz)	140	0	9
Soy7				
Burger Bits as prep	½ cup	60	0	2
Burger Mix as prep	1 serv (3.2 oz)	120	0	3
Recipe Strips as prep	¾ cup	70	0	3
Veggie Patch				
Veggie Rounds	1 (2.5 oz)	120	0	4
Veggitinos Meatballs	5 (2.8 oz)	120	0	3
Worthington				
Beef Style Meatless	⅜ in slice (1.9 oz)	110	0	3
Bolono	3 slices (2 oz)	80	0	2
Choplets	2 slices (3.2 oz)	90	0	2
Corned Beef Meatless	4 slices (2 oz)	140	0	2
Country Stew	1 cup (8.4 oz)	210	0	5
Dinner Roast	¾ in slice (3 oz)	180	<5	3
FriPats	1 patty (2.2 oz)	130	0	3
Multigrain Cutlets	2 slices (3.2 oz)	100	0	4
Numete	⅜ in slice (1.9 oz)	130	0	3
Prime Stakes	1 piece (3.2 oz)	120	0	4

FOOD	PORTION	CALS	CHOL	FIBER
Prosage Roll	⅝ in slice (1.9 oz)	140	0	2
Protose	⅜ in slice (1.9 oz)	130	0	3
Salami Meatless	3 slices (2 oz)	130	0	2
Savory Slices	3 slices (2.9 oz)	150	0	3
Smoked Beef Meatless	6 slices (2 oz)	120	0	3
Stakelets	1 piece (2.5 oz)	140	0	2
Veelets	1 patty (2.5 oz)	180	0	5
Vegetable Skallops	½ cup (3 oz)	90	0	2
Vegetable Steaks	2 pieces (2.5 oz)	80	0	3
Wham	2 slices (1.6 oz)	80	0	0
Yves				
Veggie Bologna	4 slices (2.2 oz)	70	0	0
Veggie Ground Italian	⅓ cup (2 oz)	60	0	3
Veggie Ground Round Italian	⅓ cup (1.9 oz)	60	0	3
Veggie Ground Round Original	2 oz	60	0	3
Veggie Pizza Pepperoni Slices	1 serv (1.7 oz)	70	0	3
Veggie Salami Deli Slices	1 serv (2.2 oz)	90	0	1
Zoglo's				
Crispy Vegetarian Cutlets	1 (3.5 oz)	200	0	2
Savory Vegetarian Kebabs	1 serv (2.8 oz)	135	0	2
MELON				
melon balls frzn	1 cup	55	0	–
Sunfresh				
Melon Salad In Extra Light Syrup	½ cup (4.5 oz)	45	0	2
MELON JUICE				
Ocean Spray Mega Melon	8 oz	130	0	0

MEXICAN FOOD (see SALSA, SPANISH FOOD, TORTILLA)

FOOD	PORTION	CALS	CHOL	FIBER
MILK				
CANNED				
condensed sweetened	1 oz	123	13	—
condensed sweetened	1 cup	982	104	—
evaporated	½ cup	169	37	—
evaporated skim	½ cup	99	5	—
Carnation				
Evaporated	½ cup	150	10	—
Evaporated Fat Free	2 tbsp (1 oz)	25	0	—
Evaporated Lowfat	½ cup	110	5	—
Sweetened Condensed	⅓ cup	330	10	0
DRIED				
buttermilk	1 tbsp	25	5	—
nonfat instantized	1 pkg (3.2 oz)	244	12	—
Carnation				
Nonfat	⅓ cup	80	<5	0
Saco				
Cultured Buttermilk	4 tbsp (0.8 oz)	80	4	0
Sanalac				
Powder	¼ cup (0.8 oz)	85	6	0
REFRIGERATED				
1%	1 cup	102	10	—
1%	1 qt	409	39	—
1% protein fortified	1 qt	477	39	—
1% protein fortified	1 cup	119	10	—
2%	1 cup	121	18	—
2%	1 qt	485	73	—
buttermilk	1 cup	99	9	—
buttermilk	1 qt	396	34	—
goat	1 cup	168	28	—
goat	1 qt	672	111	—
human	1 cup	171	34	—
indian buffalo	1 cup	236	46	—
low sodium	1 cup	149	33	—
nonfat	1 cup	86	4	—
nonfat	1 qt	342	18	—
nonfat protein fortified	1 qt	400	20	—
nonfat protein fortified	1 cup	100	5	—
whole	1 cup	150	33	—

FOOD	PORTION	CALS	CHOL	FIBER
BodyWise				
Nonfat	8 fl oz	100	5	0
Cool Cow				
Low Fat	1 cup (8 oz)	110	<5	0
Farmland				
1%	8 fl oz	100	10	0
2%	8 fl oz	130	20	0
Easylac 1%	8 fl oz	100	10	–
Easylac Nonfat	8 fl oz	90	5	–
Skim	8 fl oz	80	<5	0
Skim Plus	1 cup (8 oz)	110	<5	0
Friendship				
Buttermilk	8 fl oz	120	15	0
Hood				
1%	1 cup (8 oz)	110	15	0
Better Taste 2%	1 cup (8 oz)	130	20	0
Buttermilk	1 cup (8 oz)	90	<5	0
Whole	1 cup (8 oz)	150	35	0
Horizon Organic				
Fat Free	1 cup (8 oz)	80	4	0
Land O Lakes				
1% Lowfat	1 carton (10 oz)	120	15	–
Fat Free	1 carton (10 oz)	100	5	–
Whole	1 carton (10 oz)	180	45	–
Nuform				
1%	1 cup (8 oz)	120	15	0
Skim	1 cup (8 oz)	100	<5	0
NutraBalance				
LactaCare	1 pkg (8 oz)	500	0	–
Organic Valley				
Low Fat	1 cup	100	10	0
Nonfat	1 cup	80	5	0
Reduced Fat	1 cup	130	20	0
Whole	1 cup	150	30	0
Silovet				
Skim	1 cup (8 oz)	90	<5	0
Stonyfield Farm				
Organic Whole Milk	1 cup (8 oz)	180	40	0
Organic Whole Milk Vanilla	1 cup (8 oz)	230	30	0

FOOD	PORTION	CALS	CHOL	FIBER
Turkey Hill				
Cool Moos 2% Reduced Fat	1 cup	130	20	–
Cool Moos Whole Milk	1 cup	160	35	–
SHELF-STABLE				
Parmalat				
1%	1 cup (8 oz)	110	15	0
2%	1 cup (8 oz)	130	20	0
Skim	1 cup (8 oz)	90	5	0
Whole	1 cup (8 oz)	160	35	0
MILK DRINKS				
chocolate milk	1 cup	208	30	–
chocolate milk	1 qt	833	122	–
chocolate milk 1%	1 cup	158	7	–
chocolate milk 1%	1 qt	630	29	–
chocolate milk 2%	1 cup	179	17	–
strawberry flavor mix as prep w/ whole milk	9 oz	234	33	–
Body Wise				
Chocolate Nonfat Milk	1 cup (8 fl oz)	180	5	1
Hood				
Chocolate Lowfat	1 cup (8 oz)	150	10	0
Horizon Organic				
Lowfat Chocolate Milk	1 cup (8 oz)	160	10	1
Land O Lakes				
Chocolate	1 cup (8.4 oz)	200	30	0
Organic Valley				
Chocolate Milk Reduced Fat	1 cup	180	10	0
Parmalat				
Chocolate 2%	1 box (8 oz)	180	20	1
Quik				
Banana Lowfat	1 cup (8.4 oz)	200	20	0
Banana Powder	2 tbsp (0.8 oz)	90	0	0
Chocolate	1 cup (8.4 oz)	230	30	1
Chocolate Lowfat	1 carton (8.4 oz)	200	20	0

FOOD	PORTION	CALS	CHOL	FIBER
Cookies n Cream Powder	2 tbsp (0.8 oz)	100	0	1
Strawberry	1 cup (8.4 oz)	230	30	0
Strawberry Lowfat	1 carton (8.4 oz)	210	20	0
Strawberry Powder	2 tbsp (0.8 oz)	90	0	0
Turkey Hill				
Cool Moos Chocolate 1% Lowfat	1 cup	180	10	—
Cool Moos Orange Cream 1% Lowfat	1 cup	190	10	—
Cool Moos Strawberry 1% Lowfat	1 cup	160	10	—
Cool Moos Vanilla 1% Lowfat	1 cup	160	10	—
MILK SUBSTITUTES				
imitation milk	1 cup	150	tr	—
imitation milk	1 qt	600	2	—
8th Continent				
Soymilk Low Fat Chocolate	1 bottle (8 oz)	140	0	1
Soymilk Low Fat Original	1 bottle (8 oz)	80	0	tr
Soymilk Low Fat Vanilla	1 bottle (8 oz)	90	0	tr
Rice Original	2 tbsp (0.66 oz)	78	0	1
Rice Original Light	2 tbsp (0.66 oz)	66	0	1
Rice Vanilla	2 tbsp (0.66 oz)	78	0	1
Rice Vanilla Light	2 tbsp (0.66 oz)	66	0	1
Soy Carob	2 tbsp (1 oz)	90	0	2
Soy Chocolate	2 tbsp (1.1 oz)	112	0	1
Soy Light	2 tbsp (0.66 oz)	73	0	1
Soy Original	2 tbsp (0.8 oz)	100	0	0
Soy Vanilla	2 tbsp (0.7 oz)	77	0	1
Blue Diamond				
Almond Breeze Chocolate	8 oz	120	0	1
Almond Breeze Original	8 oz	60	0	1

FOOD	PORTION	CALS	CHOL	FIBER
Almond Breeze Vanilla	8 oz	90	0	1
EdenBlend				
Organic	8 oz	120	0	0
Edensoy				
Organic Light	8 oz	93	0	0
Organic Light Vanilla	8 oz	120	0	0
Galaxy				
Veggi Milk Chocolate	1 cup (8 oz)	150	0	1
Veggie Milk Original	1 cup (8 oz)	110	0	2
Hansen's				
Soy Smoothie Lemon Chiffon	8 oz	150	0	tr
Soy Smoothie Orange Dream	8 oz	150	0	tr
Harmony Farms				
Original Rice Beverage	1 cup (8 oz)	90	0	0
Harmony House				
Enriched Rice Beverage	1 cup (8 oz)	90	0	0
Enriched Soy Beverage	1 cup (8 oz)	90	0	0
Original Soy Beverage	1 cup (8 oz)	90	0	0
Health Valley				
Soo Moo	1 cup	110	0	1
NutraBalance				
NuTaste	1 pkg (8 oz)	80	0	8
Rice Dream				
Carob	1 box (8 oz)	150	0	0
Chocolate	1 box (8 oz)	170	0	2
Chocolate Enriched	1 box (8 oz)	170	0	0
Organic Original	1 box (8 oz)	120	0	0
Organic Original Enriched	1 box (8 oz)	120	0	0
Vanilla	1 box (8 oz)	130	0	0
Vanilla Enriched	1 box (8 oz)	130	0	0
Silk				
Chocolate	1 cup	140	0	0
Organic Plain	1 cup	100	0	0
Vanilla	1 bottle (11 oz)	140	0	0
Tree Of Life				
Original Rice Beverage	1 cup	90	0	0

FOOD	PORTION	CALS	CHOL	FIBER
Vitamite				
Non-Diary	1 cup (8 oz)	110	0	0
Vitasoy				
1% Low Fat Vanilla Delight	8 oz	90	0	0
Carob Supreme	8 fl oz	150	0	tr
Creamy Unsweetened	8 oz	80	0	0
Creamy Original	8 fl oz	110	0	1
Enriched Light Original	8 fl oz	60	0	0
Enriched Light Vanilla	8 fl oz	90	0	0
Green Tea Soymilk	8 oz	130	0	1
Original Creamy	8 fl oz	110	0	1
Original Light	8 fl oz	60	0	0
Rich Chocolate	8 fl oz	160	0	1
Rich Cocoa	8 fl oz	150	0	1
Vanilla Light	8 fl oz	90	0	0
Vanilla Delite	8 fl oz	120	0	1
White Wave				
Mocha	1 cup	140	0	1
MILKFISH				
baked	3 oz	162	57	.
MILKSHAKE				
chocolate	10 oz	360	37	–
strawberry	10 oz	319	31	–
thick shake chocolate	10.6 oz	356	32	–
thick shake vanilla	11 oz	350	37	–
vanilla	10 oz	314	32	–
D'Frosta Shake				
Vanilla	1 serv (13.5 oz)	340	40	1
Freeze Flip				
Fruit Shake No Fat Lactose Free Black Raspberry	1 serv (6 oz)	150	0	1
Hood				
Shake Up Chocolate	1 cup (8 oz)	240	20	0
Shake Up Strawberry	1 cup (8 oz)	220	20	0
Shake Up Vanilla	1 cup (8 oz)	220	20	0
Milky Way				
Shake	1 (10 fl oz)	390	60	0

FOOD	PORTION	CALS	CHOL	FIBER
Parmalat				
Shake A Shake Chocolate	1 box (6 oz)	180	15	1
Shake A Shake Orange Vanilla	1 box (6 oz)	110	10	0
Shake A Shake Vanilla	1 box (6 oz)	170	15	0
MILLET				
cooked	1 cup (6.1 oz)	207	0	2
MINERAL WATER (see WATER)				
MISO				
miso	½ cup	284	0	7
Eden				
Organic Genmai	1 tbsp	25	0	tr
Tekka	1 tsp	5	0	0
MOLASSES				
blackstrap	1 tbsp (0.7 oz)	47	0	—
blackstrap	1 cup (11.5 oz)	771	0	—
molasses	1 tbsp (0.7 oz)	53	0	—
molasses	1 cup (11.5 oz)	873	0	—
Brer Rabbit				
Dark	1 tbsp	60	0	—
Mott's				
Sulphured	1 tbsp	50	0	—
Unsulphured	1 tbsp	50	0	—
MONKFISH				
baked	3 oz	82	27	—
MOOSE				
roasted	3 oz	114	66	—
MOTH BEANS				
dried cooked	1 cup	207	0	—
MOUSSE				
FROZEN				
Sara Lee				
Chocolate	⅓ pkg (4.3 oz)	400	30	2

FOOD	PORTION	CALS	CHOL	FIBER
Weight Watchers				
Chocolate Mousse	1 (2.75 oz)	190	5	3
TAKE-OUT				
chocolate	½ cup (7.1 oz)	447	299	—
orange	½ cup	87	1	—
MUFFIN				
FROZEN				
Pepperidge Farm				
Blueberry	1 (2 oz)	180	30	0
Bran w/ Raisins	1 (2 oz)	180	25	0
Corn	1 (2 oz)	190	30	0
Orange Cranberry	1 (2 oz)	180	36	0
Sara Lee				
Blueberry	1 (2.2 oz)	220	15	tr
Blueberry	1 (2.2 oz)	220	15	tr
Corn	1 (2.2 oz)	260	25	1
Weight Watchers				
Chocolate Chocolate Chip	1 (2.5 oz)	190	0	4
Fat Free Banana	1 (2.5 oz)	170	0	3
Fat Free Blueberry	1 (2.5 oz)	160	0	2
MIX				
blueberry	1 (1 ¼ oz)	149	23	—
corn	1 (1.75 oz)	160	31	—
wheat bran as prep	1 (1 ¾ oz)	138	34	—
Betty Crocker				
Apple Cinnamon as prep	1	170	36	—
Apple Streusel as prep	1	210	18	—
Banana Nut as prep	1	170	18	1
Cranberry Orange as prep	1	150	18	—
Double Chocolate as prep	1	220	27	—
Golden Corn as prep	1	160	36	—
Lemon Poppyseed as prep	1	180	36	—

FOOD	PORTION	CALS	CHOL	FIBER
Sunkist Lemon Poppyseed as prep	1	190	18	—
Twice The Blueberries as prep	1	140	18	1
Wild Blueberry as prep	1	170	18	tr
Flako				
Corn	⅓ cup (1.4 oz)	160	0	1
Gold Medal				
Corn	1	160	35	0
Hodgson Mill				
Bran	¼ cup (1.3 oz)	130	0	3
Cornbread	¼ cup (1.3 oz)	130	0	3
Whole Wheat	¼ cup (1.3 oz)	130	0	3
Robin Hood				
Apple Cinnamon	1	170	35	0
Banana Nut	1	170	35	0
Blueberry	1	160	35	0
Caramel Nut	1	170	35	0
Sweet Rewards				
Low Fat Apple Cinnamon as prep	1	140	16	—
Wanda's				
Blue Corn	¼ cup (1.2 oz) mix per serv	130	0	1
READY-TO-EAT				
Blueberry	1 (2 oz)	158	17	2
oat bran wheat free	1 (2 oz)	154	0	4
Dolly Madison				
Blueberry	1 (1.75 oz)	170	0	0
Mega Banana Nut	1 (5.9 oz)	620	75	2
Mega Blueberry	1 (5.9 oz)	590	80	1
Mega Chocolate Chip	1 (5.9 oz)	620	80	2
Mega Cranberry Orange	1 (5.9 oz)	590	90	1
Mega Cream Cheese	1 (5.9 oz)	620	90	1
Dutch Mill				
Apple Oat Bran	1 (2 oz)	180	0	1
Banana Walnut	1 (2 oz)	220	5	1
Carrot	1 (2 oz)	190	30	1

FOOD	PORTION	CALS	CHOL	FIBER
Corn	1 (2 oz)	190	40	1
Cranberry Orange	1 (2 oz)	170	55	1
Raisin Bran	1 (2 oz)	230	30	3
Freihofer's				
Corn Toasters	1 (1.3 oz)	130	15	0
Hostess				
Banana Bran Low Fat	1 (2.7 oz)	240	0	2
Blueberry Low Fat	1 (2.7 oz)	230	0	1
Hearty Banana Nut	1 (5.9 oz)	620	75	2
Hearty Blueberry	1 (5.9 oz)	590	80	1
Hearty Chocolate Chip	1 (5.9 oz)	620	80	2
Hearty Cranberry Orange	1 (5.9 oz)	590	90	1
Hearty Cream Cheese	1 (5.9 oz)	620	90	1
Mini Banana Walnut	3 (1.2 oz)	160	25	0
Mini Blueberry	3 (1.2 oz)	150	25	0
Mini Chocolate Chip	3 (1.2 oz)	160	20	0
Mini Cinnamon Apple	3 (1.2 oz)	160	25	0
Mini Cinnamon Bites	3 (1.1 oz)	130	15	0
Mini Rocky Road	3 (1.2 oz)	160	20	0
Muffin Loaf Apple Spice	1 (3.7 oz)	430	80	1
Muffin Loaf Banana Nut	1 (3.8 oz)	460	60	0
Muffin Loaf Blueberry	1 (3.8 oz)	440	80	2
Muffin Loaf Chocolate Chocolate Chip	1 (3.8 oz)	400	45	2
Muffin Loaf Raspberry	1 (3.8 oz)	440	80	2
Oat Bran	1 (1.5 oz)	160	0	1
Otis Spunkmeyer				
Apple Cinnamon	1 (2 oz)	220	36	tr
Low Fat Wild Blueberry	1 (2.25 oz)	200	35	tr
Mayport Almond Poppy Seed	½ muffin (2 oz)	210	40	tr
Mayport Banana Nut	1 (2.25 oz)	270	30	tr
Mayport Cheese Streusel	½ muffin (2 oz)	220	25	tr
Mayport Chocolate Chocolate Chip	1 (2.25 oz)	260	40	1

FOOD	PORTION	CALS	CHOL	FIBER
Mayport Chocolate Chip	½ muffin (2 oz)	240	35	tr
Mayport Cinnamon Spice	½ muffin (2 oz)	230	40	1
Mayport Corn	½ muffin (2 oz)	230	50	0
Mayport Harvest Bran	1 (2.25 oz)	240	35	3
Mayport Lemon	½ muffin (2 oz)	230	40	1
Mayport Orange	½ muffin (2 oz)	230	40	tr
Mayport Pineapple	½ muffin (2 oz)	210	40	1
Mayport Wild Blueberry	1 (2.25 oz)	230	45	1
Mayport Low Fat Apple Cinnamon	1 (4 oz)	380	65	1
Mayport Low Fat Banana Nut	1 (4 oz)	350	65	1
Mayport Low Fat Chocolate Chocolate Chip	1 (4 oz)	370	65	2
Uncle Wally's				
Fat Free Apple Cinnamon Delight	1 (1.9 oz)	110	0	1
Weight Watchers				
Fat Free Apple Crisp	1 (2.5 oz)	160	0	1
Fat Free Cranberry Orange	1 (2.5 oz)	160	0	1
Fat Free Double Chocolate	1 (2.5 oz)	180	0	2
Fat Free Wild Blueberry	1 (2.5 oz)	160	0	1
Low Fat Apple Cinnamon	1 (2.5 oz)	170	0	2
Low Fat Blueberry	1 (2.5 oz)	180	0	2
Low Fat Carrot	1 (2.5 oz)	160	0	2
Low Fat Chocolate Chip	1 (2.5 oz)	180	0	2
Low Fat Cranberry Orange	1 (2.5 oz)	180	0	2
Low Fat Lemon Poppy	1 (2.5 oz)	190	0	2

FOOD	PORTION	CALS	CHOL	FIBER
TAKE-OUT				
raisin bran lowfat	1 (4 oz)	270	0	5
MULBERRIES				
fresh	1 cup	61	0	–
MULLET				
striped cooked	3 oz	127	54	–
striped raw	3 oz	99	42	–
MUNG BEANS				
dried cooked	1 cup	213	0	–
MUNGO BEANS				
dried cooked	1 cup	190	1	–
MUSHROOMS				
CANNED				
chanterelle	3.5 oz	12	0	6
pieces	½ cup	19	0	–
straw	1 cup (6.4 oz)	58	0	5
whole	1 (0.4 oz)	3	0	–
BinB				
Pieces & Stems	1 can (4.2 oz)	30	0	2
Sliced	1 can (4.2 oz)	30	0	2
Sliced With Garlic	1 can (4.2 oz)	35	0	1
Whole	1 can (4.2 oz)	30	0	2
Green Giant				
Pieces & Stems	½ cup (4.2 oz)	30	0	2
Sliced	½ cup (4.2 oz)	30	0	2
Whole	½ cup (4.2 oz)	30	0	2
DRIED				
chanterelle	1 oz	25	0	17
cloud ear	1 (5 g)	13	0	3
cloud ears	1 cup (1 oz)	80	0	20
shiitake	4 (½ oz)	44	0	–
straw	1 piece (6 g)	2	0	tr
tree ear	½ cup (0.4 oz)	36	0	–
Eden				
Shitake	6 (0.4 oz)	35	0	5
FRESH				
chanterelle	3.5 oz	11	0	6

FOOD	PORTION	CALS	CHOL	FIBER
enoki raw	1 (4 in)	2	0	—
morel	3.5 oz	9	0	7
oyster raw	1 lg (5.2 oz)	55	0	4
oyster raw	1 sm (0.5 oz)	6	0	tr
portabella	1 serv (2 oz)	14	0	—
raw	1 (½ oz)	5	0	tr
raw sliced	½ cup	9	0	tr
shitake cooked	4 (2.5 oz)	40	0	—
sliced cooked	½ cup	21	0	1
whole cooked	1 (0.4 oz)	3	0	—
Mother Earth				
Organic	4 oz	35	0	tr
FROZEN				
Empire				
Breaded	7 (2.8 oz)	90	0	1
MUSSELS				
blue raw	1 cup	129	42	—
blue raw	3 oz	73	24	—
fresh blue cooked	3 oz	147	48	—
MUSTARD				
dry mustard	1 tsp	15	0	—
yellow ready-to-use	1 tsp	5	0	—
Blanchard & Blanchard				
Mustard	1 tsp (5 g)	0	0	0
Boar's Head				
Delicatessen Style	1 tsp (5 g)	0	0	0
Honey	1 tsp (5 g)	10	0	0
Eden				
Organic Stone Ground	1 tsp	0	0	0
Hunt's				
Mustard	1 tsp (5 g)	3	0	tr
Kosciuszko				
Spicy Brown	1 tsp	5	0	—
Kraft				
Horseradish Mustard	1 tsp (5 g)	0	0	0
Mustard	1 tsp (5 g)	0	0	0
Luzianne				
Creole Mustard	1 tbsp	10	0	0

FOOD	PORTION	CALS	CHOL	FIBER
Plochman				
Dijon	1 tsp (5 g)	7	0	—
Spoonable Salad	1 tsp (5 g)	4	0	—
Squeeze Salad	1 tsp (5 g)	4	0	—
Stone Ground	1 tsp (5 g)	6	0	—
Tree Of Life				
Dijon	1 tsp (5 g)	0	0	—
Dijon Imported	1 tsp (5 g)	5	0	—
Stone Ground	1 tsp (5 g)	0	0	—
Yellow	1 tsp (5 g)	0	0	—
Wild Thyme Farms				
Chili Pepper Garlic	1 tsp	5	0	—
Dill Horseradish	1 tsp	5	0	—
MUSTARD GREENS				
fresh chopped cooked	½ cup	11	0	—
fresh raw chopped	½ cup	7	0	—
frozen chopped cooked	½ cup	14	0	—
Birds Eye				
Chopped	1 cup	30	0	2
NATTO				
natto	½ cup	187	0	—
NAVY BEANS				
CANNED				
navy	1 cup	296	0	—
DRIED				
cooked	1 cup	259	0	—
Hurst				
HamBeens w/ Ham	3 tbsp (1.2 oz)	120	0	11
NECTARINE				
fresh	1	67	0	2
Chiquita				
Fresh	1 med (4.9 oz)	70	0	2
NEUFCHATEL				
neufchatel	1 oz	74	22	—
neufchatel	1 pkg (3 oz)	221	65	—

FOOD	PORTION	CALS	CHOL	FIBER
Horizon Organic				
Neufchatel	2 tbsp	70	20	0
Organic Valley				
Neufchatel	1 oz	70	20	0
Philadelphia				
Neufchatel	1 oz	70	20	0
WisPride				
Garden Vegetable Cup	2 tbsp (1.1 oz)	60	15	0
Garlic & Herb Cup	2 tbsp (1.1 oz)	60	15	0

NOODLE DISHES (see also PASTA DINNERS)

FOOD	PORTION	CALS	CHOL	FIBER
Annie Chun				
Chow Mein Noodles w/ Garlic Black Bean Sauce	1 serv	230	0	2
Japanese Soba Noodles w/ Soy Ginger Sauce	1 serv	210	0	3
Hormel				
Microcup Meals Noodles & Chicken	1 cup (7.5 oz)	200	40	1
Hunt's				
Noodles & Chicken	1 cup (8.7 oz)	176	37	2
Noodles & Beef	1 cup (8.7 oz)	151	17	5
Kraft				
Noodle Classics Cheddar Cheese as prep	1 cup (7.4 oz)	400	70	1
Noodle Classics Savory Chicken as prep	1 cup (8.5 oz)	340	55	2
Lipton				
Noodles & Sauce Alfredo Broccoli as prep	1 cup (2.2 oz)	340	80	2
Noodles & Sauce Alfredo as prep	1 cup (2.2 oz)	330	80	2
Noodles & Sauce Beef as prep	1 cup (2.1 oz)	280	60	2
Noodles & Sauce Butter as prep	1 cup (2.2 oz)	310	70	2

FOOD	PORTION	CALS	CHOL	FIBER
Noodles & Sauce Butter & Herb as prep	1 cup (2.2 oz)	300	65	2
Noodles & Sauce Chicken Broccoli as prep	1 cup (2.1 oz)	310	70	2
Noodles & Sauce Chicken Tetrazzini as prep	1 cup (2 oz)	300	70	2
Noodles & Sauce Chicken as prep	1 cup (2.1 oz)	290	65	2
Noodles & Sauce Creamy Chicken as prep	1 cup (2.1 oz)	320	75	2
Noodles & Sauce Parmesan as prep	1 cup (2.1 oz)	330	75	2
Noodles & Sauce Sour Cream & Chives as prep	1 cup (2.2 oz)	310	70	2
Noodles & Sauce Stroganoff as prep	1 cup (2 oz)	300	70	2
Luigino's				
Stroganoff	1 pkg (8 oz)	310	55	2
Noodles By Leonardo				
Macaroni & Cheese as prep	1 cup (2.5 oz)	250	0	2
TAKE-OUT				
noodle pudding	½ cup	132	27	–

NOODLES

FOOD	PORTION	CALS	CHOL	FIBER
cellophane	1 cup	492	0	–
chow mein	1 cup (1.6 oz)	237	0	2
egg	1 cup (38 g)	145	36	–
egg cooked	1 cup (5.6 oz)	213	53	2
japanese soba cooked	1 cup (4 oz)	113	0	–
japanese somen cooked	1 cup (6.2 oz)	231	0	–
rice cooked	1 cup (6.2 oz)	192	0	2

FOOD	PORTION	CALS	CHOL	FIBER
spinach/egg cooked	1 cup (5.6 oz)	211	53	4
Annie Chun				
Chow Mein	2 oz	200	0	3
Rice	2 oz	210	0	0
Rice Hunan	2 oz	210	0	0
Rice Pad Thai	2 oz	210	0	0
Rice Pad Thai Basil	2 oz	210	0	0
Azumaya				
Spinach	1 cup	210	0	2
Thin Cut	1 cup	210	0	2
Wide Cut	1 cup	210	0	2
Chun King				
Chow Mein	½ cup (1 oz)	137	0	1
Creamette				
Egg	2 oz	221	70	—
Eden				
Kudzu	2 oz	200	0	2
Hodgson Mill				
Four Color Veggie Egg	2 oz	200	35	2
Whole Wheat Egg	2 oz	190	30	4
La Choy				
Chow Mein	½ cup (1 oz)	137	0	1
Chow Mein Crispy Wide	½ cup (1 oz)	148	0	1
Rice	½ cup (1 oz)	121	0	tr
Manischewitz				
Fine Yolk Free	1½ cups	210	0	2
Fine Egg	1½ cups	220	65	2
Nasoya				
Chinese	1 cup	210	0	2
Japanese	1 cup	210	0	2
Spinach	1 cup	210	0	2
Noodles By Leonardo				
Egg Fine	2 oz	210	80	2
Egg Medium	2 oz	210	80	2
Egg Wide	2 oz	210	80	2
San Giorgio				
Egg	2 oz	210	70	—

FOOD	PORTION	CALS	CHOL	FIBER
Shofar				
No Yolks	2 oz	210	0	3
NOPALES				
cooked	1 cup (5.2 oz)	23	0	–
raw sliced	1 cup (3 oz)	14	0	–
NUTMEG				
ground	1 tsp	12	0	–
Watkins				
Ground	¼ tsp (0.5 g)	0	0	0
NUTRITION SUPPLEMENTS				
Enlive!				
Drink All Flavors	1 box (8.1 oz)	300	<5	0
Ensure				
Supplement All Flavors	1 can (8 fl oz)	250	<5	0
Essential				
Protein Powder	1 serv (0.6 oz)	70	0	tr
Gatorade				
ReLode	1 pkt (0.75 oz)	80	0	–
GeniSoy				
Soy Natural Protein Powder	1 scoop (1 oz)	100	0	0
Glucerna				
Shakes All Flavors	1 can (8 oz)	220	<5	3
Met-Rx				
Lite	1 pkg (1.6 oz)	170	30	1
Original	1 pkg (2.5 oz)	250	15	tr
Protein Shake	1 can	200	10	2
Ultra	1 pkg (2.6 oz)	250	50	2
Nestle				
Additions	2½ tsp (0.7 oz)	100	0	0
NutraBalance				
EggPro	1 tbsp (7.5 g)	30	0	0
PermaLean				
Protein Powder Bodacious Berry	1 scoop (1 oz)	104	0	–
Protein Powder Chocoholic Chocolate	1 scoop (1 oz)	104	0	–

FOOD	PORTION	CALS	CHOL	FIBER
Pounds Off				
All Flavors	1 bar (2.1 oz)	210	0	2
NUTS MIXED *(see also individual names)*				
dry roasted w/ peanuts	1 oz	169	0	–
dry roasted w/ peanuts salted	1 oz	169	0	–
mixed nuts chocolate covered	¼ cup (1.5 oz)	240	5	2
oil roasted w/ peanuts	1 oz	175	0	–
oil roasted w/ peanuts salted	1 oz	175	0	–
oil roasted w/o peanuts	1 oz	175	0	–
oil roasted w/o peanuts salted	1 oz	175	0	–
Estee				
Fruit & Nut Mix	¼ cup	210	<5	2
Maranatha				
Cashew Macadamia Butter	2 tbsp	210	0	2
Tamari Organic	¼ cup	160	0	2
Tamari Roasted	¼ cup	160	0	2
Planters				
Cashews & Peanuts Honey Roasted	1 oz	150	0	2
Deluxe Oil Roasted	1 oz	170	0	2
Dry Roasted	1 oz	170	0	2
Honey Roasted	1 oz	140	0	2
Lightly Salted Oil Roasted	1 oz	170	0	2
No Brazils Lightly Salted Oil Roasted	1 oz	170	0	2
No Brazils Oil Roasted	1 oz	170	0	2
Oil Roasted	1 oz	170	0	2

FOOD	PORTION	CALS	CHOL	FIBER
Select Mix Cashews Almonds & Macadamias Oil Roasted	1 oz	170	0	2
Select Mix Cashews Almonds & Pecans Oil Roasted	1 oz	170	0	2
Unsalted Oil Roasted	1 oz	170	0	3

OCTOPUS

fresh steamed	3 oz	140	82	—

OHELOBERRIES

fresh	1 cup	39	0	—

OIL

almond	1 tbsp	120	0	—
almond	1 cup	1927	0	—
apricot kernel	1 cup	1927	0	—
apricot kernel	1 tbsp	120	0	—
avocado	1 cup	1927	0	—
avocado	1 tbsp	124	0	—
babassu palm	1 tbsp	120	0	—
butter oil	1 tbsp	112	33	—
butter oil	1 cup	1795	524	—
canola	1 cup	1927	0	—
canola	1 tbsp	124	0	—
coconut	1 tbsp	117	0	—
corn	1 tbsp	120	0	—
corn	1 cup	1927	0	—
cottonseed	1 cup	1927	0	—
cottonseed	1 tbsp	120	0	—
cupu assu	1 tbsp	120	0	—
grapeseed	1 tbsp	120	0	—
hazelnut	1 tbsp	120	0	—
hazelnut	1 cup	1927	0	—
mustard	1 tbsp	124	0	—
mustard	1 cup	1927	0	—
oat	1 tbsp	120	0	—
olive	1 tbsp	119	0	—

FOOD	PORTION	CALS	CHOL	FIBER
olive	1 cup	1909	0	–
palm	1 tbsp	120	0	–
palm	1 cup	1927	0	–
palm kernel	1 cup	1879	0	–
palm kernel	1 tbsp	117	0	–
peanut	1 cup	1909	0	–
peanut	1 tbsp	119	0	–
poppyseed	1 tbsp	120	0	–
rice bran	1 tbsp	120	0	–
safflower	1 tbsp	120	0	–
safflower	1 cup	1927	0	–
sesame	1 tbsp	120	0	–
sheanut	1 tbsp	120	0	–
soybean	1 tbsp	120	0	–
soybean	1 cup	1927	0	–
sunflower	1 cup	1927	0	–
sunflower	1 tbsp	120	0	–
teaseed	1 tbsp	120	0	–
tomatoseed	1 tbsp	120	0	–
vegetable	1 tbsp	120	0	–
vegetable	1 cup	1927	0	–
walnut	1 cup	1927	0	1
walnut	1 tbsp	120	0	–
wheat germ	1 tbsp	120	0	–
Bertolli				
Classico	1 tbsp	120	0	–
Extra Light	1 tbsp	120	0	–
Extra Virgin	1 tbsp	120	0	–
Crisco				
Corn Canola	1 tbsp (0.5 fl oz)	120	0	–
Oil	1 tbsp (0.5 fl oz)	120	0	–
Puritan Canola	1 tbsp (0.5 fl oz)	120	0	0
Eden				
Olive Spanish Extra Virgin	1 tbsp	120	0	0
Safflower	1 tbsp (0.5 oz)	120	0	–
House Of Tsang				
Hot Chili Sesame	1 tsp (5 g)	45	0	0
Mongolian Fire	1 tsp (5 g)	45	0	0
Pure Sesame	1 tsp (5 g)	45	0	0

FOOD	PORTION	CALS	CHOL	FIBER
Singapore Curry	1 tsp (5 g)	45	0	0
Wok Oil	1 tbsp (0.5 oz)	130	0	0
Italica				
Olive Oil	1 tbsp	120	0	—
Loriva				
5 Pepper Hot	1 tbsp	120	0	—
Avocado	1 tbsp	120	0	—
Basil Flavored	1 tbsp	120	0	—
Canola	1 tbsp	120	0	—
Canolive	1 tbsp	120	0	—
Garlic Flavored	1 tbsp	120	0	—
Grapeseed	1 tbsp	120	0	—
Olive	1 tbsp	120	0	—
Olive Organic Extra Virgin	1 tbsp	120	0	—
Peanut	1 tbsp	120	0	—
Rice Bran	1 tbsp	120	0	—
Safflower	1 tbsp	120	0	—
Sesame	1 tbsp	120	0	—
Sunflower	1 tbsp	120	0	—
Toasted Sesame	1 tbsp	120	0	—
Walnut	1 tbsp	120	0	—
Mazola				
Oil	1 tbsp (14 g)	120	0	—
Orville Redenbacher's				
Popping	1 tbsp (0.5 oz)	120	0	0
Pam				
Butter	⅓ sec spray (0.3 g)	0	0	—
Cooking Spray	⅓ sec spray (0.3 g)	0	0	—
Olive Oil	⅓ sec spray (0.3 g)	0	0	—
Planters				
Peanut	1 tbsp (0.5 oz)	120	0	—
Popcorn	1 tbsp (0.5 oz)	120	0	—
Pompeian				
Olive	1 tbsp	130	0	—
Progresso				
Olive Extra Mild	1 tbsp (0.5 oz)	120	0	0
Olive Extra Virgin	1 tbsp (0.5 oz)	120	0	0
Olive Riviera Blend	1 tbsp (0.5 oz)	120	0	0

FOOD	PORTION	CALS	CHOL	FIBER
Smart Beat				
Canola	1 tbsp	120	0	—
Tree Of Life				
Olive Extra Virgin Organic	1 tbsp (0.5 g)	130	0	—
Weight Watchers				
Butter Spray	⅓ sec spray	0	0	0
Cooking Spray	⅓ sec spray	0	0	0
OKRA				
FRESH				
raw	8 pods	36	0	—
raw sliced	½ cup	19	0	—
sliced cooked	½ cup	25	0	—
sliced cooked	8 pods	27	0	—
FROZEN				
sliced cooked	½ cup	34	0	—
sliced cooked	1 pkg (10 oz)	94	0	—
Birds Eye				
Cut	¾ cup	25	0	3
Whole	9 pods	25	0	3
McKenzie's				
Breaded Okra	1 serv (2.8 oz)	90	0	3
OLIVES				
green	4 med	15	0	tr
green	3 extra lg	15	0	tr
green olive tapenade	1 tbsp	25	0	0
ripe	1 sm	4	0	tr
ripe	1 lg	5	0	tr
ripe	1 colossal	12	0	—
ripe	1 jumbo	7	0	—
spanish stuffed	5 (0.5 oz)	15	0	0
Italia In Tavola				
Black Olives Paste	1 tbsp (0.5 oz)	20	0	—
Progresso				
Olive Salad (drained)	2 tbsp (0.8 oz)	25	0	tr
Vlasic				
Ripe Colossal Pitted	2 (0.6 oz)	20	0	0
Ripe Jumbo Pitted	3 (0.6 oz)	25	0	0

FOOD	PORTION	CALS	CHOL	FIBER
Ripe Large Pitted	4 (0.5 oz)	25	0	0
Ripe Medium Pitted	5 (0.5 oz)	25	0	0
Ripe Sliced	¼ cup (0.5 oz)	25	0	0
Ripe Small Pitted	6 (0.5 oz)	25	0	0

ONION
CANNED
chopped	½ cup	21	0	—
whole	1 (2.2 oz)	12	0	—
Boar's Head				
Sweet Vidalia In Sauce	1 tbsp	10	0	0
Watkins				
Liquid Spice	1 tbsp (0.5 oz)	120	0	0

DRIED
flakes	1 tbsp	16	0	—
powder	1 tsp	7	0	—
shallots	1 tbsp	3	0	—
Watkins				
Flakes	¼ tsp (1 g)	0	0	0

FRESH
chopped cooked	½ cup	47	0	—
raw chopped	1 tbsp	4	0	tr
raw chopped	½ cup	30	0	—
scallions raw chopped	1 tbsp	2	0	tr
scallions raw sliced	½ cup	16	0	1
shallots raw chopped	1 tbsp	7	0	—
welsh raw	3½ oz	34	0	—
Antioch Farms				
Vidalia	1 med	60	0	3

FROZEN
chopped cooked	1 tbsp	4	0	—
chopped cooked	½ cup	30	0	—
rings	7 (2.5 oz)	285	0	—
rings cooked	2 (0.7 oz)	81	0	—
whole cooked	3½ oz	28	0	—
Birds Eye				
Diced	⅔ cup	30	0	1
Pearl Onions In Real Cream Sauce	½ cup	60	10	1

FOOD	PORTION	CALS	CHOL	FIBER
Small Whole	17	30	0	1
Kineret				
Rings	6 (3 oz)	200	0	0
McKenzie's				
Onion Rounds	1 serv 3.2 oz)	220	0	6
Ore Ida				
Chopped	¾ cup (3 oz)	25	0	1
Onion Ringers	6 pieces (3 oz)	240	0	2
TAKE-OUT				
rings breaded & fried	8 to 9	275	14	—

ORANGE
CANNED
Del Monte
Mandarin In Light Syrup	½ cup (4.5 oz)	80	0	1
Dole				
FruitBowls Mandarin Oranges	1 pkg (4 oz)	70	0	0
FRESH				
california navel	1	65	0	3
california valencia	1	59	0	3
florida	1	69	0	4
peel	1 tbsp	6	0	—
sections	1 cup	85	0	4

ORANGE EXTRACT
Virginia Dare
Virginia Dare	1 tsp	22	0	—

ORANGE JUICE
canned	1 cup	104	0	—
chilled	1 cup	110	0	—
fresh	1 cup	111	0	—
frzn as prep	1 cup	112	0	1
frzn not prep	6 oz	339	0	2
orange drink	6 oz	94	0	—
After The Fall				
Juice	1 bottle (10 oz)	110	0	—
Big Juicy				
Drink	8 oz	110	0	—

FOOD	PORTION	CALS	CHOL	FIBER
Bright & Early				
Chilled	8 fl oz	120	0	–
Frozen	8 fl oz	120	0	–
Capri Sun				
Drink	1 pkg (7 oz)	100	0	0
Everfresh				
Juice	1 can (8 oz)	100	0	0
Ruby Red Orange Drink	1 can (8 oz)	130	0	0
Fresh Samantha				
Juice	1 cup (8 oz)	100	0	0
Hood				
From Concentrate	1 cup (8 oz)	120	0	–
Select	1 cup (8 oz)	120	0	–
With Calcium	1 cup (8 oz)	120	0	–
Horizon Organic				
Juice Pulp Free	8 fl oz	110	0	–
Juicy Juice				
Punch	1 box (8.45 oz)	130	0	0
Punch	1 box (4.23 oz)	60	0	0
Kool-Aid				
Drink Mix Orange as prep	1 serv (8 oz)	60	0	0
Orange Drink as prep w/ sugar	1 serv (8 oz)	100	0	0
Minute Maid				
Simply Orange 100%	8 fl oz	110	0	–
Simply Orange Calcium Fortified	8 fl oz	110	0	–
Simply Orange Grove Made	8 fl oz	110	0	–
Mott's				
100% Juice	1 box (8 oz)	130	0	–
100% Juice	8 fl oz	130	0	–
Nantucket Nectars				
100% Juice	8 oz	120	0	–
NutraShake				
Fortified	1 pkg (4 oz)	50	0	4
Ocean Spray				
100% Juice	8 oz	120	0	0

FOOD	PORTION	CALS	CHOL	FIBER
Shasta Plus				
Orange Drink	1 can (11.5 oz)	160	0	0
Snapple				
Juice	10 fl oz	130	0	–
Orangeade	8 fl oz	120	0	–
Tang				
Orange Drink as prep	1 serv (8 oz)	90	0	0
Sugar Free Orange as prep	1 serv (8 oz)	5	0	0
Tropicana				
Double Vitamin C	8 fl oz	110	0	–
Juice	8 oz	110	0	–
Ruby Red	8 oz	110	0	–
Season's Best	8 oz	110	0	–
Season's Best Homestyle	8 fl oz	110	0	–
Tropical	8 oz	110	0	–
With Calcium	8 fl oz	110	0	–
Turkey Hill				
Orangeade	1 cup	120	0	–
Veryfine				
100% Juice	1 bottle (10 oz)	150	0	2
Chillers Artric Orange	8 fl oz	130	0	0
Juice Blend	1 can (11.5 oz)	160	0	0
Orange Drink	1 bottle (10 oz)	160	0	0
OREGANO				
ground	1 tsp	5	0	–
Watkins				
Liquid Spice	1 tbsp (0.5 oz)	120	0	0

ORGAN MEATS *(see* BRAINS, GIBLETS, GIZZARD, HEART, KIDNEY, LIVER, SWEETBREADS*)*

OSTRICH				
cooked	3 oz	120	74	–
OYSTERS				
canned eastern	1 cup	170	136	–
canned eastern	3 oz	58	46	–
eastern cooked	6 med	58	46	–
eastern cooked	3 oz	117	93	–

FOOD	PORTION	CALS	CHOL	FIBER
eastern raw	6 med	58	46	–
eastern raw	1 cup	170	136	–
Bumble Bee				
Fancy Whole	2 oz	70	45	0
Smoked	½ can (1.9 oz)	120	35	0
TAKE-OUT				
breaded & fried	6 (4.9 oz)	368	109	–
oysters rockefeller	3 oysters	66	38	–
stew	1 cup	278	100	tr
PANCAKE/WAFFLE SYRUP				
low calorie	1 tbsp	12	0	0
maple	1 tbsp (0.8 oz)	52	0	–
maple	1 cup (11.1 oz)	824	0	–
pancake syrup	1 cup (11 oz)	903	0	–
pancake syrup	1 tbsp (0.7 oz)	57	0	–
pancake syrup light	1 oz	46	0	–
pancake syrup w/ butter	1 tbsp (0.7 oz)	59	1	–
pancake syrup w/ butter	1 cup (11 oz)	933	14	–
Aunt Jemima				
Butter Rich	¼ cup (2.8 oz)	210	0	–
Butterlite	¼ cup (2.5 oz)	100	0	–
Lite	¼ cup (2.5 oz)	100	0	–
Original	¼ cup (2.8 oz)	210	0	–
Estee				
Maple	¼ cup	80	0	0
Log Cabin				
Original	¼ cup	210	0	0
Mrs. Butter-worth's				
Original	¼ cup (2 oz)	230	0	–
Mrs.Richardson's				
Lite	¼ cup (2.5 oz)	100	0	–
Original Recipe	¼ cup (2.8 oz)	210	0	–
Red Wing				
Lite	¼ cup (2 oz)	100	0	0
Syrup	¼ cup (2 oz)	210	0	0

FOOD	PORTION	CALS	CHOL	FIBER
Smucker's				
Breakfast Syrup Sugar Free	¼ cup (2 oz)	30	0	–
PANCAKES				
FROZEN				
buttermilk	1 4 in diam	83	3.	–
plain	1 4 in diam	83	3	–
Aunt Jemima				
Blueberry	3 (3.4 oz)	210	15	2
Buttermilk	3 (3 oz)	180	15	2
Lowfat	3 (3.4 oz)	130	0	8
Original	3 (3.4 oz)	200	15	2
Eggo				
Buttermilk	3 (4.1 oz)	270	15	1
Jimmy Dean				
Flapstick	1 (2.5 oz)	240	20	1
Flapstick Blueberry	1 (2.5 oz)	260	15	1
MIX				
buckwheat	1 (4 in diam)	62	20	–
sugar free low sodium	1 (3 in diam)	44	0	–
whole wheat	1 (4 in diam)	92	27	–
Aunt Jemima				
Buckwheat Pancake & Waffle Mix	¼ cup (1.4 oz)	120	0	4
Buttermilk Pancake & Waffle Mix	⅓ cup (1.9 oz)	190	10	2
Original Pancake & Waffle Mix	⅓ cup (1.6 oz)	150	0	1
Pancake & Waffle Mix Regular	⅓ cup (1.9 oz)	190	15	1
Pancake & Waffle Mix Whole Wheat	¼ cup (1.4 oz)	130	0	3
Betty Crocker				
Buttermilk as prep	3	200	10	1
Original as prep	3	200	10	2
Bisquick				
Shake 'N Pour Blueberry as prep	3	210	0	1

FOOD	PORTION	CALS	CHOL	FIBER
Bruce				
Sweet Potato Pancakes	2	210	0	2
Estee				
Pancake Mix as prep	4 (4 in diam)	180	0	1
Hodgson Mill				
Buckwheat	⅓ cup (1.8 oz)	160	0	5
Hungry Jack				
Potato as prep	3 (3 in diam)	90	50	1
Robin Hood				
Buttermilk as prep	3	230	60	1
Stone-Buhr				
Buckwheat	¼ cup (1.4 oz)	130	0	3
Oat Bran	¼ cup (1.4 oz)	130	0	2
Whole Wheat	¼ cup (1.4 oz)	120	0	3
Wanda's				
Blue Corn mix per serv	⅓ cup (1.7 oz)	170	0	2
TAKE-OUT				
blueberry	1 (4 in diam)	84	21	–
plain	1 (4 in diam)	86	23	–
potato	1 (4 in diam)	78	60	tr
w/ butter & syrup	2 (8.1 oz)	520	58	–
PAPAYA				
fresh	1	117	0	–
fresh cubed	1 cup	54	0	–
Sonoma				
Dried Pieces	2 pieces (2 oz)	200	0	6
Sunfresh				
In Extra Light Syrup	½ cup (4.5 oz)	70	0	1
PAPAYA JUICE				
nectar	1 cup	142	0	–
Everfresh				
Premium Drink	1 can (8 oz)	140	0	0
Nantucket Nectars				
Cocktail	8 oz	120	0	–
PAPRIKA				
paprika	1 tsp	6	0	–
Watkins				
Ground	¼ tsp (0.5 oz)	0	0	0

FOOD	PORTION	CALS	CHOL	FIBER
PARSLEY				
dry	1 tsp	1	0	–
dry	1 tbsp	1	0	–
fresh chopped	½ cup	11	0	–
PARSNIPS				
fresh cooked	1 (5.6 oz)	130	0	–
fresh sliced cooked	½ cup	63	0	–
raw sliced	½ cup	50	0	–
PASSION FRUIT				
purple fresh	1	18	0	–
purple	1 cup	126	0	–
yellow	1 cup	149	0	–
Snapple				
Passion Supreme	10 fl oz	160	0	–
PASTA (see also NOODLES, PASTA DINNERS, PASTA SALAD)				
DRY				
corn cooked	1 cup (4.9 oz)	176	0	7
corn spaghetti	2 oz	180	0	3
elbows	1 cup	389	0	–
elbows cooked	1 cup (4.9 oz)	197	0	2
shells small cooked	1 cup (4 oz)	162	0	2
shells small protein fortified cooked	1 cup (4 oz)	189	0	–
spaghetti cooked	1 cup (4.9 oz)	197	0	2
spaghetti protein fortified cooked	1 cup (4.9 oz)	230	0	2
spinach spaghetti cooked	1 cup (4.9 oz)	182	0	–
spirals cooked	1 cup (4.7 oz)	189	0	2
vegetable cooked	1 cup (4.7 oz)	172	0	6
whole wheat cooked	1 cup (4.9 oz)	174	0	4
whole wheat spaghetti cooked	1 cup (4.9 oz)	174	0	6
Annie Chun's				
Soba Noodles	2 oz	200	0	3
Barilla				
Conchiglie Rigate	1 cup (2 oz)	200	0	2
Gemelli as prep	1 cup (2 oz)	200	0	2

FOOD	PORTION	CALS	CHOL	FIBER
Pennette Rigate	1⅓ cups (2 oz)	200	0	2
Tortelloni Porcini Mushroom	¾ cup	240	50	5
Tortelloni Ricotta & Asparagus	¾ cup	240	60	5
Tortelloni Ricotta & Spinach	¾ cup	220	40	4
Classico				
Gnocchi Di Toscana	1 cup (2 oz)	210	0	2
Creamette				
Linguini Egg	2 oz	221	70	—
Rotelle	2 oz	210	0	—
Rotini Rainbow	2 oz	210	0	—
Spaghetti Egg	2 oz	221	70	—
Spaghetti Thin	2 oz	210	0	—
Ziti	2 oz	210	0	—
Cuore				
Capellini cooked	1⅓ cup (2 oz)	190	0	3
Fusilli cooked	1⅓ cup (2 oz)	190	0	3
Tortiglioni cooked	1⅓ cup (2 oz)	190	0	3
De Bole's				
Whole Wheat Organic Elbows	2 oz	210	0	5
DeCecco				
Whole Wheat Linguine cooked	2 oz	180	<5	7
Delverde				
Spaghetti Whole Wheat	2 oz	206	0	5
Duc Amici				
Pasta Lite Low Carb Fusilli	2 oz	160	0	7
Eden				
Organic Extra Fine	2 oz	210	0	3
Organic Gemelli	2 oz	210	0	5
Organic Pesto Gemelli	2 oz	210	0	4
Organic Ribbons Saffron	2 oz	210	0	3
Organic Spaghetti Semolina	2 oz	200	0	2
Organic Spaghetti 50% Whole Grain	2 oz	210	0	4

FOOD	PORTION	CALS	CHOL	FIBER
Organic Spirals Kamut Vegetable	2 oz	210	0	6
Organic Spirals Sesame Rice	2 oz	200	0	4
Organic Spirals Mixed Grain	2 oz	210	0	7
Organic Spirals Spinach	2 oz	210	0	4
Organic Vegetable Alphabets	2 oz	200	0	2
Spirals Rye	2 oz	200	0	8
Goya				
Coditos not prep	½ cup	230	0	3
Hodgson Mill				
Four Color Veggie Bows	2 oz	200	0	1
Four Color Veggie Rotini Spirals	2 oz	200	0	1
Four Color Veggie Wagon Wheels	2 oz	200	0	1
Pastamania! Durum Wheat Fettuccine	2 oz	200	30	1
Pastamania! Fettuccine Garlic & Parsley	2 oz	200	30	1
Pastamania! Fettuccine w/ Jerusalem Artichoke	2 oz	210	0	2
Pastamania! Fettucinne w/ Mushroom	2 oz	210	35	2
Pastamania! Fusilli Tre Colore w/ Tomato & Spinach	2 oz	200	0	2
Pastamania! Pesto Fettuccine	2 oz	200	30	1
Pastamania! Sea Shell Mix	2 oz	200	0	1
Pastamania! Spinach Fettuccine	2 oz	200	40	2
Pastamania! Thin Linguine	2 oz	200	30	1

FOOD	PORTION	CALS	CHOL	FIBER
Pastamania! Tomato Spinach & Durum Wheat	2 oz	210	35	2
Spaghetti Whole Wheat	2 oz	190	0	6
La Molisana				
Radiatori	2 oz	230	0	—
Lundberg				
Spaghetti Organic Brown Rice	2 oz	210	0	3
Lupini				
Elbow uncooked	½ cup (2 oz)	190	0	5
Spaghetti Light uncooked	½ cup (2 oz)	190	0	5
Spaghetti With Triticale	½ pkg (2 oz)	190	0	6
Noodles By Leonardo				
Capellini	2 oz	200	0	2
Elbows not prep	½ cup (2 oz)	200	0	2
Fettucini	2 oz	200	0	2
Linguine not prep	½ cup (2 oz)	200	0	2
Rigatoni	2 oz	200	0	2
Rotini	2 oz	200	0	2
Shells not prep	½ cup (2 oz)	200	0	2
Spaghetti not prep	½ cup (2 oz)	200	0	2
Spaghettini	2 oz	200	0	2
Vermicelli not prep	½ cup (2 oz)	200	0	2
Pomi				
Capellini	2 oz	210	0	—
Pritikin				
Spaghetti Whole Wheat	⅛ box (2 oz)	190	0	—
Spiral	⅔ cup (2 oz)	190	0	—
Real Torino				
Tirali not prep	1 cup (2 oz)	210	0	2
Ronzoni				
Elbows	¾ cup (2 oz)	210	0	—
Fettucini	¾ cup (2 oz)	210	0	—
Fusilli	¾ cup (2 oz)	210	0	—
Lasagne	2½ pieces (2 oz)	210	0	2
Manicotti	¾ cup (2 oz)	210	0	—
Mostaccioli	¾ cup (2 oz)	210	0	—

FOOD	PORTION	CALS	CHOL	FIBER
Rigatoni	¾ cup (2 oz)	210	0	—
Rotelle uncooked	¾ cup (2 oz)	210	0	—
Rotini uncooked	¾ cup (2 oz)	210	0	—
Shells uncooked	¾ cup (2 oz)	210	0	—
Shells Jumbo	¾ cup (2 oz)	210	0	—
Spaghetti not prep	¾ cup (2 oz)	210	0	—
Tubettini	¾ cup (2 oz)	210	0	—
San Giorgio				
Bowties Egg	2 oz	210	70	—
Capellini	2 oz	210	0	2
Elbow Macaroni	2 oz	210	0	2
Fettuccine Egg	2 oz	210	70	—
Fettuccini Florentine	2 oz	210	70	—
Lasagne	2 oz	210	0	2
Linguini	2 oz	210	0	2
Mostaccioli Rigati	2 oz	210	0	—
Rigatoni	2 oz	210	0	2
Rotini	2 oz	210	0	2
Shells	2 oz	210	0	2
Spaghetti	2 oz	210	0	2
Spaghetti Thin	2 oz	210	0	2
Vermicelli	2 oz	210	0	2
Ziti Cut	2 oz	210	0	2
Soy7				
Pasta All Shapes	2 oz	200	0	2
FRESH				
cooked	2 oz	75	33	—
spinach cooked	2 oz	74	19	—
Contadina				
Angel's Hair	1¼ cup (2.8 oz)	240	90	2
Fettuccine	1¼ cup (2.9 oz)	250	85	2
Fettuccine Cholesterol Free	1 cup (2.9 oz)	240	0	2
Light Ravioli Cheese	1 cup (3.1 oz)	240	60	2
Light Ravioli Garden Vegetable	1¼ cup (3.8 oz)	290	65	3
Light Tortellini Garlic & Cheese	1 cup (3.6 oz)	280	55	3
Linguine	1¼ cup (3 oz)	260	95	2

FOOD	PORTION	CALS	CHOL	FIBER
Linguine Cholesterol Free	1¼ cup (3.1 oz)	250	0	2
Ravioli Beef And Garlic	1¼ cup (4 oz)	350	110	3
Ravioli Cheese	1 cup (3.1 oz)	280	85	2
Ravioli Chicken And Rosemary	1¼ cup (4 oz)	330	85	3
Tagliatelli Spinach	1¼ cup (3.1 oz)	270	105	4
Tortellini Spianch Three Cheese	¾ cup (3.1 oz)	280	55	3
Tortelloni Cheese	¾ cup (3 oz)	260	45	3
Tortelloni Cheese And Basil	1 cup (4 oz)	360	65	3
Tortelloni Chicken And Prosciutto	1 cup (3.8 oz)	360	75	3
Tortelloni Chicken And Vegetable	¾ cup (2.9 oz)	260	45	2
Tortelloni Spicy Italian Sausage And Bell Pepper	1 cup (3.6 oz)	330	90	3
Di Giorno				
Angel's Hair	1 cup	160	0	2
Beef & Roasted Garlic Tortellini	1 cup	340	50	1
Fettuccine	1 cup	200	0	2
Four Cheese Raviolo	1 cup	350	70	2
Herb Linguine	1 cup	200	0	2
Italian Sausage Ravioli In Green Bell Pepper Pasta	1¼ cup	350	55	3
Lemon Chicken Tortellini In Cracked Black Pepper Pasta	1 cup	270	40	1
Light Cheese Ravioli	1 cup	280	40	2
Linguine	1 cup	200	0	2
Mozzarella Garlic Tortelloni	1 cup	300	45	1
Pesto Tortelloni	1 cup	320	45	3
Portabello Mushroom Tortelloni	1 cup	310	40	3

FOOD	PORTION	CALS	CHOL	FIBER
Red Bell Pepper Fettuccine	1 cup	200	0	2
Spinach Fettuccine	1 cup	190	0	2
Sun-Dried Tomato Ravioli	1⅓ cup	380	55	3
Three Cheese Tortellini	¾ cup	250	35	2
Trios				
Ravioli Cracked Pepper Garlic Cheese	1 cup (4.3 oz)	340	50	0

PASTA DINNERS (see also PASTA SALAD)
CANNED
Chef Boyardee

FOOD	PORTION	CALS	CHOL	FIBER
99% Fat Free Beef Ravioli	1 cup (8.6 oz)	210	15	3
99% Fat Free Cheese Ravioli	1 cup (8.8 oz)	210	<5	4
Beef Ravioli	1 cup (8.6 oz)	230	20	4
Beefaroni	1 cup (8.7 oz)	260	25	5
Macaroni & Cheese	½ can (7.5 oz)	180	20	2
Mini Ravioli	1 cup (8.8 oz)	252	20	3
Spaghetti & Meat Balls	1 cup (8.4 oz)	240	25	3
Tortellini Cheese	½ can (7 oz)	230	15	5
Tortellini Meat	½ can (7 oz)	260	30	4
Franco-American				
Beef Raviolios	1 can (7.7 oz)	250	12	4
Beefy Mac	1 can (7.5 oz)	228	10	3
Elbow Macaroni & Cheese	1 can (7.5 oz)	187	7	2
Spaghetti 'N Beef	1 can (7.5 oz)	226	14	3
Spaghetti w/ Meatballs	1 can (7.2 oz)	249	14	4
Hormel				
Spaghetti & Meatballs	1 can (7.5 oz)	210	20	2
Kid's Kitchen				
Microwave Meals Cheezy Mac & Beef	1 can (7.5 oz)	260	30	1
Microwave Meals Noodle Rings & Chicken	1 cup (7.5 oz)	150	30	1

FOOD	PORTION	CALS	CHOL	FIBER
Microwave Meals Spaghetti Rings & Franks	1 cup (7.5 oz)	240	30	1
Progresso				
Beef Ravioli	1 cup (9.1 oz)	260	5	4
Cheese Ravioli	1 cup (9.1 oz)	220	<5	4
FROZEN				
Amy's				
Bowl Stuffed Pasta Shells	1 pkg (10 oz)	300	30	5
Cannelloni w/ Vegetables	1 pkg (9 oz)	330	15	6
Lasagna Cheese	1 pkg (10.25 oz)	330	35	5
Lasagna Garden Vegetable	1 pkg (10.25 oz)	290	20	5
Macaroni & Cheese	1 pkg (9 oz)	410	50	3
Macaroni & Soy Cheese	1 pkg (9 oz)	370	0	4
Pasta & Vegetable Alfredo	1 cup	220	20	4
Pasta Primavera	1 pkg (9 oz)	300	45	3
Ravioli w/ Sauce	1 pkg (8 oz)	340	25	3
Rice Mac & Cheese	1 pkg (9 oz)	140	50	3
Skillet Meals	1 cup	250	5	3
Tofu Vegetable Lasagna	1 pkg (9.5 oz)	300	0	6
Vegetable Lasagna	1 pkg (9.5 oz)	280	20	3
Banquet				
Chicken Pasta Primavera	1 meal (9.5 oz)	320	25	6
Family Size Egg Noodles w/ Beef & Brown Gravy	1 serv	150	35	2
Family Size Lasagna w/ Meat Sauce	1 cup	270	45	2
Family Size Macaroni & Cheese	1 cup	230	10	3
Fettuccine Alfredo	1 meal (9.5 oz)	350	25	4
Homestyle Noodles & Chicken	1 meal (12 oz)	390	50	7
Lasagna w/ Meat Sauce	1 meal (9.5 oz)	260	15	3
Macaroni & Cheese	1 meal (12 oz)	420	20	5

FOOD	PORTION	CALS	CHOL	FIBER
Birds Eye				
Easy Recipe Creations Basil Herb Primavera	2¼ cup	260	25	3
Easy Recipe Creations Tortellini Parmigiana	2¼ cups	240	25	4
Pasta Secrets Italian Pesto	2⅓ cups	240	5	2
Pasta Secrets Primavera	2⅓ cups	230	10	3
Pasta Secrets Ranch	2⅓ cups	300	25	2
Pasta Secrets Three Cheese	2 cups	230	5	2
Pasta Secrets White Cheddar	2 cups	240	10	2
Pasta Secrets Zesty Garlic	2 cups	240	5	2
Budget Gourmet				
Cheese Ravioli	1 meal (9.5 oz)	290	30	—
Lasagna Italian Sausage	1 meal (10 oz)	430	45	—
Lasagna Vegetable	1 meal (10.5 oz)	390	15	—
Lasagne Three Cheese	1 meal (10 oz)	390	70	—
Lasagne With Meat Sauce	1 meal (9.4 oz)	290	30	—
Linguini With Shrimp & Clams	1 meal (9.5 oz)	280	45	—
Linguini With Shrimp And Clams	1 meal (10 oz)	270	50	—
Macaroni & Cheese	1 meal (5.75 oz)	230	35	—
Macaroni & Cheese With Cheddar & Parmesan	1 meal (10.5 oz)	330	30	—
Mainicotti Cheese	1 meal (10 oz)	440	75	—
Pasta Alfredo With Broccoli	1 meal (5.5 oz)	210	30	—
Penne Pasta With Chunky Tomato Sauce & Italian Sausage	1 meal (10 oz)	320	5	—
Rigatoni In Cream Sauce With Broccoli & Chicken	1 meal (10.8 oz)	290	30	—

FOOD	PORTION	CALS	CHOL	FIBER
Spaghetti With Chunky Tomato & Meat Sauce	1 meal (10 oz)	300	35	—
Tortellini Cheese	1 meal (5.5 oz)	200	20	—
Ziti In Marinara Sauce	1 meal (6.25 oz)	200	10	—
Formagg				
Penne Pasta Alfredo	⅔ cup (5 oz)	190	0	0
Penne Pasta Primavera	⅔ cup (5 oz)	190	0	0
Vegetable Pasta & Caesar Italian Garden	⅔ cup (5 oz)	190	0	0
Green Giant				
Create A Meal Creamy Alfredo as prep	1¼ cups (10 oz)	380	75	4
Create A Meal Creamy Cheddar as prep	1½ cups (10 oz)	290	45	4
Create A Meal Creamy Chicken Noodle as prep	1¼ cups (10 oz)	350	65	3
Pasta Accents Alfredo	2 cups (5.6 oz)	210	15	4
Pasta Accents Creamy Cheddar	2⅓ cups (6.7 oz)	250	15	5
Pasta Accents Florentine	2 cups (7.3 oz)	310	20	5
Pasta Accents Garden Herb Seasoning	2 cups (6.8 oz)	230	15	7
Pasta Accents Garlic Seasoning	2 cups (6.6 oz)	260	15	5
Pasta Accents Primavera	2¼ cups (7 oz)	320	20	7
Pasta Accents White Cheddar Sauce	1¾ cups (5.6 oz)	300	20	4
Healthy Choice				
Beef Macaroni	1 meal (8.5 oz)	220	20	5
Bowls Cheese & Chicken Tortellini	1 meal (8.7 oz)	250	20	6
Breaded Chicken Breast Stips w/ Macaroni & Cheese	1 meal (8 oz)	270	40	1
Cheese Ravioli Parmigiana	1 meal (9 oz)	260	20	6
Chicken Fettuccine Alfredo	1 meal (8.5 oz)	280	35	4
Fettuccine Alfredo	1 meal (8 oz)	240	20	2

FOOD	PORTION	CALS	CHOL	FIBER
Lasagna Roma	1 meal (13.5 oz)	420	35	6
Macaroni & Cheese	1 meal (9 oz)	240	20	3
Manicotti w/ Three Cheeses	1 meal (11 oz)	300	35	5
Spaghetti & Sauce w/ Seasoned Beef	1 meal (10 oz)	260	30	5
Stuffed Pasta Shells	1 meal (10.35 oz)	370	20	5
Kid Cuisine				
Magical Macaroni & Cheese	1 meal (10.6 oz)	440	15	4
Lean Cuisine				
Cafe Classics Bow Tie Pasta & Chicken	1 pkg (9.5 oz)	220	40	5
Cafe Classics Cheese Lasagna w/ Chicken Scaloppini	1 pkg (10 oz)	270	35	4
Cafe Classics Shrimp & Angel Hair Pasta	1 pkg (10 oz)	240	45	2
Everyday Favorites	1 pkg (10 oz)	270	10	5
Everyday Favorites Alfredo Pasta Primavera	1 pkg (10 oz)	290	10	3
Everyday Favorites Angel Hair Pasta	1 pkg (10 oz)	240	5	4
Everyday Favorites Cheese Cannelloni	1 pkg (9.1 oz)	230	15	4
Everyday Favorites Cheese Ravioli	1 pkg (8.5 oz)	260	35	4
Everyday Favorites Chicken Lasagna	1 pkg (10 oz)	280	40	2
Everyday Favorites Classic Cheese Lasagna	1 pkg (11.5 oz)	290	25	4
Everyday Favorites Fettucini Alfredo	1 pkg (9.25 oz)	280	15	3
Everyday Favorites Fettucini Primavera	1 pkg (10 oz)	270	15	4
Everyday Favorites Lasagna w/ Meat Sauce	1 pkg (10.5 oz)	300	30	4

FOOD	PORTION	CALS	CHOL	FIBER
Everyday Favorites Macaroni & Cheese	1 pkg (10 oz)	290	20	2
Everyday Favorites Macaroni & Beef	1 pkg (10 oz)	270	25	4
Everyday Favorites Penne Pasta	1 pkg (10 oz)	260	0	5
Everyday Favorites Spaghetti w/ Meat Sauce	1 pkg (11.5 oz)	290	20	7
Everyday Favorites Spaghetti w/ Meatballs	1 pkg (9.5 oz)	270	20	4
Everyday Favorites Cheese Lasagna Casserole	1 pkg (9.25 oz)	270	40	3
Family Style Favorites Five Cheese Lasagna	1 serv (8 oz)	210	20	3
Skillet Sensations Chicken Alfredo	1 serv	280	30	3
Luigino's				
Pasta & Pomodoro Sauce With Meatballs	1 pkg (9 oz)	320	15	2
Cheese Ravioli & Alfredo With Broccoli Sauce	1 pkg (8.5 oz)	420	70	2
Cheese Tortellini & Alfredo Sauce With Broccoli	1 pkg (8 oz)	390	65	2
Fettuccine Alfredo	1 pkg (9.4 oz)	390	30	4
Fettuccine Alfredo	1 cup (7.5 oz)	330	20	3
Fettuccine Alfredo With Broccoli	1 pkg (9.2 oz)	360	25	4
Fettuccine Carbonara	1 pkg (9 oz)	360	35	3
Lasagna Alfredo	1 cup (6.3 oz)	300	25	2
Lasagna Alfredo	1 pkg (9 oz)	360	30	2
Lasagna Pollo	1 pkg (9 oz)	320	30	3
Lasagna With Meat Sauce	1 cup (7.2 oz)	240	15	2
Lasagna With Meat Sauce	1 pkg (9 oz)	290	20	2

FOOD	PORTION	CALS	CHOL	FIBER
Lasagna With Vegetables	1 pkg (9 oz)	290	20	2
Linguini With Clams & Sauce	1 pkg (9 oz)	270	10	2
Linguini With Red Sauce	1 pkg (9 oz)	260	0	3
Linguini With Seafood	1 pkg (9 oz)	290	0	4
Macaroni & Cheese	1 cup (7.2 oz)	310	15	2
Macaroni & Cheese	1 pkg (9 oz)	370	20	3
Marinara Sauce Penne Pasta Italian Sausage & Peppers	1 pkg (9 oz)	350	35	2
Marinara Sauce Penne Pasta Italian Sausage & Peppers	1 cup (7.4 oz)	290	30	2
Meat Ravioli & Pomodoro Sauce	1 pkg (8.5 oz)	320	50	3
Minestrone With Penne Pasta	1 cup (6.3 oz)	180	5	1
Penne Pollo	1 pkg (9 oz)	330	20	3
Penne Primavera	1 pkg (9 oz)	350	25	3
Rigatoni Pomodoro Italiano	1 pkg (9 oz)	290	0	4
Shells & Cheese With Jalapenos	1 pkg (8.5 oz)	360	30	2
Spaghetti Bolognese	1 pkg (9 oz)	270	20	4
Spaghetti Marinara	1 pkg (10 oz)	250	0	3
Spinach Ravioli & Primavera Sauce	1 pkg (8.5 oz)	360	45	2
Marie Callender's				
Cheese Ravioli In Marinara Sauce w/ Spirals & Garlic Bread	1 meal (16 oz)	750	30	11
Extra Cheese Lasagna	1 meal (15 oz)	590	50	7
Fettuccine Alfredo & Garlic Bread	1 meal (14 oz)	920	90	3
Fettuccine Alfredo Supreme	1 meal (13 oz)	450	80	4
Fettuccine Primavera w/ Tortellini	1 meal (14 oz)	750	65	6

FOOD	PORTION	CALS	CHOL	FIBER
Fettuccine w/ Broccoli & Chicken	1 meal (13 oz)	710	85	6
Lasagna w/ Meat Sauce	1 meal (15 oz)	630	75	3
Macaroni & Cheese	1 meal (12 oz)	540	50	5
Skillet Meal Chicken Alfredo	½ pkg	490	75	7
Skillet Meal Penne Pasta & Meatballs	½ pkg	600	45	4
Skillet Meal Rigatoni Vegetables In Cheese Sauce	1 cup	290	30	4
Spaghetti w/ Meat Sauce & Garlic Bread	1 meal (17 oz)	670	35	9
Stuffed Pasta Trio	1 meal (10.5 oz)	380	50	5
Morton				
Macaroni & Cheese	1 serv (8 oz)	240	20	3
Spaghetti w/ Meat Sauce	1 meal (8.5 oz)	200	5	4
Mrs. Paul's				
Seafood Rotini	9 oz	240	25	—
Palmazone				
Macaroni 'n Cheese	½ pkg (6 oz)	260	20	—
Quorn				
Fettuccine Alfredo	1 pkg (10.5 oz)	360	45	4
Lasagna	1 pkg (10.5 oz)	360	15	4
Senor Felix's				
Lasagna Southwestern	1 serv (6 oz)	160	15	2
Stouffer's				
Cheddar Pasta w/ Beef & Tomatoes	1 pkg (11 oz)	450	51	3
Cheese Manicotti	1 pkg (9 oz)	380	45	4
Cheese Ravioli	1 pkg (10.6 oz)	380	100	6
Chicken Lasagna	1 serv (7.8 oz)	320	30	4
Fettucini Alfredo	1 pkg (10 oz)	520	100	4
Fettucini Primavera	1 pkg (10 oz)	430	50	5
Five Cheese Lasagna	1 pkg (10.75 oz)	360	35	6
Grilled Chicken & Angel Hair Pasta	1 pkg (10.9 oz)	380	40	5
Homestyle Chicken Fettucini	1 pkg (10.5 oz)	390	65	3

FOOD	PORTION	CALS	CHOL	FIBER
Homestyle Chicken Parmigiana w/ Spaghetti	1 pkg (12 oz)	460	45	5
Homestyle Veal Parmigiana w/ Spaghetti	1 pkg (11.9 oz)	430	80	6
Lasagna Bake	1 pkg (10.25 oz)	370	30	6
Lasagna w/ Meat Sauce	1 pkg (10.5 oz)	370	45	4
Macaroni & Cheese	1 cup (6 oz)	320	30	3
Macaroni & Cheese w/ Broccoli	1 pkg (10.5 oz)	360	25	5
Macaroni & Beef	1 pkg (11.5 oz)	420	50	5
Noodles Romanoff	1 pkg (12 oz)	490	60	4
Pasta Shells w/ American Cheese	1 cup (6 oz)	260	20	2
Salisbury Steak w/ Macaroni & Cheese	1 serv (11.3 oz)	410	70	2
Spaghetti w/Meat Sauce	1 pkg (10 oz)	350	35	5
Spaghetti w/Meatballs	1 pkg (12.6 oz)	440	50	5
Tuna Noodle Casserole	1 pkg (10 oz)	320	40	0
Turkey Tettrazini	1 pkg (10 oz)	360	55	1
Vegetable Lasagna	1 pkg (10.5 oz)	440	35	5
Tabatchnick				
Macaroni & Cheese	7.5 oz	280	26	2
Weight Watchers				
Garden Lasagna	1 pkg (11 oz)	270	30	5
Homestyle Macaroni & Cheese	1 pkg (9 oz)	290	10	2
Smart Ones Angel Hair Pasta	1 pkg (9 oz)	180	0	4
Smart Ones Bowtie Pasta & Mushrooms Marsala	1 pkg (9.65 oz)	270	40	4
Smart Ones Chicken Fettucini	1 pkg (10 oz)	300	70	4
Smart Ones Creamy Rigatoni w/ Broccoli & Chicken	1 pkg (9 oz)	230	20	4

FOOD	PORTION	CALS	CHOL	FIBER
Smart Ones Fettucini Alfredo w/ Broccoli	1 pkg (8.5 oz)	230	20	3
Smart Ones Lasagna Florentine	1 pkg (10 oz)	200	10	5
Smart Ones Lasagna Alfredo	1 pkg (9 oz)	300	25	3
Smart Ones Lasagna w/ Meat Sauce	1 pkg (10.25 oz)	270	55	6
Smart Ones Lasagna w/ Meat Sauce	1 pkg (9 oz)	240	10	4
Smart Ones Macaroni & Cheese	1 pkg (9 oz)	220	5	4
Smart Ones Pasta & Spinach Romano	1 pkg (10.4 oz)	260	15	4
Smart Ones Pasta w/ Tomato Basil Sauce	1 pkg (9.6 oz)	260	10	3
Smart Ones Penne Pasta w/ Sun-Dried Tomatoes	1 pkg (10 oz)	280	15	3
Smart Ones Penne Pollo	1 pkg (10 oz)	290	55	3
Smart Ones Ravioli Florentine	1 pkg (8.5 oz)	220	5	4
Smart Ones Spaghetti Marinara	1 pkg (9 oz)	280	5	4
Smart Ones Spaghetti w/ Meat Sauce	1 pkg (10 oz)	280	15	4
Smart Ones Spicy Penne & Ricotta	1 pkg (10.2 oz)	280	5	4
Smart Ones Tuna Noodle Casserole	1 pkg (9.5 oz)	270	45	4
Smart Ones Zita Mozzarella	1 pkg (9 oz)	290	5	5
Yves				
Veggie Lasagna	1 pkg (10.5 oz)	300	0	4
Veggie Macaroni	1 pkg (10.5 oz)	230	0	3
Veggie Penne	1 pkg (10.5 oz)	220	0	4
MIX				
Annie's Homegrown				
Mac & Cheese Meals	1 pkg	230	10	tr

FOOD	PORTION	CALS	CHOL	FIBER
Casbah				
Pasta Fasul	1 pkg (1.6 oz)	150	0	2
Hamburger Helper				
Ravioli as prep	1 cup	280	50	1
Ravioli w/ White Cheese Topping as prep	1 cup	310	50	1
Hodgson Mill				
Macaroni & Cheese Whole Wheat	1 serv	250	<5	6
Kraft				
Deluxe Macaroni & Cheese Four Cheese Blend as prep	1 cup (6.2 oz)	320	25	1
Deluxe Macaroni & Cheese Original as prep	1 cup (6.1 oz)	320	25	1
Light Deluxe Macaroni & Cheese as prep	1 cup (6.5 oz)	290	15	1
Macaroni & Cheese All Shapes as prep	1 cup (6.9 oz)	410	10	1
Macaroni & Cheese Original as prep	1 cup (6.9 oz)	410	10	1
Macaroni & Cheese Original as prep light recipe	1 cup (6.4 oz)	290	10	2
Premium Macaroni & Cheese Cheesy Alfredo as prep	1 cup (6.9 oz)	410	10	2
Premium Macaroni & Cheese Mild White Cheddar as prep	1 cup (6.8 oz)	410	10	1
Premium Macaroni & Cheese Thick 'N Creamy as prep	1 cup (7.6 oz)	420	15	2
Premium Macaroni & Cheese Three Cheese as prep	1 cup (6.9 oz)	410	10	2
Spaghetti Classics Mild Italian as prep	1 cup (9.1 oz)	240	<5	3
Spaghetti Classics Tangy Italian as prep	1 cup (8.9 oz)	240	0	3

FOOD	PORTION	CALS	CHOL	FIBER
Spaghetti Classics Zesty Cheese as prep	1 cup (8.6 oz)	240	5	3
Spaghetti Classics w/ Meat Sauce as prep	1 cup (8.2 oz)	330	15	3
Lipton				
Pasta & Sauce Angel Hair Chicken Broccoli as prep	1 cup	260	0	2
Pasta & Sauce Angel Hair Parmesan as prep	1 cup	280	10	2
Pasta & Sauce Bow Tie Chicken Primavera as prep	1 cup	290	10	2
Pasta & Sauce Bow Tie Italian Cheese as prep	1 cup	300	15	tr
Pasta & Sauce Butter & Herbs as prep	1 cup	270	5	2
Pasta & Sauce Cheddar Broccoli as prep	1 cup	340	15	1
Pasta & Sauce Chicken Herb Parmesan as prep	1 cup	80	5	2
Pasta & Sauce Chicken Stir-Fry as prep	1 cup	270	0	2
Pasta & Sauce Creamy Garlic as prep	1 cup	350	15	1
Pasta & Sauce Creamy Mushroom as prep	1 cup	320	15	0
Pasta & Sauce Garlic & Butter Linguine as prep	1 cup	260	5	2
Pasta & Sauce Mild Cheddar Cheese as prep	1 cup	290	10	tr
Pasta & Sauce Roasted Garlic Chicken as prep	1 cup	290	10	tr
Pasta & Sauce Roasted Garlic & Olive Oil w/ Tomato as prep	1 cup	270	0	2

FOOD	PORTION	CALS	CHOL	FIBER
Pasta & Sauce Rotini Primavera as prep	1 cup	320	15	2
Pasta & Sauce Savory Herb w/ Garlic as prep	1 cup	280	5	2
Pasta & Sauce Three Cheese Rotini as prep	1 cup	320	15	tr
Melting Pot				
Terrazza Black Beans & Penne	1 cup	180	0	2
Terrazza Florentine Red Beans & Fusilli	1 cup	220	<5	2
Terrazza Red Lentils & Bow Ties	1 cup	240	40	5
Terrazza Tuscan White Beans & Gemelli	1 cup	220	<5	3
Nile Spice				
Pasta'n Sauce Mediterranean	1 pkg	210	10	2
Pasta'n Sauce Parmesan	1 pkg	200	10	1
Pasta'n Sauce Primavera	1 pkg	200	10	2
Uncle Ben				
Country Inn Pasta & Sauce Angel Hair Parmesan	1 serv (2.2 oz)	245	13	3
Country Inn Pasta & Sauce Broccoli & White Cheddar	1 serv (2.2 oz)	240	8	2
Country Inn Pasta & Sauce Butter & Herb	1 serv (2 oz)	230	10	1
Country Inn Pasta & Sauce Creamy Garlic	1 serv (2.4 oz)	261	8	2
Country Inn Pasta & Sauce Fettuccine Alfredo	1 serv (2.2 oz)	310	12	2
Country Inn Pasta & Sauce Herb Linguine	1 serv (2.2 oz)	240	5	2
Country Inn Pasta & Sauce Mushroom Fettuccine	1 serv (2.2 oz)	250	12	2

FOOD	PORTION	CALS	CHOL	FIBER
Country Inn Pasta & Sauce Vegetable Alfredo	1 serv (2.2 oz)	240	11	2
Velveeta				
Rotini & Cheese w/ Broccoli as prep	1 cup (7.2 oz)	400	50	2
Shells & Cheese Bacon as prep	1 cup (6.8 oz)	360	40	1
Shells & Cheese Original as prep	1 cup (6.6 oz)	360	40	1
Shells & Cheese Salsa as prep	1 cup (7.5 oz)	380	40	2
READY-TO-EAT				
Tyson				
Rosemary Penne	1 pkg (12.5 oz)	330	45	5
SHELF-STABLE				
Hormel				
Microcup Meals Lasagna	1 cup (7.5 oz)	250	25	1
Microcup Meals Macaroni & Cheese	1 cup (7.5 oz)	260	35	1
Microcup Meals Ravioli w/ Tomato Sauce	1 cup (7.5 oz)	220	15	2
Microcup Meals Spaghetti & Meatballs	1 cup (7.5 oz)	220	25	1
It's Pasta Anytime				
Penne With Tomato Italian Sausage Sauce	1 pkg (15.25 oz)	540	<5	12
Kid's Kitchen				
Microwave Meals Beefy Macaroni	1 cup (7.5 oz)	190	30	2
Microwave Meals Macaroni & Cheese	1 cup (7.5 oz)	260	35	1
Microwave Meals Mini Ravioli	1 cup (7.5 oz)	240	20	1
Microwave Meals Spaghetti & Meatballs	1 cup (7.5 oz)	220	25	1
Microwave Meals Spaghetti Ring & Meatballs	1 cup (7.5 oz)	250	20	3

FOOD	PORTION	CALS	CHOL	FIBER
Lunch Bucket				
Beef Ravioli In Tomato Sauce	1 pkg (7.5 oz)	180	5	3
Italian Pasta w/ Chicken	1 pkg (7.5 oz)	130	10	2
Lasagna 'n Meatsauce	1 pkg (7.5 oz)	160	5	2
Light'n Healthy Pasta'n Garden Vegetables	1 pkg (7.5 oz)	150	0	—
Macaroni 'n Beef in Meatsauce	1 pkg (7.5 oz)	180	10	8
Macaroni'n Cheese	1 pkg (7.5 oz)	190	20	2
Pasta'n Chicken	1 pkg (7.5 oz)	150	20	2
Spaghetti'n Meatsauce	1 pkg (7.5 oz)	160	5	2
My Own Meal				
Cheese Tortellini	1 pkg (10 oz)	340	15	6
TAKE-OUT				
lasagna	1 piece (2.5 in x 2.5 in)	374	107	2
macaroni & cheese	1 cup	230	24	—
manicotti	¾ cup (6.4 oz)	273	77	2
rigatoni w/ sausage sauce	¾ cup	260	59	3
spaghetti w/ meatballs & cheese	1 cup	407	104	—
PASTA MACHINE MIX				
Wanda's				
Dried Tomato	⅓ cup (1.9 oz) mix per serv	202	0	1
Durum & Semolina	⅓ cup (1.9 oz) mix per serv	199	0	1
Semolina Blend	⅓ cup (1.9 oz) mix per serv	202	0	1
Spinach	⅓ cup (1.9 oz) mix per serv	202	0	1
Whole Wheat & Semolina	⅓ cup (1.9 oz) mix per serv	198	0	4
PASTA SALAD				
MIX				
Kraft				
Herb & Garlic as prep	¾ cup (4.9 oz)	280	0	2

FOOD	PORTION	CALS	CHOL	FIBER
Pasta Salad Classic Ranch w/ Bacon as prep	¾ cup (4.7 oz)	350	10	2
Pasta Salad Creamy Ceasar as prep	¾ cup (4.8 oz)	340	15	2
Pasta Salad Garden Primavera as prep	¾ cup (5 oz)	240	<5	2
Pasta Salad Italian 97% Fat Free as prep	¾ cup (4.9 oz)	190	<5	2
Pasta Salad Parmesan Peppercorn as prep	¾ cup (4.9 oz)	360	15	2
Suddenly Salad				
Classic Pasta	¾ cup	250	0	2
Classic Pasta Reduced Fat Recipe	¾ cup	210	0	2
Garden Italian 98% Fat Free	¾ cup	140	0	2
TAKE-OUT				
elbow macaroni salad	3.5 oz	160	0	–
italian style pasta salad	3.5 oz	140	0	–
mustard macaroni salad	3.5 oz	190	0	–
pasta salad w/ vegetables	3.5 oz	140	0	–
PATE				
antipasto pate	1 can (2.25 oz)	110	5	1
goose liver smoked canned	1 tbsp (13 g)	60	20	–
mushroom anchovy pate	1 can (2.25 oz)	130	5	1
pate foie gras	1 oz	127	109	–
pork pate	1 oz	107	51	0
pork pate en croute	1 oz	91	32	tr
rabbit pate	1 oz	66	21	–
salmon pate	1 can (2.25 oz)	140	10	0
shrimp	1 can (2.25 oz)	140	25	0
smoked turkey	1 can (2.25 oz)	170	15	0

FOOD	PORTION	CALS	CHOL	FIBER
PEACH				
CANNED				
halves in heavy syrup	1 half	60	0	—
halves in light syrup	1 half	44	0	—
halves juice pack	1 half	34	0	—
halves water pack	1 half	18	0	—
spiced in heavy syrup	1 fruit	66	0	—
spiced in heavy syrup	1 cup	180	0	—
Del Monte				
Fruit Cup Diced Extra Light Syrup	1 pkg (4 oz)	50	0	1
Fruit Cup Diced In Heavy Syrup	1 serv (4 oz)	80	0	1
Fruit Cup Fruit Naturals Diced	1 pkg (4 oz)	50	0	1
Fruit Pleasures Raspberry Flavor	½ cup (4.5 oz)	80	0	1
Fruit To Go Banana Berry Peaches	1 pkg (4 oz)	70	0	1
Fruitrageous Peachy Pie	1 pkg (4 oz)	80	0	1
Fruitrageous Wild Raspberry Flavor	1 pkg (4 oz)	80	0	1
Halves Ginger Flavor	½ cup (4.5 oz)	90	0	1
Halves In Extra Light Syrup	½ cup (4.4 oz)	60	0	1
Halves In Heavy Syrup	½ cup (4.5 oz)	100	0	1
Halves Melba In Heavy Syrup	½ cup (4.5 oz)	100	0	1
Slice Fruit Natural	½ cup (4.4 oz)	60	0	1
Sliced In Extra Light Syrup	½ cup (4.4 oz)	60	0	1
Sliced In Heavy Syrup	½ cup (4.5 oz)	100	0	1
Sliced Natural Raspberry Flavor	½ cup (4.4 oz)	80	0	1
Sliced Natural Harvest Spice Flavor	½ cup (4.5 oz)	80	0	1

FOOD	PORTION	CALS	CHOL	FIBER
Whole Spiced In Heavy Syrup	½ cup (4.2 oz)	100	0	1
DRIED				
halves	10	311	0	11
halves	1 cup	383	0	13
halves cooked w/ sugar	½ cup	139	0	—
halves cooked w/o sugar	½ cup	99	0	—
Del Monte				
Sun Dried	⅓ cup (1.4 oz)	90	0	5
Sonoma				
Pieces	3–5 pieces (1.4 oz)	120	0	1
FRESH				
peach	1	37	0	1
sliced	1 cup	73	0	—
Chiquita				
Peach	1 med (3.4 oz)	40	0	2
FROZEN				
slices sweetened	1 cup	235	0	—
PEACH JUICE				
nectar	1 cup	134	0	—
Nantucket Nectars				
The Original	8 oz	120	0	—
Snapple				
Dixie Peach	10 fl oz	140	0	—
PEANUT BUTTER				
chunky	1 cup	1520	0	17
chunky	2 tbsp	188	0	2
chunky w/o salt	2 tbsp	188	0	2
chunky w/o salt	1 cup	1520	0	17
smooth	2 tbsp	188	0	2
smooth	1 cup	1517	0	15
smooth w/o salt	2 tbsp	188	0	2
smooth w/o salt	1 cup	1517	0	15
Crazy Richard's				
Natural Creamy	2 tbsp (1.1 oz)	190	0	2
Estee				
Creamy Low Sodium	2 tbsp (1 oz)	190	0	2

FOOD	PORTION	CALS	CHOL	FIBER
Jif				
Apple Cinnamon	2 tbsp (1.3 oz)	200	0	2
Berry Blend	2 tbsp (1.2 oz)	200	0	1
Chocolate Silk	2 tbsp (1.3 oz)	190	0	1
Creamy	2 tbsp (1.1 oz)	190	0	2
Extra Crunchy	2 tbsp (1.1 oz)	190	0	2
Reduced Fat Creamy	2 tbsp (1.3 oz)	190	0	2
Reduced Fat Crunchy	2 tbsp (1.3 oz)	190	0	2
Simply	2 tbsp (1.1 oz)	190	0	2
Maranatha				
Salted	2 tbsp	190	0	2
P.B.				
Slices	1 slice (1 oz)	170	0	1
Peanut Wonder				
Low Sodium	2 tbsp	100	0	0
Regular	2 tbsp	100	0	0
Red Wing				
Creamy	2 tbsp (1.1 oz)	200	0	2
Crunchy	2 tbsp (1.1 oz)	200	0	2
Reese's				
Peanut Butter Chips	1 tbsp (0.5 oz)	80	0	—
Skippy				
Creamy	2 tbsp	190	0	2
Creamy w/ 2 slices white bread	1 sandwich	340	0	—
Reduced Fat Creamy	2 tbsp	190	0	1
Tropical Source				
Chips Dairy Free	13 pieces (1.5 oz)	80	0	0
PEANUTS				
chocolate coated	10 (1.4 oz)	208	4	—
chocolate coated	1 cup (5.2 oz)	773	13	—
cooked	½ cup	102	0	—
dry roasted	1 cup	855	0	12
dry roasted w/ salt	30 nuts (1 oz)	170	0	2
Estee				
Candy Coated	¼ cup	200	<5	1
Frito Lay				
Honey Roasted	1 serv (1.5 oz)	270	0	3
Hot	1 serv (1.1 oz)	190	0	2

FOOD	PORTION	CALS	CHOL	FIBER
Salted	1 oz	200	0	2
Lance				
Honey Toasted	1 pkg (1⅜ oz)	220	0	3
Roasted	1 pkg (1¼ oz)	190	0	4
Salted	1 pkg (1⅛ oz)	200	0	4
Salted Long Tube	¼ cup (1 oz)	180	0	3
Little Debbie				
Salted	¼ cup (1 oz)	160	0	2
Pennant				
Oil Roasted	1 oz	170	0	3
Planters				
Cocktail Lightly Salted Oil Roasted	1 oz	170	0	2
Cocktail Oil Roasted	1 oz	170	0	3
Cocktail Unsalted Oil Roasted	1 oz	170	0	2
Dry Roasted	1 oz	160	0	3
Fun Size! Oil Roasted	2 pkg (1 oz)	170	0	2
Heat Hot Spicy Oil Roasted	1 pkg (1.7 oz)	290	0	4
Heat Hot Spicy Oil Roasted	1 oz	160	0	2
Heat Hot Spicy Oil Roasted	1 pkg (2 oz)	330	0	5
Heat Mild Spicy Oil Roasted	1 oz	160	0	2
Honey Roasted	1 oz	160	0	2
Honey Roasted Dry Roasted	1 pkg (1.7 oz)	260	0	3
Lightly Salted Dry Roasted	1 oz	160	0	3
Lightly Salted Dry Roasted	1 pkg (1.75 oz)	290	0	4
Lightly Salted Oil Roasted	1 pkg (1.8 oz)	300	0	4
Munch'N Go Singles Heat Hot Spicy Oil Roasted	1 pkg (2.5 oz)	410	0	6
Reduced Fat Honey Roasted	⅓ cup (1 oz)	130	0	2

FOOD	PORTION	CALS	CHOL	FIBER
Salted Oil Roasted	1 pkg (1 oz)	170	0	2
Spanish Oil Roasted	1 oz	170	0	2
Spanish Raw	1 oz	150	0	3
Sweet N Crunchy	1 oz	140	0	2
Unsalted Dry Roasted	1 oz	160	0	3
Tom's				
Double Coated	1 pkg (1.35 oz)	220	0	1
Toasted	1 pkg (1.4 oz)	240	0	2
Weight Watchers				
Honey Roasted	1 pkg (0.7 oz)	100	0	2
PEAR				
CANNED				
halves in heavy sirup	1 cup	188	0	—
halves in heavy syrup	1 half	68	0	—
halves in light syrup	1 half	45	0	—
halves juice pack	1 cup	123	0	—
halves water pack	1 half	22	0	—
Del Monte				
Fruit Cup Diced In Heavy Syrup	1 pkg (4 oz)	80	0	1
Fruit Cup Diced Extra Light Syrup	1 pkg (4 oz)	50	0	1
Fruit To Go Peachy Peaches	1 pkg (4 oz)	70	0	1
Halves Fruit Naturals	½ cup (4.4 oz)	60	0	1
Halves In Extra Light Syrup	½ cup (4.4 oz)	60	0	1
Halves In Heavy Syrup	½ cup (4.5 oz)	100	0	1
Orchard Select Sliced Bartlett	½ cup (4.4 oz)	80	0	2
Sliced In Extra Light Syrup	½ cup (4.5 oz)	60	0	1
DRIED				
halves	10	459	0	—
halves	1 cup	472	0	—
halves cooked w/ sugar	½ cup	196	0	—

FOOD	PORTION	CALS	CHOL	FIBER
halves cooked w/o sugar	½ cup	163	0	—
Sonoma				
Pieces	3-4 pieces (1.4 oz)	120	0	3
FRESH				
asian	1 (4.3 oz)	51	0	—
pear	1	98	0	4
sliced w/ skin	1 cup	97	0	4
Chiquita				
Pear	1 med (5.8 oz)	100	0	4
PEAR JUICE				
nectar	1 cup	149	0	—
PEAS				
CANNED				
green	½ cup	59	0	—
green low sodium	½ cup	59	0	—
Del Monte				
Sweet	½ cup (4.4 oz)	60	0	4
Sweet No Salt Added	½ cup (4.4 oz)	60	0	4
Sweet Very Young Small	½ cup (4.4 oz)	60	0	4
Green Giant				
Sweet	½ cup (4.3 oz)	60	0	4
Sweet 50% Less Sodium	½ cup (4.3 oz)	60	0	3
LeSueur				
Early Peas	½ cup (4.2 oz)	60	0	3
Early Peas 50% Less Sodium	½ cup (4.2 oz)	60	0	4
Sweet	½ cup (4.2 oz)	60	0	3
Sweet 50% Less Sodium	½ cup (4.2 oz)	60	0	4
Owatonna				
Early June or Sweet	½ cup	70	0	—
S&W				
Petite	½ cup (4.4 oz)	70	0	4
Small	½ cup (4.4 oz)	70	0	4
Veg-All				
Tender Sweet	½ cup	60	0	3
DRIED				
split cooked	1 cup	231	0	—

FOOD	PORTION	CALS	CHOL	FIBER
Bascom's				
Yellow Split as prep	½ cup	110	0	—
Hurst				
HamBeens Green Split Peas w/ Ham	1 serv	120	0	4
FRESH				
green cooked	½ cup	67	0	—
green raw	½ cup	58	0	—
snap peas cooked	½ cup	34	0	2
snap peas raw	½ cup	30	0	2
FROZEN				
green cooked	½ cup	63	0	—
snap peas cooked	1 pkg (10 oz)	132	0	—
snap peas cooked	½ cup	42	0	—
Birds Eye				
Butter Peas	½ cup	110	0	4
Crowder	½ cup	120	0	4
Field Peas w/ Snaps	⅔ cup	130	0	4
Green	½ cup	70	0	5
Purple Hull Peas	½ cup	110	0	4
Sugar Snap	½ cup	40	0	2
Tiny Tender	¾ cup	40	0	2
GREEN GIANT				
Butter Sauce	¾ cup (4 oz)	100	<5	5
Butter Sauce LeSueur Baby Peas	¾ cup (4 oz)	100	<5	4
Harvest Fresh LeSueur Baby	⅔ cup (3.2 oz)	70	0	4
Harvest Fresh Sugar Snap	⅔ cup (3.2 oz)	50	0	3
Harvest Fresh Sweet	⅔ cup (3.3 oz)	60	0	4
LaSueur Baby Sweet	⅔ cup (2.8 oz)	60	0	5
LaSueur Early June	⅔ cup (2.8 oz)	80	0	5
LaSueur Early June w/ Mushrooms	¾ cup (3 oz)	60	0	4
Select Sugar Snap	¾ cup (2.8 oz)	35	0	3
Sweet	⅔ cup (3.1 oz)	70	0	4
La Choy				
Snow Pea Pods	½ pkg (3 oz)	35	0	2

FOOD	PORTION	CALS	CHOL	FIBER
Tree Of Life				
Peas	⅔ cup (3.1 oz)	70	0	4
SHELF-STABLE				
TastyBite				
Agra Peas & Greens	½ pkg (5 oz)	260	0	1

PECANS

FOOD	PORTION	CALS	CHOL	FIBER
dry roasted	1 oz	187	0	—
dry roasted salted	1 oz	187	0	—
halves dry roasted w/ salt	20 (1 oz)	200	0	3
halves dried	1 cup	721	0	7
oil roasted	1 oz	195	0	—
oil roasted salted	1 oz	195	0	—
Planters				
Chips	1 pkg (2 oz)	390	0	7
Gold Measure Halves	1 pkg (2 oz)	390	0	3
Halves	1 oz	190	0	2
Honey Roasted	1 oz	180	0	2
Pieces	1 oz	190	0	2
Pieces	1 pkg (2 oz)	390	0	3

PECTIN

FOOD	PORTION	CALS	CHOL	FIBER
powder	¼ pkg (0.4 oz)	39	0	—
powder	1 pkg (1.75 oz)	163	0	—
Slim Set				
Packet	1 pkg	208	0	14
Powder	1 tbsp	3	0	tr
Sure Jell				
For Lower Sugar Recipes	1 tsp (2.8 g)	20	0	0
Fruit Pectin	1 tsp (3.6 g)	20	0	0

PEPEAO

FOOD	PORTION	CALS	CHOL	FIBER
dried	½ cup	36	0	—
raw sliced	1 cup	25	0	—

PEPPER

FOOD	PORTION	CALS	CHOL	FIBER
black	1 tsp	5	0	—
cayenne	1 tsp	6	0	—
red	1 tsp	6	0	—
white	1 tsp	7	0	—

FOOD	PORTION	CALS	CHOL	FIBER
Lawry's				
Lemon	1 tsp	6	0	tr
Watkins				
Black	¼ tbsp (0.5 g)	0	0	0
Cajun	¼ tbsp (0.5 g)	0	0	0
Cracked Black	¼ tbsp (0.5 g)	0	0	0
Dijon	¼ tbsp (0.5 g)	0	0	0
Garlic Peppercorn Blend	¼ tbsp (1 g)	0	0	0
Herb	¼ tbsp (0.5 g)	0	0	0
Italian	¼ tbsp (0.5 g)	0	0	0
Lemon	¼ tbsp (1 g)	0	0	0
Mexican	¼ tbsp (0.5 g)	0	0	0
Red Pepper Flakes	¼ tsp (0.5 oz)	0	0	0
Royal Pepper Blend	¼ tbsp (0.5 g)	0	0	0
PEPPERS				
CANNED				
chili green	1 cup (5.5 oz)	29	0	2
chili green hot chopped	½ cup	17	0	—
chili red hot	1 (2.6 oz)	18	0	—
chili red hot chopped	½ cup	17	0	—
green halves	½ cup	13	0	—
jalapeno chopped	½ cup	17	0	—
red halves	½ cup	13	0	—
Chi-Chi's				
Chilies Diced Green	2 tbsp (1.2 oz)	10	0	0
Chilies Green Whole	¾ pepper (1 oz)	10	0	0
Hebrew National				
Filet	¼ pepper (1 oz)	9	0	—
Hot Cherry	⅓ pepper (1 oz)	11	0	—
Red Filet	¼ pepper (1 oz)	9	0	—
Old El Paso				
Green Chilies Chopped	2 tbsp (1 oz)	5	0	1
Green Chilies Whole	1 (1.2 oz)	10	0	1
Jalapenos Peeled	3 (1 oz)	10	0	1
Jalapenos Pickled	2 (0.9 oz)	5	0	0
Jalapenos Slices	2 tbsp (1.1 oz)	15	0	1
Progresso				
Cherry Sliced & So Hot	2 tbsp (1 oz)	25	0	1

FOOD	PORTION	CALS	CHOL	FIBER
Hot Cherry	1 (1 oz)	10	0	tr
Pepper Salad (drained)	2 tbsp (1 oz)	15	0	tr
Roasted	1 piece (1 oz)	10	0	0
Sweet Fried w/ Onions	2 tbsp (0.9 oz)	20	0	1
Tuscan	3 (1 oz)	10	0	1
Rosarita				
Chilies Diced Green	2 tbsp (1 oz)	6	0	1
Chilies Green Strips	¼ cup (1.2 oz)	5	0	1
Chilies Whole Green	2 tbsp (1.2 oz)	5	0	1
Jalapeno Whole w/ Escabeche	¼ cup (1.2 oz)	8	0	1
Jalapenos Diced	2 tbsp (1 oz)	5	0	1
Jalapenos Nacho Sliced	2 tbsp (1 oz)	2	0	tr
Rosoff's				
Sweet	¼ pepper (1 oz)	9	0	—
Schorr's				
Filet Peppers	1 oz	9	0	—
Trappey				
Jalapeno Hot Sliced	21 slices (1 oz)	4	tr	1
Jalapeno Whole	2 peppers (1 oz)	11	tr	1
Vlasic				
Hot Sliced Cherry	1 oz	5	0	—
Jalapeno Sliced	1 oz	10	0	—
Mild Cherry	1 oz	5	0	—
Pepper Rings Hot	1 oz	5	0	—
Pepper Rings Mild	1 oz	5	0	—
DRIED				
ancho	1 (0.6 oz)	48	0	4
green	1 tbsp	1	0	—
pasilla	1 (7 g)	24	0	2
red	1 tbsp	1	0	—
FRESH				
banana	1 cup (4.4 oz)	33	0	4
banana	1 (4 in) (1.2 oz)	9	0	1
chili green hot	1	18	0	—
chili green hot chopped	½ cup	30	0	—
chili red chopped	½ cup	30	0	—
chili red hot	1 (1.6 oz)	18	0	—
green	1 (2.6 oz)	20	0	1
green chopped	½ cup	13	0	1

FOOD	PORTION	CALS	CHOL	FIBER
green chopped cooked	½ cup	19	0	—
green cooked	1 (2.6 oz)	20	0	—
habanero chile	1 tsp	9	0	1
hungarian	1 (0.9 oz)	8	0	0
jalapeno	1 (0.5 oz)	4	0	tr
jalapeno sliced	1 cup (3.2 oz)	27	0	3
red	1 (2.6 oz)	20	0	1
red chopped	½ cup	13	0	1
red chopped cooked	½ cup	19	0	—
red cooked	1 (2.6 oz)	20	0	—
serrano	1 (6 g)	2	0	tr
serrano chopped	1 cup (3.7 oz)	34	0	4
yellow	10 strips	14	0	—
yellow	1 (6.5 oz)	50	0	—
Chiquita				
Pepper	1 med (5.2 oz)	30	0	2
FROZEN				
green chopped	1 oz	6	0	—
red chopped	1 oz	6	0	—
Birds Eye				
Diced Green	¾ cup	20	0	2
PERCH				
FRESH				
cooked	3 oz	99	98	—
cooked	1 fillet (1.6 oz)	54	53	—
ocean perch atlantic cooked	3 oz	103	46	—
ocean perch atlantic cooked	1 fillet (1.8 oz)	60	27	—
ocean perch atlantic raw	3 oz	80	36	—
raw	3 oz	77	76	—
FROZEN				
Van De Kamp's				
Battered Fillets	2 (4 oz)	300	25	0
PERSIMMONS				
dried japanese	1	93	0	—
fresh	1	32	0	—
fresh japanese	1	118	0	—

FOOD	PORTION	CALS	CHOL	FIBER
Sonoma				
Dried	6-8 pieces (1.4 oz)	140	0	3
PHEASANT				
roasted	3.5 oz	215	120	0
PHYLLO				
phyllo dough	1 oz	85	0	—
phyllo dough sheet	1	57	0	—
Ekizian				
Sheets	½ lb	865	123	—
Fillo Factory				
Fillo Dough Spelt Vegan	3 sheets (2 oz)	180	0	4
Fillo Dough Vegan	3 sheets (2 oz)	170	0	1
Fillo Dough Whole Wheat Vegan	3 sheets (2 oz)	190	0	3
Pastry Shells Vegan	3 (0.4 oz)	45	0	0
PICANTE (see SALSA)				
PICKLES				
dill	1 (2.3 oz)	12	0	—
dill low sodium	1 (2.3 oz)	12	0	1
dill low sodium sliced	1 slice	1	0	tr
dill sliced	1 slice	1	0	tr
gerkins	1 oz	6	0	—
kosher dill	1 (2.3 oz)	12	0	1
polish dill	1 (2.3 oz)	12	0	1
quick sour	1 (1.2 oz)	4	0	—
quick sour low sodium	1 (1.2 oz)	4	0	—
quick sour sliced	1 slice	1	0	—
sweet	1 (1.2 oz)	41	0	tr
sweet gherkin	1 sm (½ oz)	20	0	—
sweet low sodium	1 (1.2 oz)	41	0	tr
sweet sliced	1 slice	7	0	tr
Claussen				
Bread 'N Butter Chips	4 slices (1 oz)	20	0	0
Deli Style Hearty Garlic Whole	½ (1 oz)	5	0	0
Kosher Dill Spears	1 spear (1.2 oz)	5	0	0
Kosher Dills Halves	1 half (1 oz)	5	0	0
Kosher Dills Mini	1 (0.8 oz)	5	0	0

FOOD	PORTION	CALS	CHOL	FIBER
Kosher Dills Whole	½ (1 oz)	5	0	0
New York Deli Style Half Sours Whole	½ (1 oz)	5	0	0
Sandwich Slices Bread 'N Butter	2 (1.2 oz)	25	0	0
Sandwich Slices Deli Style Hearty Garlic	2 (1.2 oz)	5	0	0
Sandwich Slices Kosher Dills	2 (1.2 oz)	5	0	0
Super Slices For Burgers	1 (0.8 oz)	5	0	0
Hebrew National				
Half Sour	½ pickle (1 oz)	4	0	—
Kosher	⅓ pickle (1 oz)	4	0	—
Kosher Barrel Cured Dill	1 pkg	23	0	—
Kosher Barrel Cured Hot Dill	1 pkg	23	0	—
Kosher Chips	3 slices (1 oz)	4	0	—
Kosher Halves	⅓ pickle (1 oz)	4	0	—
Kosher Large	⅓ pickle (1 oz)	4	0	—
Kosher Spears	½ spear (1 oz)	4	0	—
Sour Garlic	⅓ pickle (1 oz)	3	0	—
Rosoff's				
Half Sour	⅓ pickle (1 oz)	4	0	—
Half Sour Spears	½ spear (1 oz)	4	0	—
Kosher	⅓ pickle (1 oz)	4	0	—
Kosher Halves	⅓ pickle (1 oz)	4	0	—
Schorr's				
Garlic	⅓ pickle (1 oz)	3	0	—
Half Sour	½ spear (1 oz)	4	0	—
Half Sour	⅓ pickle (1 oz)	4	0	—
Kosher Deli	½ pickle (1 oz)	4	0	—
Kosher Halves	⅓ pickle (1 oz)	4	0	—
Kosher Spears	½ spear (1 oz)	4	0	—
Kosher Whole	⅓ pickle (1 oz)	4	0	—
Vlasic				
Hamburger Dill Chips	1 oz	5	0	—
Kosher Cross Cuts	1 oz	5	0	—
Kosher Spears	1 oz	5	0	—
Kosher Whole	1 oz	5	0	—

FOOD	PORTION	CALS	CHOL	FIBER
Sweet Butter Chips	1 oz	30	0	—
Sweet Gerkins	1 oz	35	0	—
Whole Dills	1 oz	5	0	—
PIE				
FROZEN				
apple	⅛ of 9 in pie (4.4 oz)	297	0	2
blueberry	⅛ of 9 in pie (4.4 oz)	289	0	—
cherry	⅛ of 9 in pie (4.4 oz)	325	0	1
chocolate creme	⅛ of 8 in pie (4 oz)	344	6	—
coconut creme	⅛ of 7 in pie (2.2 oz)	191	0	1
lemon meringue	⅙ of 8 in pie (4.5 oz)	303	51	1
peach	⅙ of 8 in pie (4.1 oz)	261	0	—
Amy's				
Apple	1 serv (4 oz)	240	25	2
Kineret				
Apple Homestyle	⅙ pie (4 oz)	313	0	1
Mrs. Smith's				
Apple	1 slice (4.3 oz)	350	0	3
Banana Cream	¼ of 8 in pie (3.4 oz)	250	0	1
Blueberry	1 slice (4.6 oz)	330	0	3
Cappuccino	1 slice (4.2 oz)	300	0	2
Cherry	1 slice (4.3 oz)	320	0	2
Cherry Crumb	1 slice (4.2 oz)	320	0	1
Chocolate Cream	1 slice (4.6 oz)	340	15	2
Chocolate Mint Cream	1 slice (4.3 oz)	360	0	2
Coconut Custard	1 slice (4.4 oz)	260	70	tr
Cookies 'N Cream	1 slice (4.3 oz)	360	0	2
Dutch Apple	1 slice (4.4 oz)	330	0	2
French Silk	1 slice (4.4 oz)	560	55	1
Key West Line	1 slice (4.3 oz)	430	15	1
Lemon Cream	1 slice (5 oz)	440	0	tr
Lemonade	1 slice (4.3 oz)	340	0	1
Mince	1 slice (4.6 oz)	380	0	2
Mixed Berry	1 slice (4.2 oz)	300	0	2
Peach	1 slice (4.6 oz)	320	0	2
Peach Lattice	1 slice (4.2 oz)	290	0	2
Peanut Butter Silk	1 slice (4.6 oz)	600	55	2
Pecan	1 slice (4.8 oz)	560	65	2
Pumpkin Custard	1 slice (4.6 oz)	270	40	2

FOOD	PORTION	CALS	CHOL	FIBER
Raspberry	1 slice (4.6 oz)	330	0	1
S'Mores Cream	1 slice (4.3 oz)	360	0	2
Strawberry Banana	1 slice (4.3 oz)	330	0	1
Sweet Potato Custard	1 slice (4.6 oz)	340	40	2
Sara Lee				
Apple 45% Reduced Fat	⅛ pie (4.5 oz)	290	<5	2
Chocolate Silk	⅕ pie (4.8 oz)	500	<5	<2
Coconut Cream	⅕ pie (4.8 oz)	480	0	2
Homestyle Apple	⅛ pie (4.6 oz)	340	0	1
Homestyle Blueberry	⅛ pie (4.6 oz)	360	0	2
Homestyle Cherry	⅛ pie (4.6 oz)	320	0	2
Homestyle Dutch Apple	⅛ pie (4.6 oz)	350	0	2
Homestyle Mince	⅛ pie (4.6 oz)	390	0	3
Homestyle Peach	⅛ pie (4.6 oz)	320	0	2
Homestyle Pecan	⅛ pie (4.2 oz)	520	45	3
Homestyle Pumpkin	⅛ pie (4.6 oz)	260	30	2
Homestyle Raspberry	⅛ pie (4.6 oz)	380	<5	2
Lemon Meringue	⅙ pie (5 oz)	350	0	5
Weight Watchers				
Mississippi Mud	1 piece (2.45 oz)	160	5	1
MIX				
Jell-O				
No Bake Chocolate Silk as prep	⅛ pie (4.4 oz)	320	5	tr
SNACK				
apple	1 (3 oz)	266	13	—
cherry	1 (3 oz)	266	13	—
lemon	1 (3 oz)	266	13	—
Dolly Madison				
Apple	1 (4.5 oz)	480	15	2
Blueberry	1 (4.5 oz)	480	20	2
Cherry	1 (4.5 oz)	470	20	1
Chocolate Pudding	1 (4.5 oz)	530	30	1
Lemon	1 (4.5 oz)	500	20	0
Peach	1 (4.5 oz)	480	25	1
Pecan	1 (3 oz)	360	70	1
Pecan Fried	1 (4.5 oz)	530	10	1
Pineapple	1 (4.5 oz)	460	15	1
Hostess				
Apple	1 (4.5 oz)	480	15	2

FOOD	PORTION	CALS	CHOL	FIBER
Blackberry	1 (4.5 oz)	520	15	2
Blueberry	1 (4.5 oz)	480	20	2
Cherry	1 (4.5 oz)	470	20	1
French Apple	1 (4.5 oz)	480	15	2
Lemon	1 (4.5 oz)	500	20	0
Peach	1 (4.5 oz)	480	25	1
Pineapple	1 (4.5 oz)	460	15	1
Strawberry	1 (4.5 oz)	510	15	2
Lance				
Pecan	1 (3 oz)	350	25	3
Tastykake				
Apple	1 (4 oz)	270	0	1
Blueberry	1 (4 oz)	300	0	1
Cherry	1 (4 oz)	290	0	tr
Coconut Creme	1 (4 oz)	370	55	1
French Apple	1 (4.2 oz)	310	0	1
Lemon	1 (4 oz)	300	40	tr
Peach	1 (4 oz)	280	0	1
Pineapple	1 (4 oz)	290	20	1
Pineapple Cheese	1 (4 oz)	320	20	1
Pumpkin	1 (4 oz)	340	35	1
Strawberry	1 (3.5 oz)	320	0	1
Tastyklair	1 (4 oz)	400	90	0
Tom's				
Apple	1 pkg (3 oz)	330	5	1
Banana Marshmallow	1 pkg (2.75 oz)	320	0	0
Cherry	1 pkg (3 oz)	320	5	1
Chocolate Marshmallow	1 pkg (2.75 oz)	320	0	tr
TAKE-OUT				
apple	⅛ of 9 in pie (5.4 oz)	411	0	3
banana cream	⅛ of 9 in pie (5.2 oz)	398	75	—
blueberry	⅛ of 9 in pie (5.2 oz)	360	0	—
butterscotch	⅛ of 9 in pie (4.5 oz)	355	78	—
cherry	⅛ of 9 in pie (6.3 oz)	486	0	—
coconut creme	⅛ of 9 in pie (4.7 oz)	396	77	—
coconut custard	⅛ of 8 in pie (3.6 oz)	271	36	—
custard	⅛ of 9 in pie (4.5 oz)	262	87	2
lemon meringue	⅛ of 9 in pie (4.5 oz)	362	68	2
mince	⅛ of 9 in pie (5.8 oz)	477	0	—
pecan	⅛ of 8 in pie (4 oz)	452	36	4

FOOD	PORTION	CALS	CHOL	FIBER
pumpkin	⅛ of 8 in pie (3.8 oz)	229	22	3
vanilla cream	⅛ of 9 in pie (4.4 oz)	350	78	—

PIE CRUST
FROZEN
puff pastry baked	1 shell (1.4 oz)	223	0	—
Pepperidge Farm				
Puff Pastry Sheets	⅙ sheet (1.4 oz)	170	0	0
Puff Pastry Shell	1 (1.6 oz)	190	0	0
Puff Pastry Squares	1 sq (2 oz)	240	0	0
Pet-Ritz				
Deep Dish	⅙ pie (0.7 oz)	90	<5	0
Regular	⅙ pie (0.6 oz)	80	<5	0
Tart Shells	1 (1 oz)	130	0	0
MIX				
as prep	9 in crust (5.6 oz)	801	0	—
as prep	⅛ of 9 in pie (0.7 oz)	100	0	—
Betty Crocker				
Pie Crust as prep	⅙ crust	110	0	—
Flako				
Mix	¼ cup (0.9 oz)	130	5	1
READY-TO-EAT				
chocolate cookie crumb	9 in crust (7.7 oz)	1130	3	—
chocolate cookie crumb	⅛ of 9 in pie (1 oz)	139	0	—
graham cracker	9 in crust (8.4 oz)	1181	0	—
graham cracker	⅛ of 9 in pie (1 oz)	148	0	—
vanilla wafer cracker crumbs	9 in crust (6.1 oz)	937	69	—
vanilla wafer cracker crumbs	⅛ of 9 in pie (0.8 oz)	119	9	—
Honey Maid				
Graham	⅙ crust (1 oz)	140	0	tr
Keebler				
Graham Single Serve	1 (0.8 oz)	120	0	tr
Reduced Fat Graham	⅛ pie (0.7 oz)	90	0	0
Nabisco				
Nilla	⅙ crust (1 oz)	140	<5	0
Oreo				
Crumb Crust	⅙ crust (1 oz)	140	0	tr

FOOD	PORTION	CALS	CHOL	FIBER
REFRIGERATED				
All Ready				
Crust	⅛ pie (0.9 oz)	120	5	0
PIE FILLING				
apple	1 can (21 oz)	599	0	6
apple	⅛ can (2.6 oz)	74	0	1
cherry	⅛ can (2.6 oz)	85	0	–
cherry	1 can (21 oz)	683	0	–
pumpkin pie mix	1 cup	282	0	–
Comstock				
MoreFruit Light Cherry	⅓ cup (2.9 oz)	60	0	0
Red Ruby Cherry	⅓ cup (3.1 oz)	90	0	1
Libby				
Pumpkin Pie Mix	⅓ cup	90	0	2
Smucker's				
Pie Glaze Strawberry	2 oz	80	0	–
PIEROGI				
pierogi	¾ cup (4.4 oz)	307	49	–
Empire				
Potato Cheese	3 (4.6 oz)	260	5	5
Potato Onion	3 (4.6 oz)	250	0	4
Golden				
Potato Cheese	3 (4 oz)	250	35	–
Health Is Wealth				
Potato & Cheddar	2 (2.8 oz)	140	0	3
Potato & Onion	2 (2.8 oz)	140	0	3
Mrs. T's				
Jalapeno & Cheddar	3 (4.2 oz)	190	10	2
Potato & American Cheese	3 (4.2 oz)	220	15	2
Potato & Cheddar	3 (4.2 oz)	190	10	2
Potato & Onion	3 (4.2 oz)	180	0	2
Potato & Roasted Garlic	3 (4.2 oz)	190	5	2
Rogies Cheddar & Bacon	7 (3 oz)	140	5	1
Rogies Jalapeno & Cheddar	7 (3 oz)	120	5	1
Rogies Potato & Cheddar	7 (3 oz)	130	5	1

FOOD	PORTION	CALS	CHOL	FIBER
PIG'S EARS AND FEET				
ear simmered	1	184	100	0
feet pickled	1 lb	921	417	0
feet pickled	1 oz	58	26	0
feet simmered	3 oz	165	85	0
Hormel				
Pickled Feet	2 oz	80	45	0
Pickled Hocks	2 oz	110	45	0
PIGEON				
w/ skin & bone	3.5 oz	169	110	–
PIGEON PEAS				
dried cooked	½ cup	102	0	–
dried cooked	1 cup	204	0	–
PIGNOLIA (*see* PINE NUTS)				
PIKE				
northern cooked	½ fillet (5.4 oz)	176	78	–
northern cooked	3 oz	96	43	–
northern raw	3 oz	75	33	–
roe raw	1 oz	37	103	–
walleye baked	3 oz	101	94	–
walleye fillet baked	4.4 oz	147	137	–
PILLNUTS				
canarytree dried	1 oz	204	0	–
PIMIENTOS				
canned	1 tbsp	3	0	–
canned	1 slice	0	0	–
Dromedary				
Peeled	½ tsp (4 g)	0	0	0
Unpeeled	½ tsp (4 g)	0	0	0
PINE NUTS				
pignolia dried	1 oz	146	0	–
pignolia dried	1 tbsp	51	0	–
pinyon dried	1 oz	161	0	–
Progresso				
Pignoli	1 jar (1 oz)	170	0	0

FOOD	PORTION	CALS	CHOL	FIBER
PINEAPPLE				
CANNED				
chunks in heavy syrup	1 cup	199	0	–
chunks juice pack	1 cup	150	0	–
crushed in heavy syrup	1 cup	199	0	–
slices in heavy syrup	1 slice	45	0	–
slices in light syrup	1 slice	30	0	–
slices juice pack	1 slice	35	0	–
slices water pack	1 slice	19	0	–
tidbits in heavy syrup	1 cup	199	0	–
tidbits in juice	1 cup	150	0	–
tidbits in water	1 cup	79	0	–
Del Monte				
Chunks in Heavy Syrup	½ cup (4.3 oz)	90	0	1
Chunks In Its Own Juice	½ cup (4.3 oz)	70	0	1
Crushed In Heavy Syrup	½ cup (4.3 oz)	90	0	1
Crushed In Its Own Juice	½ cup (4.3 oz)	70	0	1
Fruit Cup Tidbits	1 pkg (4 oz)	50	0	1
Sliced In Heavy Syrup	2 slices (4.1 oz)	90	0	1
Sliced In Its Own Juice	½ cup (4 oz)	60	0	1
Spears In Its Own Juice	½ cup (4.3 oz)	70	0	1
Tidbits In Its Own Juice	½ cup (4.3 oz)	70	0	1
Wedges In Its Own Juice	½ cup (4.3 oz)	70	0	1
Dole				
Chunks Juice Pack	½ cup	60	0	1
Sunfresh				
In Extra Light Syrup	½ cup (4.6 oz)	80	0	0
DRIED				
Sonoma				
Pieces	2 pieces (1.4 oz)	140	0	2
FRESH				
diced	1 cup	77	0	2
slice	1 slice	42	0	1
Bonita Hill				
Golden Extra Sweet	2 slices (3.9 oz)	60	0	1
FROZEN				
chunks sweetened	½ cup	104	0	–
PINEAPPLE JUICE				
canned	1 cup	139	0	–

FOOD	PORTION	CALS	CHOL	FIBER
frzn as prep	1 cup	129	0	–
frzn not prep	6 oz	387	0	–
After The Fall				
Mandarin Pineapple	1 can (12 oz)	150	0	0
Bright & Early				
Frozen	8 fl oz	120	0	–
Del Monte				
Juice	6 fl oz	80	0	0
Dole				
Chilled	8 oz	130	0	–
PINK BEANS				
dried cooked	1 cup	252	0	–
PINTO BEANS				
CANNED				
pinto	1 cup	186	0	–
Chi-Chi's				
Pinto Beans	½ cup (4.3 oz)	100	0	3
Eden				
Organic Spicy	½ cup (4.6 oz)	125	0	2
Green Giant				
Pinto Beans	½ cup (4.4 oz)	110	0	5
Old El Paso				
Pinto Beans	½ cup (4.6 oz)	110	0	7
Progresso				
Pinto Beans	½ cup (4.6 oz)	110	0	7
DRIED				
cooked	1 cup	235	0	–
Hurst				
HamBeens w/ Ham	3 tbsp (1.2 oz)	120	0	6
FROZEN				
cooked	3 oz	152	0	–
PISTACHIOS				
dried	1 cup	739	0	14
dry roasted	1 oz	172	0	–
dry roasted salted	1 oz	172	0	–
dry roasted salted	1 cup	776	0	–
dry roasted w/ salt	47 nuts (1 oz)	160	0	3

FOOD	PORTION	CALS	CHOL	FIBER
Lance				
Pistachios	1 pkg (1⅛ oz)	90	0	2
Planters				
Munch'N Go Singles Shelled Dry Roasted	1 pkg (2 oz)	330	0	6
Red Salted Dry Roasted	1 pkg	160	0	3
Uncolored Dry Roasted	½ cup	160	0	3
Sonoma				
Salted Shelled	¼ cup (1 oz)	190	0	3
PITANGA				
fresh	1 cup	57	0	—
fresh	1	2	0	—
PIZZA (see also PIZZA DOUGH, PIZZA SAUCE)				
Amy's				
Cheese	⅓ pie	300	15	2
Mushroom & Olive	⅓ pie	250	10	2
Pesto	⅓ pie	310	10	2
Pocket Sandwich Cheese Pizza	1 (4.5 oz)	300	15	4
Pocket Sandwich Vegetarian Pizza	1 (4.5 oz)	250	10	4
Roasted Vegetable	⅓ pie	260	0	2
Snacks Cheese	5–6 pieces	180	10	2
Soy Cheese	⅓ pie	290	0	2
Spinach	⅓ pie	300	15	2
Veggie Combo	⅓ pie	280	10	2
Appian Way				
Pizza Mix Thick Crust	⅓ pie (4.2 oz)	290	10	2
Pizza Mix Thin Crust	⅓ pie (4.1 oz)	250	0	2
Banquet				
Pepperoni	1 pie (6.75 oz)	490	35	5
Pizza Snack Cheese	6 pieces (7.5 oz)	200	20	2
Pizza Snack Pepperoni	6 pieces (7.5 oz)	230	20	2
Pizza Snack Pepperoni & Sausage	6 pieces (7.5 oz)	210	20	2
Celeste				
Italian Bread Deluxe	1 (5.1 oz)	290	15	3
Italian Bread Garlic & Herb Zesty Chicken	1 (5 oz)	260	20	3

FOOD	PORTION	CALS	CHOL	FIBER
Italian Bread Pepperoni	1 (5 oz)	320	20	3
Italian Bread Zesty Four Cheese	1 (4.6 oz)	300	25	3
Large Cheese	¼ pie (4.4 oz)	320	25	3
Large Deluxe	¼ pie (5.5 oz)	350	20	4
Large Pepperoni	¼ pie (4.7 oz)	350	20	3
Large Suprema With Meat	⅕ pie (4.6 oz)	290	15	3
Large Zesty Four Cheese	¼ pie (4.4 oz)	330	30	3
Small Cheese	1 (7.5 oz)	540	45	4
Small Deluxe	1 (8.2 oz)	540	25	6
Small Hot & Zesty Four Cheese	1 (7 oz)	530	50	4
Small Original Four Cheese	1 (7 oz)	540	50	4
Small Pepperoni	1 (6.7 oz)	520	25	4
Small Sausage	1 (7.5 oz)	530	25	5
Small Suprema Vegetable	1 (7.5 oz)	480	5	5
Small Suprema With Meat	1 (9 oz)	580	30	7
Small Zesty Four Cheese	1 (7 oz)	530	50	4
Croissant Pocket				
Stuffed Sandwich Pepperoni Pizza	1 piece (4.5 oz)	350	30	3
Di Giorno				
Rising Crust 12 inch Four Cheese	⅙ pie (4.9 oz)	320	25	3
Rising Crust 12 inch Italian Sausage	⅙ pie (5.3 oz)	360	35	3
Rising Crust 12 inch Pepperoni	⅙ pie (5.2 oz)	370	35	3
Rising Crust 12 inch Supreme	⅙ pie (5.8 oz)	380	40	3
Rising Crust 12 inch Three Meat	⅙ pie (5.4 oz)	380	40	3
Rising Crust 12 inch Vegetable	⅙ pie (5.6 oz)	310	20	3

FOOD	PORTION	CALS	CHOL	FIBER
Rising Crust 8 inch Chicken Supreme	⅓ pie (4.8 oz)	270	30	2
Rising Crust 8 inch Four Cheese	⅓ pie (4 oz)	260	20	2
Rising Crust 8 inch Italian Sausage	⅓ pie (4.4 oz)	300	25	2
Rising Crust 8 inch Pepperoni	⅓ pie (4.2 oz)	300	30	2
Rising Crust 8 inch Spinach	⅓ pie (4.3 oz)	250	15	3
Rising Crust 8 inch Supreme	⅓ pie (4.7 oz)	310	30	2
Rising Crust 8 inch Three Meat	⅓ pie (4.4 oz)	310	30	2
Rising Crust 8 inch Vegetable	⅓ pie (4.6 oz)	250	15	2
Empire				
3 Pack	1 (3 oz)	210	20	7
Bagel	1 (2 oz)	150	15	0
English Muffin	1 (2 oz)	130	15	1
Pizza	½ pie (5 oz)	340	30	2
Health Is Wealth				
Pizza Munchees	6 (3 oz)	190	0	1
Healthy Choice				
French Bread Cheese	1 piece (6 oz)	340	15	5
French Bread Pepperoni	1 piece (6 oz)	340	20	6
French Bread Sausage	1 piece (6 oz)	320	25	5
French Bread Supreme	1 piece (6.35 oz)	330	20	6
French Bread Vegetable	1 piece (6 oz)	280	10	5
Hot Pocket				
Stuffed Sandwich Pepperoni & Sausage Pizza	1 (4.5 oz)	340	30	3
Stuffed Sandwich Pepperoni Pizza	1 (4.5 oz)	350	30	2
Jack's				
Great Combinations 12 inch Bacon Cheeseburger	¼ pie (4.7 oz)	360	45	2

FOOD	PORTION	CALS	CHOL	FIBER
Great Combinations 12 inch Double Cheese	¼ pie (4.9 oz)	380	50	2
Great Combinations 12 inch Pepperoni	¼ pie (5.2 oz)	410	40	3
Great Combinations 12 inch Pepperoni & Mushrooms	¼ pie (4.8 oz)	340	35	2
Great Combinations 12 inch Sausage	¼ pie (5.4 oz)	390	40	3
Great Combinations 12 inch Sausage & Mushroom	¼ pie (4.9 oz)	310	30	3
Great Combinations 12 inch Sausage & Pepperoni	¼ pie (4.8 oz)	350	40	2
Great Combinations 12 inch Supreme	¼ pie (5.2 oz)	350	40	5
Great Combinations 9 inch Double Cheese	½ pie (5.5 oz)	430	55	3
Great Combinations 9 inch Pepperoni & Sausage	½ pie (5.1 oz)	380	40	3
Naturally Rising 12 inch Bacon Cheeseburger	⅙ pie (5 oz)	350	40	2
Naturally Rising 12 inch Canadian Bacon	⅙ pie (4.9 oz)	280	30	2
Naturally Rising 12 inch Cheese	⅙ pie (4.5 oz)	290	25	2
Naturally Rising 12 inch Combination w/ Sausage & Pepperoni	⅙ pie (5.2 oz)	360	40	2
Naturally Rising 12 inch Pepperoni	⅙ pie (4.9 oz)	350	40	2
Naturally Rising 12 inch Pepperoni Supreme	⅙ pie (5.1 oz)	340	35	2
Naturally Rising 12 inch Sausage	⅙ pie (5.1 oz)	340	35	2

FOOD	PORTION	CALS	CHOL	FIBER
Naturally Rising 12 inch Spicy Italian Sausage	⅙ pie (5.1 oz)	330	40	2
Naturally Rising 12 inch The Works	⅙ pie (5.3 oz)	330	35	2
Naturally Rising 9 inch Cheese	⅓ pie (4.7 oz)	300	25	2
Naturally Rising 9 inch Combination w/ Sausage & Pepperoni	¼ pie (4.2 oz)	300	35	2
Naturally Rising 9 inch Pepperoni	⅓ pie (5.2 oz)	360	40	2
Naturally Rising 9 inch Sausage	⅓ pie (5.4 oz)	360	35	2
Naturally Rising 9 inch The Works	¼ pie (4.5 oz)	280	30	2
Original 12 inch Canadian Bacon	¼ pie (4.4 oz)	280	30	2
Original 12 inch Cheese	⅓ pie (5 oz)	360	30	3
Original 12 inch Hamburger	¼ pie (4.4 oz)	300	35	2
Original 12 inch Pepperoni	¼ pie (4.3 oz)	330	35	2
Original 12 inch Sausage	¼ pie (4.3 oz)	300	30	2
Original 12 inch Spicy Italian Sausage	¼ pie (4.3 oz)	290	35	2
Original 9 inch Pepperoni	½ pie (5 oz)	380	40	3
Original 9 inch Sausage	½ pie (5.1 oz)	360	35	3
Pizza Bursts Combination Sausage & Pepperoni	6 pieces (3 oz)	250	20	2
Pizza Bursts Pepperoni	6 pieces (3 oz)	260	20	2
Pizza Bursts Sausage	6 pieces (3 oz)	250	20	2
Pizza Bursts Supercheese	6 pieces (3 oz)	250	20	2
Pizza Bursts Supreme	6 pieces (3 oz)	250	20	2
Kid Cuisine				
Backpacking Pizza Snack	6 pieces	230	20	1

FOOD	PORTION	CALS	CHOL	FIBER
Big League Hamburger	1 meal (8.3 oz)	400	35	5
Fire Chief Cheese	1 pie (5.2 oz)	340	20	2
Pirate Pizza w/ Cheese	1 meal (8 oz)	430	30	5
Poolside Pepperoni	1 (5.2 oz)	380	35	2
Kineret				
Bagel Pizza	2 (4 oz)	300	30	1
Slice	1 (4.9 oz)	490	20	2
Lean Cuisine				
Everyday Favorites French Bread Cheese	1 pkg (6 oz)	320	15	4
Everyday Favorites French Bread Deluxe	1 pkg (6.1 oz)	290	25	3
Everyday Favorites French Bread Pepperoni	1 pkg (5.25 oz)	300	25	3
Everyday Favorites French Bread Sun Dried Tomatoes	1 serv (6 oz)	340	20	3
Lean Pockets				
Stuffed Sandwich Pizza Deluxe	1 (4.5 oz)	270	25	2
Marie Callender's				
French Bread Cheese	1 (7.2 oz)	530	60	4
French Bread Pepperoni	1 (7.5 oz)	570	65	4
French Bread Supreme	1 (7.5 oz)	510	50	4
Old El Paso				
Pizza Burrito Cheese	1 (3.5 oz)	320	20	0
Pizza Burrito Pepperoni	1 (3.5 oz)	260	20	0
Pizza Burrito Sausage	1 (3.5 oz)	260	15	0
Pepperidge Farm				
Gourmet Crust Cheese	1 (4.4 oz)	390	90	6
Gourmet Crust Pepperoni	1 (4.5 oz)	420	90	5
Stouffer's				
French Bread Bacon Cheddar	1 piece (5.7 oz)	430	25	4
French Bread Cheese	1 piece (5.2 oz)	370	15	3
French Bread Cheeseburger	1 piece (6 oz)	420	30	3
French Bread Deluxe	1 piece (6.2 oz)	430	20	3

FOOD	PORTION	CALS	CHOL	FIBER
French Bread Double Cheese	1 piece (5.9 oz)	400	25	4
French Bread Pepperoni	1 piece (5.6 oz)	430	15	3
French Bread Pepperoni & Mushroom	1 piece (6.1 oz)	440	30	5
French Bread Sausage	1 piece (6 oz)	420	20	3
French Bread Sausage & Pepperoni	1 piece (6.25 oz)	470	25	3
French Bread Three Meat	1 piece (6.25 oz)	460	35	5
French Bread Vegetable Deluxe	1 piece (6.4 oz)	380	20	4
French Bread White Pizza	1 piece (5.1 oz)	460	20	5
Tombstone				
Double Top Pepperoni	⅛ pie (4.5 oz)	340	45	2
Double Top Sausage	⅛ pie (4.6 oz)	320	40	2
Double Top Sausage & Pepperoni	⅛ pie (4.6 oz)	340	45	2
Double Top Supreme	⅛ pie (4.7 oz)	330	40	2
Double Top Two Cheese	⅛ pie (5.2 oz)	380	50	2
For One ½ Less Fat Cheese	1 pie (6.5 oz)	460	20	3
For One ½ Less Fat Vegetable	1 pie (7.2 oz)	360	10	5
For One Extra Cheese	1 pie (6.9 oz)	520	50	3
For One Pepperoni	1 pie (6.9 oz)	550	55	3
For One Supreme	1 pie (7.5 oz)	550	55	3
Light Supreme	⅕ pie (4.8 oz)	270	20	3
Light Vegetable	⅕ pie (4.6 oz)	240	10	3
Original 12 inch Canadian Bacon	¼ pie (5.5 oz)	350	35	3
Original 12 inch Deluxe	⅕ pie (4.8 oz)	310	30	3
Original 12 inch Extra Cheese	¼ pie (5.1 oz)	350	30	3
Original 12 inch Hamburger	⅕ pie (4.4 oz)	310	30	2
Original 12 inch Pepperoni	¼ pie (5.3 oz)	400	40	3

FOOD	PORTION	CALS	CHOL	FIBER
Original 12 inch Sausage	⅓ pie (4.4 oz)	300	30	2
Original 12 inch Sausage & Mushroom	⅓ pie (4.6 oz)	300	30	3
Original 12 inch Sausage & Pepperoni	⅓ pie (4.4 oz)	320	30	2
Original 12 inch Supreme	⅓ pie (5.1 oz)	320	30	2
Original 9 inch Deluxe	⅓ pie (4.4 oz)	280	25	2
Original 9 inch Extra Cheese	½ pie (5.6 oz)	380	30	3
Original 9 inch Hamburger	⅓ pie (4 oz)	280	25	2
Original 9 inch Pepperoni	⅓ pie (4 oz)	300	30	2
Original 9 inch Pepperoni & Sausage	⅓ pie (4.1 oz)	300	30	2
Original 9 inch Sausage	⅓ pie (4 oz)	280	25	2
Original 9 inch Sausage	⅓ pie (4.4 oz)	310	30	2
Oven Rising Italian Sausage	⅙ pie (5.1 oz)	320	30	2
Oven Rising Pepperoni	⅙ pie (4.9 oz)	340	35	2
Oven Rising Supreme	⅙ pie (5.1 oz)	320	30	2
Oven Rising Three Cheese	⅙ pie (4.8 oz)	320	35	2
Oven Rising Three Meat	⅙ pie (5.1 oz)	340	35	2
Thin Crust Four Meat Combo	¼ pie (5 oz)	380	45	2
Thin Crust Italian Sausage	¼ pie (5 oz)	370	45	2
Thin Crust Pepperoni	¼ pie (4.8 oz)	400	50	2
Thin Crust Supreme	¼ pie (5 oz)	380	45	2
Thin Crust Supreme Taco	¼ pie (5.1 oz)	370	50	2
Thin Crust Three Cheese	¼ pie (4.7 oz)	360	45	2
Weight Watchers				
Smart Ones Deluxe Combo	1 (6.57 oz)	380	40	6

FOOD	PORTION	CALS	CHOL	FIBER
Smart Ones Pepperoni	1 (5.56 oz)	390	45	4
TAKE-OUT				
cheese	12 in pie	1121	74	—
cheese	⅛ of 12 in pie	140	9	—
cheese deep dish individual	1 (5.5 oz)	460	20	2
cheese meat & vegetables	12 in pie	1472	165	—
cheese meat & vegetables	⅛ of 12 in pie	184	21	—
pepperoni	12 in pie	1445	115	—
pepperoni	⅛ of 12 in pie	181	14	—

PIZZA DOUGH

FOOD	PORTION	CALS	CHOL	FIBER
crust	1 slice (1.7 oz)	130	0	1
Betty Crocker				
Italian Herb Crust Mix	¼ crust (1.6 oz)	180	0	1
Boboli				
Shell + Sauce	⅙ sm shell (2.6 oz)	170	5	1
Shell + Sauce	⅛ lg shell (2.6 oz)	170	5	1
Thin Crust	⅓ crust (2 oz)	160	0	1
House of Pasta				
Frozen	⅛ of 14 in pie (1.9 oz)	140	0	1
Pillsbury				
Crust	⅓ crust (2 oz)	150	0	tr
Robin Hood				
Crust	¼ crust	160	0	1
Sassafras				
Cornmeal Pizza Crust	1 slice (1.4 oz)	140	0	1
Italian Pizza Crust Mix	1 slice (1.4 oz)	140	0	1
Wanda's				
Crust Mix Oregano & Basil	⅒ pie (1.4 oz)	149	0	1
Crust Mix Oregano & Basil Whole Wheat	⅒ pie (1.4 oz)	141	0	5
Watkins				
Crust Mix	⅛ pkg (1.8 oz)	180	0	2

PIZZA SAUCE

FOOD	PORTION	CALS	CHOL	FIBER
Boboli				
Sauce	¼ cup (2.5 oz)	40	0	1

FOOD	PORTION	CALS	CHOL	FIBER
Sauce	1 pkg (1.2 oz)	20	0	1
Hunt's				
Fully Prepared	¼ cup (2.2 oz)	21	0	2
Pizza Sauce	¼ cup (2.2 oz)	27	0	2
Prima Choice Supper Heavy	¼ cup (2.2 oz)	28	0	3
Muir Glen				
Organic	¼ cup (2.2 oz)	40	0	2
Progresso				
Pizza Sauce	¼ cup (2.1 oz)	20	0	1
Ragu				
Quick Traditional	3 tbsp (1.7 oz)	35	0	—
PLANTAINS				
fresh uncooked	1 (6.3 oz)	218	0	—
sliced cooked	½ cup	89	0	—
Chifles				
Plantain Chips	1 pkg (2 oz)	170	0	2
PLUMS				
CANNED				
purple in heavy syrup	3	119	0	—
purple in heavy syrup	1 cup	320	0	—
purple in light syrup	1 cup	158	0	—
purple in light syrup	3	83	0	—
purple juice pack	3	55	0	—
purple juice pack	1 cup	146	0	—
purple water pack	3	39	0	—
purple water pack	1 cup	102	0	—
Eden				
Umeboshi Paste	1 tsp	5	0	0
Umeboshi Plums	1	5	0	0
FRESH				
plum	1	36	0	—
sliced	1 cup	91	0	—
Chiquita				
Purple	2 med (4.6 oz)	80	0	2
POI				
poi	½ cup	134	0	—

FOOD	PORTION	CALS	CHOL	FIBER
POKEBERRY SHOOTS				
cooked	½ cup	16	0	–
fresh	½ cup	18	0	–
POLENTA				
Aurora				
Ready-To-Use	½ cup (5 oz)	110	0	1
Frieda's				
Dried Tomato	4 oz	80	0	2
Italian Herb	4 oz	80	0	2
Mexicana	4 oz	80	0	2
Original	4 oz	80	0	2
Wild Mushroom	4 oz	80	0	2
Melissa's				
Original	4 oz	80	0	2
POLLACK				
altantic fillet baked	5.3 oz	178	137	–
atlantic baked	3 oz	100	77	–
POMEGRANATE				
fresh	1	104	0	–
Cortas				
Concentrated Juice	1 tbsp (0.6 oz)	40	0	0
POMPANO				
florida cooked	3 oz	179	54	–
florida raw	3 oz	140	43	–
POPCORN (*see also* POPCORN CAKES)				
air-popped	1 cup (0.3 oz)	31	0	2
carmel coated w/ peanuts	⅔ cup (1 oz)	114	0	1
cheese	1 cup (0.4 oz)	58	1	1
oil popped	1 cup (0.4 oz)	55	0	1
Barrel O' Fun				
Baked Curl	1 oz	150	0	0
Caramel Corn	1 oz	115	0	1
Corn Pop	1 oz	190	0	0
Popcorn	1 oz	160	0	1
White Cheddar Pops	1 oz	170	0	0

FOOD	PORTION	CALS	CHOL	FIBER
Chester's				
Butter	3 cups	160	0	2
Caramel Craze	¾ cup	130	0	1
Cheddar Cheese	3 cups	190	<5	3
Microwave Butter	5 cups	200	0	4
Cracker Jack				
Fat Free Butter Toffee	¾ cup	110	0	1
Fat Free Caramel	¾ cup	110	0	1
Original	½ cup (1 oz)	120	0	1
Estee				
Caramel	1 cup	120	0	1
Herr's				
Regular	3 cups (1 oz)	140	0	3
Husman's				
Cheese Corn	2¼ cups (1 oz)	160	<5	1
Jolly Time				
America's Best 94% Fat Free	1 cup	20	0	1
Blast O Butter	1 cup	45	0	1
Blast O Butter Light	1 cup	30	0	1
Butter Licious	1 cup	35	0	1
Butter Licious Light	1 cup	30	0	tr
Crispy & White	1 cup	40	0	1
Crispy & White Light	1 cup	25	0	1
Healthy Pop 94% Fat Free	1 cup	20	0	1
White Air Popped	5 cups	100	0	6
Yellow Air Popped	5 cups	100	0	6
Lance				
Cheese	1 pkg (0.6 oz)	90	0	2
Plain	1 pkg (0.5 oz)	70	0	1
White Cheddar	1 pkg (0.6 oz)	100	0	1
White Cheddar	1 pkg (0.9 oz)	150	0	1
Louise's				
Fat-Free Apple Cinnamon	1 oz	100	0	1
Fat-Free Buttery Toffee	1 oz	100	0	1
Fat-Free Caramel	1 oz	100	0	1
Newman's Own				
Microwave Butter Flavor	3½ cups	170	0	3

FOOD	PORTION	CALS	CHOL	FIBER
Microwave Light Butter	3½ cups	110	0	3
Microwave Light Natural	3½ cups	110	0	3
Microwave Natural	3½ cups	170	0	3
Popcorn unpopped	3 tbsp	110	0	7
Orville Redenbacher's				
Gourmet Original	3 cups	92	0	5
Hot Air	3 cups	92	0	5
Microwave Butter	3 cups	168	0	4
Microwave Butter No Salt Added	3 cups	176	0	4
Microwave Butter Light	3 cups	122	0	5
Microwave Caramel	1 serv	179	0	3
Microwave Golden Cheddar	1 serv	169	0	3
Microwave Natural	3 cups	164	0	4
Microwave Natural No Salt Added	3 cups	174	0	5
Microwave Natural Light	3 cups	118	0	5
Microwave Smartpop	1 serv	96	0	5
Microwave Smartpop Butter Snack Size	1 bag	155	0	0
Microwave Snack Size Butter	1 bag	287	0	6
Microwave Snack Size Butter Light	1 bag	183	0	7
Microwave White Cheddar	1 serv	169	0	3
Redenbudders Microwave Herb & Garlic	1 serv	176	0	4
Redenbudders Microwave Zesty Butter	1 serv	177	0	4
Redenbudders Movie Theater Butter Light	1 serv	113	0	5
Redenbudders Movie Theater Microwave Butter	1 serv	176	0	4

FOOD	PORTION	CALS	CHOL	FIBER
Smart Pop Movie Theater Butter	1 serv	92	0	5
White	3 cups	92	0	5
Planters				
Fiddle Faddle Caramel Fat Free	1 cup (1 oz)	110	0	1
Pop Secret				
94% Fat Free Butter	1 cup (5 g)	20	0	tr
94% Fat Free Natural	1 cup (5 g)	20	0	tr
Butter	1 cup (7 g)	35	0	tr
Cheddar Cheese	1 cup (6 g)	30	0	tr
Jumbo Pop Butter	1 cup (7 g)	40	0	tr
Jumbo Pop Movie Theater Butter	1 cup (7 g)	40	0	tr
Light Butter	1 cup (5 g)	20	0	tr
Light Movie Theater Butter	1 cup (5 g)	25	0	tr
Light Natural	1 cup (5 g)	25	0	tr
Movie Theater Butter	1 cup (7 g)	40	0	tr
Nacho Cheese	1 cup (6 g)	30	0	tr
Natural	1 cup (7 g)	35	0	tr
Pop Chips	1½ cups (1 oz)	130	0	1
Real Butter	1 cup (7 g)	35	0	tr
Smartfood				
Butter	3 cups	150	5	1
Low Fat Toffee Crunch	¾ cup	110	0	1
Reduced Fat Golden Butter	3⅓ cups	130	0	4
Reduced Fat White Cheddar	3 cups	140	<5	3
White Cheddar	2 cups	190	5	2
Snyder's Of Hanover				
Butter	⅝ oz	110	0	0
Tom's				
Caramel Corn	1 pkg (1.6 oz)	180	0	2
Utz				
Au Natural	3 cups (1 oz)	120	0	5
Butter	2 cups (1 oz)	170	0	3
Cheese	2 cups (1 oz)	150	5	3
Hulless Puff'N Corn	2 cups (1 oz)	180	0	0

FOOD	PORTION	CALS	CHOL	FIBER
Hulless Puff'N Corn Hot Cheese	1 pkg (1.75 oz)	290	0	0
Hulless Pull'N Corn Cheese	2 cups (1 oz)	170	<5	0
White Cheddar	2 cups (1 oz)	150	<5	3
Weight Watchers				
Butter	1 pkg (0.66 oz)	90	0	3
Butter Toffee	1 pkg (0.9 oz)	110	0	1
Caramel	1 pkg (0.9 oz)	100	0	1
Microwave	1 pkg (1 oz)	100	0	7
White Cheddar Cheese	1 pkg (0.66 oz)	90	0	2

POPCORN CAKES
Mother's

FOOD	PORTION	CALS	CHOL	FIBER
Butter Flavor	1 (0.3 oz)	35	0	0
Unsalted	1 (0.3 oz)	35	0	0
Orville Redenbacher's				
BBQ Mini	8 (0.5 oz)	55	0	1
Butter	2 (0.6 oz)	134	tr	2
Butter Mini	8 (0.5 oz)	56	1	1
Caramel	1 (0.4 oz)	34	0	1
Caramel Mini	7 (0.5 oz)	50	tr	1
Nacho Cheese Mini	8 (0.5 oz)	56	1	1
Peanut Crunch Mini	7 (0.5 oz)	55	tr	1
White Cheddar	2 (0.6 oz)	63	tr	2
White Cheddar Mini	8 (0.5 oz)	56	tr	1
Quaker				
Blueberry Crunch	1 (0.5 oz)	50	0	—
Butter Mini	6 (0.5 oz)	50	0	2
Butter Popped	1 (0.3 oz)	35	0	—
Caramel	1 (0.5 oz)	50	0	—
Caramel Mini	5 (0.5 oz)	50	0	1
Cheddar Cheese Mini	6 (0.5 oz)	50	0	1
Lightly Salted Mini	7 (0.5 oz)	50	0	2
Monterey Jack	1 (0.4 oz)	40	0	—
Strawberry Crunch	1 (0.5 oz)	50	0	—
White Cheddar	1 (0.4 oz)	40	0	—

POPOVER

FOOD	PORTION	CALS	CHOL	FIBER
home recipe as prep w/ 2% milk	1 (1.4 oz)	87	46	—

FOOD	PORTION	CALS	CHOL	FIBER
popover home recipe as prep w/ whole milk	1 (1.4 oz)	90	47	—

POPPY SEEDS
poppy seeds	1 tsp	15	0	—

PORK *(see also HAM, PORK DISHES)*
CANNED
Hormel
Pickled Tidbits	2 oz	100	45	0

FRESH
boston blade roast lean & fat cooked	3 oz	229	73	0
boston blade steak lean & fat cooked	3 oz	220	81	0
center loin roast lean bone in cooked	3 oz	169	67	0
center loin choplean bone in cooked	3 oz	172	72	0
center rib chop lean & fat bone in cooked	3 oz	213	62	0
center rib roast lean & fat bone in cooked	3 oz	217	62	0
fresh ham rump lean roasted	3 oz	175	82	0
fresh ham rump lean & fat roasted	3 oz	214	82	0
fresh ham shank lean roasted	3 oz	183	78	0
fresh ham shank lean & fat roasted	3 oz	246	78	0
fresh ham whole lean roasted	3 oz	179	80	0
fresh ham whole lean roasted diced	1 cup	285	127	0
fresh ham whole lean & fat roasted	3 oz	232	80	0
fresh ham whole lean & fat roasted diced	1 cup	369	127	0
ground cooked	3 oz	252	80	0

FOOD	PORTION	CALS	CHOL	FIBER
leg loin & shoulder lean only roasted	3 oz	198	79	—
loin chop lean bone in braised	3 oz	191	71	0
loin chop lean bone in broiled	3 oz	199	71	0
loin roast lean bone in roasted	3 oz	210	79	0
loin whole lean & fat braised	3 oz	203	68	0
loin whole lean & fat broiled	3 oz	206	68	0
loin whole lean & fat roasted	3 oz	211	70	0
lungs braised	3 oz	84	329	0
pancreas cooked	3 oz	186	268	0
ribs country style lean & fat braised	3 oz	252	74	0
shoulder arm picnic lean & fat roasted	3 oz	269	80	0
shoulder whole lean & fat roasted	3 oz	248	77	0
shoulder whole lean & fat roasted diced	1 cup	394	122	0
shoulder whole lean roasted	3 oz	196	77	0
shoulder whole lean roasted diced	1 cup	311	122	0
sirloin chop lean & fat bone in braised	3 oz	208	70	0
sirloin roast lean & fat bone in cooked	3 oz	222	74	0
spareribs braised	3 oz	338	103	0
spleen braised	3 oz	127	428	0
tail simmered	3 oz	336	110	0
tenderloin lean roasted	3 oz	139	67	0
top loin chop boneless lean & fat cooked	3 oz	198	64	0
top loin roast bonless lean & fat cooked	3 oz	192	66	0

FOOD	PORTION	CALS	CHOL	FIBER
Freirich				
Porkette	4 oz	220	70	0
Hormel				
Extra Lean Loin Lemon Garlic	1 serv (4 oz)	130	45	0
Oscar Mayer				
Sweet Morsel Smoked Boneless Pork Shoulder Butt	3 oz	180	50	0
READY-TO-EAT				
Tyson				
Pork Pattie	1 (3.8 oz)	200	40	3
PORK DISHES				
Jimmy Dean				
BBQ Pork Rib Sandwich	1 (5.4 oz)	440	55	1
Smithfield				
Pulled Pork w/ Barbecue Sauce	2 oz	90	20	–
Thomas E. Wilson				
Lemon Pepper Pork Roast	1 serv (3 oz)	110	30	0
TAKE-OUT				
pork roast	2 oz	70	40	–
POT PIE				
Amy's				
Broccoli	1 (7.5 oz)	430	45	4
Country Vegetable	1 (7.5 oz)	370	40	4
Shepherd's	1 (8 oz)	160	0	5
Vegetable	1 (7.5 oz)	420	50	4
Vegetable Non Dairy	1 (7.5 oz)	320	0	4
Banquet				
Beef	1 (7 oz)	400	30	1
Cheesy Potato & Broccoli w/ Ham	1 (7 oz)	410	25	2
Chicken	1 (7 oz)	380	40	1
Chicken & Broccoli	1 (7 oz)	350	35	2
Family Size Hearty Chicken	1 cup	460	35	2
Macaroni & Cheese	1 pkg (6.5 oz)	210	10	1

FOOD	PORTION	CALS	CHOL	FIBER
Turkey	1 (7 oz)	370	45	3
Vegetable Cheese	1 (7 oz)	340	10	1
Empire				
Chicken	1 (8.1 oz)	440	30	11
Turkey	1 (8.1 oz)	470	25	11
Healthy Choice				
Colonial Chicken	1 (9.5 oz)	310	45	5
Lean Cuisine				
Everyday Favorites Chicken Pie	1 pkg (9.5 oz)	300	30	—
Everyday Favorites Vegetable Eggroll	1 pkg (9 oz)	300	0	4
Marie Callender's				
Beef	1 (9.5 oz)	680	20	1
Chicken	1 (9.5 oz)	680	20	3
Chicken & Broccoli	1 (9.5 oz)	670	25	4
Chicken Au Gratin	1 (9.5 oz)	690	30	4
Turkey	1 (9.5 oz)	680	15	5
Morton				
Macaroni & Cheese	1 (6.5 oz)	210	10	1
Vegetable w/ Beef	1 (7 oz)	340	20	2
Vegetable w/ Chicken	1 (7 oz)	320	25	2
Vegetable w/ Turkey	1 (7 oz)	310	25	2
Mrs. Paterson's				
Aussie Pie Chicken	1 (5.5 oz)	460	90	2
Aussie Pie Chicken Low Fat	1 (5.5 oz)	380	35	1
Aussie Pie Philly Steak	1 (5.5 oz)	420	40	2
Stouffer's				
Beef Pie	1 pkg (10 oz)	450	65	3
Chicken Pie	1 pkg (10 oz)	540	25	4
Turkey	1 pkg (10 oz)	530	65	3
Swanson				
Beef	1 (7 oz)	376	22	5
Chicken	1 (7 oz)	416	19	2
Turkey	1 (7 oz)	440	18	2
TAKE-OUT				
beef	⅓ of 9 in pie (7.4 oz)	515	42	—
chicken	⅓ of 9 in pie (8.1 oz)	545	56	—

FOOD	PORTION	CALS	CHOL	FIBER
POTATO (see also CHIPS, KNISH, PANCAKES)				
CANNED				
potatoes	½ cup	54	0	—
Del Monte				
New Sliced	⅔ cup (5.4 oz)	60	0	2
New Whole	2 med (5.5 oz)	60	0	2
Hormel				
Au Gratin & Bacon	1 can (7.5 oz)	250	25	2
S&W				
Whole Small	2 (5.5 oz)	60	0	2
FRESH				
baked skin only	1 skin (2 oz)	115	0	2
baked w/ skin	1 (6.5 oz)	220	0	—
baked w/o skin	1 (5 oz)	145	0	2
baked w/o skin	½ cup	57	0	1
boiled	½ cup	68	0	1
microwaved	1 (7 oz)	212	0	—
microwaved w/o skin	½ cup	78	0	—
raw w/o skin	1 (3.9 oz)	88	0	—
PurelyIdaho				
Oven Roasts	1 serv (3 oz)	70	0	2
Yukon Gold				
Fresh	1 (5.3 oz)	110	0	—
FROZEN				
french fries	10 strips	111	0	2
french fries thick cut	10 strips	109	0	—
potato puffs	½ cup	138	0	—
potato puffs as prep	1	16	0	—
Birds Eye				
Baby Gourmet	7 (4 oz)	100	0	1
Whole	3	50	0	1
Budget Gourmet				
Baked With Broccoli And Cheese	1 pkg (10.5 oz)	300	30	—
Cheddared Potatoes	1 pkg (5.5 oz)	260	35	—
Cheddared Potatoes With Broccoli	1 pkg (5 oz)	150	20	—
Three Cheese Potatoes	1 pkg (5.75 oz)	220	30	—
Empire				
Crinkle Cut French Fries	½ cup (3 oz)	90	0	7

FOOD	PORTION	CALS	CHOL	FIBER
Latkes Potato Pancakes	1 (2 oz)	80	0	8
Latkes Mini Potato Pancakes	2 (2 oz)	90	0	6
Fillo Factory				
Petite Fillo Puffs Potato & Herb	7 (4.6 oz)	280	15	1
Golden				
Potato Pancakes	1 (1.33 oz)	71	4	—
Healthy Choice				
Cheddar Broccoli Potatoes	1 meal (10.5 oz)	330	25	6
Kineret				
Crinkle Cut	18 pieces (3 oz)	120	0	2
Kugel	1 piece (2.5 oz)	150	30	1
Latkes	1 (1.5 oz)	90	0	2
Latkes Mini	10 (3 oz)	160	0	2
Lean Cuisine				
Everyday Favorites Deluxe Cheddar Potato	1 pkg (10.4 oz)	250	20	5
Everyday Favorites Roasted Potatoes w/ Broccoli	1 pkg (10.25 oz)	260	15	7
MicroMagic				
French Fries Low Fat	1 pkg (3 oz)	130	0	3
Oh Boy!				
Stuffed With Cheddar Cheese	1 (5 oz)	130	<5	2
Stuffed With Real Bacon	1 (6 oz)	120	5	4
Ore Ida				
Cheddar Browns	1 patty (3 oz)	90	<5	1
Cottage Fries	14 pieces (3 oz)	130	0	1
Crispers!	17 pieces (3 oz)	220	0	2
Crispers! Nacho	10 pieces (3 oz)	170	0	2
Crispers! Texas	3 oz	170	0	2
Crispy Crowns!	12 pieces (3 oz)	100	0	2
Crispy Crunchies	12 pieces (3 oz)	160	0	2
Deep Fries Crinkle Cuts	18 pieces (3 oz)	160	0	2
Deep Fries French Fries	22 pieces (3 oz)	160	0	2

FOOD	PORTION	CALS	CHOL	FIBER
Dinner Fries Country Style	8 pieces (3 oz)	110	0	1
Fast Fries	23 pieces (3 oz)	140	0	2
Fast Fries Ranch	22 pieces (3 oz)	150	0	1
Golden Crinkles	16 pieces (3 oz)	120	0	2
Golden Fries	16 pieces (3 oz)	120	0	1
Golden Patties	1 (2.5 oz)	140	0	1
Golden Twirls	28 pieces (3 oz)	160	0	2
Hash Browns Country Style	1 cup (2.6 oz)	60	0	1
Hash Browns Shredded	1 patty (3 oz)	70	0	1
Hash Browns Southern Style	¾ cup (3 oz)	70	0	2
Hot Tots	9 pieces (3 oz)	150	0	2
Mashed Natural Butter	½ cup (2.1 oz)	80	<5	tr
Microwave Crinkle Cuts	1 pkg (3.5 oz)	180	0	2
Microwave Hash Browns	1 patty (2 oz)	110	0	tr
Microwave Tater Tots	1 pkg (3.75 oz)	190	0	2
O'Brien Potatoes	¾ cup (3 oz)	60	0	2
Pixie Crinkles	33 pieces (3 oz)	140	0	3
Shoestrings	38 pieces (3 oz)	150	0	2
Snackin' Fries	1 pkg (5 oz)	180	0	3
Snackin' Fries Extra Zesty	1 pkg (5 oz)	180	0	4
Tater ABC's	10 pieces (3 oz)	190	0	2
Tater Tots	9 pieces (3 oz)	160	0	2
Tater Tots Bacon	9 pieces (3 oz)	150	0	1
Tater Tots Onion	9 pieces (3 oz)	150	0	2
Toaster Hash Browns	2 patties (3.5 oz)	190	0	1
Topped Broccoli & Cheese	½ (6 oz)	150	10	4
Topped Salsa & Cheese	½ (5.5 oz)	160	10	3
Twice Baked Butter	1 (5 oz)	200	0	4
Twice Baked Cheddar Cheese	1 (5 oz)	190	0	3
Twice Baked Ranch	1 (5 oz)	180	0	3
Twice Baked Sour Cream & Chives	1 (5 oz)	180	0	3
Waffle Fries	15 pieces (3 oz)	140	0	2

FOOD	PORTION	CALS	CHOL	FIBER
Wedges With Skin	9 pieces (3 oz)	110	0	2
Zesties!	12 pieces (3 oz)	160	0	1
Stouffer's				
Au Gratin	½ cup (5.75 oz)	130	15	1
Scalloped	½ cup (5.75 oz)	140	<5	2
Tree Of Life				
Organic French Fries	20 pieces (3 oz)	110	0	1
Weight Watchers				
Smart Ones Baked Broccoli & Cheese	1 pkg (10 oz)	250	20	6
MIX				
au gratin as prep	½ cup	160	29	—
instant mashed flakes as prep w/ whole milk & butter	½ cup	118	15	—
instant mashed flakes not prep	½ cup	78	0	—
instant mashed granules as prep w/ whole milk & butter	½ cup	114	15	—
instant mashed granules not prep	½ cup	372	0	—
scalloped	½ cup	105	14	—
Betty Crocker				
Au Gratin Low Fat Recipe	½ cup	110	<5	1
Au Gratin as prep	½ cup	150	5	1
Cheddar & Bacon	½ cup	150	<5	1
Cheddar & Bacon Low Fat Recipe	½ cup	120	0	1
Cheddar & Sour Cream	½ cup	130	5	1
Chicken & Vegetable	⅔ cup	140	<5	2
Chicken & Vegetable Low Fat Recipe	⅔ cup	120	<5	2
Hash Browns	½ cup	190	0	3
Homestyle Broccoli Au Gratin	½ cup	140	<5	2
Homestyle Broccoli Au Gratin Low Fat Recipe	½ cup	110	0	2

FOOD	PORTION	CALS	CHOL	FIBER
Homestyle Cheddar Cheese	½ cup	120	<5	1
Homestyle Cheddar Cheese Stove Top Recipe	½ cup	140	5	1
Homestyle Cheesy Scalloped	½ cup	140	<5	2
Homestyle Cheesy Scalloped Low Fat Recipe	½ cup	110	<5	3
Julienne	½ cup	150	<5	1
Mashed Butter & Herb	½ cup	160	5	1
Mashed Butter & Herb Reduced Fat Recipe	½ cup	130	<5	1
Mashed Chicken & Herb	½ cup	150	<5	1
Mashed Chicken & Herb Reduced Fat Recipe	½ cup	120	0	1
Mashed Four Cheese	½ cup	150	<5	2
Mashed Four Cheese Reduced Fat Recipe	½ cup	120	0	2
Mashed Potato Buds	⅔ cup	160	<5	1
Mashed Potato Buds Reduced Fat Recipe	⅔ cup	120	0	1
Mashed Roasted Garlic	½ cup	150	<5	2
Mashed Roasted Garlic Reduced Fat Recipe	½ cup	130	0	2
Mashed Sour Cream & Chives	½ cup	150	5	1
Mashed Sour Cream & Chives Reduced Fat Recipe	½ cup	120	<5	1
Potato Shakers Original	⅔ cup	140	<5	2
Potato Shakers Original Low Fat Recipe	⅔ cup	120	<5	2
Ranch	½ cup	160	<5	2
Scalloped	½ cup	150	<5	1
Scalloped Low Fat Recipe	⅔ cup	110	0	1
Sour Cream'n Chive	½ cup	160	5	2

FOOD	PORTION	CALS	CHOL	FIBER
Three Cheese	½ cup	150	<5	1
Twice Baked Cheddar & Bacon Low Fat Recipe	⅔ cup	130	<5	1
Twice Baked Cheddar & Bacon as prep	⅔ cup	210	85	1
Hungry Jack				
Au Gratin as prep	½ cup	150	10	1
Cheddar & Bacon as prep	½ cup	150	10	2
Cheesy Scalloped as prep	½ cup	150	10	1
Creamy Scalloped as prep	½ cup	150	10	2
Mashed Butter Flavored as prep	½ cup	150	<5	1
Mashed Garlic Flavored as prep	½ cup	150	<5	1
Mashed Parsley Butter as prep	½ cup	150	<5	1
Mashed Sour Cream 'n Chives as prep	½ cup	150	<5	1
Mashed Potato Flakes as prep	½ cup	160	3	1
Sour Cream & Chives as prep	½ cup	160	15	1
Idaho				
Mashed Potato Granules as prep	½ cup	160	<5	2
Shake 'N Bake				
Perfect Potatoes Crispy Cheddar	⅛ pkg (7 g)	30	5	0
Perfect Potatoes Herb & Garlic	⅛ pkg (7 g)	20	0	0
Perfect Potatoes Home Fries	⅛ pkg (7 g)	20	0	0
Perfect Potatoes Parmesan Peppercorn	⅛ pkg (7 g)	25	<5	0
Perfect Potatoes Savory Onion	⅛ pkg (7 g)	20	0	0

FOOD	PORTION	CALS	CHOL	FIBER
REFRIGERATED				
Simply Potatoes				
Au Gratin	¼ pkg (3 oz)	130	21	—
Hash Browns	½ pkg (4 oz)	100	0	—
Hash Browns Onion	⅓ pkg (4 oz)	120	0	—
Hash Browns Southwest Style	⅓ pkg (4 oz)	100	0	—
Mashed	⅓ pkg (4 oz)	90	0	—
Scalloped	¼ pkg (3 oz)	100	17	—
SHELF-STABLE				
Lunch Bucket				
Scalloped w/ Ham Chunks	1 pkg (7.5 oz)	170	10	3
Micro Cup Meals				
Microcup Meals Scalloped Potatoes w/ Ham	1 cup (7.5 oz)	240	35	2
TastyBite				
Bombay Potatoes	½ pkg (5 oz)	190	0	6
Mumbai Pav Bhaji	½ pkg (5 oz)	229	0	7
Simla Potatoes	½ pkg (5 oz)	180	0	1
TAKE-OUT				
au gratin w/ cheese	½ cup	178	18	—
baked topped w/ cheese sauce	1	475	19	—
baked topped w/ cheese sauce & bacon	1	451	30	—
baked topped w/ cheese sauce & broccoli	1	402	20	—
baked topped w/ cheese sauce & chili	1	481	31	—
baked topped w/ sour cream & chives	1	394	23	—
french fries	1 reg	235	0	—
french fries	1 lg	355	0	—
hash brown	½ cup (2.5 oz)	151	9	—
indian yogurt potatoes	1 serv	315	18	0
mashed	½ cup	111	2	—
mustard potato salad	3.5 oz	120	0	—
o'brien	1 cup	157	7	—

FOOD	PORTION	CALS	CHOL	FIBER
potato pancakes	1 (1.3 oz)	101	35	—
potato salad	½ cup	179	86	—
potato salad w/ vegetables	3.5 oz	120	0	—
scalloped	½ cup	127	7	—
twice backed w/ cheese	1 half (10 oz)	392	54	4
POTATO STARCH				
potato starch	1 oz	96	0	—
POUT				
ocean baked	3 oz	86	57	—
ocean fillet baked	4.8 oz	139	91	—
PRETZELS				
dutch twist	4 (2.1 oz)	229	0	2
pretzels	1 oz	108	0	1
rods	4 (2 oz)	229	0	2
sticks	10	10	tr	—
sticks	120 (2 oz)	229	0	2
twist	1 (½ oz)	65	tr	—
twists	10 (2.1 oz)	229	0	2
whole wheat	2 sm (1 oz)	103	0	—
whole wheat	2 med (2 oz)	205	0	—
Bachman				
Thin'n Right	12 (1 oz)	120	0	1
Barrel O' Fun				
Mini	1 oz	110	0	1
Sticks	1 oz	110	0	1
Twists	1 oz	110	0	1
Estee				
Chocolate Covered	7	130	0	tr
Dutch	2 (1.1 oz)	130	0	1
Unsalted	23 (1 oz)	120	0	1
Formagg				
Pretzel Nuts	1 oz	120	0	tr
Gardetto's				
Mustard	1 pkg (0.5 oz)	50	0	tr
Herr's				
Hard Sourdough	1 (1 oz)	100	0	2

FOOD	PORTION	CALS	CHOL	FIBER
Lance				
Pretzels	1 pkg (1.25 oz)	140	0	tr
Little Debbie				
Mini Twists	1 pkg (1.2 oz)	140	0	1
Manischewitz				
Bagel Pretzels Original	4 (1 oz)	110	0	1
Mister Salty				
Chips	16 (1 oz)	110	0	tr
Dutch	2 (1.1 oz)	120	0	1
Fat Free Chips	16 (1 oz)	100	0	1
Mini	22 (1 oz)	110	0	1
Sticks Fat Free	47 (1 oz)	110	0	1
Twist Fat Free	9 (1 oz)	110	0	1
Mr. Phipps				
Chips Lower Sodium	16 (1 oz)	120	0	tr
Chips Original	16 (1 oz)	120	0	tr
Chips Original Fat-Free	16 (1 oz)	100	0	tr
Nabisco				
Air Crisps Fat Free	23 pieces (1 oz)	110	0	tr
Nestle				
Flipz Milk Chocolate Covered	9 pieces (1 oz)	130	<5	tr
Flipz White Fudge Covered	9 pieces (1 oz)	130	0	0
Newman's Own				
Salted Rounds Organic	1 pkg (1.4 oz)	150	0	1
Planters				
Twists	1 pkg (1.5 oz)	160	0	1
Twists	1 oz	100	0	1
Quinlan				
Beers	1 oz	110	0	1
Hard Sourdough	1 oz	110	0	1
Logs	1 oz	110	0	1
Nuggets	1 oz	110	0	1
Rods	1 oz	110	0	1
Sticks	1 oz	110	0	1
Thins	1 oz	110	0	1
Rold Gold				
Crispy's Thins	4 (1 oz)	110	0	1
Fat Free Honey Mustard	17 (1 oz)	110	0	1

FOOD	PORTION	CALS	CHOL	FIBER
Fat Free Sticks	48 (1 oz)	110	0	1
Fat Free Thins	12 pieces (1 oz)	110	0	1
Fat Free Tiny Twists	18 pieces (1 oz)	110	0	1
Honey Mustard	16 (1 oz)	110	0	1
Rods	3 (1 oz)	110	0	1
Sharp Cheddar	22 (1 oz)	110	0	1
Sour Dough Nuggets	11 (1 oz)	110	0	1
Snyder's Of Hanover				
Dips White Fudge	1 oz	130	0	0
Hard Sourdough	1 oz	100	0	1
Hard Sourdough Unsalted	1 oz	100	0	1
Logs	1 oz	110	0	tr
Mini	1 oz	120	0	tr
Mini Unsalted	1 oz	110	0	tr
Nibblers	1 oz	120	0	tr
Nibblers Honey Mustard & Onions	1 oz	130	0	tr
Nibblers Oat Bran	1 oz	130	0	3
Nibblers Unsalted	1 oz	120	0	tr
Oat Bran	1 oz	100	0	2
Old Fashioned Dipping Stix	1 oz	100	0	1
Old Tyme	1 oz	310	0	—
Old Tyme Unsalted	1 oz	120	0	1
Olde Tyme	1 oz	120	0	1
Olde Tyme Stix	1 oz	120	0	1
Pieces Buttermilk Ranch	1 oz	130	0	tr
Pieces Cheddar Cheese	1 oz	190	0	tr
Pieces Honey Mustard & Onions	1 oz	140	0	tr
Pieces Peppered Pizza	1 oz	150	0	tr
Rods	1 oz	120	0	tr
Snaps	24 (1 oz)	120	0	tr
Thin	1 oz	130	0	tr
Whole Wheat Honey	1 oz	120	0	2
Utz				
Country Store Stix	5 (1 oz)	110	0	1
Fat Free Hard	1 (0.8 oz)	90	0	tr

FOOD	PORTION	CALS	CHOL	FIBER
Fat Free Hard No Salt Added	1 (0.8 oz)	90	0	tr
Fat Free Sour Dough Nuggets	10 (1 oz)	100	0	1
Fat Free Stix	14 (1 oz)	100	0	1
Fat Free Thin	10 (1 oz)	100	0	1
Honey Mustard & Onion Rods	⅓ cup (1 oz)	130	0	tr
	3 (1 oz)	120	0	1
Specials	5 (1 oz)	110	0	1
Specials Extra Dark	5 (1 oz)	110	0	1
Specials Unsalted	5 (1 oz)	110	0	1
Wheels	20 (1 oz)	100	0	1
Weight Watchers				
Oat Bran Nuggets	1 pkg (1.5 oz)	170	0	3

PRUNE JUICE

canned	1 cup	181	0	3

PRUNES

canned in heavy syrup	5	90	0	—
canned in heavy syrup	1 cup	245	0	—
dried	10	201	0	6
dried	1 cup	385	0	12
dried cooked w/ sugar	½ cup	147	0	7
dried cooked w/o sugar	½ cup	113	0	6
Del Monte				
Pitted	¼ cup (1.4 oz)	120	0	3
Unpitted	⅓ cup (1.4 oz)	110	0	1
Sonoma				
Pitted	¼ cup (1.4 oz)	120	0	3
Sunsweet				
Orange Essence Pitted Prunes	6 (1.4 oz)	100	0	3

PUDDING

MIX

banana as prep w/ 2% milk	½ cup (4.9 oz)	142	9	-
banana as prep w/ whole milk	½ cup (4.9 oz)	157	17	—
chocolate	½ cup (5 oz)	150	9	—

FOOD	PORTION	CALS	CHOL	FIBER
chocolate as prep w/ whole milk	½ cup (5 oz)	158	17	–
coconut cream	½ cup (4.9 oz)	148	9	–
instant banana as prep w/ 2% milk	½ cup (5.2 oz)	152	9	–
instant banana as prep w/ whole milk	½ cup (5.2 oz)	167	17	–
instant chocolate	½ cup (5.2 oz)	149	9	–
instant chocolate as prep w/ whole milk	½ cup (5.2 oz)	164	17	–
instant lemon	½ cup (5.2 oz)	155	9	–
instant vanilla	½ cup (5 oz)	147	9	–
lemon	½ cup (5.1 oz)	163	77	–
rice as prep w/ whole milk	½ cup (5.1 oz)	175	17	–
tapioca	½ cup (5 oz)	147	9	–
tapioca as prep w/ whole milk	½ cup (5 oz)	161	17	–
vanilla as prep w/ 2% milk	½ cup (4.9 oz)	141	9	–
vanilla as prep w/ whole milk	½ cup (4.9 oz)	155	17	–
Betty Crocker				
Rice as prep	1 serv	200	9	–
Jell-O				
Americana Rice as prep w/ skim milk	½ cup (5.2 oz)	140	<5	0
Americana Tapioca as prep w/ skim milk	½ cup (5.1 oz)	130	<5	0
Banana Cream as prep w/ 2% milk	½ cup (5.1 oz)	140	10	0
Butterscotch as prep w/ 2% milk	½ cup (5.2 oz)	160	10	0
Chocolate as prep w/ 2% milk	½ cup (5.2 oz)	150	10	tr
Chocolate Fudge as prep w/ 2% milk	½ cup (5.2 oz)	150	10	1
Coconut Cream as prep w/ 2% milk	½ cup (5.1 oz)	150	10	tr

FOOD	PORTION	CALS	CHOL	FIBER
Fat Free Chocolate as prep w/ skim milk	½ cup (5.2 oz)	130	<5	0
Fat Free Vanilla as prep w/ skim milk	½ cup (5.1 oz)	130	<5	0
Instant Banana Cream as prep w/ 2% milk	½ cup (5.2 oz)	150	10	0
Instant Butterscotch as prep w/ 2% milk	½ cup (5.2 oz)	150	10	0
Instant Chocolate as prep w/ 2% milk	½ cup (5.2 oz)	160	10	tr
Instant Chocolate Fudge as prep w/ 2% milk	½ cup (4.2 oz)	160	10	tr
Instant Coconut Cream as prep w/ 2% milk	½ cup (4.2 oz)	160	10	tr
Instant French Vanilla as prep w/ 2% milk	½ cup (4.2 oz)	150	10	0
Instant Lemon as prep w/ 2% milk	½ cup (4.2 oz)	150	10	0
Instant Pistachio as prep w/ 2% milk	½ cup (4.2 oz)	160	10	0
Instant Vanilla as prep w/ 2% milk	½ cup (4.2 oz)	150	10	0
Instant Fat Free Chocolate as prep w/ skim milk	½ cup (5.3 oz)	140	<5	tr
Instant Fat Free Devil's Food as prep w/ skim milk	½ cup (5.3 oz)	140	<5	tr
Instant Fat Free Sugar Free Banana as prep w/ skim milk	½ cup (4.6 oz)	70	<5	0
Instant Fat Free Sugar Free Butterscotch as prep w/ skim milk	½ cup (4.6 oz)	70	<5	0
Instant Fat Free Sugar Free Chocolate Fudge as prep w/ skim milk	½ cup (4.7 oz)	80	<5	tr
Instant Fat Free Sugar Free Chocolate as prep w/ skim milk	½ cup (4.6 oz)	80	<5	tr

FOOD	PORTION	CALS	CHOL	FIBER
Instant Fat Free Sugar Free Vanilla as prep w/ skim milk	½ cup (4.6 oz)	70	<5	0
Instant Fat Free Sugar Free White Chocolate as prep w/ skim milk	½ cup (4.6 oz)	70	<5	0
Instant Fat Free Vanilla as prep w/ skim milk	½ cup (5.2 oz)	140	<5	0
Instant Fat Free White Chocolate as prep w/ skim milk	½ cup (5.2 oz)	140	<5	0
Lemon as prep	½ cup (4.4 oz)	140	75	0
Milk Chocolate as prep w/ 2% milk	½ cup (5.2 oz)	150	10	tr
Sugar Free Chocolate as prep w/ 2% milk	½ cup (4.6 oz)	90	10	tr
Sugar Free Vanilla as prep w/ 2% milk	½ cup (4.5 oz)	80	10	0
Vanilla as prep w/ 2% milk	½ cup (5.1 oz)	150	9	0
Louisiana Purchase				
Bread	1 serv (1.3 oz)	150	0	2
Lundberg				
Elegant Rice Cinnamon Raisin	½ cup (3.9 oz)	70	0	1
Elegant Rice Coconut	½ cup (3.9 oz)	70	0	1
Elegant Rice Honey Almond	½ cup (3.9 oz)	70	0	1
Uncle Ben's				
Rice Pudding Cinnamon & Raisins as prep	½ cup (1.5 oz)	160	0	1
READY-TO-EAT				
chocolate	1 pkg (5 oz)	189	5	–
lemon	1 pkg (5 oz)	177	0	–
vanilla	1 pkg (4 oz)	146	8	–
Handi-Snacks				
Banana	1 serv (3.5 oz)	120	0	0
Butterscotch	1 serv (3.5 oz)	120	0	0
Chocolate	1 serv (3.5 oz)	130	0	tr
Chocolate Fudge	1 serv (3.5 oz)	130	0	tr

FOOD	PORTION	CALS	CHOL	FIBER
Fat Free Chocolate	1 serv (3.5 oz)	90	0	0
Fat Free Vanilla	1 serv (3.5 oz)	90	0	0
Tapioca	1 serv (3.5 oz)	120	0	0
Vanilla	1 serv (3.5 oz)	120	0	0
Healthy Choice				
Low Fat Chocolate Raspberry	½ cup (3.5 oz)	102	0	0
Low Fat Chocolate Almond	½ cup (3.5 oz)	109	0	0
Low Fat Double Chocolate Fudge	½ cup (3.5 oz)	101	0	0
Low Fat French Vanilla	½ cup (3.5 oz)	98	0	0
Low Fat Tapioca	½ cup (3.5 oz)	101	1	0
Hunt's				
Snack Pack Banana	1 serv (3.5 oz)	119	2	0
Snack Pack Butterscotch	1 serv (3.5 oz)	130	2	0
Snack Pack Chocolate	1 serv (3.5 oz)	143	1	0
Snack Pack Chocolate Fudge	1 serv (3.5 oz)	147	1	0
Snack Pack Chocolate Marshmallow	1 serv (3.5 oz)	134	1	0
Snack Pack Fat Free Chocolate	1 serv (3.5 oz)	86	1	0
Snack Pack Fat Free Tapioca	1 serv (3.5 oz)	82	0	0
Snack Pack Fat Free Vanilla	1 serv (3.5 oz)	81	0	0
Snack Pack Lemon	1 serv (3.5 oz)	124	0	0
Snack Pack Milk Chocolate Variety	1 serv (3.5 oz)	143	2	0
Snack Pack Swirl Chocolate Caramel	1 serv (3.5 oz)	143	1	0
Snack Pack Swirl Chocolate Peanut Butter	1 serv (3.5 oz)	146	2	0
Snack Pack Swirl Smores	1 serv (3.5 oz)	136	1	0
Snack Pack Tapioca	1 serv (3.5 oz)	125	1	0
Snack Pack Toppers Chocolate Fudge w/ Rainbow Sprinkles	1 serv (4 oz)	164	tr	tr

FOOD	PORTION	CALS	CHOL	FIBER
Snack Pack Toppers Chocolate w/ Dinosaurs	1 serv (4 oz)	161	tr	tr
Snack Pack Toppers Chocolate w/ Fun Chips	1 serv (4 oz)	176	1	tr
Snack Pack Toppers Vanilla w/ Chocolate Sprinkles	1 serv (4 oz)	164	tr	tr
Snack Pack Vanilla	1 serv (3.5 oz)	135	1	0
Imagine				
Banana	1 pkg (4 oz)	150	0	0
Butterscotch	1 pkg (4 oz)	150	0	0
Chocolate	1 pkg (4 oz)	170	0	1
Lemon	1 pkg (4 oz)	150	0	1
Jell-O				
Chocolate	1 serv (4 oz)	160	0	0
Chocolate Vanilla Swirls	1 serv (4 oz)	160	0	0
Fat Free Chocolate	1 serv (4 oz)	100	0	tr
Fat Free Chocolate Vanilla Swirl	1 serv (4 oz)	100	0	tr
Fat Free Chocolate Fudge & Caramel	1 serv (4 oz)	100	0	0
Fat Free Devil's Food	1 serv (4 oz)	100	0	tr
Fat Free Rocky Road	1 serv (4 oz)	100	0	tr
Fat Free Tapioca	1 serv (4 oz)	100	0	0
Fat Free Vanilla	1 serv (4 oz)	100	0	0
Tapioca	1 serv (4 oz)	140	0	0
Vanilla	1 serv (4 oz)	160	0	0
Kozy Shack				
Banana	1 pkg (4 oz)	130	10	1
Chocolate	1 pkg (4 oz)	140	5	1
Light Chocolate	1 pkg (4 oz)	110	5	1
Light Vanilla	1 pkg (4 oz)	110	10	0
Rice	1 pkg (4 oz)	130	17	1
Tapioca	1 pkg (4 oz)	140	5	0
Vanilla	1 pkg (4 oz)	130	10	1
NutraBalance				
Low Lactose All Flavors	1 serv (4 oz)	225	0	—

FOOD	PORTION	CALS	CHOL	FIBER
Swiss Miss				
Butterscotch	1 pkg (4 oz)	156	1	0
Chocolate	1 pkg (4 oz)	166	1	0
Chocolate Fudge	1 pkg (4 oz)	175	1	0
Fat Free Chocolate	1 pkg (4 oz)	98	0	0
Fat Free Chocolate Fudge	1 pkg (4 oz)	101	0	0
Fat Free Tapioca	1 pkg (4 oz)	98	0	0
Fat Free Vanilla	1 pkg (4 oz)	93	0	0
Fat Free Parfait Vanilla Chocolate	1 pkg (4 oz)	96	0	0
Lemon Meringue Pie	1 pkg (4 oz)	150	0	—
Milk Chocolate	1 pkg (4 oz)	166	1	0
Parfait Vanilla Chocolate	1 pkg (4 oz)	164	1	0
Swirl Chocolate Caramel	1 pkg (4 oz)	169	1	1
Swirl Chocolate Vanilla	1 pkg (4 oz)	169	1	0
Swirl Chocolate Vanilla Chocolate	1 pkg (4 oz)	169	1	0
Tapioca	1 pkg (4 oz)	138	1	0
Vanilla	1 pkg (4 oz)	156	1	0
TAKE-OUT				
bread pudding	½ cup (4.4 oz)	212	83	—
bread w/ raisins	½ cup	180	77	—
chocolate	½ cup (5.5 oz)	221	17	—
corn	⅔ cup	181	122	—
rice w/ raisins	½ cup	246	136	4
tapioca	½ cup (5.3 oz)	189	124	—
vanilla	½ cup (4.3 oz)	130	17	—
yorkshire	1 serv (3 oz)	177	57	tr
PUDDING POPS				
chocolate	1 (1.6 oz)	72	1	—
vanilla	1 (1.6 oz)	75	1	—
PUMMELO				
fresh	1	228	0	—
sections	1 cup	71	0	—

FOOD	PORTION	CALS	CHOL	FIBER
PUMPKIN				
CANNED				
pumpkin	½ cup	41	0	–
Libby				
Solid Pack	½ cup	40	0	5
Owatonna				
Pumpkin	½ cup	40	0	–
FRESH				
cooked mashed	½ cup	24	0	–
flowers cooked	½ cup	10	0	–
flowers raw	1	0	0	–
leaves cooked	½ cup	7	0	–
leaves raw	½ cup	4	0	–
raw cubed	½ cup	15	0	–
SEEDS				
dried	1 oz	154	0	–
roasted	1 oz	148	0	–
roasted	1 cup	1184	0	–
salted & roasted	1 oz	148	0	–
salted & roasted	1 cup	1184	0	–
whole roasted	1 oz	127	0	–
whole roasted	1 cup	285	0	–
whole salted roasted	1 oz	127	0	–
whole salted roasted	1 cup	285	0	–
PURSLANE				
cooked	1 cup	21	0	–
fresh	1 cup	7	0	–
QUICHE				
TAKE-OUT				
lorraine	⅛ of 8 in pie	600	285	–
QUINCE				
fresh	1	53	0	–
QUINOA				
quinoa not prep	1 cup (6 oz)	636	0	10
RABBIT				
domestic w/o bone roasted	3 oz	167	70	–

FOOD	PORTION	CALS	CHOL	FIBER
wild w/o bone stewed	3 oz	147	104	—

RADICCHIO
raw shredded	½ cup	5	0	—

RADISHES
chinese dried	½ cup	157	0	—
chinese raw	1 (12 oz)	62	0	—
chinese raw sliced	½ cup	8	0	—
chinese sliced cooked	½ cup	13	0	—
daikon dried	½ cup	157	0	—
daikon raw	1 (12 oz)	62	0	—
daikon raw sliced	½ cup	8	0	—
daikon sliced cooked	½ cup	13	0	—
red raw	10	7	0	—
red sliced	½ cup	10	0	—
white icicle raw	1 (½ oz)	2	0	—
white icicle raw sliced	½ cup	7	0	—
Eden				
Daikon Dried Shredded	2 tbsp	45	0	3
Daikon Pickled	2 slices	5	0	0
TAKE-OUT				
moo namul saengche korean salad	1 serv (3.7 oz)	34	0	2

RAISINS
chocolate coated	10 (0.4 oz)	39	0	—
chocolate coated	1 cup (6.7 oz)	741	5	—
golden seedless	1 cup	437	0	8
seedless	1 cup	434	0	8
seedless	1 tbsp	27	0	—
Cinderella				
Seedless	½ cup	250	0	—
Del Monte				
Golden	¼ cup (1.4 oz)	130	0	2
Raisins	¼ cup (1.4 oz)	130	0	2
Raisins	1 box (0.5 oz)	45	0	tr
Raisins	1 box (1.5 oz)	140	0	3
Raisins	1 box (1 oz)	90	0	2
Yogurt Raisins Strawberry	1 pkg (0.9 oz)	110	0	tr

FOOD	PORTION	CALS	CHOL	FIBER
Yogurt Raisins Vanilla	1 pkg (1 oz)	120	0	tr
Yogurt Raisins Vanilla	3 tbsp (1 oz)	130	0	1
Yogurt Raisins Vanilla	1 pkg (0.9 oz)	110	0	tr
Dole				
CinnaRaisins	1 pkg (1 oz)	95	0	2
Estee				
Chocolate Covered	¼ cup	180	<5	1
Mariana				
Fruitn Yogurt Milk Chocolate Covered Raisins	32 pieces (1 oz)	130	0	2
Nestle				
Chocolate Covered	1⅓ tbsp	70	0	tr
Sonoma				
Monukka Thompson	¼ cup (1.4 oz)	130	0	2
Tree Of Life				
Organic	¼ cup (1.4 oz)	130	0	2
RASPBERRIES				
canned in heavy syrup	½ cup	117	0	—
fresh	1 cup	61	0	—
fresh	1 pint	154	0	—
frozen sweetened	1 cup	256	0	—
frozen sweetened	1 pkg (10 oz)	291	0	—
Birds Eye				
Red	5 oz	90	0	5
Tree Of Life				
Organic	⅔ cup (5 oz)	50	0	2
RASPBERRY JUICE				
Crystal Geyser				
Juice Squeeze Mountain Raspberry	1 bottle (12 fl oz)	135	0	—
Crystal Light				
Raspberry Ice Drink	1 serv (8 oz)	5	0	0
Raspberry Ice Drink Mix as prep	1 serv (8 oz)	5	0	0
Dole				
Country Raspberry	8 fl oz	140	0	—
Kool-Aid				
Drink Mix as prep	1 serv (8 oz)	60	0	0

FOOD	PORTION	CALS	CHOL	FIBER
Raspberry Drink as prep w/ sugar	1 serv (8 oz)	100	0	0
Splash Blue Raspberry Drink	1 serv (8 oz)	120	0	0

RED BEANS
CANNED
Green Giant

| Red Beans | ½ cup (4.5 oz) | 100 | 0 | 6 |

Hunt's

| Small | ½ cup (4.5 oz) | 89 | 0 | 6 |

Van Camp

| Red Beans | ½ cup (4.6 oz) | 90 | 0 | 5 |

DRIED
Hurst

| HamBeens w/ Ham | 1 serv | 120 | 0 | 10 |

MIX
Bean Cuisine

| Pasta & Beans Barcelona Red With Radiatore | 1 serv | 210 | 0 | 4 |

RELISH

cranberry orange	½ cup	246	0	—
hamburger	1 tbsp	19	0	—
hamburger	½ cup	158	0	—
hot dog	½ cup	111	0	—
hot dog	1 tbsp	14	0	—
sweet	½ cup	159	0	—
sweet	1 tbsp	19	0	—

Claussen

| Sweet Pickle | 1 tbsp (0.5 oz) | 15 | 0 | 0 |

Green Giant

| Corn | 1 tbsp (0.6 oz) | 20 | 0 | 0 |

Old El Paso

| Jalapeno | 1 tbsp (0.5 oz) | 5 | 0 | 0 |

Vlasic

| Fancy Sweet | 1 tbsp | 15 | 0 | — |

RHUBARB

| fresh | ½ cup | 13 | 0 | — |

FOOD	PORTION	CALS	CHOL	FIBER
frozen	½ cup	60	0	—
frzn as prep w/ sugar	½ cup	139	0	—
RICE *(see also* RICE CAKES, WILD RICE)				
brown long grain cooked	1 cup (6.8 oz)	216	0	4
brown medium grain cooked	1 cup (6.8 oz)	218	0	4
glutinous cooked	1 cup (6.1 oz)	169	0	2
starch	1 oz	98	0	—
white long grain cooked	1 cup (5.5 oz)	205	0	1
white long grain instant cooked	1 cup (5.8 oz)	162	0	1
white medium grain cooked	1 cup (6.5 oz)	242	0	1
white short grain cooked	1 cup (6.5 oz)	242	0	—
Amy's				
Bowls Brown Rice & Vegetables	1 pkg (10 oz)	240	0	5
Birds Eye				
Rice & Broccoli In Cheese Sauce	1 pkg	290	15	2
White & Wild w/ Green Beans	1 cup (6.6 oz)	180	10	2
Budget Gourmet				
Oriental Rice With Vegetables	1 pkg (5.75 oz)	230	20	—
Rice Pilaf With Green Beans	1 pkg (5.5 oz)	230	10	—
Carolina				
Red Beans & Rice as prep	¼ pkg	190	0	6
Casbah				
Jambalaya	1 pkg (1.4 oz)	130	0	1
La Fiesta	1 pkg (1.59 oz)	170	0	0
Nutted Pilaf as prep	1 cup	220	0	1
Pilaf as prep	1 cup	200	0	tr
Spanish Pilaf as prep	1 cup	200	0	1
Thai Yum	1 pkg (1.7 oz)	180	0	1

FOOD	PORTION	CALS	CHOL	FIBER
Chun King				
Fried Rice Mix	½ cup (1.4 oz)	126	0	1
Goodman's				
Rice & Vermicelli For Beef	¾ cup	160	5	0
Rice & Vermicelli For Chicken	¾ cup	160	0	1
Goya				
Arroz Amarillo	¼ cup (1.6 oz)	170	0	1
Green Giant				
Rice & Broccoli	1 pkg (10 oz)	320	15	2
Rice Medley	1 pkg (10 oz)	240	5	2
Rice Pilaf	1 pkg (10 oz)	230	5	3
White & Wild	1 pkg (10 oz)	250	0	3
Kitchen Del Sol				
Mediterranean Paella Costa Brave as prep	½ cup (1.2 oz)	130	0	1
Mediterranean Sunny Lemon Pilaf as prep	½ cup (1.2 oz)	110	0	1
Mediterranean Tomato & Basil With Pine Nuts	½ cup (1 oz)	110	0	1
La Choy				
Fried Rice	1 cup (4.9 oz)	236	0	2
Lipton				
Golden Saute Onion Mushroom	½ cup (2.1 oz)	240	0	2
Oriental Stir Fry as prep	1 cup	270	0	1
Rice & Sauce Alfredo Broccoli as prep	1 cup	320	15	1
Rice & Sauce Beef as prep	1 cup	270	0	1
Rice & Sauce Cajun Style as prep	1 cup	270	0	1
Rice & Sauce Cajun Style w/ Beans as prep	1 cup	310	0	7
Rice & Sauce Cheddar Broccoli as prep	1 cup	280	5	1
Rice & Sauce Chicken & Parmesan Risotto as prep	1 cup	270	0	tr

FOOD	PORTION	CALS	CHOL	FIBER
Rice & Sauce Chicken Broccoli as prep	1 cup	280	0	2
Rice & Sauce Chicken Flavor as prep	1 cup	280	5	1
Rice & Sauce Creamy Chicken as prep	1 cup	290	0	1
Rice & Sauce Herb & Butter as prep	1 cup	280	10	tr
Rice & Sauce Medley as prep	1 cup	270	5	2
Rice & Sauce Mushroom as prep	1 cup	270	0	1
Rice & Sauce Mushroom & Herb as prep	1 cup	290	0	1
Rice & Sauce Oriental as prep	1 cup	280	0	2
Rice & Sauce Pilaf as prep	1 cup	260	0	1
Rice & Sauce Scampi Style as prep	1 cup	270	5	1
Rice & Sauce Spanish as prep	1 cup	270	0	2
Rice & Sauce Teriyaki as prep	1 cup	270	0	1
Roasted Chicken as prep	1 cup	260	0	1
Salsa Style as prep	1 cup	220	0	2
Southwestern Chicken Flavor as prep	1 cup	260	0	1
Luigino's				
Fried Rice Chicken	1 pkg (8 oz)	250	55	2
Fried Rice Pork	1 pkg (8 oz)	250	60	2
Fried Rice Pork & Shrimp	1 pkg (8 oz)	250	55	2
Fried Rice Shrimp	1 pkg (8 oz)	220	60	2
Risotto Parmesano	1 pkg (8 oz)	360	50	2
Lundberg				
One-Step Curry	1 cup (7.4 oz)	160	0	5
Risotto Tomato Basil	1 serv	140	0	1

FOOD	PORTION	CALS	CHOL	FIBER
Melting Pot				
Risotto Melanese w/ Saffron	1 cup	210	0	0
Risotto Primavera	1 cup	200	0	1
Risotto Sun-Dried Tomatoes & Peas	1 cup	200	0	1
Risotto Three Cheese	1 cup	200	5	0
Risotto Wild Mushroom	1 cup	200	0	2
Minute				
Boil-In-Bag White as prep	1 cup (5.7 oz)	190	0	tr
Instant Brown as prep	⅔ cup	170	0	2
Instant White as prep	1 cup (5.7 oz)	160	0	tr
Long Grain & Wild Seasoned w/ Herbs as prep	1 cup (7.8 oz)	230	0	1
Near East				
Barley Pilaf as prep	1 cup	220	0	5
Beef Pilaf as prep	1 cup	220	0	1
Curry Rice as prep	1 cup	220	0	1
Lentil Pilaf as prep	1 cup	210	0	0
Long Grain & Wild as prep	1 cup	220	0	2
Pilaf Brown Rice as prep	1 cup	220	0	2
Pilaf Chicken as prep	1 cup	220	0	1
Pilaf Kosher as prep	1 cup	220	0	1
Spanish Pilaf as prep	1 cup	230	0	1
Old El Paso				
Mexican	½ cup (4 oz)	410	0	3
Spanish	1 cup (8.6 oz)	130	0	2
Pritikin				
Mexican	⅓ cup (2 oz)	200	0	–
Oriental	⅓ cup (2 oz)	190	0	–
Success				
Broccoli & Cheese	½ cup	130	0	tr
Brown	1 cup	150	0	2
Brown & Wild Mix	½ cup	120	0	2
Classic Chicken	½ cup	90	0	1
Long Grain & Wild	½ cup	120	0	tr

FOOD	PORTION	CALS	CHOL	FIBER
Pilaf	½ cup	120	0	1
Spanish	½ cup	120	0	1
TastyBite				
Pilaf Curried Vegetable	½ pkg (4.5 oz)	180	0	9
Pilaf Green Peas	½ pkg (4.5 oz)	208	0	4
Pilaf Vegetable Kofta	½ pkg (4.5 oz)	229	0	7
Uncle Ben				
Boil-In-Bag	1 serv (0.9 oz)	94	0	tr
Brown	1 serv (1.6 oz)	158	0	1
Brown & Wild Fast Cooking	1 serv (1.3 oz)	120	tr	1
Country Inn Broccoli Almondine	1 serv (1.2 oz)	124	tr	1
Country Inn Broccoli & White Cheddar	1 serv (1.2 oz)	131	3	1
Country Inn Broccoli Au Gratin	1 serv (1.1 oz)	116	2	1
Country Inn Chicken Stock	1 serv (1.2 oz)	123	3	1
Country Inn Chicken With Wild Rice	1 serv (1.1 oz)	108	1	1
Country Inn Creamy Chicken & Mushroom	1 serv (1.3 oz)	138	2	1
Country Inn Creamy Chicken & Wild Rice	1 serv (1.3 oz)	135	4	1
Country Inn Green Bean Almondine	1 serv (1.2 oz)	128	2	1
Country Inn Herbed Au Gratin	1 serv (1.2 oz)	119	3	1
Country Inn Homestyle Chicken & Vegetables	1 serv (1.3 oz)	139	7	1
Country Inn Rice Florentine	1 serv (1.2 oz)	212	3	1
Country Inn Vegetable Pilaf	1 serv (1.2 oz)	115	1	1
In An Instant	1 serv (1.1 oz)	111	0	tr
Long Grain & Wild Chicken Stock Sauce	1 serv (1.3 oz)	133	5	1
Long Grain & Wild Fast Cooking	1 serv (1 oz)	101	1	1

FOOD	PORTION	CALS	CHOL	FIBER
Long Grain & Wild Garden Vegetable Blend	1 serv (1.3 oz)	128	1	1
Long Grain & Wild Original	1 serv (1 oz)	96	tr	1
White Converted	1 serv (1.2 oz)	123	0	tr
Van Camp				
Spanish	½ cup (4.5 oz)	90	0	2
Watkins				
Brown & Wild	¼ cup (1.6 oz)	160	0	3
Calico Medley	¼ cup (1.6 oz)	160	0	4
East/West Medley	¼ cup (1.6 oz)	160	0	5
Heartland Medley	¼ cup (1.6 oz)	160	0	4
Minnesota Medley	¼ cup (1.6 oz)	160	0	2
White & Wild	¼ cup (1.6 oz)	160	0	1
Zatarain's				
Dirty Rice Mix as prep w/o meat and oil	½ cup	130	0	0
Red Beans & Rice as prep w/o oil	½ cup	100	0	4
TAKE-OUT				
nasi goreng indonesian rice & vegetables	1 cup (4.9 oz)	130	0	1
paella	1 serv (7 oz)	308	92	3
pilaf	½ cup	84	22	3
risotto w/ asparagus	1 cup	170	15	1
spanish	¾ cup	363	35	—

RICE CAKES (see also POPCORN CAKES)

FOOD	PORTION	CALS	CHOL	FIBER
Estee				
Banana Nut	5	60	0	0
Cinnamon Spice	5	60	0	0
Granny Smith Apple	5	60	0	0
Mixed Berry	5	60	0	0
Peanut Butter Crunch	5	60	0	tr
Lundberg				
Nutra Farmed Brown Rice	1 (0.7 oz)	70	0	—
Nutra Farmed Sesame Tamari	1 (0.7 oz)	70	0	2

FOOD	PORTION	CALS	CHOL	FIBER
Organic Koku Sesame	1 (0.7 oz)	80	0	2
Mother's				
Mini Apple	5 (0.5 oz)	50	0	0
Mini Caramel	5 (0.5 oz)	50	0	0
Mini Cinnamon	5 (0.5 oz)	50	0	0
Mini Plain Unsalted	7 (0.5 oz)	60	0	0
Multigrain Lightly Salted	1 (0.3 oz)	35	0	0
Rye Unsalted	1 (0.3 oz)	35	0	1
Wheat Unsalted	1 (0.3 oz)	35	0	1
Pritikin				
Mini Apple Crisp	5 (0.5 oz)	50	0	—
Multigrain	1 (0.3 oz)	35	0	—
Multigrain Unsalted	1 (0.3 oz)	35	0	—
Plain	1 (0.3 oz)	35	0	—
Plain Unsalted	1 (0.3 oz)	35	0	—
Sesame Low Sodium	1 (0.3 oz)	35	0	—
Sesame Unsalted	1 (0.3 oz)	35	0	—
Quaker				
Apple Cinnamon	1 (0.5 oz)	50	0	—
Banana Crunch	1 (0.5 oz)	50	0	—
Cinnamon Crunch	1 (0.5 oz)	50	0	—
Mini Apple Cinnamon	5 (0.5 oz)	50	0	—
Mini Banana Nut	5 (0.5 oz)	50	0	—
Mini Butter Popped Corn	6 (0.5 oz)	50	0	—
Mini Caramel Corn	5 (0.5 oz)	50	0	—
Mini Chocolate Crunch	5 (0.5 oz)	50	0	—
Mini Cinnamon Crunch	5 (0.5 oz)	50	0	—
Mini Honey Nut	5 (0.5 oz)	50	0	—
Mini Monterey Jack	6 (0.5 oz)	50	0	—
Mini White Cheddar	6 (0.5 oz)	50	0	—
Salt-Free	1 (0.3 oz)	35	0	—
Salted	1 (0.3 oz)	35	0	—
Weight Watchers				
Apple Cinnamon	1 oz	110	0	1
Butter	1 oz	110	0	1
Caramel	1 oz	110	0	1
White Cheddar	1 oz	100	0	1

FOOD	PORTION	CALS	CHOL	FIBER
ROCKFISH				
pacific cooked	1 fillet (5.2 oz)	180	66	–
pacific cooked	3 oz	103	38	–
pacific raw	3 oz	80	29	–
ROE (see also individual fish names)				
fish	1 oz	11	30	–
fresh baked	3 oz	173	408	–
fresh baked	1 oz	58	136	–
ROLL				
FROZEN				
New York				
Garlic	1 (2 oz)	210	0	1
Sara Lee				
Deluxe Cinnamon Rolls w/o Icing	1 (2.7 oz)	370	40	1
READY-TO-EAT				
bialy	1 (2.2 oz)	138	0	1
brioche sweet roll	1 (3.5 oz)	410	190	3
brown & serve	1 (1 oz)	85	0	–
cinnamon raisin	1 (2¾ in)	223	40	1
dinner	1 (1 oz)	85	0	–
french	1 (1.3 oz)	105	0	–
hamburger multi-grain	1 (1½ oz)	113	0	2
hamburger reduced calorie	1 (1½ oz)	84	0	3
hard	1 (3½ in)	167	0	–
hotdog reduced calorie	1 (1½ oz)	84	0	3
hotdog whole wheat	1 (1.5 oz)	110	0	2
kaiser	1 (3½ in)	167	0	–
oat bran	1 (1.2 oz)	78	0	1
rye	1 (1 oz)	81	0	–
submarine	1 (4.7 oz)	155	tr	–
wheat	1 (1 oz)	77	0	–
whole wheat	1 (1 oz)	75	0	–
Alvarado St. Bakery				
Burger Buns	1 (2.2 oz)	140	0	3
Hot Dog Buns	1 (2.2 oz)	140	0	3

FOOD	PORTION	CALS	CHOL	FIBER
August Bros.				
Kaiser	1	170	0	2
Onion	1	160	0	2
Sesame Cubano	1	170	0	2
Bread Du Jour				
Cracked Wheat	1 (1.2 oz)	100	0	1
Italian	1 (1.2 oz)	90	0	0
Sourdough	1 (1.2 oz)	90	0	0
Country Kitchen				
Frankfurt	1	120	0	—
Freihofer's				
Brown 'N Serve	1 (1 oz)	80	0	1
Pepperidge Farm				
Brown & Serve Club	1 (1.6 oz)	120	0	2
Dinner Rolls Finger Poppy	1 (0.9 oz)	80	<5	tr
Parker House	1 (0.9 oz)	80	<5	tr
San Francisco				
Sourdough	1 (1.8 oz)	180	0	3
Stroehmann				
Hamburger	1 (1.4 oz)	100	0	tr
Hamburger Potato	1 (1.9 oz)	140	0	tr
Hot Dog	1 (1.4 oz)	100	0	tr
Hot Dog Potato	1 (1.9 oz)	140	0	tr
The Baker				
Honey Cinnamon Raisin	1 (2 oz)	150	0	4
Wonder				
Brown & Serve	1 (1 oz)	80	0	0
Brown & Serve Sourdough	1 (1 oz)	70	0	0
Brown & Serve Wheat	1 (1 oz)	80	0	0
Bun	1 (3 oz)	220	0	1
Club French	1 (1.6 oz)	120	0	0
Club Grain	1 (1.6 oz)	120	0	1
Club Sourdough	1 (1.6 oz)	120	0	0
Dinner	2 (1.6 oz)	130	0	1
Dinner Honey Rich	1 (1.3 oz)	100	0	0
Dinner Wheat	2 (1.6 oz)	140	0	1
Hamburger	1 (2.5 oz)	190	0	1

FOOD	PORTION	CALS	CHOL	FIBER
Hamburger	1 (2 oz)	150	0	1
Hamburger	1 (2.5 oz)	180	0	2
Hamburger	1 (1.5 oz)	110	0	0
Hamburger Wheat	1 (1.9 oz)	140	0	2
Hamburger Wheat	1 (1.5 oz)	120	0	1
Hoagie French	1 (3 oz)	220	0	1
Hoagie Grain	1 (3 oz)	220	0	2
Hoagie Sourdough	1 (3 oz)	220	0	1
Hot Dog	1 (2 oz)	160	0	0
Kaiser	1 (2.2 oz)	180	0	1
Kaiser Hoagie	1 (3 oz)	220	0	1
Multigrain	1 (1.8 oz)	140	0	1
Potato Bun	1 (1.5 oz)	110	0	1
Steak	1 (2.5 oz)	190	0	1
REFRIGERATED				
crescent	1 (1 oz)	98	0	–
Pillsbury				
Apple Cinnamon	1 (1.5 oz)	150	0	tr
Caramel	1 (1.7 oz)	170	0	tr
Cinnamon w/ Icing	1 (1.5 oz)	150	0	tr
Cinnamon w/ Icing Reduced Fat	1 (1.5 oz)	140	0	tr
Cinnamon Raisin w/ Icing	1 (1.7 oz)	170	0	tr
Cornbread Twists	1 (1.4 oz)	140	0	0
Crecents Reduced Fat	1 (1 oz)	100	0	0
Crescent	1 (1 oz)	110	0	0
Dinner	1 (1.4 oz)	110	0	1
Dinner Wheat	1 (1.4 oz)	110	0	1
Orange Sweet Roll w/ Icing	1 (1.7 oz)	150	0	tr

ROSE APPLE
fresh	3.5 oz	32	0	–

ROSE HIP
fresh	1 oz	26	0	–

ROSELLE
fresh	1 cup	28	0	–

FOOD	PORTION	CALS	CHOL	FIBER
ROSEMARY				
dried	1 tsp	4	0	–
ROUGHY				
orange baked	3 oz	75	22	–
RUTABAGA				
cooked mashed	½ cup	41	0	–
raw cubed	½ cup	25	0	–
SABLEFISH				
baked	3 oz	213	53	–
fillet baked	5.3 oz	378	95	–
smoked	1 oz	72	18	–
smoked	3 oz	218	55	–
SAFFLOWER				
seeds dried	1 oz	147	0	–
SAFFRON				
saffron	1 tsp	2	0	–
SAGE				
ground	1 tsp	2	0	–
Watkins				
Sage	¼ tsp (0.5 g)	0	0	0
SALAD				
MIX				
Dole				
All American Toss	2 cups (3.5 oz)	50	<5	2
American Blend	1½ cups (3 oz)	15	0	1
Classic	1½ cups (3 oz)	15	0	1
Classic Romaine Blend	1½ cups (3 oz)	15	0	1
Coleslaw	1½ cups (3 oz)	25	0	2
European Special Blend	2 cups (3 oz)	15	0	1
Garlic Caesar Complete w/ Dressing	1½ cups (3.5 oz)	180	5	1
Greek Marinade	1½ cups (3.5 oz)	100	<5	1
Greener Selection	1½ cups (3 oz)	15	0	1
Light Caesar Complete w/ Dressing	1½ cups (3.5 oz)	60	0	2

FOOD	PORTION	CALS	CHOL	FIBER
Light Herb Ranch Complete w/ Dressing	1½ cups (3.5 oz)	50	5	2
Light Roasted Garlic Caesar Complete w/ Dressing	1½ cups (3.5 oz)	60	0	1
Light Zesty Italian Complete w/ Dressing	1½ cups (3.5 oz)	50	0	1
Mediterranean Marinade	2 cups (3.5 oz)	90	0	1
Oriental Complete w/ Dressing	1½ cups (3.5 oz)	120	0	2
Romano Complete w/ Dressing	1½ cups (3.5 oz)	150	0	2
Sunflower Ranch Complete w/ Dressing	1½ cups (3.5 oz)	160	5	2
Tomato & Mozzarella Medley	2 cups (3.5 oz)	60	5	2
Triple Cheese Toss	2 cups (3.5 oz)	80	15	1
Earthbound Farm				
Baby Caesar Mix	1 pkg (5 oz)	25	0	2
Baby Greens w/ Low Fat Honey Dijon Vinaigrette & Tomato Croutons	1 serv (3.5 oz)	90	0	2
Caesar w/ Garlic Croutons	1 serv (3.5 oz)	170	10	1
Italian Salad Organic	1⅔ cups (2.9 oz)	15	0	1
Mixed Baby Greens Organic	1 pkg (4 oz)	30	0	2
Organic Baby Greens w/ Vinaigrette & Garlic Croutons	1 serv (3.5 oz)	230	0	1
Organic Baby Spinach w/ Sesame Soy Vinaigrette & Peanuts	1 serv (3.5 oz)	150	0	2
Organic Italian Salad w/ Blue Cheese Dressing & Walnuts	1 serv (3.5 oz)	190	15	1
Romaine Blend Organic	1⅔ cups (2.9 oz)	15	0	1

FOOD	PORTION	CALS	CHOL	FIBER
Fresh Express				
American Salad	1½ cups (3 oz)	20	0	1
Caesar Salad	1½ cups (3 oz)	140	10	1
European Salad	1½ cups (3 oz)	20	0	1
Fancy Field Greens	1½ cups (3 oz)	15	0	2
Garden Salad	1½ cups (3 oz)	20	0	1
Italian Salad	1½ cups (3 oz)	20	0	1
Oriental Salad	1½ cups (3 oz)	120	0	1
Original Iceberg Garden w/ Zip	1½ cups (3 oz)	15	0	1
Riviera Salad	1½ cups (3 oz)	10	0	1
Spinach Salad	1½ cups (3 oz)	130	0	3
Veggie Lover's	1½ cups (3 oz)	20	0	1
Suddenly Salad				
Caesar	¾ cup	220	0	1
Caesar Low Fat Recipe	¾ cup	170	0	1
Italian Pepperoni	1 cup	190	0	2
Italian Pepperoni Low Fat Recipe	1 cup	180	0	2
Ranch & Bacon	¾ cup	330	15	1
Ranch & Bacon Low Fat Recipe	¾ cup	180	<5	1
Weight Watchers				
Caesar Salad	1 serv (3.5 oz)	60	0	1
Caesar Salad w/ Cookies	1 pkg (4.3 oz)	160	0	3
European Salad	1 serv (3.5 oz)	60	0	2
European Salad w/ Cookies	1 pkg (4.3 oz)	160	0	2
Garden Salad	1 serv (3.5 oz)	60	0	1
Garden Salad w/ Cookies	1 pkg (4 oz)	120	0	2
TAKE-OUT				
caesar	2 cups (5 oz)	235	10	1
chef w/o dressing	1½ cups	386	244	—
tossed w/o dressing	¾ cup	16	0	—
tossed w/o dressing	1½ cups	32	0	—
tossed w/o dressing w/ cheese & egg	1½ cups	102	98	—
tossed w/o dressing w/ chicken	1½ cups	105	72	—

FOOD	PORTION	CALS	CHOL	FIBER
tossed w/o dressing w/ pasta & seafood	1½ cups (14.6 oz)	380	50	–
tossed w/o dressing w/ shrimp	1½ cups	107	180	–
waldorf	½ cup	79	8	1

SALAD DRESSING
MIX
Et Tu
Caesar Salad Kit	1 serv	140	5	0

Good Seasons
Cheese Garlic as prep	2 tbsp (1 oz)	140	0	0
Fat Free Honey Mustard as prep	2 tbsp (1.2 oz)	20	0	0
Fat Free Italian as prep	2 tbsp (1.1 oz)	10	0	0
Fat Free Ranch as prep	2 tbsp (1.2 oz)	20	0	0
Fat Free Zesty Herb as prep	2 tbsp (1.1 oz)	10	0	0
Garlic & Herbs as prep	2 tbsp (1 oz)	140	0	0
Gourmet Caesar as prep	2 tbsp (1.1 oz)	150	0	0
Gourmet Parmesan Italian as prep	2 tbsp (1.1 oz)	150	0	0
Honey French as prep	2 tbsp (1.2 oz)	160	0	0
Honey Mustard as prep	2 tbsp (1.1 oz)	150	0	0
Italian as prep	2 tbsp (1 oz)	140	0	0
Mexican Spice as prep	2 tbsp (1.1 oz)	140	0	0
Mild Italian as prep	2 tbsp (1.1 oz)	150	0	0
Oriental Sesame as prep	2 tbsp (1.1 oz)	150	0	0
Reduced Calorie Italian as prep	2 tbsp (1 oz)	50	0	0
Reduced Calorie Zesty Italian as prep	2 tbsp (1 oz)	50	0	0
Roasted Garlic as prep	2 tbsp (1.1 oz)	150	0	0
Zesty Italian as prep	2 tbsp (1 oz)	140	0	0

READY-TO-EAT
french reduced calorie	1 tbsp	22	1	–
italian reduced calorie	1 tbsp	16	1	–
russian reduced calorie	1 tbsp	23	1	–
sesame seed	1 tbsp	68	0	–

FOOD	PORTION	CALS	CHOL	FIBER
thousand island reduced calorie	1 tbsp	24	2	—
Annie Chun				
Lemongrass	2 tbsp	60	0	0
Sesame Cilantro	1 tbsp	4	0	0
Benecol				
Creamy Italian	2 tbsp	100	0	0
French	2 tbsp (0.8 oz)	130	0	0
Ranch	2 tbsp	130	0	0
Thousand Island	2 tbsp	130	0	0
Estee				
Creamy French	2 tbsp (1 oz)	10	0	—
Italian	2 tbsp	5	0	0
Kraft				
⅓ Less Fat Catalina	2 tbsp (1.2 oz)	80	0	0
⅓ Less Fat Cucumber Ranch	2 tbsp (1.1 oz)	60	0	0
⅓ Less Fat Italian	2 tbsp (1.1 oz)	70	0	0
⅓ Less Fat Ranch	2 tbsp (1.1)	110	10	0
⅓ Less Fat Thousand Island	2 tbsp (1.2 oz)	70	10	0
Bacon & Tomato	2 tbsp (1.1 oz)	140	<5	0
Buttermilk Ranch	2 tbsp (1.1 oz)	150	<5	0
Caesar Italian	2 tbsp (1.1 oz)	100	0	0
Caesar Ranch	2 tbsp (1.1 oz)	110	10	0
Catalina	2 tbsp (1.1 oz)	120	0	0
Catalina With Honey	2 tbsp (1.1 oz)	130	0	0
Classic Caesar	2 tbsp (1.1 oz)	110	10	0
Coleslaw	2 tbsp (1.1 oz)	130	15	0
Creamy French	2 tbsp (1.1 oz)	160	0	0
Creamy Garlic	2 tbsp (1.1 oz)	110	0	0
Creamy Italian	2 tbsp (1.1 oz)	110	0	0
Cucumber Ranch	2 tbsp (1.1 oz)	140	0	0
Free Blue Cheese	2 tbsp (1.2 oz)	45	0	1
Free Caesar Italian	2 tbsp (1.2 oz)	25	0	0
Free Catalina	2 tbsp (1.2 oz)	35	0	tr
Free Classic Caesar	2 tbsp (1.2 oz)	45	0	tr
Free Creamy Italian	2 tbsp (1.2 oz)	50	0	tr
Free French	2 tbsp (1.2 oz)	45	0	tr
Free Garlic Ranch	2 tbsp (1.2 oz)	45	0	1

FOOD	PORTION	CALS	CHOL	FIBER
Free Honey Dijon	2 tbsp (1.2 oz)	45	0	1
Free Italian	2 tbsp (1.2 oz)	20	0	0
Free Peppercorn Ranch	2 tbsp (1.2 oz)	45	0	tr
Free Ranch	1 tbsp (1.2 oz)	50	0	1
Free Red Wine Vinegar	2 tbsp (1.1 oz)	15	0	0
Free Thousand Island	2 tbsp (1.2 oz)	40	0	1
Garlic Ranch	2 tbsp (1.1 oz)	180	10	0
Herb Vinaigrette	2 tbsp (1.1 oz)	140	0	0
Honey Dijon	2 tbsp (1.1 oz)	110	0	0
Honey Mustard	2 tbsp (1.1 oz)	110	0	0
House Italian w/ Olive Oil Blend	2 tbsp (1.1 oz)	120	<5	0
Peppercorn Ranch	2 tbsp (1 oz)	170	10	0
Pesto Italian	2 tbsp (1.1 oz)	90	0	0
Ranch	2 tbsp (1 oz)	170	10	0
Roka Blue Cheese	2 tbsp (1.1 oz)	130	<5	tr
Russian	2 tbsp (1.2 oz)	130	0	0
Sour Cream & Onion Ranch	2 tbsp (1 oz)	170	10	0
Thousand Island	2 tbsp (1.1 oz)	110	10	0
Thousand Island With Bacon	2 tbsp (1.1 oz)	130	0	0
Tomato & Herb Italian	2 tbsp (1.1 oz)	100	0	0
Zesty Italian	2 tbsp (1.1 oz)	110	0	0
LaMartinique				
Blue Cheese Vinaigrette	2 tbsp	160	5	0
Poppy Seed	2 tbsp	170	0	0
Marzetti				
Bacon Spinach Salad	2 tbsp	80	1	15
Blue Cheese	2 tbsp	160	20	0
Buttermilk & Herb	2 tbsp	180	3	0
Buttermilk Bacon Ranch	2 tbsp	180	10	0
Buttermilk Blue Cheese	2 tbsp	160	10	0
Buttermilk Parmesan Pepper	2 tbsp	170	10	0
Buttermilk Parmesan Ranch	2 tbsp	160	10	0
Buttermilk Ranch	2 tbsp	180	4	0
Buttermilk Veggie Dip	2 tbsp	170	3	0
Caesar	2 tbsp	150	0	0

FOOD	PORTION	CALS	CHOL	FIBER
Caesar Ranch	2 tbsp	190	5	0
California French	2 tbsp	160	0	0
Celery Seed	2 tbsp	160	0	0
Chunky Blue Cheese	2 tbsp	150	25	0
Classic Caesar Ranch	2 tbsp	190	5	0
Country French	2 tbsp	150	10	0
Cracked Peppercorn	2 tbsp	140	30	0
Creamy Garlic Italian	2 tbsp	160	15	0
Creamy Italian	2 tbsp	150	15	0
Crispy Celery Seed	2 tbsp	160	0	0
Dijon Honey Mustard	2 tbsp	140	20	0
Dijon Ranch	2 tbsp	170	25	0
Dutch Sweet'N Sour	2 tbsp	160	0	0
Fat Free California French	2 tbsp	45	0	0
Fat Free Honey Dijon	2 tbsp	60	0	1
Fat Free Honey French	2 tbsp	45	0	0
Fat Free Italian	2 tbsp	15	0	0
Fat Free Peppercorn Ranch	2 tbsp	30	0	1
Fat Free Ranch	2 tbsp	30	0	1
Fat Free Raspberry	2 tbsp	70	0	0
Fat Free Slaw	2 tbsp	45	15	0
Fat Free Sweet & Sour	2 tbsp	45	0	0
Fat Free Thousand Island	2 tbsp	35	0	0
Garden Ranch	2 tbsp	180	3	0
Gusto Italian	2 tbsp	120	0	0
Honey Dijon	2 tbsp	140	15	0
Honey Dijon Ranch	2 tbsp	150	25	0
Honey French	2 tbsp	160	0	0
Honey French Blue Cheese	2 tbsp	160	0	0
House Caesar	2 tbsp	150	5	0
Italian With Olive Oil	2 tbsp	120	0	0
Light Blue Cheese	2 tbsp	60	15	0
Light Buttermilk Ranch	2 tbsp	90	10	0
Light California French	2 tbsp	80	0	0
Light Chunky Blue Cheese	2 tbsp	80	15	0

FOOD	PORTION	CALS	CHOL	FIBER
Light French	2 tbsp	40	0	0
Light French	2 tbsp	40	0	0
Light Honey French	2 tbsp	80	0	0
Light Italian	2 tbsp	60	0	0
Light Ranch	2 tbsp	90	5	0
Light Red Wine Vinegar & Oil	2 tbsp	20	0	0
Light Slaw	2 tbsp	60	30	0
Light Sweet & Sour	2 tbsp	100	0	0
Light Thousand Island	2 tbsp	70	20	0
Old Fashioned Poppyseed	2 tbsp	140	10	0
Olde Venice Italian	2 tbsp	130	0	0
Olde World Caesar	2 tbsp	150	5	0
Parmesan Pepper	2 tbsp	160	10	0
Peppercorn Ranch	2 tbsp	180	10	0
Poppyseed	2 tbsp	160	15	0
Potato Salad Dressing	2 tbsp	120	35	0
Ranch	2 tbsp	180	3	0
Red Wine Vinegar & Oil	2 tbsp	130	0	0
Romano Cheese Caesar	2 tbsp	150	15	0
Romano Italian	2 tbsp	160	0	0
Savory Italian	2 tbsp	110	0	0
Slaw	2 tbsp	170	30	0
Southern Slaw	2 tbsp	100	20	0
Sweet & Saucy	2 tbsp	140	0	0
Sweet & Sour	2 tbsp	160	0	0
Thousand Island	2 tbsp	150	25	0
Vintage Champagne	2 tbsp	150	0	0
Wilde Raspberry	2 tbsp	150	0	0
Nasoya				
Creamy Dill	2 tbsp	70	0	0
Creamy Italian	2 tbsp	60	0	0
Garden Herb	2 tbsp	70	0	0
Sesame Garlic	2 tbsp	60	0	0
Thousand Island	2 tbsp	70	0	0
Newman's Own				
Balsamic Vinaigrette	2 tbsp (1.1 oz)	90	0	0
Caesar	2 tbsp (1.1 oz)	150	<5	0
Light Italian	2 tbsp (1.1 oz)	20	0	0

FOOD	PORTION	CALS	CHOL	FIBER
Olive Oil & Vinegar	2 tbsp (1 oz)	150	0	0
Ranch	2 tbsp (1 oz)	180	<5	0
Old Dutch				
Sweet & Sour	2 tbsp	50	0	0
Paul's				
No-Fat Raspberry & Balsamic	2 tbsp	20	0	—
No-Oil Orange & Basil	2 tbsp	15	0	0
Pfeiffer				
1000 Island	2 tbsp	140	20	0
California French	2 tbsp	140	0	0
French	2 tbsp	150	10	0
Honey Dijon	2 tbsp	140	15	0
Lite Italian	2 tbsp	50	0	0
Ranch	2 tbsp	180	3	0
Savory Italian	2 tbsp	110	0	0
Pritikin				
Dijon Balsamic Vinaigrette	2 tbsp (1 oz)	3	0	—
French	2 tbsp (1 oz)	35	0	—
Honey Dijon	2 tbsp (1 oz)	45	0	—
Honey French	2 tbsp (1 oz)	40	0	—
Italian	2 tbsp (1 oz)	20	0	—
Raspberry Vinaigrette	2 tbsp (1 oz)	45	0	—
Red Wing				
"K" Dressing	1 tbsp (0.5 oz)	70	5	0
Chunky Blue Cheese	2 tbsp (1 oz)	130	0	0
Creamy Ranch	2 tbsp (1 oz)	150	15	0
French Traditional	2 tbsp (1 oz)	130	0	0
Italian Traditional	2 tbsp (1 oz)	100	0	0
Spicy Sweet French	2 tbsp (1 oz)	130	0	0
Thousand Island Thick & Rich	2 tbsp (1 oz)	110	15	0
Seven Seas				
⅓ Less Fat Creamy Italian	2 tbsp (1.1 oz)	60	0	0
⅓ Less Fat Italian w/ Olive Oil Blend	2 tbsp (1.1 oz)	45	0	0
⅓ Less Fat Ranch	2 tbsp (1.1 oz)	100	0	0

FOOD	PORTION	CALS	CHOL	FIBER
⅓ Less Fat Red Wine Vinegar & Oil	2 tbsp (1.1 oz)	45	0	0
⅓ Less Fat Viva Italian	2 tbsp (1.1 oz)	45	0	0
2 Cheese Italian	2 tbsp (1.1 oz)	70	0	0
Chunky Blue Cheese	2 tbsp (1.1 oz)	130	<5	tr
Classic Caesar	2 tbsp (1.1 oz)	100	0	0
Creamy Italian	2 tbsp (1.1 oz)	120	0	0
Free Ranch	2 tbsp (1.2 oz)	45	0	1
Free Red Wine Vinegar	2 tbsp (1.1 oz)	15	0	0
Free Sour Cream & Onion Ranch	2 tbsp (1.2 oz)	50	0	1
Free Viva Italian	2 tbsp (1.1 oz)	10	0	1
Green Goddess	2 tbsp (1.1 oz)	130	0	0
Herbs & Spices	2 tbsp (1.1 oz)	90	0	0
Ranch	2 tbsp (1.1 oz)	160	<5	0
Red Wine Vinegar & Oil	2 tbsp (1.1 oz)	90	0	0
Viva Italian	2 tbsp (1.1 oz)	90	0	0
Viva Russian	2 tbsp (1.1 oz)	150	0	0
Walden Farms				
Fat Free Balsamic Vinaigrette	2 tbsp (1 oz)	15	0	0
Fat Free Bleu Cheese	2 tbsp (1 oz)	25	8	0
Fat Free Caesar	2 tbsp (1 oz)	25	0	0
Fat Free Creamy Italian With Parmesan	1 tbsp (1 oz)	25	0	0
Fat Free French Style	2 tbsp (1 oz)	25	0	0
Fat Free Honey Dijon	2 tbsp (1 oz)	25	0	0
Fat Free Italian	2 tbsp (1 oz)	10	0	0
Fat Free Ranch	2 tbsp (1 oz)	25	0	0
Fat Free Raspberry Vinaigrette	2 tbsp (1 oz)	20	0	0
Fat Free Russian	2 tbsp (1 oz)	30	5	0
Fat Free Sodium Free Italian	2 tbsp (1 oz)	10	0	0
Fat Free Sugar Free Italian	2 tbsp (1 oz)	0	0	0
Fat Free Thousand Island	2 tbsp (1 oz)	35	5	0
Italian With Sun Dried Tomato	2 tbsp (1 oz)	15	0	0

FOOD	PORTION	CALS	CHOL	FIBER
Ranch With Sun Dried Tomato	2 tbsp (1 oz)	25	0	0
Weight Watchers				
Fat Free Caesar	1 pkg (0.75 oz)	5	0	0
Fat Free Caesar	2 tbsp	10	0	0
Fat Free Creamy Italian	2 tbsp	30	0	0
Fat Free French Style	2 tbsp	40	0	0
Fat Free Honey Dijon	2 tbsp	45	0	0
Fat Free Italian	2 tbsp	10	0	0
Fat Free Ranch	1 pkg (0.75 oz)	25	0	0
Fat Free Ranch	2 tbsp	35	0	0
Wishbone				
Caesar	2 tbsp (1 oz)	90	5	0
Chunky Blue Cheese	2 tbsp (1 oz)	150	0	0
Classic House Italian	2 tbsp (1 oz)	140	5	0
Classic Olive Oil Italian	2 tbsp (1 oz)	60	0	0
Creamy Caesar	2 tbsp (1 oz)	180	10	0
Creamy Italian	2 tbsp (1 oz)	110	0	0
Creamy Roasted Garlic	2 tbsp (1 oz)	110	0	0
Deluxe French	2 tbsp (1 oz)	120	0	0
Fat Free Chunky Blue Cheese	2 tbsp (1 oz)	35	0	tr
Fat Free Creamy Italian	2 tbsp (1 oz)	35	0	tr
Fat Free Creamy Roasted Garlic	2 tbsp (1 oz)	40	0	0
Fat Free Deluxe French	2 tbsp (1 oz)	30	0	tr
Fat Free Honey Dijon	2 tbsp (1 oz)	45	0	0
Fat Free Italian	2 tbsp (1 oz)	10	0	0
Fat Free Parmesan & Onion	2 tbsp (1 oz)	45	0	tr
Fat Free Ranch	2 tbsp (1 oz)	40	0	tr
Fat Free Red Wine Vinaigrette	2 tbsp (1 oz)	35	0	0
Fat Free Sweet N' Spicy French	2 tbsp (1 oz)	30	0	0
Fat Free Thousand Island	2 tbsp (1 oz)	35	0	tr
Italian	2 tbsp (1 oz)	80	0	0
Lite French	2 tbsp (1 oz)	50	5	0
Lite Italian	2 tbsp (1 oz)	15	0	0

FOOD	PORTION	CALS	CHOL	FIBER
Lite Ranch	2 tbsp (1 oz)	100	5	0
Olive Oil Vinaigrette	2 tbsp (1 oz)	60	0	0
Oriental	2 tbsp (1 oz)	70	0	0
Parmesan & Onion	2 tbsp (1 oz)	110	5	0
Ranch	2 tbsp (1 oz)	160	10	0
Red Wine Vinaigrette	2 tbsp (1 oz)	80	0	0
Robusto Italian	2 tbsp (1 oz)	90	0	0
Russian	2 tbsp (1 oz)	110	0	0
Sweet N' Spicy French	2 tbsp (1 oz)	140	0	0
Thousand Island	2 tbsp (1 oz)	140	10	0
TAKE-OUT				
vinegar & oil	1 tbsp	72	0	—
SALMON				
CANNED				
chum w/ bone	1 can (13.9 oz)	521	144	—
chum w/ bone	3 oz	120	33	—
sockeye w/ bone	1 can (12.9 oz)	566	161	—
sockeye w/ bone	3 oz	130	37	—
FRESH				
atlantic baked	3 oz	155	60	—
chinook baked	3 oz	196	72	—
chum baked	3 oz	131	81	—
coho cooked	½ fillet (5.4 oz)	286	76	—
coho cooked	3 oz	157	42	—
coho raw	3 oz	124	33	—
pink baked	3 oz	127	57	—
sockeye cooked	3 oz	183	74	—
sockeye cooked	½ fillet (5.4 oz)	334	135	—
sockeye raw	3 oz	143	53	—
SMOKED				
chinook	3 oz	99	20	—
chinook	1 oz	33	7	—
Lascco				
Nova Sliced	2 oz	60	20	0
Nathan's				
Nova	2 oz	80	30	0
TAKE-OUT				
roulette w/ spinach stuffing	1 serv (4 oz)	160	45	tr

FOOD	PORTION	CALS	CHOL	FIBER
salmon cake	1 (3 oz)	241	104	–
SALSA				
black bean & corn	2 tbsp (1 oz)	15	0	tr
cirtus	2 tbsp (1 oz)	10	0	0
Chi-Chi's				
Con Queso	2 tbsp (1.1 oz)	90	15	0
Hot	2 tbsp (1 oz)	10	0	0
Medium	2 tbsp (1 oz)	10	0	0
Mild	2 tbsp (1 oz)	10	0	0
Picante Hot	2 tbsp (1 oz)	10	0	0
Picante Medium	2 tbsp (1 oz)	10	0	0
Picante Mild	2 tbsp (1 oz)	10	0	0
Verde Medium	2 tbsp (1.2 oz)	15	0	0
Verde Mild	2 tbsp (1.2 oz)	15	0	0
Guiltless Gourmet				
Roasted Red Pepper	2 tbsp (1 oz)	10	0	0
Southwestern Grill	2 tbsp (1 oz)	10	0	0
Heluva Good Cheese				
Cheese & Salsa	2 tbsp (1.1 oz)	80	10	0
Thick & Chunky Hot	2 tbsp (1.2 oz)	10	0	0
Thick & Chunky Mild	2 tbsp (1.2 oz)	10	0	0
Hot Cha Cha				
Medium	2 tbsp (1 oz)	5	0	–
Hunt's				
Alfresco All Varieties	2 tbsp (1.1 oz)	10	0	tr
Hot	2 tbsp (1.1 oz)	27	0	1
Medium	2 tbsp (1.1 oz)	27	0	1
Mild	2 tbsp (1.1 oz)	27	0	1
Picante All Varieties	2 tbsp (1.1 oz)	11	0	tr
Squeeze Mild & Medium	2 tbsp (1.1 oz)	27	0	1
Louise's				
Fat Free BBQ Black Bean	1 oz	10	0	0
Fat Free Black Bean	1 oz	10	0	0
Fat Free Medium	1 oz	10	0	1
Fat Free Mild	1 oz	10	0	1
Fat Free Nacho Queso	1 oz	15	0	0

FOOD	PORTION	CALS	CHOL	FIBER
Muir Glen				
Black Bean & Corn Medium	2 tbsp (1.1 oz)	15	0	tr
Chipotle Medium	2 tbsp (1.1 oz)	10	0	0
Fire Roasted Tomato Medium	2 tbsp (1.1 oz)	10	0	0
Garlic Cilantro Medium	2 tbsp (1.1 oz)	10	0	0
Habanero Hot	2 tbsp (1.1 oz)	10	0	0
Organic Medium	2 tbsp (1.1 oz)	10	0	0
Organic Mild	2 tbsp (1.1 oz)	10	0	0
Roasted Garlic Medium	2 tbsp (1.1 oz)	10	0	0
Newman's Own				
Bandito Hot	2 tbsp (1.1 oz)	10	0	tr
Bandito Medium	2 tbsp (1.1 oz)	10	0	tr
Bandito Mild	2 tbsp (1.1 oz)	10	0	tr
Peach	2 tbsp (1.1 oz)	25	0	1
Pineapple	2 tbsp (1.1 oz)	15	0	1
Roasted Garlic	2 tbsp (1.1 oz)	10	0	1
Old El Paso				
Green Chili Medium	2 tbsp (1 oz)	10	0	tr
Homestyle	2 tbsp (1 oz)	5	0	0
Homestyle Mild	2 tbsp (1 oz)	5	0	0
Picante Hot	2 tbsp (1 oz)	10	0	0
Picante Medium	2 tbsp (1 oz)	10	0	0
Picante Mild	2 tbsp (1 oz)	10	0	0
Picante Thick'n Chunky Hot	2 tbsp (1 oz)	10	0	0
Picante Thick'n Chunky Medium	2 tbsp (1 oz)	10	0	0
Picante Thick'n Chunky Mild	2 tbsp (1 oz)	10	0	0
Pico De Gallo Hot	2 tbsp (1 oz)	5	0	tr
Pico De Gallo Medium	1 tbsp (1 oz)	5	0	tr
Salsa Verde	2 tbsp (1 oz)	10	0	0
Thick'n Chunky Hot	2 tbsp (1 oz)	10	0	0
Thick'n Chunky Medium	2 tbsp (1 oz)	10	0	0
Thick'n Chunky Mild	2 tbsp (1 oz)	10	0	0
Pace				
Picante Mild or Medium	2 tbsp	10	0	0

FOOD	PORTION	CALS	CHOL	FIBER
Thick & Chunky Mild or Medium	2 tbsp	10	0	0
Rosarita				
Extra Chunky Medium	2 tbsp (1 oz)	7	0	tr
Green Tomatillo Medium	2 tbsp (1 oz)	8	0	1
Picante Zesty Jalapeno Hot	2 tbsp (1 oz)	8	0	1
Picante Zesty Jalapeno Medium	2 tbsp (1 oz)	9	0	1
Picante Zesty Jalapeno Mild	2 tbsp (1 oz)	8	0	tr
Roasted Mild	2 tbsp (1 oz)	10	0	1
Traditional Medium	2 tbsp (1 oz)	7	0	1
Traditional Mild	2 tbsp (1 oz)	7	0	1
Snyder's Of Hanover				
Mild	2 tbsp	10	0	0
Taco Bell				
Smooth 'N Zesty Picante Medium	2 tbsp (1.1 oz)	15	0	tr
Smooth 'N Zesty Picante Mild	2 tbsp (1.1 oz)	15	0	tr
Thick 'N Chunky Salsa Hot	2 tbsp (1.1 oz)	15	0	tr
Thick 'N Chunky Salsa Medium	2 tbsp (1.1 oz)	15	0	tr
Thick 'N Chunky Salsa Mild	2 tbsp (1.1 oz)	15	0	tr
Tostitos				
Con Queso	2.3 oz	80	<10	<2
Hot	2.3 oz	30	0	2
Low Fat Con Queso	2.5 oz	80	<10	tr
Medium	2.3 oz	30	0	2
Mild	2.3 oz	30	0	2
Restaurant Style	2.2 oz	30	0	<2
Ultimate Garden	2.4 oz	30	0	2
Tree Of Life				
Medium	2 tbsp (1 oz)	10	0	–
Mild	2 tbsp (1 oz)	10	0	–

FOOD	PORTION	CALS	CHOL	FIBER
Utz				
Chunky	2 tbsp (1 fl oz)	60	0	4
Watkins				
Salsa Seasoning Blend	⅛ tsp (0.5 g)	0	0	0
Tropical	2 tbsp (1 oz)	60	0	0
SALSIFY				
fresh sliced cooked	½ cup	46	0	–
raw sliced	½ cup	55	0	–
SALT SUBSTITUTES				
Cardia				
Salt Alternative	1 pkg (0.6 g)	0	0	–
Eden				
Shiso Leaf Powder	1 tsp	0	0	2
Estee				
Salt-It	¼ tsp	0	0	0
Halsosalt				
All Flavors	¼ tsp (7 g)	1	0	–
Morton				
Salt Substitute	¼ tsp (1.2 g)	tr	0	–
Mrs. Dash				
Onion & Herb	⅛ tsp (0.02 oz)	2	0	–
NoSalt				
Salt Alternative	1 pkg (0.75 g)	0	0	–
Papa Dash				
Lite Salt	½ tsp (1 g)	0	0	–
SALT/SEASONED SALT				
salt	1 tbsp (18 g)	0	0	–
salt	1 tsp (6 g)	0	0	–
Eden				
Atlantic Sea Salt	¼ tsp	0	0	0
Brittany Sea Salt	¼ tsp	0	0	0
Morton				
Garlic	1 tsp	3	0	–
Iodized	1 tsp	tr	0	–
Kosher	1 tsp	0	0	–
Lite	¼ tsp (1.4 g)	tr	0	–
Nature's Season Seasoning Blend	1 tsp	3	0	–

FOOD	PORTION	CALS	CHOL	FIBER
Non-Iodized	1 tsp	0	0	–
Seasoned	1 tsp	4	0	–
Watkins				
Bacon Cheese Salt	¼ tbsp (1 g)	0	0	0
Butter Salt	¼ tbsp (1 g)	0	0	0
Cheese Salt	¼ tbsp (1 g)	0	0	0
Garlic Salt	¼ tsp (1 g)	0	0	0
Salt & Vinegar Seasoning	¼ tsp (1 g)	0	0	0
Seasoning Salt	¼ tsp (1 g)	0	0	0
Sour Cream & Onion Salt	¼ tbsp (1 g)	0	0	0

SANDWICHES

FOOD	PORTION	CALS	CHOL	FIBER
Amy's				
Pocket Sandwich Broccoli & Cheese	1 (4.5 oz)	270	15	3
Pocket Sandwich Roasted Vegetables	1 (4.5 oz)	220	0	4
Pocket Sandwich Tofu Scramble	1 (4 oz)	160	0	tr
Pocket Sandwich Vegetable Pie	1 (5 oz)	300	0	3
Toaster Pops Grilled Cheese	1	180	20	0
Croissant Pocket				
Stuffed Sandwich Chicken Broccoli & Cheddar	1 piece (4.5 oz)	300	35	5
Stuffed Sandwich Ham & Cheddar	1 piece (4.5 oz)	360	45	5
Healthy Choice				
Bread Stuffs Chicken & Broccoli	1 (6.1 oz)	310	25	2
Bread Stuffs Ham & Cheese w/ Broccoli	1 (6.1 oz)	320	20	1
Bread Stuffs Italian Style Meatball	1 (6.1 oz)	330	20	4
Bread Stuffs Philly Beef Steak	1 (6.1 oz)	310	20	3

FOOD	PORTION	CALS	CHOL	FIBER
Hot Pocket				
Stuffed Sandwich Barbecue	1 (4.5 oz)	340	25	1
Stuffed Sandwich Beef & Cheddar	1 (4.5 oz)	360	50	tr
Stuffed Sandwich Beef Fajita	1 (4.5 oz)	360	40	5
Stuffed Sandwich Chicken & Cheddar With Broccoli	1 (4.5 oz)	300	30	tr
Stuffed Sandwich Ham & Cheese	1 (4.5 ox)	340	45	4
Stuffed Sandwich Turkey & Ham With Cheese	1 (4.5 oz)	320	35	1
Lean Pockets				
Stuffed Sandwich Beef & Broccoli	1 (4.5 oz)	250	50	7
Stuffed Sandwich Chicken Fajita	1 (4.5 oz)	260	40	3
Stuffed Sandwich Chicken Parmesan	1 (4.5 oz)	260	25	1
Stuffed Sandwich Glazed Chicken Supreme	1 (4.5 oz)	240	30	1
Stuffed Sandwich Turkey & Ham With Cheddar	1 (4.5 oz)	260	35	4
Stuffed Sandwich Turkey Broccoli & Cheese	1 (4.5 oz)	260	35	4
Smucker's				
Uncrustables Grape	1 (2 oz)	200	0	2
TAKE-OUT				
chicken fillet plain	1	515	60	—
chicken fillet w/ cheese lettuce mayonnaise & tomato	1	632	76	—
croque monsieur	1 (12.4 oz)	765	152	2

FOOD	PORTION	CALS	CHOL	FIBER
fish fillet w/ tartar sauce & cheese	1	524	68	–
fried egg w/ cheese	1	340	291	–
fried egg w/ cheese & ham	1	348	245	–
ham w/ cheese	1	353	58	–
roast beef submarine sandwich w/ tomato lettuce & mayonnaise	1	411	73	–
roast beef w/ cheese	1	402	77	–
roast beef plain	1	346	52	–
steak w/ tomato lettuce salt & mayonnaise	1	459	73	–
submarine w/ salami ham cheese lettuce tomato onion & oil	1	456	35	–
tuna salad submarine sandwich w/ lettuce & oil	1	584	47	–

SAPODILLA
fresh	1	140	0	–
fresh cut up	1 cup	199	0	–

SAPOTES
fresh	1	301	0	–

SARDINES
CANNED
atlantic in oil w/ bone	2	50	34	–
atlantic in oil w/ bone	1 can (3.2 oz)	192	131	–
pacific in tomato sauce w/ bone	1 can (13 oz)	658	225	–
pacific in tomato sauce w/ bone	1	68	23	–

Bumble Bee
In Hot Sauce	½ can (2 oz)	109	30	0
In Mustard	½ can (2 oz)	88	35	0
In Oil	½ can (2 oz)	125	39	0
In Water	½ can (2 oz)	83	60	0

FOOD	PORTION	CALS	CHOL	FIBER
Port Clyde				
In Louisiana Hot Sauce	1 can (3.75 oz)	170	105	0
In Mustard Sauce	1 can (3.75 oz)	150	110	1
In Soybean Oil Select Small	1 can (3.3 oz)	220	115	0
In Soybean Oil With Hot Chilies	1 can (3.3 oz)	155	80	0
In Soybean Oil drained	1 can (3.3 oz)	220	115	0
In Spring Water	1 can (3.3 oz)	170	140	0
In Tomato Sauce	1 can (3.75 oz)	150	100	0

SAUCE *(see also* BARBECUE SAUCE, GRAVY, PIZZA SAUCE, SPAGHETTI SAUCE*)*
JARRED

FOOD	PORTION	CALS	CHOL	FIBER
fish sauce vietnamese nuoc mam	1 tbsp	6	0	0
hoisin	1 tbsp	35	0	tr
oyster	1 tbsp	8	0	0
teriyaki	1 oz	30	0	—
teriyaki	1 tbsp	15	0	—
Annie Chun				
Shiitake Mushroom	1 tbsp	15	0	0
Thai Peanut	2 tbsp	120	0	1
Armour				
Chili Hot Dog	¼ cup (2.2 oz)	120	20	0
Meatless Sloppy Joe Sauce	¼ cup (2.2 oz)	30	0	0
Boar's Head				
Ham Glaze Brown Sugar & Spice	2 tbsp (1.4 oz)	120	0	0
Cheez Whiz				
Cheese	2 tbsp (1.2 oz)	90	20	0
Cheese Jalapeno Pepper	2 tbsp (1.2 oz)	90	25	0
Cheese Mild Salsa	2 tbsp (1.2 oz)	100	25	0
Chi-Chi's				
Enchilada	¼ cup (2.1 oz)	30	0	0
Taco	1 tbsp (0.5 oz)	10	0	0
Chun King				
Sweet And Sour	2 tbsp (1.2 oz)	58	0	0
Teriyaki	1 tbsp (0.6 oz)	17	0	0

FOOD	PORTION	CALS	CHOL	FIBER
Teriyaki Hot	1 tbsp (0.6 oz)	17	0	0
Del Monte				
Seafood Cocktail	¼ cup (2.7 oz)	100	0	0
Sloppy Joe Hickory Flavor	¼ cup (2.4 oz)	70	0	0
Sloppy Joe Original	¼ cup (2.4 oz)	70	0	0
Fritos				
Texas-Style Chili Hearty Topping	2.3 oz	50	10	1
Utimate Taco Hearty Topping	2.3 oz	50	10	1
Gebhardt				
Enchilada Sauce	¼ cup (2.2 oz)	35	0	1
Hot Dog Chili Sauce	¼ cup (2.2 oz)	60	1	2
Hot Sauce	1 tsp (5 g)	1	0	0
Green Giant				
Sloppy Joe	¼ cup (2.6 oz)	50	0	2
Sloppy Joe as prep w/ meat	1 serv (4.4 oz)	200	45	2
Heluva Good Cheese				
Cocktail	¼ cup (1.6 oz)	40	0	–
Hormel				
Not-So-Sloppy-Joe Sauce	¼ cup (2.2 oz)	70	0	1
House Of Tsang				
Bangkok Padang	1 tbsp (0.6 oz)	45	0	0
Hoisin	1 tsp (6 g)	15	0	0
Mandarin Marinade	1 tbsp (0.6 oz)	25	0	0
Saigon Sizzle	1 tbsp (0.6 oz)	40	0	0
Spicy Brown Bean	1 tsp (6 g)	15	0	0
Stir Fry Classic	1 tbsp (0.6 oz)	25	0	0
Stir Fry Sweet & Sour	1 tbsp (0.6 oz)	30	0	0
Stir Fry Szechuan Spicy	1 tbsp (0.6 oz)	20	0	0
Sweet & Sour Concentrate	1 tsp (6 g)	10	0	0
Teriyaki Korean	1 tbsp (0.6 oz)	30	0	0
Hunt's				
Light w/ Mushrooms	½ cup (4.4 oz)	42	0	2
Steak	1 tbsp (0.6 oz)	10	0	tr

FOOD	PORTION	CALS	CHOL	FIBER
Just Rite				
Hot Dog	¼ cup (2.2 oz)	50	2	2
Kraft				
Cocktail	¼ cup (2.3 oz)	60	0	1
Fat Free Tartar Sauce	2 tbsp (1.1 oz)	25	0	0
Lemon & Herb Tartar Sauce	2 tbsp (1 oz)	150	15	0
Reduced Fat Sandwich Spread	1 tbsp (0.5 oz)	35	0	0
Sandwich Spread	1 tbsp (0.5 oz)	50	<5	0
Sweet'n Sour	2 tbsp (1.2 oz)	60	0	0
Tartar	2 tbsp (1.1 oz)	90	10	2
La Choy				
Duck Sauce Sweet & Sour	2 tbsp (1.3 oz)	61	0	0
Sweet & Sour	2 tbsp (1.2 oz)	58	0	0
Teriyaki	1 tbsp (0.6 oz)	17	0	0
Lawry's				
Teriyaki Marinade	2 tbsp	72	0	tr
Lea & Perrins				
Worcestershire	1 tsp	5	0	–
Manwich				
BBQ Sloppy Joe	¼ cup (2.2 oz)	57	0	1
Bold	¼ cup (2.2 oz)	62	0	1
Mexican	¼ cup (2.2 oz)	27	0	1
Original	¼ cup (2.2 oz)	32	0	1
Taco Season	¼ cup (2.2 oz)	27	0	1
Thick & Chunky	¼ cup (2.3 oz)	44	0	1
Marzetti				
Teriyaki Stir-Fry	2 tbsp	80	0	0
Mrs. Dash				
Steak	1 tbsp (0.4 oz)	17	0	–
Newman's Own				
Spicy Simmer Sauce Diavolo	½ cup (4.4 oz)	70	0	3
Old El Paso				
Enchilada Hot	¼ cup (2 oz)	30	0	0
Enchilada Mild	¼ cup (2 oz)	25	0	0
Green Chili Enchilada Sauce	¼ cup (2.1 oz)	30	0	0

FOOD	PORTION	CALS	CHOL	FIBER
Taco Hot	1 tbsp (0.5 oz)	5	0	0
Taco Medium	1 tbsp (0.5 oz)	5	0	0
Taco Mild	1 tbsp (0.5 oz)	5	0	0
Taco Sauce	1 tbsp (0.5 oz)	5	0	0
Taco Sauce Extra Chunky Medium	1 tbsp (0.5 oz)	5	0	0
Taco Sauce Extra Chunky Mild	1 tbsp (0.5 oz)	5	0	0
Open Range				
Hot Dog Chili	¼ cup (2.2 oz)	61	3	2
Ortega				
Taco Western Style	1 oz	8	0	–
Enchilada Sauce	¼ cup	36	0	0
Taco Sauce	¼ cup	32	0	0
Progresso				
Alfredo	½ cup (4.4 oz)	200	50	1
Red Wing				
Chili Sauce	1 tbsp (0.6 oz)	20	0	0
Seafood Cocktail	¼ cup (2 oz)	90	0	0
Sauce Arturo				
Original	¼ cup (2.2 fl oz)	50	0	0
Simmer Chef				
Golden Honey Mustard	½ cup (4 fl oz)	150	0	1
Hearty Onion & Mushroom	½ cup (4 fl oz)	50	0	1
Tabasco				
Caribbean Steak Sauce	1 tbsp (0.6 oz)	15	0	0
Garlic Basting Sauce	1 tbsp (0.6 oz)	20	0	0
Habanero Sauce	1 tsp (0.2 oz)	5	0	0
Hot Sauce w/ Garlic	1 tsp (0.2 oz)	0	0	0
Jalepeno Pepper Sauce	1 tbsp	15	0	tr
New Orleans Steak Sauce	1 tbsp (0.6 oz)	15	0	0
Pepper Sauce	1 tsp (0.2 oz)	0	0	0
Taco Bell				
Taco Sauce Medium	2 tbsp (1.1 oz)	15	0	tr
Taco Sauce Mild	2 tbsp (1.1 oz)	15	0	tr
The Restaurant Hot Sauce	1 tsp (5 g)	0	0	0

FOOD	PORTION	CALS	CHOL	FIBER
Tostitos				
Beef Fiesta Nacho	2.4 oz	120	10	tr
Chicken Quesadilla Topping	2.5 oz	90	10	tr
Watkins				
Inferno Hot Pepper Sauce	2 tbsp (1 oz)	35	0	1
Steak Sauce	1 tbsp (0.5 oz)	20	0	0
Wild Thyme Farms				
Chili Ginger Honey	1 tbsp	30	0	—
MIX				
cheese as prep w/ milk	1 cup	307	53	—
curry as prep w/ milk	1 cup	270	35	—
mushroom as prep w/ milk	1 cup	228	34	—
sourcream as prep w/ milk	1 cup	509	91	—
stroganoff as prep	1 cup	271	38	—
sweet & sour as prep	1 cup	294	0	—
teriyaki as prep	1 cup	131	0	—
white as prep w/ milk	1 cup	241	34	—
Durkee				
A La King as prep	1 cup	60	0	0
Cheese as prep	¼ cup	25	2	0
Hollandaise as prep	2 tbsp	10	0	0
White as prep	¼ cup	20	0	0
French's				
Cheese as prep	¼ cup	25	0	0
Hollandaise as prep	2 tbsp	10	0	0
Manwich				
Mix	¼ oz	22	0	tr
McCormick				
Chicken Dijon Blend	1⅔ tbsp (10 g)	40	<5	—
Hollandaise Blend	2 tsp (4 g)	15	15	—
Watkins				
Beef Marinade	¼ tbsp (2 g)	5	0	0
Calypso Hot Pepper Sauce	1 tsp (5 g)	10	0	0
Caribbean Red Pepper Sauce	1 tsp (5 g)	10	0	0

FOOD	PORTION	CALS	CHOL	FIBER
Chicken & Pork Marinade	¼ tbsp (2 g)	5	0	0
Fish & Seafood Marinade	¼ tbsp (2 g)	10	0	0
Meat Magic	1 tsp (6 g)	10	0	0
SHELF-STABLE				
Cheez Whiz				
Cheese Squeezable	2 tbsp (1.2 oz)	100	15	0
TAKE-OUT				
bearnaise	1 oz	177	21	tr
SAUERKRAUT				
canned	½ cup	22	0	–
B&G				
Sauerkraut	2 tbsp (1 oz)	6	0	1
Boar's Head				
Sauerkraut	2 tbsp (1 oz)	5	0	tr
Claussen				
Sauerkraut	¼ cup (1.1 oz)	5	0	1
Del Monte				
Bavarian Style	2 tbsp (1 oz)	15	0	0
Sauerkraut	2 tbsp (1 oz)	0	0	1
Eden				
Organic	½ cup	25	0	3
Hebrew National				
Gallon Kraut	½ cup	25	0	–
S&W				
Canned	2 tbsp (1 oz)	5	0	0
Red Cabbage	2 tbsp (1 oz)	15	0	0
SAUSAGE				
bratwurst pork cooked	1 link (3 oz)	256	51	–
brotwurst pork & beef	1 link (2.5 oz)	226	44	–
chipolata	3.5 oz	342	66	0
chorizo	3.5 oz	499	70	tr
italian pork cooked	1 (3 oz)	268	65	–
kielbasa pork	1 oz	88	19	–
knockwurst pork & beef	1 (2.4 oz)	209	39	–
polish pork	1 (8 oz)	739	158	–
pork cooked	1 link (½ oz)	48	11	–
vienna canned	7 (4 oz)	315	59	–

FOOD	PORTION	CALS	CHOL	FIBER
vienna canned	1 (½ oz)	45	8	—
Aidells				
Andouille Cajun Cooked	1 (3.5 oz)	220	40	—
Burmese Curry Cooked	1 (3.5 oz)	220	20	—
Chicken & Apple Fresh	1 (1.9 oz)	110	20	—
Chicken & Apple Smoked	1 (3.5 oz)	220	30	0
Chicken & Turkey New Mexico Smoked	1 (3.5 oz)	220	40	—
Chicken & Turkey Thai Fresh	1 (3.5 oz)	200	35	—
Chicken & Turkey Thai Smoked	1 (3.5 oz)	220	30	—
Chicken & Turkey With Sun-Dried Tomatoes & Basil Fresh	1 (3.5 oz)	200	35	—
Chicken & Turkey With Sun-Dried Tomatoes & Basil Smoked	1 (3.5 oz)	200	30	—
Creole Hot Cooked	1 (3.5 oz)	220	30	—
Duck & Turkey Smoked	1 (3.5 oz)	220	60	—
Hunter's Cooked	1 (3.5 oz)	240	35	—
Italian Hot Fresh	1 (3.5 oz)	230	40	—
Italian Mild Fresh	1 (3.5 oz)	230	40	—
Lamb & Beef With Rosemary Fresh	1 (3.5 oz)	220	35	—
Lemon Chicken Cooked	1 (3.5 oz)	220	35	—
Mexican Chorizo Beef Fresh	1 (3.5 oz)	400	70	—
Whiskey Fennel Cooked	1 (3.5 oz)	230	65	—
Armour				
Vienna Sausage 25% Less Fat	3 (1.9 oz)	130	50	0
Vienna Sausage 50% Less Fat	3 (1.9 oz)	90	40	0
Vienna Sausage Chicken & Beef	3 (1.9 oz)	120	65	0
Vienna Sausage Hot'n Spicy	3 (2.1 oz)	150	50	0

FOOD	PORTION	CALS	CHOL	FIBER
Vienna Sausage In BBQ Sauce	3 (2.1 oz)	150	50	0
Vienna Sausage In Beef Stock	3 (1.9 oz)	150	50	0
Vienna Sausage Jalapeno In Beef Stock	3 (1.9 oz)	170	50	0
Banner				
Sausage Stomachs	2 oz	90	95	0
Sausage Tripe	2 oz	90	85	0
Bilinski's				
Chicken & Vegetable	1 (3 oz)	80	40	tr
Chicken Italian With Peppers & Onions	1 (3 oz)	120	80	–
Boar's Head				
Bratwurst	1 (4 oz)	300	75	0
Hot Smoked	1 (3.2 oz)	280	55	0
Kielbasa	2 oz	120	50	0
Knockwurst	1 (4 oz)	310	50	0
Brown'N Serve				
Turkey	3 (2.1 oz)	120	35	0
Healthy Choice				
Low Fat Smoked	2 oz	70	25	1
Low Fat Smoked Polska Kielbasa	2 oz	70	25	1
Hebrew National				
Beef Knocks	1 (3 oz)	260	55	–
Polish Beef	1 link	240	50	–
Hormel				
Kielbasa	2 oz	150	40	–
Light & Lean 97 Dinner Smoked	2 oz	60	20	0
Pickled Hot	6 (2 oz)	140	40	0
Pickled Smoked	6 (2 oz)	140	40	0
Smoked Summer	2 oz	200	55	0
Vienna	2 oz	140	45	0
Vienna Chicken	2 oz	110	55	0
Jimmy Dean				
Brick Sausage	2.5 oz	270	55	0
Bulk	2.5 oz	300	55	0

FOOD	PORTION	CALS	CHOL	FIBER
Hickory Smoked Dinner Sausage	2 oz	170	35	0
Pattie Pre-Cooked	1 (1.9 oz)	230	45	0
Polska Kielbaska	2 oz	170	35	0
Sage Pattie	1 (2 oz)	200	45	0
Sausage Pattie Raw	1 (2 oz)	200	40	0
Skinless Link	2 (2 oz)	200	45	0
Skinless Link	4 (2 oz)	200	45	0
Little Sizzlers				
Brown & Serve	3 links (2.1 oz)	190	45	0
Brown & Serve	2 patties (1.8 oz)	190	40	0
Cooked	2 patties (1.8 oz)	230	45	0
Cooked	3 links (1.8 oz)	230	45	0
Heat & Serve Pork cooked	3 links (1.8 oz)	230	45	0
Louis Rich				
Polska Kielbasa	2 oz	90	35	0
Turkey Hot	2.5 oz	120	55	0
Turkey Original	2.5 oz	120	55	0
Turkey Smoked	2 oz	90	30	0
Mr. Turkey				
Breakfast	2.5 oz	130	65	—
Hearty Blend Polish Kielbasa	1 oz	70	23	—
Hearty Blend Smoked	1 oz	70	23	—
Hot Smoked	1 oz	45	15	—
Italian Smoked	1 oz	45	15	—
Polish Kielbasa	1 oz	45	15	—
Smoked	1 oz	45	15	—
Old Smokehouse				
Summer Sausage	2 oz	200	55	0
Oscar Mayer				
Pork cooked	2 links (1.7 oz)	170	40	0
Smokies Beef	1 (1.5 oz)	120	30	0
Smokies Cheese	1 (1.5 oz)	130	30	0
Smokies Link	1 (1.5 oz)	130	25	0
Smokies Little	6 (2 oz)	170	35	0
Smokies Little Cheese	6 (2 oz)	180	40	0

FOOD	PORTION	CALS	CHOL	FIBER
Perdue				
Hot Italian Turkey Cooked	1 link (2.4 oz)	150	60	—
Sweet Italian Turkey Cooked	1 link (2.4 oz)	150	60	—
Rudy's Farm				
Italian Hot	2.5 oz	240	50	0
Italian Mild	2.5 oz	240	50	0
Italian Mild Natural Casing	1 (2 oz)	190	40	0
Morning Right Link	3 (2.9 oz)	150	40	0
Morning Right Pattie	2 (2.9 oz)	150	40	0
Pattie Pre-Cooked	1 (1.4 oz)	100	35	1
Smoked	4 (2.1 oz)	200	40	0
Sweet Link	1 (3.9 oz)	380	80	0
Shady Brook				
Turkey Breakfast	2 oz	80	35	—
Turkey Hot Italian	2 oz	100	40	—
Turkey Old World Style	4 oz	190	65	—
Turkey Sweet Italian	2 oz	100	40	—
Shofar				
Knockwurst Beef	1 (3 oz)	260	50	0
Turkey Store				
Breakfast	2 links (2 oz)	140	45	—
Wampler				
Breakfast Turkey	2 (2.4 oz)	110	45	—
Italian Turkey	1 (2.7 oz)	120	50	—
TAKE-OUT				
pork	1 patty (1 oz)	100	22	—
pork	1 link (0.5 oz)	48	11	—
SAUSAGE DISHES				
Jimmy Dean				
Italian Sausage & Mozzarella Sandwich	1 (4.5 oz)	380	40	2
TAKE-OUT				
italian sausage w/ peppers & onions	1 cup	210	70	—

FOOD	PORTION	CALS	CHOL	FIBER
SAUSAGE SUBSTITUTES				
nonmeat sausage	1 patty (38 g)	97	0	–
nonmeat sausage	1 link (25 g)	64	0	–
Boca Burgers				
Breakfast Patties	1 (1.3 oz)	70	0	2
GardenSausage				
Patty	1 (2.5 oz)	140	5	5
Lightlife				
Gimme Lean	2 oz	70	0	1
Lean Links Breakfast	1 (1.2 oz)	60	0	0
Lean Links Italian	1 (1.4 oz)	60	0	0
Light	2 patties (2.3 oz)	80	0	1
Loma Linda				
Linketts	1 (1.2 oz)	70	0	1
Little Links	2 (1.6 oz)	90	0	2
Morningstar Farms				
Breakfast Links	2 (1.6 oz)	60	0	2
Breakfast Patties	1 (1.3 oz)	80	0	2
Grillers	1 patty (2.2 oz)	140	0	3
Sausage Style Recipe Crumbles	⅔ cup (1.9 oz)	90	0	2
Natural Touch				
Vegan Sausage Crumbles	½ cup (1.9 oz)	60	0	2
Worthington				
Leanies	1 link (1.4 oz)	100	0	1
Prosage Links	2 (1.6 oz)	60	0	2
Saucettes	1 link (1.3 oz)	90	0	1
Super Links	1 (1.7 oz)	110	0	1
Veja Links	1 (1.1 oz)	50	0	0
Yves				
Veggie Breakfast Links	1 (1.6 oz)	60	0	2
Veggie Breakfast Patties	1 (2 oz)	70	0	2
SAVORY				
ground	1 tsp	4	0	–
SCALLOP				
raw	3 oz	75	28	–
TAKE-OUT				
breaded & fried	2 lg	67	19	–

FOOD	PORTION	CALS	CHOL	FIBER
SCONE				
Finnegan's				
Cranberry	1 (2.7 oz)	90	0	1
Irish Raisin	1 (2.7 oz)	90	0	1
Health Valley				
Apple Kiwi	1	180	0	5
Cinnamon Raisin	1	180	0	5
Cranberry Orange	1	180	0	5
Mountain Blueberry	1	180	0	5
Pineapple Banana	1	180	0	5
TAKE-OUT				
apricot	1	232	34	–
blueberry	1 (3 oz)	270	10	2
orange poppy	1 (3 oz)	260	30	2
raisin	1 (3 oz)	270	10	2
SEA BASS (see BASS)				
SEA CUCUMBER				
dried	1 oz	74	17	0
fresh	1 oz	20	14	0
SEA TROUT (see TROUT)				
SEAWEED				
agar dried	1 oz	87	0	–
agar fresh	1 oz	tr	0	–
hijiki dried	1 tbsp	9	0	1
irishmoss fresh	1 oz	14	0	–
kelp fresh	1 oz	12	0	–
kombu fresh	1 oz	12	0	–
laver fresh	1 oz	10	0	–
nori fresh	1 oz	10	0	–
nori sheet dried	1 (8 x 8 in)	5	0	1
seahair dried	1 tbsp	13	0	tr
spirulina dried	1 oz	83	0	–
spirulina fresh	1 oz	7	0	–
tangle fresh	1 oz	12	0	–
wakame fresh	1 oz	13	0	–
Maine Coast				
Alaria	⅓ cup (7 g)	18	0	2
Dulse	⅓ cup (7 g)	18	0	2

FOOD	PORTION	CALS	CHOL	FIBER
Kelp	⅓ cup (7 g)	17	0	3
Kelp Crunch	1 bar (1 oz)	129	0	2
Kelp Crunch Peanut-Raisin	1 bar (1 oz)	129	0	2
Laver	⅓ cup (7 g)	22	0	3
Sea Seasoning Dulse	1 g	3	0	—
Sea Seasoning Dulse With Celery	1 g	3	0	—
Sea Seasoning Dulse With Garlic	1 g	3	0	—
Sea Seasoning Dulse With Sesame	1 g	3	0	—
Sea Seasoning Kelp	1 g	3	0	—
Sea Seasoning Kelp With Cayenne	1 g	3	0	—
Sea Seasoning Nori	1 g	3	0	—
Sea Seasoning Nori With Ginger	1 g	3	0	—

SEITAN *(see WHEAT)*

SEMOLINA

dry	1 cup (5.9 oz)	601	0	7

SESAME

seeds	1 tsp	16	0	—
sesame butter	1 tbsp	95	0	1
sesame crunch candy	1 oz	146	0	—
sesame crunch candy	20 pieces (1.2 oz)	181	0	—
tahini from roasted & toasted kernels	1 tbsp	89	0	—
tahini from stone ground kernels	1 tbsp	86	0	—
tahini from unroasted kernels	1 tbsp	85	0	—
Casbah				
Tahini Sauce Mix as prep	¼ cup	160	0	tr
Eden				
Organic Seaweed Gomasio	1 serv (1.5 oz)	10	0	0

FOOD	PORTION	CALS	CHOL	FIBER
Organic Gomasio	½ tsp	10	0	tr
Organic Gomasio Garlic	½ tsp	10	0	tr
Joyva				
Tahini	2 tbsp (1 oz)	200	0	1
Maranatha				
Raw Tahini	2 tbsp	190	0	3
Roasted Tahini	2 tbsp	210	0	2
Planters				
Nut Mix	1 oz	150	0	2
Stone-Buhr				
Seeds Raw	4 tsp (1 oz)	180	0	1
SESBANIA				
flower	1	1	0	—
flowers	1 cup	5	0	—
flowers cooked	1 cup	23	0	—
SHAD				
roe raw	1 oz	37	103	—
SHARK				
batter-dipped & fried	3 oz	194	50	—
raw	3 oz	111	43	—
SHELLFISH *(see individual names,* SHELLFISH SUBSTITUTES*)*				
SHELLFISH SUBSTITUTES				
crab imitation	3 oz	87	17	—
scallop imitation	3 oz	84	18	—
shrimp imitation	3 oz	86	31	—
surimi	3 oz	84	25	—
surimi	1 oz	28	8	—
Louis Kemp				
Crab Delights	½ cup (3 oz)	90	10	2
Lobster Delights	½ cup (3 oz)	80	10	0
Scallop Delights	13 pieces (3 oz)	80	10	0
Ocean Magic				
Imitation King Crab	3 oz	80	15	—
SHELLIE BEANS				
canned	½ cup	37	0	—

FOOD	PORTION	CALS	CHOL	FIBER
SHERBET				
orange	½ cup (4 fl oz)	132	5	–
orange	½ gal	2158	113	–
orange	1 bar (2.75 fl oz)	91	3	–
orange home recipe	½ cup	120	9	–
Breyers				
Fat Free Orange	½ cup (3 oz)	110	0	0
Fat Free Rainbow	½ cup (3 oz)	110	0	0
Fat Free Raspberry	½ cup (3 oz)	120	0	0
Fat Free Tropical	½ cup (3 oz)	110	0	0
Orange	½ cup (3 oz)	120	5	0
Rainbow	½ cup (3 oz)	120	5	0
Raspberry	½ cup (3 oz)	120	5	0
Tropical	½ cup (3 oz)	120	5	0
Hood				
Lime Orange Lemon	½ cup (3.1 oz)	120	<5	0
Orange	½ cup (3.1 oz)	120	<5	0
Rainbow Swirl	½ cup (3.1 oz)	120	<5	0
Raspberry Orange Lime	½ cup (3.1 oz)	120	<5	0
Sealtest				
Lime	½ cup (3 oz)	130	5	0
Orange	½ cup (3 oz)	130	5	0
Rainbow Orange Red Raspberry Lime	½ cup (3 oz)	130	5	0
Red Raspberry	½ cup (3 oz)	130	5	0
Turkey Hill				
Fruit Rainbow	½ cup	120	5	–
Orange Grove	½ cup	120	5	–
SHRIMP				
canned	3 oz	102	147	–
canned	1 cup	154	222	–
chinese shrimp paste	1 tbsp	15	45	–
cooked	3 oz	84	166	–
cooked	4 large	22	43	–
raw	4 large	30	43	–
raw	3 oz	90	130	–
Bumble Bee				
Medium	⅓ can (2 oz)	45	115	0
Orleans Tiny Cocktail	½ can (3 oz)	44	114	0

FOOD	PORTION	CALS	CHOL	FIBER
Gorton's				
Popcorn Garlic & Herb	22 pieces (3.6 oz)	270	90	–
Popcorn Original	20 pieces (3.2 oz)	240	65	–
Van De Kamp's				
Breaded Butterfly	7 (4 oz)	280	55	2
Breaded Popcorn	20 (4 oz)	270	35	1
Breaded Whole	7 (4 oz)	240	50	2
TAKE-OUT				
breaded & fried	3 oz	206	150	–
jambalaya	¾ cup	188	50	8
SMELT				
rainbow cooked	3 oz	106	76	–
rainbow raw	3 oz	83	60	–
SNACKS				
cheese puffs	1 oz	157	1	tr
corn puffs cheese	1 bag (8 oz)	1256	9	2
corn twists cheese	1 oz	157	1	tr
corn twists cheese	1 bag (8 oz)	1256	9	2
oriental mix	1 oz	155	0	–
pork skins	1 oz	154	27	–
pork skins barbecue	1 oz	152	33	–
trail mix	1 oz	131	0	–
trail mix	1 cup (5.3 oz)	693	0	–
trail mix tropical	1 oz	115	0	–
Baken-ets				
BBQ	9 (0.5 oz)	70	10	tr
Hot N'Spicy	7 (0.5 oz)	70	20	tr
Hot N'Spicy Cracklins	8 (0.5 oz)	80	20	tr
Regular	9 (0.5 oz)	80	20	tr
Regular Cracklins	8 (0.5 oz)	40	15	tr
Barbara's Bakery				
Cheese Puffs Bakes	1½ cups (1 oz)	160	0	0
Cheese Puffs Jalapeno	¾ cup (1 oz)	150	0	0
Cheese Puffs Original	¾ cup (1 oz)	150	0	0
Big Dipper				
Bagel Chips Lowfat Barbeque	12 (1 oz)	110	0	1
Bagel Chips Lowfat Garlic	12 (1 oz)	120	0	1

FOOD	PORTION	CALS	CHOL	FIBER
Bagel Chips Lowfat Original	12 (1 oz)	110	0	1
Bugles				
Baked Cheddar Cheese	1½ cups (1 oz)	130	0	0
Baked Original	1½ cups (1 oz)	130	0	0
Baked Original	1 pkg (1.4 oz)	170	0	tr
Nacho	1⅓ cups (1 oz)	160	0	0
Nacho	1 pkg (0.9 oz)	130	0	0
Original	1 pkg (1.5 oz)	230	0	tr
Original	1⅓ cups (1 oz)	160	0	tr
Ranch	1⅓ cups (1 oz)	160	0	tr
Smokin BBQ	1⅓ cups (1 oz)	150	0	0
Sour Cream & Onion	1⅓ cups (1 oz)	160	0	0
Cheetos				
Crunchy	21 pieces (1 oz)	160	0	tr
Curls	15 pieces (1 oz)	150	0	1
Flamin' Hot	21 pieces (1 oz)	160	0	tr
Nacho Cheese	23 pieces (1 oz)	160	0	tr
Puffed Balls	38 pieces (1 oz)	150	0	tr
Puffs	29 pieces (1 oz)	160	0	tr
Zig Zags	17 pieces (1 oz)	170	<5	tr
Chex Mix				
Bold'n Zesty	1 pkg (1.7 oz)	230	0	3
Cheddar Cheese	1 pkg (1.7 oz)	220	0	2
Hot'n Spicy	⅔ cup (1 oz)	130	0	2
Hot'n Spicy	1 pkg (1.7 oz)	210	0	3
Traditional	1 pkg (1.7 oz)	210	0	2
Combos				
Cheddar Cheese Cracker	1 pkg (1.7 oz)	250	5	1
Cheddar Cheese Cracker	1 oz	140	5	0
Cheddar Cheese Pretzel	1 oz	130	0	0
Cheddar Cheese Pretzel	1 pkg (1.8 oz)	240	5	1
Chili Cheese w/ Corn Shell	1 oz	140	0	1
Chili Cheese w/ Corn Shell	1 pkg (1.7 oz)	230	5	2
Mustard Pretzel	1 pkg (1.8 oz)	230	0	1
Mustard Pretzel	1 oz	130	0	1
Nacho Cheese Pretzel	1 pkg (1.7 oz)	230	0	1

FOOD	PORTION	CALS	CHOL	FIBER
Nacho Cheese Pretzel	1 oz	130	0	1
Nacho Cheese w/ Tortilla Shell	1 oz	140	0	1
Nacho Cheese w/ Tortilla Shell	1 pkg (1.7 oz)	230	0	1
Peanut Butter Cracker	1 oz	140	0	1
Pepperoni & Cheese Pizza	1 pkg (1.7 oz)	240	5	1
Pepperoni & Cheese Pizza	1 oz	140	5	0
Pizzeria Pretzel	1 pkg (1.8 oz)	230	0	1
Pizzeria Pretzel	1 oz	130	0	1
Tortilla Ranch	1 oz	140	5	1
Tortilla Ranch	1 bag (1.7 oz)	240	5	1
Cornnuts				
Original	1 pkg (2 oz)	260	0	4
Dakota Gourmet				
Amazing Corn Classic	1 pkg (1 oz)	360	0	5
Amazing Corn Cool Ranch	1 pkg (1 oz)	367	2	5
Amazing Corn Mesquite BBQ	1 pkg (1 oz)	369	0	5
Heart Smart Toasted Corn	⅓ cup (1 oz)	110	0	3
Toasted Corn Heart Smart	1 pkg (1.75 oz)	177	0	2
Trail Mix Heart Smart	1 pkg (1.75 oz)	172	0	3
Eden				
Rice Puffs Five Flavor Arare	1 oz	110	0	2
Energy Food Factory				
Poprice Cheddar Cheese	½ oz	60	0	–
Poprice Herb & Garlic	½ oz	50	0	–
Poprice Lite	½ oz	50	0	–
Poprice Original No Salt	½ oz	45	0	–
Frito Lay				
Funyuns	13 (1 oz)	140	0	tr
Munchos	16 (1 oz)	160	0	1
Munchos BBQ	14 (1 oz)	160	0	1

FOOD	PORTION	CALS	CHOL	FIBER
Hapi				
Chili Bits	½ cup (1 oz)	110	0	1
Health Valley				
Cheddar Lites Green Onion	1¾ cups	120	5	1
Cheddar Lites Original	1¾ cups	120	5	1
Corn Puffs Caramel	2 cups	120	0	1
Low Fat Potato Puffs Cheddar Cheese	1½ cups	110	5	1
Low Fat Potato Puffs Garlic w/ Cheese	1½ cups	260	0	1
Low Fat Potato Puffs Zesty Ranch	1½ cups	110	0	1
Innovative Foods				
Roasted Sweet Corn	1 pkg (0.8 oz)	76	0	2
Lance				
Cheese Balls	1 pkg (1 oz)	150	0	0
Crunchy Cheese Twists	1 pkg (1.25 oz)	190	0	0
Gold-N-Chees	1 pkg (1 oz)	130	0	1
Onion Rings	1 pkg (0.9 oz)	100	0	1
Pork Skins	1 pkg (0.4 oz)	65	10	0
Pork Skins BBQ	1 pkg (0.4 oz)	60	10	0
Maranatha				
High Energy Mix	¼ cup	120	0	2
Organic Harvest Mix	¼ cup	150	0	2
Organic Nature Mix	¼ cup	150	0	2
Snack Attack Mix	¼ cup	140	0	2
Tail Mix Organic Raw	¼ cup	140	0	2
Trail Mix Deluxe	¼ cup	150	0	2
Trail Mix Navajo	¼ cup	140	0	4
Trail Mix Olympic w/ Chocolate	¼ cup	140	0	2
Trail Mix Organic Delight	¼ cup	150	0	2
Mr. Peanut				
Peanut Butter Crisps Graham	12 pieces (1.1 oz)	150	0	2
Old Dutch Foods				
Baked Cheese Curls	2 cups (1.1 oz)	180	0	tr
Cheese Puffcorn Curls	2 cups (1.1 oz)	170	0	0

FOOD	PORTION	CALS	CHOL	FIBER
Pita Puffs				
Barbeque	35 (1 oz)	120	0	1
Lowfat Garlic	35 (1 oz)	110	0	1
Lowfat Original	35 (1 oz)	110	0	1
Lowfat Salsa	35 (1 oz)	110	0	1
Pizza	35 (1 oz)	120	0	1
Ranch	35 (1 oz)	120	0	1
Planters				
Cheez Balls	1 oz	150	2	1
Cheez Balls	1 pkg (1 oz)	150	2	1
Cheez Curls	1 pkg (1.2 oz)	190	2	1
Cheez Mania Original	42 pieces (1 oz)	150	<5	1
Heat Snack Mix	1 oz	140	0	2
Pumpkorn				
Caramel	⅓ cup	150	0	2
Chili	⅓ cup	150	0	2
Curry	⅓ cup	150	0	2
Maple Vanilla	⅓ cup	150	0	2
Mesquite	⅓ cup	150	0	2
Original	⅓ cup	150	0	2
Robert's American Gourmet				
Pirate's Booty Puffed Rice & Corn w/ Cheddar	1 oz	120	0	4
Rold Gold				
Snack Mix Colossal Cheddar	1 pkg (1 oz)	140	0	1
Snyder's Of Hanover				
Cheese Twists	1 oz	230	0	0
Fried Pork Skins	1 oz	80	30	0
Fried Pork Skins Barbecue	1 oz	80	20	0
Kruncheez	1.25 oz	200	0	tr
Onion Toasters	1 oz	188	0	tr
Utz				
Caramel Corn Clusters	1⅛ cups (1 oz)	120	0	tr
Cheese Balls	50 (1 oz)	150	0	tr
Cheese Curls	18 (1 oz)	150	0	tr
Cheese Curls Crunchy	30 (1 oz)	160	0	0

FOOD	PORTION	CALS	CHOL	FIBER
Cheese Curls Reduced Fat	32 (1 oz)	140	<5	2
Onion Rings	41 (1 oz)	140	0	0
Party Mix	¾ cup (1 oz)	140	0	1
Pork Cracklins	0.5 oz	90	15	—
Pork Cracklins Hot & Spicy	0.5 oz	80	15	—
Pork Rinds	0.5 oz	80	15	—
Pork Rinds BBQ	0.5 oz	80	15	—
Weight Watchers				
Cheese Curls	1 pkg (0.5 oz)	70	0	0
SNAIL				
cooked	3 oz	233	110	—
raw	3 oz	117	55	—
TAKE-OUT				
escargot cooked	5	25	15	0
SNAPPER				
cooked	3 oz	109	40	—
cooked	1 fillet (6 oz)	217	80	—
raw	3 oz	85	31	—
SODA				
club	12 oz	0	0	—
cola	12 oz	151	0	—
cream	12 oz	191	0	—
diet cola	12 oz	2	0	—
diet cola w/ equal	12 oz	2	0	—
diet cola w/ saccharin	12 oz	2	0	—
ginger ale	12 oz can	124	0	—
grape	12 oz	161	0	—
lemon lime	12 oz	149	0	—
orange	12 oz	177	0	—
pepper type	12 oz	151	0	—
quinine	12 oz	125	0	—
root beer	12 oz	152	0	—
tonic water	12 oz	125	0	—
7 Up				
Diet	8 oz	0	0	—
Original	1 can	140	0	—

FOOD	PORTION	CALS	CHOL	FIBER
A & W				
Root Beer	1 can (12 oz)	170	0	–
After The Fall				
Raspberry Ginger Ale	1 can (12 oz)	150	0	0
Barrelhead				
Root Beer	8 fl oz	110	0	0
Barritts				
Ginger Beer	1 bottle (12 oz)	200	0	–
Best Health				
Root Beer	1 bottle (12 oz)	165	0	–
Vanilla Cream	1 bottle (12 oz)	170	0	–
Burst				
Cola Strawberry	8 fl oz	117	0	–
Canada Dry				
Birch Beer Brown	8 fl oz	110	0	0
Birch Beer Clear	8 fl oz	110	0	0
Black Cherry Wishniak	8 fl oz	130	0	0
Cactus Cooler	8 fl oz	110	0	0
California Strawberry	8 fl oz	110	0	0
Club	8 fl oz	0	0	0
Club Sodium Free	8 fl oz	0	0	0
Concord Grape	8 fl oz	120	0	0
Diet Ginger Ale	8 fl oz	0	0	0
Diet Ginger Ale Cherry	8 fl oz	0	0	0
Diet Ginger Ale Cranberry	8 fl oz	0	0	0
Diet Ginger Ale Lemon	8 fl oz	5	0	0
Diet Tonic Water	8 fl oz	0	0	0
Diet Tonic Water Twist Of Lime	8 fl oz	0	0	0
Ginger Ale	1 can (12 oz)	140	0	0
Ginger Ale Cherry	8 fl oz	110	0	0
Ginger Ale Cranberry	8 fl oz	100	0	0
Ginger Ale Golden	8 fl oz	100	0	0
Ginger Ale Lemon	8 fl oz	100	0	0
Half & Half	8 fl oz	110	0	0
Hi-Spot	8 fl oz	110	0	0
Island Lime	8 fl oz	140	0	0
Jamaica Cola	8 fl oz	110	0	0
Lemon Sour	8 fl oz	100	0	0

FOOD	PORTION	CALS	CHOL	FIBER
Peach	8 fl oz	120	0	0
Pina Pineapple	8 fl oz	110	0	0
Seltzer	8 fl oz	0	0	0
Seltzer Cherry	8 fl oz	0	0	0
Seltzer Cranberry Lime	8 fl oz	0	0	0
Seltzer Grapefruit	8 fl oz	0	0	0
Seltzer Lemon Lime	8 fl oz	0	0	0
Seltzer Mandarin Orange	8 fl oz	0	0	0
Seltzer Peach	8 fl oz	0	0	0
Seltzer Raspberry	8 fl oz	0	0	0
Seltzer Strawberry	8 fl oz	0	0	0
Seltzer Tropical	8 fl oz	0	0	0
Sunripe Orange	8 fl oz	140	0	0
Tahitian Treat	8 fl oz	150	0	0
Tonic Water	8 fl oz	90	0	0
Tonic Water Twist Of Lime	8 fl oz	100	0	0
Vanilla Cream	8 fl oz	120	0	0
Vichy Water	8 fl oz	0	0	0
Wild Cherry	8 fl oz	110	0	0
Clearly Canadian				
Soda	8 fl oz	0	0	—
Coca-Cola				
Cherry	8 fl oz	104	0	—
Classic	1 can (12 oz)	140	0	—
Classic Caffeine-Free	8 fl oz	97	0	—
Coke II	8 fl oz	105	0	—
Diet	1 can (12 oz)	0	0	—
Diet Cherry	8 fl oz	1	0	—
Diet Coke Caffeine-free	8 fl oz	1	0	—
Cott				
Cola	8 fl oz	110	0	0
Ginger Ale	8 fl oz	90	0	0
Grape	8 fl oz	130	0	0
Orange	8 fl oz	140	0	0
Pineapple	8 fl oz	130	0	0
Punch	8 fl oz	130	0	0
Seltzer	8 fl oz	0	0	0

FOOD	PORTION	CALS	CHOL	FIBER
Crush				
Cherry	8 fl oz	140	0	0
Grape	8 fl oz	110	0	0
Orange	8 fl oz	140	0	0
Orange Diet	8 fl oz	0	0	0
Pineapple	8 fl oz	140	0	0
Tropical Fruit Punch	1 bottle (10 fl oz)	180	0	0
Tropical Fruit Punch	1 can (11.5 fl oz)	200	0	–
Diet Rite				
Black Cherry Salt/Sodium Free	8 fl oz	2	0	–
Cola	8 fl oz	1	0	–
Cola Caffeine/ Sugar Free	8 fl oz	1	0	–
Cola Salt/Sodium Free	8 fl oz	1	0	–
Fruit Punch Salt/Sodium Free	8 fl oz	2	0	–
Golden Peach Salt/Sodium Free	8 fl oz	2	0	–
Key Lime Salt/Sodium Free	8 fl oz	7	0	–
Pink Grapefruit Salt/Sodium Free	8 fl oz	2	0	–
Red Raspberry Salt/Sodium Free	8 fl oz	3	0	–
Tangerine Salt/Sodium Free	8 fl oz	2	0	–
White Grape Salt/Sodium Free	8 fl oz	1	0	–
Dr Pepper				
Diet	1 oz	tr	0	–
Original	1 can (12 oz)	150	0	–
Dr. Nehi				
Soda	8 fl oz	100	0	–
Fanta				
Ginger Ale	8 fl oz	86	0	–
Grape	8 fl oz	117	0	–
Orange	8 fl oz	118	0	–
Root Beer	8 fl oz	111	0	–

FOOD	PORTION	CALS	CHOL	FIBER
Fresca				
Soda	8 fl oz	3	0	—
Hansen's				
Black Cherry	8 fl oz	110	0	—
Diet All Flavors	1 can	0	0	—
Ginger Beer	8 fl oz	100	0	—
Natural Black Cherry	1 can	160	0	—
Natural Cherry Vanilla	1 can	140	0	—
Natural Creamy Rootbeer	1 can	160	0	—
Natural Ginger Ale	1 can	140	0	—
Natural Grapefruit	1 can	130	0	—
Natural Key Lime	1 can	130	0	—
Natural Kiwi Strawberry	1 can	130	0	—
Natural Mandarin Lime	1 can	130	0	—
Natural Orange Mango	1 can	170	0	—
Natural Raspberry	1 can	130	0	—
Natural Tangerine	1 can	160	0	—
Natural Tropical Passion	1 can	160	0	—
Natural Vanilla Cola	1 can	140	0	—
Orange Creme	8 fl oz	110	0	—
Sangria	8 fl oz	110	0	—
Sarsaparilla	8 fl oz	110	0	—
Sparkling Orangeade	8 fl oz	100	0	—
Vanilla Creme	8 fl oz	110	0	—
Health Valley				
Ginger Ale	1 bottle	160	0	0
Rootbeer Old Fashioned	1 bottle	160	0	0
Sarsaparilla Rootbeer	1 bottle	160	0	0
Hires				
Cream	8 fl oz	130	0	0
Cream Soda Diet	8 fl oz	0	0	0
Original Mocha	8 fl oz	100	0	0
Original Mocha Diet	8 fl oz	5	0	0
Root Beer	8 fl oz	130	0	0
Root Beer Diet	8 fl oz	0	0	0
IBC				
Root Beer	1 can	160	0	—
Kick				
Soda	8 fl oz	120	0	—

FOOD	PORTION	CALS	CHOL	FIBER
Like				
Cola	1 oz	13	0	–
Lucozade				
Soda	7 oz	136	0	0
Mello Yellow				
Diet	8 fl oz	4	0	–
Soda	8 fl oz	119	0	–
Mountain Dew				
Diet	8 fl oz	2	0	–
Soda	8 fl oz	118	0	–
Mr. PiBB				
Diet	8 fl oz	1	0	–
Soda	6 oz	97	0	–
Mug				
Cream	8 fl oz	122	0	–
Diet Cream	8 fl oz	2	0	–
Diet Root Beer	8 fl oz	1	0	–
Root Beer	8 fl oz	141	0	–
Nehi				
Cream	8 fl oz	120	0	–
Fruit Punch	8 fl oz	120	0	–
Ginger Ale	8 fl oz	90	0	–
Grape	8 fl oz	120	0	–
Orange	8 fl oz	130	0	–
Peach	8 fl oz	130	0	–
Pineapple	8 fl oz	130	0	–
Quinine Water	8 fl oz	90	0	–
Root Beer	8 fl oz	120	0	–
Strawberry	8 fl oz	120	0	–
Wild Red	8 fl oz	120	0	–
Old Colony				
Grape	8 fl oz	140	0	0
Pennsylvania Dutch				
Birch Beer	8 fl oz	110	0	–
Pepsi				
Blue Berry Cola Fusion	8 fl oz	100	0	–
Caffeine Free	8 fl oz	105	0	–
Diet	1 can (12 oz)	0	0	–
Diet Caffeine Free	8 fl oz	1	0	–
Regular	1 can (12 oz)	150	0	–

FOOD	PORTION	CALS	CHOL	FIBER
Ramblin' Root Beer				
Ramblin' Root Beer	8 fl oz	120	0	–
Razing Razberry				
Cola	8 fl oz	117	0	–
Royal Crown				
Caffeine Free Cola	8 fl oz	110	0	–
Cherry	8 fl oz	110	0	–
Cola	8 fl oz	100	0	–
Diet	8 fl oz	1	0	–
Diet Caffeine Free	8 fl oz	1	0	–
Diet Cranberry Apple Salt/Sodium Free	8 fl oz	2	0	–
Diet Cranberry Salt/Sodium Free	8 fl oz	2	0	–
Saranac				
Diet Root Beer	1 bottle (12 oz)	35	0	–
Ginger Beer	1 bottle (12 oz)	160	0	–
Root Beer	1 bottle (12 oz)	180	0	–
Schweppes				
Bitter Lemon	8 fl oz	110	0	0
Club	8 fl oz	0	0	0
Club Sodium Free	8 fl oz	0	0	0
Diet Ginger Ale	8 fl oz	0	0	0
Diet Ginger Ale Dry Grape	8 fl oz	2	0	0
Diet Ginger Ale Raspberry	8 fl oz	0	0	0
Ginger Ale	8 fl oz	90	0	0
Ginger Ale Dry Grape	8 fl oz	100	0	0
Ginger Ale Raspberry	8 fl oz	100	0	0
Ginger Beer	8 fl oz	100	0	0
Grape	8 fl oz	130	0	0
Grapefruit	8 fl oz	110	0	0
Lemon Sour	8 fl oz	110	0	0
Lemon-Lime	8 fl oz	100	0	0
Seltzer Black Berry	8 fl oz	0	0	0
Seltzer Lemon	8 fl oz	0	0	0
Seltzer Lemon Lime	8 fl oz	0	0	0
Seltzer Lime	8 fl oz	0	0	0
Seltzer Orange	8 fl oz	0	0	0

FOOD	PORTION	CALS	CHOL	FIBER
Seltzer Peaches & Cream	8 fl oz	0	0	0
Seltzer Raspberry	8 fl oz	0	0	0
Tonic Citrus	8 fl oz	90	0	0
Tonic Cranberry	8 fl oz	90	0	0
Tonic Raspberry	8 fl oz	90	0	0
Tonic Water Diet	8 fl oz	0	0	0
Shasta				
Black Cherry	1 can (12 oz)	170	0	0
Caffeine Free Cola	1 can (12 oz)	160	0	–
Cherry Cola	1 can (12 oz)	160	0	–
Club Soda	1 can (12 oz)	0	0	–
Cola	1 can (12 oz)	170	0	0
Creme	1 can (12 oz)	190	0	0
Diet Black Cherry	1 can (12 oz)	0	0	0
Diet Caffeine Free Cola	1 can (12 oz)	0	0	0
Diet Cherry Cola	1 can (12 oz)	0	0	0
Diet Cola	1 can (12 oz)	0	0	0
Diet Creme	1 can (12 oz)	0	0	0
Diet Doc Shasta	1 can (12 oz)	0	0	0
Diet Ginger Ale	1 can (12 oz)	0	0	0
Diet Grape	1 can (12 oz)	0	0	0
Diet Grapefruit	1 can (12 oz)	0	0	0
Diet Grapefruit	1 can (12 oz)	0	0	0
Diet Kiwi-Strawberry	1 can (12 oz)	0	0	0
Diet Lemon-Lime Twist	1 can (12 oz)	0	0	0
Diet Orange	1 can (12 oz)	0	0	0
Diet Pineapple-Orange	1 can (12 oz)	0	0	0
Diet Raspberry Creme	1 can (12 oz)	0	0	0
Diet Red Pop	1 can (12 oz)	0	0	0
Diet Root Beer	1 can (12 oz)	0	0	0
Diet Strawberry	1 can (12 oz)	0	0	0
Diet Strawberry-Peach	1 can (12 oz)	0	0	0
Doc Shasta	1 can (12 oz)	160	0	0
Fruit Punch	1 can (12 oz)	200	0	0
Ginger Ale	1 can (12 oz)	130	0	0
Grape	1 can (12 oz)	190	0	0
Kiwi-Strawberry	1 can (12 oz)	170	0	0
Lemon-Lime Twist	1 can (12 oz)	150	0	0
Moon Mist	1 can (12 oz)	180	0	0

FOOD	PORTION	CALS	CHOL	FIBER
Orange	1 can (12 oz)	200	0	0
Peach	1 can (12 oz)	170	0	0
Pineapple	1 can (12 oz)	200	0	0
Pineapple-Orange	1 can (12 oz)	180	0	0
Quinine/Tonic	1 can (12 oz)	130	0	0
Raspberry Creme	1 can (12 oz)	170	0	0
Red Pop	1 can (12 oz)	170	0	0
Root Beer	1 can (12 oz)	170	0	0
Strawberry	1 can (12 oz)	190	0	0
Strawberry-Peach	1 can (12 oz)	170	0	0
Slice				
Diet Lemon Lime	8 fl oz	5	0	—
Diet Mandarin	8 fl oz	5	0	—
Lemon Lime	8 fl oz	100	0	—
Mandarin Orange	8 fl oz	128	0	—
Red	8 fl oz	128	0	—
Snapple				
Amazin' Grape	8 fl oz	120	0	—
Cherry Lime Ricky	8 fl oz	110	0	—
Creme D'Vanilla	8 fl oz	130	0	—
French Cherry	8 fl oz	120	0	—
Kiwi Peach	8 fl oz	120	0	—
Kiwi Strawberry	8 fl oz	130	0	—
Mango Madness	8 fl oz	130	0	—
Passion Supreme	8 fl oz	120	0	—
Peach Melba	8 fl oz	120	0	—
Raspberry	8 fl oz	120	0	—
Seltzer Black Cherry	8 fl oz	0	0	—
Seltzer Lemon Lime	8 fl oz	0	0	—
Seltzer Original	8 fl oz	0	0	—
Seltzer Tangerine	8 fl oz	0	0	—
Tru Root Beer	8 fl oz	110	0	—
Sprite				
Diet	8 fl oz	3	0	—
Soda	8 fl oz	100	0	—
Stewart's				
Root Beer	1 bottle (12 oz)	160	0	—
Sundrop				
Cherry	8 fl oz	130	0	0
Diet	8 fl oz	5	0	0

FOOD	PORTION	CALS	CHOL	FIBER
Soda	8 fl oz	140	0	0
Sunkist				
Cactus Cooler	8 fl oz	110	0	0
Cherry	8 fl oz	140	0	0
Diet Citrus	8 fl oz	0	0	0
Diet Orange	8 fl oz	5	0	0
Fruit Punch	8 fl oz	130	0	0
Orange	1 can	190	0	0
Peach	8 fl oz	120	0	0
Pineapple	8 fl oz	140	0	0
Strawberry	8 fl oz	140	0	0
TAB				
Soda	8 fl oz	1	0	—
Tropical Chill				
Cola	8 fl oz	117	0	—
Diet	8 fl oz	1	0	—
Upper 10				
Diet	8 fl oz	3	0	—
Diet Salt/Sodium Free	8 fl oz	3	0	—
Salt Free	8 fl oz	100	0	—
Soda	8 fl oz	100	0	—
Wink				
Diet	8 fl oz	5	0	0
Soda	8 fl oz	130	0	0
Yoo-Hoo				
Original	9 fl oz	150	0	tr
SOLE				
cooked	3 oz	99	58	—
cooked	1 fillet (4.5 oz)	148	86	—
raw	3.5 oz	90	50	—
Van De Kamp's				
Lightly Breaded Fillets	1 (4 oz)	220	40	0
Natural Fillets	1 (4 oz)	110	50	0
TAKE-OUT				
battered & fried	3.2 oz	211	31	—
breaded & fried	3.2 oz	211	31	—
SORGHUM				
sorghum	1 cup (6.7 oz)	651	0	—

FOOD	PORTION	CALS	CHOL	FIBER
SOUFFLE				
lemon chilled	1 cup	176	2	—
raspberry chilled	1 cup	173	3	—
spinach	1 cup	218	184	—
SOUP				
CANNED				
Select Italian Style Wedding	1 cup	120	10	2
asparagus cream of as prep w/ milk	1 cup	161	22	—
asparagus cream of as prep w/ water	1 cup	87	5	—
beef broth ready-to-serve	1 can (14 oz)	27	1	—
beef broth ready-to-serve	1 cup	16	tr	—
beef noodle as prep w/ water	1 cup	84	5	—
black bean turtle soup	1 cup	218	0	—
black bean as prep w/ water	1 cup	116	0	—
celery cream of as prep w/ milk	1 cup	165	32	—
celery cream of as prep w/ water	1 cup	90	15	—
celery cream of not prep	1 can (10¾ oz)	219	34	—
cheese as prep w/ milk	1 cup	230	48	—
cheese as prep w/ water	1 cup	155	30	—
cheese not prep	1 can (11 oz)	377	72	—
chicken broth as prep w/ water	1 cup	39	1	—
chicken cream of as prep w/ milk	1 cup	191	27	—
chicken cream of as prep w/ water	1 cup	116	10	—
chicken gumbo as prep w/ water	1 cup	56	5	—

FOOD	PORTION	CALS	CHOL	FIBER
chicken noodle as prep w/ water	1 cup	75	7	–
chicken rice as prep w/ water	1 cup	251	7	–
clam chowder manhattan as prep w/ water	1 cup	77	3	–
clam chowder new england as prep w/ water	1 cup	95	5	–
clam chowder new england as prep w/ milk	1 cup	163	22	–
consomme w/ gelatin not prep	1 can (10½ oz)	71	0	–
consomme w/ gelatin as prep w/ water	1 cup	29	0	–
escarole ready-to-serve	1 cup	27	2	–
french onion as prep w/ water	1 cup	57	0	–
gazpacho ready-to-serve	1 cup	57	0	–
minestrone as prep w/water	1 cup	83	2	–
mushroom cream of as prep w/ milk	1 cup	203	20	–
mushroom cream of as prep w/ water	1 cup	129	2	–
oyster stew as prep w/ milk	1 cup	134	32	–
oyster stew as prep w/ water	1 cup	59	14	–
pepperpot as prep w/ water	1 cup	103	10	–
potato cream of as prep w/ milk	1 cup	148	22	–
potato cream of as prep w/ water	1 cup	73	5	–

FOOD	PORTION	CALS	CHOL	FIBER
scotch broth as prep w/ water	1 cup	80	5	–
split pea w/ ham as prep w/ water	1 cup	189	8	–
tomato as prep w/ milk	1 cup	160	17	–
tomato as prep w/ water	1 cup	86	0	–
vegetarian vegetable as prep w/ water	1 cup	72	0	–
vichyssoise	1 cup	148	22	–
Amy's				
Organic Barley	1 cup	50	0	2
Organic Black Bean Vegetable	1 cup	110	0	5
Organic Cream Of Mushroom	1 cup	120	5	2
Organic Cream Of Tomato	1 cup	100	10	4
Organic Lentil	1 cup	130	0	9
Organic Minestrone	1 cup	90	0	3
Organic No Chicken Noodle Soup	1 cup	90	0	2
Organic Vegetable	1 cup	35	0	1
Boston Market				
Chicken Broth Reduced Sodium	1 cup	15	0	0
Butterball				
Chicken Broth Reduced Sodium 99% Fat Free	1 cup	10	0	0
Campbell's				
98% Fat Free Cream Of Chicken as prep	1 cup	80	10	0
Bean With Bacon as prep	1 cup	168	3	8
Beef Barley as prep	1 cup	81	10	2
Cheddar Cheese	1 cup	100	10	1
Cheddar Cheese as prep	1 cup	134	19	1
Chicken Vegetable as prep	1 cup	74	9	1
Chicken & Pasta With Garden Vegetables	1 cup (8.4 oz)	90	5	1
Chicken Gumbo as prep	1 cup	55	5	1

FOOD	PORTION	CALS	CHOL	FIBER
Chunky Savory Chicken w/ White & Wild Rice	1 cup	140	25	2
Chunky Classic Chicken Noodle	1 cup (8.4 oz)	130	20	1
Clam Chowder New England as prep	1 cup	89	3	1
Classic Chicken Noodle	1 cup	80	15	1
Classic Chicken Rice	1 cup (8.4 oz)	80	5	1
Classics Beef Noodle	1 cup	70	15	1
Consomme as prep	1 cup	24	tr	tr
Cream Of Asparagus as prep	1 cup	72	2	1
Cream Of Mushroom as prep	1 cup	108	2	2
Cream Of Celery as prep	1 cup	107	2	1
Cream Of Chicken as prep	1 cup	120	10	1
Cream Of Potato as prep	1 cup	102	7	1
Fiesta Tomato as prep	1 cup	72	1	1
Garden Vegetable as prep	1 cup	69	3	1
Green Pea as prep	1 cup	173	1	4
Healthy Request Chicken Noodle as prep	1 cup	70	15	0
Healthy Request Chicken Rice as prep	1 cup	60	10	tr
Healthy Request Cream Of Mushroom as prep	1 cup	66	4	1
Healthy Request Cream Of Chicken & Broccoli as prep	1 cup	78	6	1
Healthy Request Cream Of Chicken as prep	1 cup	70	10	tr
Healthy Request Hearty Pasta w/ Vegetables	1 cup	87	1	2
Healthy Request Tomato as prep	1 cup	91	1	2
Healthy Request Vegetable as prep	1 cup	84	1	2

FOOD	PORTION	CALS	CHOL	FIBER
Home Cookin' Chicken Vegetable	1 cup (8.4 oz)	130	10	3
Home Cookin' Chicken Rice	1 cup	110	10	2
Home Cookin' Chicken With Egg Noodles	1 cup (8.4 oz)	90	15	1
Home Cookin' Oriental Noodles w/ Vegetables	1 cup (8.4 oz)	100	10	3
Italian Tomato as prep	1 cup	105	1	4
Low Sodium Chicken Broth	1 can (10.75 oz)	27	2	tr
Low Sodium Chicken w/ Noodles	1 can (10.75 oz)	162	40	2
Low Sodium Chunky Vegetable Beef	1 can (10.75 oz)	159	39	3
Low Sodium Cream of Mushroom	1 can (10.75 oz)	200	12	2
Low Sodium Green Pea	1 can (10.75 oz)	235	4	6
Low Sodium Tomato w/ Pieces	1 can (10.75 oz)	170	6	3
Minestrone as prep	1 cup	81	1	2
Ready To Serve Bean w/Bacon 'N Ham	1 can (10.5 oz)	274	13	11
Ready To Serve Chicken Noodle	1 cup	80	15	1
Ready To Serve Chicken w/ Rice	1 can (10.5 oz)	122	11	2
Ready-To-Serve Vegetable Beef	1 can (10.5 oz)	143	10	5
Savory Tomato & Dill as prep	1 cup	99	tr	2
Select Chicken & Pasta With Roasted Garlic	1 cup (8.4 oz)	100	10	2
Select Chicken Rice	1 cup	110	10	2
Select Fiesta Vegetable	1 cup (8.4 oz)	120	0	3
Select Herbed Chicken w/ Roasted Vegetables	1 cup	90	15	1
Select Mushroom w/ White & Wild Rice	1 cup	90	0	2

FOOD	PORTION	CALS	CHOL	FIBER
Select Roasted Chicken w/ Rotini & Penne Pasta	1 cup	110	10	1
Select Rosemary Chicken w/ Roasted Potatoes	1 cup	110	10	2
Select Split Pea w/ Ham	1 cup (8.4 oz)	170	10	6
Select Tuscany-Style Minestrone	1 cup (8.4 oz)	190	5	5
Simply Home Chicken Noodle	1 cup (8.4 oz)	80	10	1
Simply Home Chicken w/ Rice	1 cup (8.4 oz)	100	5	1
Soup At Hand Blended Vegetable Medley	1 pkg (10.75 oz)	110	10	4
Tomato as prep	1 cup	80	0	2
Vegetable Beef as prep	1 cup	68	8	2
Vegetarian Vegetable as prep	1 cup	79	0	2
Gold's				
Russian Borscht	8 oz	70	0	2
Health Valley				
5 Bean Vegetable	1 cup	250	0	10
Beef Broth Fat Free	1 cup	20	0	0
Beef Broth Fat Free No Salt	1 cup	20	0	0
Black Bean & Vegetable	1 cup	110	0	9
Chicken Broth	1 cup	45	25	0
Chicken Broth Fat Free	1 cup	30	0	0
Chicken Broth No Salt	1 cup	45	25	0
Country Corn & Vegetable	1 cup	70	0	7
Garden Vegetable	1 cup	80	0	4
Italian Plus Carotene	1 cup	80	0	6
Lentil & Carrot	1 cup	100	0	10
Organic Black Bean	1 cup	110	0	10
Organic Lentil No Salt	1 cup	90	0	9
Organic Minestrone	1 cup	100	0	8
Organic Mushroom Barley No Salt	1 cup	60	0	5

FOOD	PORTION	CALS	CHOL	FIBER
Organic Potato Leek	1 cup	70	0	3
Organic Potato Leek No Salt	1 cup	70	0	3
Organic Split Pea	1 cup	110	0	8
Organic Split Pea No Salt	1 cup	110	0	8
Organic Tomato	1 cup	90	0	4
Organic Vegetable No Salt	1 cup	80	0	6
Pasta Bolognese	1 cup	100	0	4
Pasta Cacciatore	1 cup	100	0	4
Pasta Romano	1 cup	100	0	4
Real Italian Minestrone	1 cup	90	0	8
Rotini & Vegetable	1 cup	100	0	4
Split Pea & Carrots	1 cup	110	0	4
Super Broccoli Carotene	1 cup	70	0	7
Tomato Vegetable	1 cup	80	0	5
Vegetable Barley	1 cup	90	0	4
Vegetable Power Carotene	1 cup	70	0	6
Healthy Choice				
Bean & Ham	1 cup (8.7 oz)	166	4	7
Beef & Potato	1 cup (8.5 oz)	116	5	tr
Broccoli Cheddar	1 cup (8.4 oz)	116	4	2
Chicken Corn Chowder	1 cup (8.8 oz)	176	8	2
Chicken Pasta	1 cup (8.6 oz)	119	6	1
Chicken Rice	1 cup (8.4 oz)	119	6	3
Chili Beef	1 cup (9.1 oz)	189	12	5
Clam Chowder	1 cup (8.8 oz)	123	12	2
Classic Italian Bean and Pasta	1 cup (8 oz)	100	0	3
Country Vegetable	1 cup (8.6 oz)	112	0	3
Cream Of Mushroom	1 cup (8.8 oz)	77	tr	1
Cream Of Celery as prep	1 cup	73	3	3
Cream Of Chicken Vegetable	1 cup (8.9 oz)	127	10	1
Cream Of Roasted Chicken as prep	1 cup	80	4	3
Cream Of Roasted Garlic as prep	1 cup	57	2	3

FOOD	PORTION	CALS	CHOL	FIBER
Garden Tomato Herbs as prep	1 cup	80	0	3
Garden Vegetable	1 cup (8.6 oz)	108	tr	6
Hearty Chicken	1 cup (8.7 oz)	136	21	3
Lentil	1 cup (8.7 oz)	135	tr	5
Minestrone	1 cup (8.6 oz)	107	1	5
Old Fashion Chicken Noodle	1 cup (8.8 oz)	137	9	1
Split Pea & Ham	1 cup (8.8 oz)	164	7	5
Tomato Garden	1 cup (8.6 oz)	101	1	5
Turkey Wild Rice	1 cup (8.4 oz)	72	3	3
Vegetable Beef	1 cup (8.8 oz)	96	2	2
Herb-Ox				
Beef Liquid	2 tsp (0.4 oz)	20	0	0
Chicken Liquid	2 tsp (0.4 oz)	15	0	0
Imagine				
Creamy Broccoli	1 serv (8 oz)	70	0	2
Creamy Butternut Squash	1 serv (8 oz)	120	0	2
Creamy Mushroom	1 serv (8 oz)	80	0	2
Creamy Potato Leek	1 serv (8 oz)	90	0	2
Creamy Sweet Corn	1 serv (8 oz)	100	0	1
Creamy Tomato	1 serv (8 oz)	90	0	2
Vegetable Broth	1 serv (8 oz)	45	0	1
Zesty Gazpacho	1 serv (8 oz)	80	0	tr
Natural Choice				
Orangic Vegan Classic Tomato	1 cup	100	0	2
Organic Vegan Classic Mushroom	1 cup	50	0	2
Organic Vegan Country Corn	1 cup	100	0	3
Organic Vegan Kabocha Squash	1 cup	60	0	1
Organic Vegan Southern Greens	1 cup	80	0	2
Organic Vegan Split Pea	1 cup	120	0	7
Organic Vegan Vegetable Curry	1 cup	110	0	2

FOOD	PORTION	CALS	CHOL	FIBER
Old El Paso				
Black Bean w/ Bacon	1 cup (8.6 oz)	160	5	7
Chicken Vegetable	1 cup (8.4 oz)	110	15	0
Chicken w/ Rice	1 cup (8.4 oz)	90	15	0
Garden Vegetable	1 cup (8.4 oz)	110	<5	0
Hearty Beef	1 cup (8.4 oz)	120	25	0
Hearty Chicken Noodle	1 cup (8.4 oz)	110	25	0
Pacific				
Free Range Organic Chicken Broth	1 cup	5	0	–
Pritikin				
Chicken & Rice	1 cup (8.8 oz)	80	5	–
Chicken Broth	1 cup (8.5 oz)	15	0	–
Chicken Pasta	1 cup (8.6 oz)	100	5	–
Hearty Vegetable	1 cup (8.8 oz)	90	0	–
Lentil	1 cup (8.4 oz)	130	0	–
Minestrone	1 cup (8.8 oz)	90	0	–
Split Pea	1 cup (9.2 oz)	140	0	–
Three Bean Chili	½ cup (4.5 oz)	90	0	–
Vegetable Broth	1 cup (8.3 oz)	20	0	–
Vegetarian Vegetables	1 cup (9 oz)	100	0	–
Progresso				
99% Fat Free Beef Barley	1 cup (8.5 oz)	140	20	3
99% Fat Free Beef Vegetable	1 cup (8.5 oz)	160	10	3
99% Fat Free Chicken Noodle	1 cup (8.3 oz)	90	20	1
99% Fat Free Chicken Rice w/ Vegetables	1 cup (8.4 oz)	110	10	1
99% Fat Free Creamy Mushroom Chicken	1 cup (8.3 oz)	90	10	1
99% Fat Free Lentil	1 cup (8.5 oz)	130	0	6
99% Fat Free Minestrone	1 cup (8.5 oz)	130	0	4
99% Fat Free Roasted Chicken w/ Italian Style Vegetable	1 cup (8 oz)	90	10	1
99% Fat Free Split Pea	1 cup (8.9 oz)	170	0	5

FOOD	PORTION	CALS	CHOL	FIBER
99% Fat Free Tomato Garden Vegetable	1 cup (8.6 oz)	100	0	2
99% Fat Free Vegetable	1 cup (8.4 oz)	70	0	2
99% Fat Free White Cheddar Potato	1 cup (8.6 oz)	140	5	2
Basil Rotini Tomato	1 cup (8.9 oz)	120	<5	2
Bean & Ham	1 cup (8.4 oz)	160	10	8
Beef Barley	1 cup (8.5 oz)	130	25	3
Beef Minestrone	1 cup (8.5 oz)	140	10	3
Beef Noodle	1 cup (8.5 oz)	140	30	1
Beef Vegetable & Rotini	1 cup (8.4 oz)	130	25	4
Cheese & Herb Tortellini Tomato	1 cup (8.6 oz)	140	<5	2
Chickarina	1 cup (8.3 oz)	130	20	tr
Chicken Minestrone	1 cup (8.4 oz)	110	15	2
Chicken Vegetable	1 cup (8.4 oz)	90	15	2
Chicken & Wild Rice	1 cup (8.4 oz)	100	15	1
Chicken Barley	1 cup (8.5 oz)	110	15	3
Chicken Broth	1 cup (8.2 oz)	20	0	0
Chicken Noodle	1 cup (8.4 oz)	90	25	tr
Chicken Rice w/ Vegetable	1 cup (8.4 oz)	90	10	1
Clam & Rotini Chowder	1 cup (8.8 oz)	190	10	0
Escarole In Chicken Broth	1 cup (8.1 oz)	25	<5	1
Green Split Pea	1 cup (8.6 oz)	170	5	5
Hearty Black Bean	1 cup (8.5 oz)	170	<5	10
Hearty Penne In Chicken Broth	1 cup (8.4 oz)	80	0	tr
Hearty Tomato	1 cup (8.7 oz)	100	0	1
Herb Rotini Vegetable	1 cup (9.1 oz)	120	0	4
Homestyle Chicken w/ Vegetable	1 cup (8.4 oz)	90	15	tr
Italian Herb Shells Minestrone	1 cup (9.1 oz)	120	0	4
Lentil	1 cup (8.5 oz)	140	0	7
Macaroni & Bean	1 cup (8.6 oz)	160	<5	6
Manhattan Clam Chowder	1 cup (8.4 oz)	110	10	3
Meatballs & Pasta Pearls	1 cup (8.3 oz)	140	15	0

FOOD	PORTION	CALS	CHOL	FIBER
Minestrone	1 cup (8.4 oz)	120	0	5
Minestrone Parmesan	1 cup (8.3 oz)	100	0	3
New England Clam Chowder	1 cup (8.4 oz)	190	15	1
Oregano Penne Italian Style Vegetable	1 cup (8.7 oz)	90	0	1
Peppercorn Penne Vegetable	1 cup (9.1 oz)	100	0	2
Potato Broccoli & Cheese	1 cup (8.8 oz)	160	<5	1
Potato Ham & Cheese	1 cup (8.6 oz)	170	10	1
Roasted Garlic Pasta Lentil	1 cup (9.3 oz)	120	0	5
Rotisserie Seasoned Chicken	1 cup (8.5 oz)	100	15	2
Spicy Chicken & Penne	1 cup (8.5 oz)	110	15	1
Split Pea w/ Ham	1 cup (8.4 oz)	150	15	5
Tomato	1 cup (8.5 oz)	100	0	1
Tomato Basil	1 cup (8.8 oz)	100	0	1
Tomato Vegetable	1 cup (8.5 oz)	90	0	4
Tortellini In Chicken Broth	1 cup (8.3 oz)	70	10	2
Turkey Noodle	1 cup (8.4 oz)	90	20	tr
Turkey Rice w/ Vegetables	1 cup (8.5 oz)	110	15	1
Vegetable	1 cup (8.4 oz)	90	<5	2
White Meat Roasted Chicken Rotini	1 cup (8.1 oz)	80	15	tr
Swanson				
Beef Broth	1 cup	19	tr	1
Beef Broth Onion Seasoned	1 cup (8.4 oz)	20	0	tr
Chicken Broth 100% Fat Free	1 cup	15	0	–
Chicken Broth Seasoned Italian Herbs	1 cup (8.4 oz)	20	<5	tr
Vegetble Broth	1 cup	19	1	0
Ultra Slim-Fast				
Chicken Alfredo Pasta	1 cup (8.3 oz)	132	10	2

FOOD	PORTION	CALS	CHOL	FIBER
Walnut Acres				
Organic Country Corn Chowder	1 cup (8.8 oz)	150	10	2
Weight Watchers				
Chicken & Rice	1 can (10.5 oz)	110	10	4
Chicken Noodle	1 can (10.5 oz)	150	30	4
Minestrone	1 can (10.5 oz)	130	5	6
Vegetable	1 can (10.5 oz)	130	0	6
FROZEN				
Nature's Entree				
Chowder	1 pkg (12 oz)	230	15	5
Tortellini Minestrone	1 pkg (12 oz)	360	10	5
Tabatchnick				
Barley Mushroom	1 serv (7.5 oz)	70	0	3
Barley Mushroom No Salt Added	1 serv (7.5 oz)	70	0	3
Broccoli Cream Of	1 serv (7.5 oz)	90	5	3
Cabbage	1 serv (7.5 oz)	60	0	2
Chicken w/ Dumplings	1 serv (7.5 oz)	70	20	1
Corn Chowder	1 serv (7.5 oz)	150	5	1
Minestrone	1 serv (7.5 oz)	150	0	10
New England Potato	1 serv (7.5 oz)	150	9	2
New York Chicken	1 serv (7.5 oz)	35	0	0
Old Fashion Potato	1 serv (7.5 oz)	70	0	2
Pea	1 serv (7.5 oz)	180	0	11
Pea No Salt Added	1 serv (7.5 oz)	180	0	11
Spinach Cream Of	1 serv (7.5 oz)	90	5	2
Vegetable	1 serv (7.5 oz)	110	0	4
Vegetable No Salt Added	1 serv (7.5 oz)	110	0	4
Wisconsin Cheddar Vegetable	1 serv (7.5 oz)	140	13	1
Yankee Bean	1 serv (7.5 oz)	160	0	11
MIX				
asparagus cream of as prep w/ water	1 cup	59	tr	—
beef broth	1 pkg (0.2 oz)	14	1	—
beef broth as prep w/ water	1 cup	19	1	—
beef broth cube	1 cube (3.6 g)	6	tr	—

FOOD	PORTION	CALS	CHOL	FIBER
beef broth cube as prep w/ water	1 cup	8	tr	—
celery cream of as prep w/ water	1 cup	63	1	—
chicken broth	1 pkg (0.2 oz)	16	1	—
chicken broth as prep w/ water	1 cup	21	1	—
chicken broth cube	1 cube (4.8 g)	9	1	—
chicken broth cube, as prep w/ water	1 cup	13	1	—
chicken cream of as prep w/ water	1 cup	107	3	—
chicken noodle as prep w/ water	1 cup	53	3	—
french onion not prep	1 pkg (1.4 oz)	115	2	—
leek as prep w/ water	1 cup	71	3	—
onion as prep w/ water	1 cup	28	0	—
tomato as prep w/ water	1 cup	102	1	—
Armour				
Bouillon Cubes Beef	1 (4 g)	5	0	0
Bouillon Cubes Chicken	1 (4 g)	5	0	0
Azumaya				
Thin Cut Noodle	1 cup	120	0	tr
Wide Cut Noodle	1 cup	120	0	tr
Bean Cuisine				
13 Bean Bouillabisse	1 cup	220	0	5
Island Black Bean	1 cup	210	0	7
Lots of Lentil	1 cup	230	0	5
Mesa Maize	1 cup	160	0	6
White Bean Provencal	1 cup	250	0	11
Casbah				
Black Bean	1 pkg (1.7 oz)	170	0	9
Split Pea	1 pkg (2.3 oz)	230	0	10
Sweet Corn Chowder	1 pkg (1.2 oz)	125	0	2
Vegetarian Chili	1 pkg (1.8 oz)	170	0	7
Cup-a-Soup				
Broccoli & Cheese as prep	1 serv (6 oz)	70	5	tr

FOOD	PORTION	CALS	CHOL	FIBER
Chicken Vegetable as prep	1 serv (6 oz)	50	10	0
Chicken Broth as prep	1 serv (6 oz)	20	0	0
Chicken Broth w/ Pasta Fat Free as prep	1 serv (6 oz)	45	0	0
Chicken Noodle as prep	1 serv (6 oz)	50	10	0
Cream Of Chicken as prep	1 serv (6 oz)	70	0	tr
Creamy Chicken Vegetable as prep	1 serv (6 oz)	80	0	tr
Creamy Mushroom as prep	1 serv (6 oz)	60	0	0
Green Pea as prep	1 serv (6 oz)	80	0	3
Hearty Chicken Noodle as prep	1 serv (6 oz)	60	15	0
Ring Noodle as prep	1 serv (6 oz)	50	10	0
Spring Vegetable as prep	1 serv (6 oz)	45	10	tr
Tomato as prep	1 serv (6 oz)	100	5	tr
Goodman's				
Cup Of Soup Beef	1 pkg (1½ cups)	180	45	2
Cup Of Soup Chicken Noodle	1 pkg (1½ cups)	180	45	2
Cup Of Soup Vegetable	1 pkg (1½ cups)	180	40	2
Matzo Ball & Soup	1 cup	40	0	1
Matzo Ball & Soup 50% Less Salt	1 serv	50	0	1
Noodleman	1 cup	45	10	0
Noodleman Low Sodium	1 cup	50	10	1
Onion	1 cup	30	0	1
Onion Low Sodium	1 cup	30	0	1
Health Valley				
Chicken Noodles w/ Vegetables	1 serv	110	0	3
Corn Chowder w/ Tomatoes	1 serv	100	0	3
Creamy Potato w/ Broccoli	1 serv	70	0	3

FOOD	PORTION	CALS	CHOL	FIBER
Garden Split Pea w/ Carrots	1 serv	130	0	2
Lentil w/ Couscous	1 serv	130	0	5
Pasta Italiano	1 serv	140	0	3
Pasta Marinara	1 serv	100	0	1
Pasta Parmesan	1 serv	100	0	1
Spicy Black Bean w/ Couscous	1 serv	130	0	5
Zesty Black Bean w/ Rice	1 serv	100	0	4
Herb-Ox				
Beef Bouillon	1 cube (3.5 g)	5	0	0
Beef Instant Bouillon Powder	1 tsp (4 g)	5	0	0
Beef Instant Broth & Seasoning Pack	1 pkg (4.5 g)	5	0	0
Beef Instant Broth & Seasoning Pack Low Sodium	1 pkg (4 g)	10	0	0
Chicken Bouillon	1 cube (4 g)	5	0	0
Chicken Instant Bouillon Powder	1 tsp (4 g)	5	0	0
Chicken Instant Broth & Seasoning Pack	1 pkg (4 g)	5	0	0
Chicken Instant Broth & Seasoning Pack Low Sodium	1 pkg (4 g)	10	0	0
Vegetable Bouillon	1 cube (4 g)	5	0	0
Hodgson Mill				
Choice Bean not prep	¼ cup (1.5 oz)	150	0	11
Hurst				
15 Bean Soup Beef	1 serv (6 oz)	120	0	9
15 Bean Soup Cajun	1 serv	120	0	9
15 Bean Soup Chicken	1 serv (6 oz)	120	0	9
15 Bean Soup Chili	1 serv (6 oz)	120	0	9
15 Bean Soup Ham	1 serv	120	0	9
HamBeens Great Northern Bean	1 serv	120	0	11
HamBeens Navy Bean	1 serv	120	0	11

FOOD	PORTION	CALS	CHOL	FIBER
Pasta Fagioli	1 serv	120	0	9
Spanish American Pinto Bean	1 serv	120	0	6
Spanish-American Black Bean	1 serv	120	0	8
Knorr				
Black Bean Cup-A-Soup as prep	1 pkg	200	0	9
Chicken Noodle Instant as prep	6 fl oz	25	5	–
Hearty Minestrone Cup-A-Soup as prep	1 pkg	150	2	1
Lentil Cup-A-Soup as prep	1 pkg	220	0	6
Navy Bean Cup-A-Soup as prep	1 pkg	140	0	5
Potato Leek Cup-A-Soup as prep	1 pkg	120	0	1
Vegetable Cup-A-Soup as prep	1 pkg	100	0	0
Kojel				
Hearty Potato w/ Vegetables Instant	1 serv (6 fl oz)	60	0	2
Noodle Soup Chicken Flavor Instant	1 serv (6 fl oz)	70	0	2
Split Pea Instant	1 serv (6 fl oz)	60	0	3
Tomato Instant	1 serv (6 fl oz)	50	0	1
Vegetable Chicken Couscous Instant	1 serv (6 fl oz)	80	0	2
Lipton				
Chicken Noodle w/ White Chicken Meat as prep	1 cup	80	15	0
Extra Noodle w/Chicken Broth as prep	1 cup	90	25	tr
Giggle Noodle w/ Chicken Broth as prep	1 cup	70	20	0
Recipe Secrets Beefy Mushroom	1½ tbsp (0.4 oz)	35	0	0

FOOD	PORTION	CALS	CHOL	FIBER
Recipe Secrets Beefy Onion	1 tbsp (0.3 oz)	25	0	0
Recipe Secrets Fiesta Herb w/ Red Pepper as prep	1 cup	30	0	0
Recipe Secrets Golden Herb w/ Lemon as prep	1 cup	35	0	0
Recipe Secrets Golden Onion	1⅔ tbsp (0.5 oz)	50	0	0
Recipe Secrets Italian Herb w/ Tomato as prep	1 cup	40	0	0
Recipe Secrets Onion as prep	1 cup	20	0	tr
Recipe Secrets Onion Mushroom as prep	1 cup	30	0	0
Recipe Secrets Savory Herb w/ Garlic as prep	1 cup	30	0	0
Recipe Secrets Vegetable as prep	1 cup	30	0	1
Ring-O-Noodle w/ Chicken Broth as prep	1 cup	70	15	0
Soup Secrets Chicken 'N Onion as prep	1 cup	120	5	1
Soup Secrets Chicken w/ Pasta & Beans as prep	1 cup	110	5	3
Soup Secrets Country Chicken w/ Pasta & Herbs as prep	1 cup	100	5	1
Soup Secrets Honestyle Lentil w/ Bow Tie Pasta as prep	1 cup	130	0	5
Soup Secrets Minestrone as prep	1 cup	110	0	4
Spiral Pasta w/ Chicken Broth as prep	1 cup	60	0	0

FOOD	PORTION	CALS	CHOL	FIBER
Maruchan				
Instant Lunch Oriental Noodles Beef	1 pkg (2.25 oz)	290	1	—
Instant Lunch Oriental Noodles Chicken	1 pkg (2.25 oz)	290	4	2
Instant Lunch Oriental Noodles Chicken Mushroom	1 pkg (2.25 oz)	280	0	—
Instant Lunch Oriental Noodles Mushroom	1 pkg (2.25 oz)	290	0	—
Instant Lunch Oriental Noodles Pork	1 pkg (2.25 oz)	290	0	—
Instant Lunch Oriental Noodles Shrimp	1 pkg (2.25 oz)	290	8	—
Instant Lunch Oriental Noodles Toast Onion	1 pkg (2.25 oz)	270	0	—
Instant Lunch Oriental Noodles Vegetable Beef	1 pkg (2.25 oz)	290	0	—
Instant Wonton Chicken	1 pkg (1.49 oz)	200	5	—
Instant Wonton Hot & Sour	1 pkg (1.49 oz)	200	0	—
Instant Wonton Oriental	1 pkg (1.49 oz)	190	0	—
Instant Wonton Pork	1 pkg (1.49 oz)	200	0	—
Instant Wonton Shrimp	1 pkg (1.49 oz)	200	10	—
Oriental Noodle Picante Style Beef	1 pkg (2.25 oz)	290	0	—
Oriental Noodle Picante Style Chicken	1 pkg (2.25 oz)	290	5	—
Oriental Noodle Picante Style Shrimp	1 pkg (2.25 oz)	300	5	—
Ramen Beef	½ pkg (1.5 oz)	190	0	—
Ramen Chicken	½ pkg (1.5 oz)	190	0	—
Ramen Chicken Mushroom	½ pkg (1.5 oz)	190	0	—
Ramen Chili	½ pkg (1.5 oz)	190	0	—
Ramen Mushroom	½ pkg (1.5 oz)	190	0	—
Ramen Oriental	½ pkg (1.5 oz)	190	0	—
Ramen Pork	½ pkg (1.5 oz)	190	0	—
Ramen Shrimp	½ pkg (1.5 oz)	190	tr	—

FOOD	PORTION	CALS	CHOL	FIBER
Wonton Beef	⅓ pkg (0.68 oz)	90	0	—
Wonton Chicken	⅓ pkg (0.67 oz)	90	0	—
Wonton Pork	⅓ pkg (0.68 oz)	90	0	—
Wonton Vegetable	⅓ pkg (0.7 oz)	90	0	—
Morga				
Vegetable Bouillon No Salt Added	½ cube (5 g)	25	0	0
Vegetable Broth Fat Free	1 tsp (4 g)	10	0	0
Nile Spice				
Couscous Almondine	1 pkg	200	0	2
Couscous Garbanzo	1 pkg	220	0	2
Couscous Lentil Curry	1 pkg	200	0	4
Couscous Minestrone	1 pkg	180	0	2
Couscous Parmesan	1 pkg	200	10	2
Homestyle Black Bean	1 pkg	190	0	2
Homestyle Chicken Flavored Vegetable	1 pkg	120	5	4
Homestyle Lentil	1 pkg	180	0	3
Homestyle Minestrone	1 pkg	160	0	4
Homestyle Red Beans & Rice	1 pkg	190	0	3
Homestyle Split Pea	1 pkg	200	0	6
Homestyle Sweet Corn Chowder	1 pkg	120	0	0
Italian Tomato	1 pkg	140	10	2
Potato Leek	1 pkg	150	20	2
Potato Romano	1 pkg	140	15	3
Ramen Noodle				
Beef Low Fat as Prep	1 pkg (2.2 oz)	216	1	2
Beef as prep	1 pkg (2.2 oz)	280	tr	3
Chicken Low Fat as prep	1 pkg (2.2 oz)	216	tr	2
Chicken as prep	1 pkg (2.2 oz)	279	1	6
Oriental Low Fat as prep	1 pkg (2.2 oz)	217	0	2
Shrimp Low Fat as prep	1 pkg (2.2 oz)	218	5	3
Shrimp as prep	1 pkg (2.2 oz)	294	1	3
Tomato as prep	1 pkg (2.2 oz)	295	tr	2
Thai Kitchen				
Rice Noodle Bowl Roasted Garlic	1 bowl	170	0	0

FOOD	PORTION	CALS	CHOL	FIBER
Rice Noodle Bowl Spring Onion	1 bowl	170	0	0
Weight Watchers				
Instant Beef Broth	1 pkg (0.16 oz)	10	0	0
Instant Chicken Broth	1 pkg (0.16 oz)	10	0	0
SHELF-STABLE				
Annie Chun				
Ginger Chicken	1 cup	30	0	0
Shiitake Mushroom	1 cup	25	0	0
Traditional Miso	1 cup	35	0	1
Campbell's				
Soup At Hand Blended Vegetable Medley	1 pkg (10.75 oz)	110	10	4
Hormel				
Micro Cup Bean & Ham	1 cup (7.5 oz)	190	15	7
Micro Cup Beef Vegetable	1 cup (7.5 oz)	90	10	1
Micro Cup Broccoli Cheese w/ Ham	1 cup (7.5 oz)	170	40	1
Micro Cup Chicken & Rice	1 cup (7.5 oz)	110	15	1
Micro Cup Chicken Noodle	1 cup (7.5 oz)	110	35	0
Micro Cup New England Clam Chowder	1 cup (7.5 oz)	130	25	1
Micro Cup Potato Cheese w/ Ham	1 cup (7.5 oz)	190	50	1
Lunch Bucket				
Chicken Noodle	1 pkg (7.25 oz)	80	10	0
Country Vegetable	1 pkg (7.25 oz)	60	0	3
TastyBite				
Tom Yum	½ pkg (5.3 oz)	92	0	1
TAKE-OUT				
beef stew soup	1 cup (8.8 oz)	221	60	–
black bean turtle soup	1 cup	241	0	–
brunswick stew soup	1 cup (8.5 oz)	232	71	–
corn & cheese chowder	¾ cup	215	66	3
gazpacho	1 cup	46	0	–
greek lemon	¾ cup	63	83	2
hot & sour	1 serv (14 oz)	173	87	1

FOOD	PORTION	CALS	CHOL	FIBER
onion soup gratinee	1 serv	492	77	4
pasta e fagioll	1 cup (8.8 oz)	194	3	–
ratatouille	1 cup (7.5 oz)	266	0	–
thai lemon grass	1 bowl	100	65	–
vietnamese pho beef noodle	1 serv (7.8 oz)	480	46	1
zupa koprowa polish dill soup	1 bowl	54	55	–
SOUR CREAM				
sour cream	1 cup (8 oz)	493	102	–
sour cream	1 tbsp (0.4 oz)	26	5	–
Breakstone's				
Free	2 tbsp (1.1 oz)	35	<5	0
Reduced Fat	2 tbsp (1.1 oz)	45	15	0
Sour Cream	2 tbsp (1 oz)	60	20	0
Friendship				
Light	2 tbsp (1 oz)	35	10	0
Sour Cream	2 tbsp (1 oz)	60	20	0
Heluva Good Cheese				
Fat-Free	2 tbsp (1.1 oz)	20	0	0
Light	2 tbsp (1.1 oz)	40	10	0
Sour Cream	2 tbsp (1.1 oz)	60	20	0
Hood				
Fat Free	2 tbsp (1 oz)	20	0	0
Light	2 tbsp (1 oz)	40	10	0
Sour Cream	2 tbsp (1 oz)	60	20	0
Knudsen				
Free	2 tbsp (1.1 oz)	35	<5	0
Hampshire	2 tbsp (1 oz)	60	25	0
Light	2 tbsp (1.1 oz)	50	10	0
Land O Lakes				
Fat Free	2 tbsp (1.1 oz)	25	<5	0
Light	2 tbsp (1 oz)	40	10	0
Sour Cream	2 tbsp (1 oz)	60	15	0
Naturally Yours				
No Fat	2 tbsp (1 fl oz)	15	0	–
SOUR CREAM SUBSTITUTES				
nondairy	1 cup	479	0	–
nondairy	1 oz	59	0	–

FOOD	PORTION	CALS	CHOL	FIBER
Tofutti				
Better Than Sour Cream Sour Supreme	1 oz	50	0	–
SOURSOP				
fresh	1	416	0	–
fresh cut up	1 cup	150	0	–
SOY *(see also CHEESE SUBSTITUTES, ICE CREAM FROZEN DESSERTS, MILK SUBSTITUTES, MISO, SOY SAUCE, SOYBEANS, TEMPEH, TOFU, YOGURT FROZEN)*				
lecithin	1 tbsp	104	0	–
soy milk	1 cup	79	0	–
GeniSoy				
Soy Nuts Deep Sea Salted	1 oz	120	0	5
Soy Nuts Old Hickory Smoked	1 oz	120	0	5
Soy Nuts Praline	55 pieces (1 oz)	120	0	2
Soy Nuts Unsalted	1 oz	120	0	5
Soy Nuts Zesty Barbeque	1 oz	120	0	5
Health Trip				
Soynut Butter Honey Sweet	2 tbsp	170	0	1
Soynut Butter Original	2 tbsp	180	0	1
Soynut Butter Unsalted	2 tbsp	180	0	1
I.M. Healthy				
SoyNut Butter Chocolate	2 tbsp (1.1 oz)	190	0	4
SoyNut Butter Honey Creamy	2 tbsp (1.1 oz)	170	0	2
SoyNut Butter Original Creamy	2 tbsp (1.1 oz)	170	0	1
SoyNut Butter Unsweetened Chunky	2 tbsp (1.1 oz)	160	0	5
SoyNut Butter Unsweetened Creamy	2 tbsp (1.1 oz)	160	0	5
Loma Linda				
Soyagen All Purpose	¼ cup (1 oz)	130	0	3

FOOD	PORTION	CALS	CHOL	FIBER
Soyagen Carob	¼ cup (1 oz)	130	0	2
Soyagen No Sucrose	¼ cup (1 oz)	130	0	3
Natural Touch				
Roasted Soy Butter	2 tbsp (1.1 oz)	170	0	1
Revival				
Chocolate Soy Nuts!	12–14 pieces (0.5 oz)	70	2	tr
Soy Shake Plain as prep w/ water	1 pkg (1 oz)	110	0	0
Soy Shakes Chocolate Daydream Equal as prep w/ water	1 pkg (1.2 oz)	130	0	2
Soy Shakes Chocolate Daydream Unsweetened as prep w/ water	1 pkg (1.2 oz)	130	0	2
Soy Shakes Chocolate Daydreams as prep w/ water	1 pkg (2.2 oz)	240	0	2
Soy Shakes Vanilla Pleasures Equal as prep w/ water	1 pkg (1.2 oz)	120	0	0
Soy Shakes Vanilla Pleasures Unsweetened as prep w/ water	1 pkg (1.2 oz)	120	0	0
Soy Shakes Vanilla Pleasures as prep w/ water	1 pkg (2 oz)	220	0	0
Soy Wonder				
Creamy	2 tbsp	170	0	1
Crunchy	2 tbsp	170	0	1
SOY SAUCE				
shoyu	1 tbsp	9	0	–
soy sauce	1 tbsp	7	0	–
tamari	1 tbsp	11	0	–
Chun King				
Lite	1 tbsp (0.5 oz)	15	0	0
Soy Sauce	1 tbsp (0.6 oz)	11	0	0

FOOD	PORTION	CALS	CHOL	FIBER
Eden				
Organic Shoyu Reduced Sodium	1 tbsp	10	0	0
Organic Tamari	1 tbsp	15	0	0
Ponzu Sauce	1 tbsp	5	0	0
Shoyu	1 tbsp	15	0	0
House Of Tsang				
Dark	1 tbsp (0.6 oz)	10	0	0
Ginger Flavored	1 tbsp (0.6 oz)	20	0	0
Light	1 tbsp (0.6 oz)	5	0	0
Low Sodium	1 tbsp (0.6 oz)	5	0	0
Low Sodium Ginger	1 tbsp (0.6 oz)	10	0	0
Low Sodium Mushroom	1 tbsp (0.6 oz)	10	0	0
Just Rite				
Soy Sauce	1 tbsp (0.5 oz)	11	0	0
Ka-Me				
Chinese Light	1 tbsp (0.5 fl oz)	5	0	0
Kikkoman				
Lite	1 tbsp (0.5 oz)	10	0	–
Soy Sauce	1 tbsp (0.5 oz)	10	0	0
La Choy				
Lite	1 tbsp (0.5 oz)	15	0	0
Soy Sauce	1 tbsp (0.6 oz)	11	0	0
Tree Of Life				
Shoyu	1 tbsp (0.5 oz)	15	0	–
Tamari Wheat Free	1 tbsp (0.5 oz)	15	0	–
SOYBEANS				
dried cooked	1 cup	298	0	–
dry roasted	½ cup	387	0	–
green cooked	½ cup	127	0	4
honey toasted	¼ cup (1 oz)	130	0	0
roasted	½ cup	405	0	–
roasted & toasted	1 oz	129	0	–
roasted & toasted	1 cup	490	0	–
roasted & toasted salted	1 oz	129	0	–
roasted & toasted salted	1 cup	490	0	–
sprouts raw	½ cup	43	0	–

FOOD	PORTION	CALS	CHOL	FIBER
sprouts steamed	½ cup	38	0	–
sprouts stir fried	1 cup	125	0	–
Dakota Gourmet				
Soy Nuts	1 oz	129	0	1
Eden				
Organic Black	½ cup (4.6 oz)	120	0	7
Seapoint Farms				
Edamame Organic	½ cup (2.6 oz)	100	0	4
Edamame In Pods frzn.	½ cup (2.6 oz)	100	0	4
Edamame Rice Bowl Kung Pao Vegetable	1 pkg (12 oz)	420	0	6
Edamame Rice Bowl Szechwan Vegetables	1 pkg (12 oz)	420	0	6
Edamame Rice Bowl Teriyaki Vegetable	1 pkg (12 oz)	430	0	5
Edamame Rice Bowl Vegetable Fried Rice	1 pkg (11 oz)	220	40	1
Edamame Shelled	½ cup (2.6 oz)	100	0	4

SPAGHETTI (see PASTA, PASTA DINNERS, PASTA SALAD, SPAGHETTI SAUCE)

SPAGHETTI SAUCE
JARRED

FOOD	PORTION	CALS	CHOL	FIBER
marinara sauce	1 cup	171	0	–
spaghetti sauce	1 cup	272	0	–
Amy's				
Family Marinara	½ cup	50	0	3
Garlic Mushroom	½ cup	120	5	3
Puttanesca	½ cup	40	0	1
Tomato Basil	½ cup	80	0	3
Wild Mushroom	½ cup	60	0	2
Classico				
Beef & Pork	4 fl oz	80	10	–
Four Cheese	4 fl oz	70	<5	–
Ripe Olives & Mushrooms	4 fl oz	50	0	–
Spicy Red Pepper	4 fl oz	50	0	–
Sweet Peppers & Onions	4 fl oz	50	0	–
Tomato & Basil	4 fl oz	60	0	–

FOOD	PORTION	CALS	CHOL	FIBER
Colavita				
Garden Style	½ cup (4.4 oz)	60	0	3
Contadina				
Italian	¼ cup	15	0	1
Sauce	¼ cup	20	0	tr
Thick & Zesty	¼ cup	15	0	1
Del Monte				
Chunky Garlic & Herb	½ cup (4.4 oz)	60	0	1
Chunky Italian Herb	½ cup (4.4 oz)	60	0	1
Tomato & Basil	½ cup (4.4 oz)	70	0	3
Traditional	½ cup (4.4 oz)	60	0	3
With Garlic & Onion	½ cup (4.4 oz)	80	0	2
With Green Peppers & Mushrooms	½ cup (4.4 oz)	80	0	3
With Meat	½ cup (4.4 oz)	60	4	3
With Mushrooms	½ cup (4.4 oz)	60	0	2
Eden				
Organic Lightly Seasoned	½ cup (4.4 oz)	80	0	3
Enrico's				
Fat Free Organic Basil	½ cup (4 oz)	50	0	4
Fat Free Organic Garlic	½ cup (4 oz)	50	0	5
Fat Free Organic Hot Pepper	½ cup (4 oz)	50	0	5
Fat Free Organic Mushroom	½ cup (4 oz)	60	0	7
Fat Free Organic Traditional	½ cup (4 oz)	45	0	6
Francesco Rinaldi				
Alfredo	¼ cup (2.1 oz)	70	15	0
Chunky Garden Mushroom & Onion	½ cup (4.4 oz)	80	0	3
Chunky Garden Tomato Garlic & Onion	½ cup (4.4 oz)	80	0	3
Dolce Sweet & Tasty Tomato	½ cup (4.4 oz)	110	0	3
Dolce Three Cheese	½ cup (4.4 oz)	90	0	3
Dulce Super Mushroom	½ cup (4.4 oz)	110	0	3
Hearty Diavolo	½ cup (4.4 oz)	70	0	3

FOOD	PORTION	CALS	CHOL	FIBER
Hearty Mushroom Pepper & Onion	½ cup (4.4 oz)	80	0	3
Hearty Tomato & Basil	½ cup (4.4 oz)	80	0	4
Puttanesca	½ cup (4.3 oz)	70	0	tr
Tomato Alfredo	¼ cup (2.1 oz)	60	10	0
Traditional Meat Flavored	½ cup (4.4 oz)	90	4	3
Traditional Mushroom	1.2 cup (4.4 oz)	90	0	3
Traditional No Salt Added	½ cup (4.4 oz)	70	0	tr
Traditional Original	½ cup (4.4 oz)	90	0	3
Traditional Original	½ cup (4.4 oz)	90	0	3
Vodka Sauce	¼ cup (2.1 oz)	60	10	0
Healthy Choice				
Chunky Italian Vegetable	½ cup (4.4 oz)	40	0	2
Chunky Mushroom	½ cup (4.4 oz)	42	0	2
Garlic & Herbs	½ cup (4.4 oz)	49	0	2
Garlic Lovers Garlic & Mushroom	½ cup (4.4 oz)	44	0	2
Garlic Lovers Roasted Garlic	½ cup (4.4 oz)	52	0	3
Garlic Lovers Roasted Garlic & Sun Dried Tomato	½ cup (4.4 oz)	52	0	3
Super Chunky Mushroom & Sweet Peppers	½ cup (4.4 oz)	43	0	2
Super Chunky Tomato Mushroom & Garlic	½ cup (4.4 oz)	45	0	2
Super Chunky Vegetable Primavera	½ cup (4.4 oz)	43	0	2
Traditional	½ cup (4.4 oz)	48	0	2
With Mushrooms	½ cup (4.4 oz)	48	0	2
Hunt's				
Angela Mia Marinara	¼ cup (2.2 oz)	24	0	2
Chunky	½ cup (4.4 oz)	38	0	2
Chunky Italian Sausage	½ cup (4.5 oz)	72	2	3
Chunky Italian Style Vegetable	½ cup (4.4 oz)	63	0	2

FOOD	PORTION	CALS	CHOL	FIBER
Chunky Marinara	½ cup (4.4 oz)	61	0	2
Chunky Tomato Garlic & Onion	½ cup (4.4 oz)	63	0	2
Classic Four Cheese	½ cup (4.4 oz)	50	0	3
Classic Garlic & Herb	½ cup (4.4 oz)	53	0	3
Classic Parmesan	½ cup (4.4 oz)	49	1	3
Classic Tomato & Basil	½ cup (4.4 oz)	48	0	2
Family Favorites Seasoned Diced Tomato Sauce	½ cup (4.3 oz)	50	0	2
Homestyle Meat Flavored	½ cup (4.4 oz)	51	0	3
Homestyle Mushrooms	½ cup (4.4 oz)	48	0	3
Homestyle Traditional	½ cup (4.4 oz)	49	0	3
Light Meat Flavored	½ cup (4.4 oz)	45	2	3
Light w/ Garlic & Herb	½ cup (4.5 oz)	40	0	3
Original Meat Flavored	½ cup (4.4 oz)	68	1	3
Original Traditional	½ cup (4.4 oz)	67	0	3
Original w/ Mushrooms	½ cup (4.4 oz)	62	0	3
Original w/ Italian Cheese & Garlic	½ cup (4.5 oz)	64	1	3
Tomato Bits	½ cup (4.5 oz)	49	0	3
Traditional Light	½ cup (4.4 oz)	40	0	1
Mama Rizzo's				
Mushroom Onion	½ cup (4.3 oz)	60	0	1
Pepper Mushroom Onion	½ cup (4.3 oz)	60	0	1
Pepper Primavera Vegetable	½ cup (4.2 oz)	50	0	2
Pepper Tomato Basil Garlic	½ cup (4.7 oz)	60	0	1
Primavera Vegetable	½ cup (4.2 oz)	50	0	2
Tomato Basil Garlic	½ cup (4.6 oz)	60	0	2
Muir Glen				
Organic Balsamic Roasted Onion	½ cup (4.4 oz)	50	0	0
Organic Cabernet Marinara	½ cup (4.4 oz)	50	0	0
Organic Chunky Herb	½ cup (4.4 oz)	50	0	0

FOOD	PORTION	CALS	CHOL	FIBER
Organic Garden Vegetable	½ cup (4.4 oz)	50	0	0
Organic Garlic & Onion	½ cup (4.4 oz)	55	0	0
Organic Garlic Roasted Garlic	½ cup (4.4 oz)	50	0	0
Organic Green Olive	½ cup (4.4 oz)	60	0	0
Organic Italian Herb	½ cup (4.4 oz)	55	0	0
Organic Mushroom Marinara	½ cup (4.4 oz)	45	0	0
Organic Portabello Mushroom	½ cup (4.4 oz)	50	0	0
Organic Sun Dried Tomato	½ cup (4.4 oz)	55	0	1
Organic Tomato Basil	½ cup (4.4 oz)	50	0	0
Newman's Own				
Marinara Ventian	½ cup (4.4 oz)	60	0	3
Marinara Ventian w/ Mushrooms	½ cup (4.4 oz)	60	0	3
Pasta Sauce Bambolina	½ cup (4.5 oz)	100	0	5
Pasta Sauce Roasted Garlic & Red & Green Peppers	½ cup (4.7 oz)	70	0	4
Pasta Sauce Say Cheese	½ cup (4.4 oz)	90	<5	3
Sockarooni	½ cup (4.4 oz)	60	0	3
Prego				
Pasta Bake Sauce Tomato Garlic & Basil	1 serv (3.4 oz)	80	0	2
Traditional	½ cup (4.2 oz)	140	0	2
Pritikin				
Chunky Garden	½ cup (4 oz)	50	0	–
Marinara	½ cup (4 oz)	60	0	–
Original	½ cup (4 oz)	60	0	–
Progresso				
Marinara	½ cup (4.3 oz)	80	<5	2
Meat Flavored	½ cup (4.4 oz)	100	5	3
Sauce	½ cup (4.4 oz)	100	<5	2
Ragu				
Chunky Garden Style Tomato Garlic & Onion	½ cup (4.5 oz)	110	0	2

FOOD	PORTION	CALS	CHOL	FIBER
Fino Italian Garden Medley	½ cup (4.5 oz)	90	0	2
Fino Italian Garlic & Basil	½ cup (4.5 oz)	90	0	2
Fino Italian Parmesan	½ cup (4.5 oz)	100	<5	2
Fino Italian Sliced Mushroom	½ cup (4.5 oz)	90	0	2
Fino Italian Tomato & Herb	½ cup (4.5 oz)	90	0	2
Fino Italian Zesty Tomato	½ cup (4.5 oz)	90	0	2
Gardenstyle Chunky Garden Combination	½ cup (4.5 oz)	120	0	3
Gardenstyle Chunky Green & Red Pepper	½ cup (4.5 oz)	120	0	2
Gardenstyle Chunky Mushroom & Green Pepper	½ cup (4.5 oz)	120	0	3
Gardenstyle Chunky Mushroom & Onion	½ cup (4.5 oz)	120	0	3
Gardenstyle Super Mushroom	½ cup (4.5 oz)	120	0	3
Gardenstyle Super Vegetable Primavera	½ cup (4.5 oz)	110	0	4
Homestyle Mushroom	½ cup (4.5 oz)	120	0	3
Homestyle Tomato & Herb	½ cup (4.5 oz)	120	0	3
Homestyle With Meat	½ cup (4.5 oz)	130	<5	3
Light Chunky Mushroom	½ cup (4.4 oz)	50	0	2
Light Garden Harvest	½ cup (4.4 oz)	50	0	2
Light No Sugar Added	½ cup (4.4 oz)	60	0	3
Light Tomato & Herb	½ cup (4.4 oz)	50	0	2
Old World Style Marinara	½ cup (4.4 oz)	90	0	3
Old World Style Mushrooms	½ cup (4.4 oz)	80	0	3
Old World Style Traditional	½ cup (4.4 oz)	80	0	3

FOOD	PORTION	CALS	CHOL	FIBER
Old World Style With Meat	½ cup (4.4 oz)	90	<5	3
Thick & Hearty Mushroom	½ cup (4.5 oz)	120	0	3
Thick & Hearty Spaghetti Sauce	4 oz	100	0	–
Thick & Hearty Tomato & Herb	½ cup (4.5 oz)	120	0	3
Thick & Hearty With Meat	1.2 cup (4.5 oz)	130	<5	3
Sara Lee				
Chunky Garden Mushroom & Peppers	½ cup (4.4 oz)	80	0	3
Tree Of Life				
Pasta Sauce	½ cup (4 oz)	50	0	–
Pasta Sauce Fat Free Classic	½ cup (3.9 oz)	40	0	0
Pasta Sauce Fat Free Mushroom & Basil	½ cup (3.9 oz)	30	0	0
Pasta Sauce Fat Free Onion & Garlic	½ cup (3.9 oz)	30	0	0
Pasta Sauce Fat Free Sweet Pepper	½ cup (3.9 oz)	30	0	0
Pasta Sauce No Salt Added	½ cup (3.9 oz)	50	0	–
MIX				
Durkee				
Spaghetti Sauce as prep	½ cup	15	0	0
With Mushrooms as prep	½ cup	15	0	0
French's				
Italian as prep	½ cup	16	0	0
Mushroom as prep	½ cup	20	2	0
Thick as prep	½ cup	10	0	0
McCormick				
Alfredo Pasta Blend as prep	½ cup	60	10	0
Pasta Rosa Blend	1 tbsp (10 g)	40	<5	0

FOOD	PORTION	CALS	CHOL	FIBER
REFRIGERATED				
Contadina				
Alfredo	½ cup (4.2 fl oz)	400	80	0
Four Cheese Sauce w/ White Wine & Shallots	½ cup (4.2 fl oz)	320	70	0
Light Alfredo	½ cup (4.2 fl oz)	190	40	0
Light Chunky Tomato	½ cup (4.4 fl oz)	45	0	3
Light Garden Vegetable	½ cup (4.4 fl oz)	45	0	3
Marinara	½ cup (4.4 fl oz)	80	0	2
Pesto With Basil	¼ cup (2 oz)	310	10	0
Pesto With Sun Dried Tomatoes	¼ cup (2 oz)	250	0	3
Plum Tomato With Basil	½ cup (4.4 fl oz)	70	0	3
Spicy Italian Sausage & Bell Pepper	½ cup (4.4 fl oz)	100	40	3
Di Giorno				
Alfredo	¼ cup (2.2 oz)	180	25	0
Basil Pesto	¼ cup (2.2 oz)	320	15	tr
Four Cheese	¼ cup (2.2 oz)	160	30	0
Garlic Pesto	¼ cup (2.1 oz)	340	15	tr
Light Alfredo Sauce	¼ cup (2.4 oz)	140	30	0
Marinara	½ cup (4.5 oz)	70	0	2
Plum Tomato Cream Sauce	½ cup (4.4 oz)	160	40	2
Plum Tomato & Mushroom	½ cup (4.4 oz)	60	0	2
Roasted Red Bell Pepper Cream Sauce	¼ cup (2.3 oz)	140	35	0
SPANISH FOOD				
CANNED				
Chi-Chi's				
Pico De Gallo	2 tbsp (1.2 oz)	10	0	0
Derby				
Tamales	3 (6.5 oz)	253	23	4
Gebhardt				
Enchiladas	2 (5.7 oz)	258	25	3
Tamales	2 (5.7 oz)	268	28	3
Tamales Jumbo	2 (6.9 oz)	332	34	3

FOOD	PORTION	CALS	CHOL	FIBER
Hormel				
Tamales Beef	3 (7.5 oz)	280	35	3
Tamales Chicken	3 (7.5 oz)	210	50	2
Tamales Hot Spicy Beef	3 (7.5 oz)	280	35	3
Tamales Jumbo Beef	2 (6.9 oz)	270	35	3
Old El Paso				
Tamales	3 (7.2 oz)	330	30	5
Rosarita				
Enchilada Sauce Mild	¼ cup (2.1 oz)	23	0	0
Van Camp				
Tamales	2 (5 oz)	210	20	3
FROZEN				
Amy's				
Black Bean Vegetable Enchilada	1 (4.75 oz)	130	0	2
Bowls Santa Fe Enchilada	1 pkg (10 oz)	340	5	10
Burrito Bean & Cheese	1 (6 oz)	280	10	6
Burrito Bean & Rice Non-Dairy	1 (6 oz)	270	0	5
Burrito Black Bean Vegetable	1 (6 oz)	320	0	4
Burrito Breakfast	1 (6 oz)	210	0	5
Cheese Enchilada	1 (4.75 oz)	210	35	2
Mexican Tamale Pie	1 (8 oz)	150	0	4
Banquet				
Chimichanga Meal	1 meal (9.5 oz)	500	20	9
Enchilada Beef	1 pkg (11 oz)	370	20	6
Enchilada Cheese	1 pkg (11 oz)	360	20	6
Enchilada Chicken	1 pkg (11 oz)	350	25	9
Enchilada Beef & Tamale Combo	1 pkg (11 oz)	450	30	9
Mexican Style Enchilada Combo	1 meal (11 oz)	360	20	9
Chi-Chi's				
Burro Beef	1 pkg (15.9 oz)	590	55	11
Burro Chicken	1 pkg (15.9 oz)	540	55	10
Chimichanga Beef	1 pkg (15.9 oz)	630	55	10
Chimichanga Chicken	1 pkg (15.9 oz)	580	50	10

FOOD	PORTION	CALS	CHOL	FIBER
Enchilada Chicken Suprema	1 pkg (15.9 oz)	600	70	11
Enchilida Baja	1 pkg (15.9 oz)	590	50	15
Health Is Wealth				
Burrito Munchees	10 (5 oz)	310	5	6
Mexican Munchees	2 (1 oz)	49	0	1
Healthy Choice				
Chicken Enchilada Supreme	1 meal (11.3 oz)	300	40	4
Chicken Enchiladas Suiz	1 meal (10 oz)	280	40	5
Chicken Breast Con Queso Burrito	1 meal (10.55 oz)	350	35	6
Jimmy Dean				
Burrito Breakfast Bacon	1 (4 oz)	260	70	1
Burrito Breakfast Sausage	1 (4 oz)	250	45	2
Lean Cuisine				
Everyday Favorites Chicken Enchilada Suiza	1 pkg (9 oz)	280	25	3
Old El Paso				
Burrito Bean & Cheese	1 (4.9 oz)	290	15	3
Burrito Beef & Bean Hot	1 (5 oz)	320	15	3
Burrito Beef & Bean Medium	1 (5 oz)	320	15	3
Burrito Beef & Bean Mild	1 (5 oz)	330	15	4
Chimichanga Beef	1 (4.5 oz)	370	10	3
Chimichanga Chicken	1 (4.5 oz)	350	20	2
Patio				
Beef & Cheese Enchiladas Chili 'N Beans	1 meal (15.5 oz)	670	60	12
Beef Enchiladas Chili 'N Beans	1 meal (15.5 oz)	540	50	12
Burrito Bean & Cheese	1 (5 oz)	300	15	4
Burrito Beef & Bean Hot	1 (5 oz)	320	25	4
Burrito Beef & Bean Mild	1 (5 oz)	330	20	4
Burrito Chicken	1 (5 oz)	290	20	2
Burritos Beef & Bean Medium	1 (5 oz)	310	20	4

FOOD	PORTION	CALS	CHOL	FIBER
Burritos Beef & Bean Red Chili Pepper Red Hot	1 (5 oz)	320	20	4
Enchilada Beef	1 meal (12 oz)	320	25	9
Enchilada Cheese	1 meal (12 oz)	370	25	7
Enchilada Chicken	1 meal (12 oz)	400	35	8
Fiesta	1 meal (12 oz)	350	25	7
Mexican Style	1 meal (13.25 oz)	470	20	10
Rudy's Farm				
Burrito Beef/Bean	1 (5 oz)	326	15	5
Burrito Hot Beef/Bean	1 (5 oz)	305	11	5
Senor Felix's				
Burrito Black Bean	1 (10 oz)	540	40	7
Burrito Black Bean Soy	1 (5 oz)	240	0	3
Burrito Chicken	1 (10 oz)	520	65	3
Burrito Hot Potato	1 (10 oz)	560	40	5
Burrito Soy Hot	1 (10 oz)	520	0	5
Burritos Charbroiled Chicken	1 + 4 tsp sauce (6.7 oz)	320	20	7
Burritos Sonora Style	1 + 4 tsp sauce (6.7 oz)	280	10	3
Burritos Yucatan Style	1 + 4 tsp sauce (6.7 oz)	310	10	5
Empanadas Chicken	1 (4.7 oz)	340	30	13
Empanadas Corn & Rice	1 (4.7 oz)	280	25	6
Empanadas Pumpkin & Mushroom	1 (4.7 oz)	260	25	6
Empanadas Spinach & Ricotta	1 (4.7 oz)	260	30	6
Enchilada Red Pepper	1 (10 oz)	420	25	8
Enchilada Soy Verda	1 (10 oz)	430	0	6
Enchilada Supreme Soy Cheese	1 (10 oz)	460	0	6
Enchilada Verde	1 (5 oz)	423	25	6
Tamales Blue Corn & Soy Cheese	2 + 4 tsp sauce (5.7 oz)	240	15	3
Tamales Chicken	2 + 4 tsp sauce (5.7 oz)	240	20	8
Tamales Gourmet Vegetarian	2 + 4 tsp sauce	240	20	8

FOOD	PORTION	CALS	CHOL	FIBER
Taquitos Blue Corn Soy	3 + 4 tsp sauce (5.2 oz)	230	0	3
Taquitos Chicken	2 + 4 tsp sauce (5.7 oz)	240	15	3
Stouffer's				
Chicken Enchilada	1 serv (4.8 oz)	230	30	3
Today's Tamales				
Cheese & Chili	1 pkg (7 oz)	390	30	6
Del Sol	1 pkg (6.5 oz)	310	0	15
Original Bean	1 pkg (7 oz)	330	0	10
Spicy Taco	1 pkg (7 oz)	310	0	10
Tyson				
Beef Fajita	3½ pieces (12.5 oz)	550	20	6
Chicken Fajita	3½ pieces (13.1 oz)	460	45	6
Weight Watchers				
Smart Ones Chicken Enchiladas Suiza	1 pkg (9 oz)	270	50	2
Smart Ones Santa Fe Style Rice & Beans	1 pkg (10 oz)	290	20	6
MIX				
Gebhardt				
Menudo Mix	¼ tsp (0.4 g)	1	0	tr
Old El Paso				
Burrito Seasoning Mix	2 tsp (6 g)	20	0	1
Dinner Kit Burrito as prep	1	280	66	3
Dinner Kit Soft Taco as prep	2	380	63	3
Dinner Kit Taco as prep	2	270	60	4
Enchilada Sauce Mix	2 tsp (4 g)	10	0	tr
Taco Mix 40% Less Sodium	2 tsp (6 g)	20	0	0
Taco Seasoning Mix	2 tsp (6 g)	20	0	0
Taco Bell				
Home Originals Chicken Fajita Dinner as prep	2 (6.9 oz)	340	40	3
Home Originals Chicken Fajita Seasoning Mix	1 tbsp (8 g)	25	0	2
Home Originals Soft Taco Dinner as prep	2 (6.3 oz)	410	60	2

FOOD	PORTION	CALS	CHOL	FIBER
Home Originals Taco Dinner as prep	2 (4.4 oz)	280	50	2
Home Originals Taco Seasoning Mix	2 tsp (6 g)	20	0	tr
Home Originals Ultimate Bean Burrito Dinner as prep	1 (4.4 oz)	200	0	3
Home Originals Ultimate Nachos as prep	12 pieces (4.6 oz)	240	0	4
READY-TO-EAT				
taco shell baked	1 med (0.5 oz)	61	0	tr
taco shell baked w/o salt	1 med (½ oz)	61	0	tr
Chi-Chi's				
Taco Shells White Corn	2 (1.2 oz)	170	0	2
Taco Shells Yellow Corn	2 shells (1.2 oz)	170	0	2
Gebhardt				
Taco Shells	3 (1.1 oz)	155	0	3
La Mexicana				
Flour Burritos	1 (1.6 oz)	160	0	2
Old El Paso				
Taco Shells Mini	7 (1.1 oz)	160	0	2
Taco Shells Regular	3 (1.1 oz)	170	0	2
Taco Shells Super	2 (1.3 oz)	190	0	2
Taco Shells White Corn	3 (1.1 oz)	170	0	2
Tostaco Shells	1 (0.8 oz)	130	0	1
Tostada Shells	3 (1.1 oz)	160	0	2
Rosarita				
Taco Shells	3 (1.1 oz)	155	0	3
Tostada Shells	2 (1 oz)	125	37	0
Taco Bell				
Home Originals Taco Shells	3 (1.1 oz)	150	0	2
TAKE-OUT				
burrito w/ apple	1 sm (2.6 oz)	231	3	–
burrito w/ apple	1 lg (5.4 oz)	484	7	–
burrito w/ beans	2 (7.6 oz)	448	5	–
burrito w/ beans & cheese	2 (6.5 oz)	377	27	–

FOOD	PORTION	CALS	CHOL	FIBER
burrito w/ beans & chili peppers	2 (7.2 oz)	413	33	–
burrito w/ beans & meat	2 (8.1 oz)	508	48	–
burrito w/ beans cheese & beef	2 (7.1 oz)	331	125	–
burrito w/ beans cheese & chili peppers	2 (11.8 oz)	663	158	–
burrito w/ beef	2 (7.7 oz)	523	65	–
burrito w/ beef & chili peppers	2 (7.1 oz)	426	54	–
burrito w/ beef cheese & chili peppers	2 (10.7 oz)	634	170	–
burrito w/ cherry	1 sm (2.6 oz)	231	3	–
burrito w/ cherry	1 lg (5.4 oz)	484	7	–
chimichanga w/ beef	1 (6.1 oz)	425	9	–
chimichanga w/ beef & cheese	1 (6.4 oz)	443	51	–
chimichanga w/ beef & red chili peppers	1 (6.7 oz)	424	9	–
chimichanga w/ beef cheese & red chili peppers	1 (6.3 oz)	364	50	–
enchilada eggplant	1	142	7	–
enchilada w/ cheese	1 (5.7 oz)	320	44	–
enchilada w/ cheese & beef	1 (6.7 oz)	324	40	–
enchirito w/ cheese beef & beans	1 (6.8 oz)	344	49	–
frijoles w/ cheese	1 cup (5.9 oz)	226	36	–
nachos w/ cheese	6 to 8 (4 oz)	345	18	–
nachos w/ cheese & jalapeno peppers	6 to 8 (7.2 oz)	607	83	–
nachos w/ cheese beans ground beef & peppers	6 to 8 (8.9 oz)	568	21	–
nachos w/ cinnamon & sugar	6 to 8 (3.8 oz)	592	39	–
taco	1 sm (6 oz)	370	57	–
taco salad	1½ cups	279	44	–

FOOD	PORTION	CALS	CHOL	FIBER
taco salad w/ chili con carne	1½ cups	288	4	—
tostada w/ beans & cheese	1 (5.1 oz)	223	30	—
tostada w/ beans beef & cheese	1 (7.9 oz)	334	75	—
tostada w/ beef & cheese	1 (5.7 oz)	315	41	—
tostada w/ guacamole	2 (9.2 oz)	360	39	—

SPICES (see individual names, HERBS/SPICES)

SPINACH
CANNED
spinach	½ cup	25	0	—
Del Monte				
Chopped	½ cup (4 oz)	30	0	2
No Salt Added	½ cup (4 oz)	30	0	2
Whole Leaf	½ cup (4 oz)	30	0	2
S&W				
Spinach	½ cup (4.5 oz)	30	0	2
FRESH				
cooked	½ cup	21	0	2
malabar cooked	1 cup (1.5 oz)	10	0	1
mustard chopped cooked	½ cup	14	0	—
mustard raw chopped	½ cup	17	0	—
new zealand chopped cooked	½ cup	11	0	—
new zealand raw	½ cup	4	0	—
raw chopped	½ cup	6	0	1
raw chopped	1 pkg (10 oz)	46	0	—
Dole				
Baby Spinach	3½ cups (3 oz)	35	0	4
Fresh Express				
Spinach	1½ cups (3 oz)	40	0	5
FROZEN				
Snacks Spinach Feta	5–6 pieces	170	15	2
cooked	½ cup	27	0	—
Birds Eye				
Chopped	⅓ cup	20	0	2

FOOD	PORTION	CALS	CHOL	FIBER
Creamed	½ cup	100	35	1
Cut Leaf	1 cup	20	0	2
Budget Gourmet				
Au Gratin	1 pkg (5.5 oz)	160	25	–
Green Giant				
Butter Sauce	½ cup (3.4 oz)	40	<5	2
Creamed	½ cup (3.8 oz)	80	0	2
Cut Leaf	¾ cup (2.6 oz)	25	0	3
Harvest Fresh	½ cup (3.5 oz)	25	0	2
Health Is Wealth				
Spinach Munchees	2 (1 oz)	60	0	1
Spinach Feta Munchees	2 (1 oz)	70	5	1
Stouffer's				
Creamed	1 serv (4.5 oz)	160	15	2
Souffle	1 serv (4 oz)	150	120	0
Tabatchnick				
Creamed	7.5 oz	60	5	2
Tree Of Life				
Organic	1 cup (3 oz)	20	0	2
SHELF-STABLE				
TastyBite				
Kashmir Spinach	½ pkg (5 oz)	170	35	3
TAKE-OUT				
indian saag	1 serv	28	0	1
spanakopita spinach pie	1 cup (6 oz)	196	30	4

SPINACH JUICE

FOOD	PORTION	CALS	CHOL	FIBER
juice	7 oz	14	0	–

SPORTS DRINKS (see ENERGY DRINKS)

SPROUTS

FOOD	PORTION	CALS	CHOL	FIBER
kidney bean	½ cup	27	0	–
kidney bean cooked	1 lb	152	0	–
lentil sprouts	½ cup	40	0	–
mung bean	½ cup	16	0	–
mung bean canned	½ cup	8	0	–
mung bean cooked	½ cup	13	0	–
navy bean	½ cup	35	0	–
navy bean cooked	3½ oz	78	0	–
pea	½ cup	77	0	–

FOOD	PORTION	CALS	CHOL	FIBER
pinto bean	3½ oz	62	0	–
pinto bean cooked	3½ oz	22	0	–
radish	½ cup	8	0	–
Chun King				
Bean Sprouts	1 cup (3 oz)	11	0	1
Fresh Alternatives				
BroccoSprouts	½ cup (1 oz)	10	0	1
Deli Blend	½ cup (1 oz)	10	0	tr
Salad Blend	½ cup (1 oz)	10	0	tr
Sandwich Blend	½ cup (1 oz)	5	0	tr
La Choy				
Bean Sprouts	1 cup (2.9 oz)	11	0	1
TAKE-OUT				
mung bean stir fried	½ cup	31	0	–
SQUAB				
boneless baked	3.5 oz	175	75	0
breast w/o skin raw	1 (3.5 oz)	135	91	–
SQUASH (*see also* ZUCCHINI)				
seeds dried	1 oz	154	0	–
seeds whole roasted	1 oz	127	0	–
CANNED				
crookneck sliced	½ cup	14	0	–
FRESH				
acorn cooked mashed	½ cup	41	0	3
acorn cubed baked	½ cup	57	0	2
butternut baked	½ cup	41	0	2
crookneck raw sliced	½ cup	12	0	1
crookneck sliced cooked	½ cup	18	0	1
hubbard baked	½ cup	51	0	3
hubbard cooked mashed	½ cup	35	0	3
scallop raw sliced	½ cup	12	0	1
scallop sliced cooked	½ cup	14	0	1
spaghetti cooked	½ cup	23	0	2
Nature's Pasta				
Spaghetti Squash	1 cup (5.5 oz)	20	0	2

FOOD	PORTION	CALS	CHOL	FIBER
FROZEN				
butternut cooked mashed	½ cup	47	0	3
crookneck sliced cooked	½ cup	24	0	–
Birds Eye				
Cooked Squash	½ cup	50	0	4
Sliced Yellow	⅔ cup	15	0	1
SEEDS				
dried	1 cup	747	0	–
roasted	1 cup	1184	0	–
roasted	1 oz	148	0	–
salted & roasted	1 oz	148	0	–
salted & roasted	1 cup	1184	0	–
whole roasted	1 cup	285	0	–
whole salted roasted	1 cup	285	0	–
whole salted roasted	1 oz	127	0	–
SQUID				
fried	3 oz	149	221	–
raw	3 oz	78	198	–
SQUIRREL				
roasted	3 oz	147	103	–
STARFRUIT				
fresh	1	42	0	–
Sonoma				
Dried	7–9 pieces (1.4 oz)	140	0	0
STRAWBERRIES				
CANNED				
in heavy syrup	½ cup	117	0	–
FRESH				
strawberries	1 cup	45	0	4
strawberries	1 pint	97	0	–
FROZEN				
sweetened sliced	1 cup	245	0	–
sweetened sliced	1 pkg (10 oz)	273	0	–
unsweetened	1 cup	52	0	–
whole sweetened	1 pkg (10 oz)	223	0	–
whole sweetened	1 cup	200	0	–

FOOD	PORTION	CALS	CHOL	FIBER
Birds Eye				
In Syrup	½ cup	120	0	1
Lite Syrup	1 pkg (10 oz)	120	0	1
Whole	½ cup	100	0	1
Tree Of Life				
Organic	¾ cup (5 oz)	50	0	2
STRAWBERRY JUICE				
Capri Sun				
Strawberry Cooler Drink	1 pkg (7 oz)	90	0	0
Kool-Aid				
Drink as prep w/ sugar	1 serv (8 oz)	100	0	0
Drink Mix as prep	1 serv (8 oz)	60	0	0
Veryfine				
Juice-Ups	8 fl oz	140	0	0
STUFFING/DRESSING				
bread as prep w/ water & fat	½ cup	251	tr	–
bread as prep w/ water egg & fat	½ cup	107	75	–
cornbread as prep	½ cup	179	0	–
Kellogg's				
Croutettes Mix	1 cup (1.2 oz)	120	0	0
Pepperidge Farm				
Corn Bread	¾ cup (1.5 oz)	170	0	2
Herb Seasoned	¾ cup (1.5 oz)	170	0	3
Herb Seasoned Cubed	¾ cup (1.3 oz)	140	0	2
One Step Chicken	½ cup (1.2 oz)	140	<5	tr
One Step Southwestern Corn Bread	½ cup (1.2 oz)	150	0	tr
One Step Turkey	½ cup (1.2 oz)	150	<5	tr
Stove Top				
Chicken as prep w/ margarine	½ cup (3.6 oz)	170	0	tr
Cornbread as prep w/ margarine	½ cup (3.6 oz)	170	0	1
Flexible Serve Chicken as prep w/ margarine	½ cup (3.3 oz)	170	0	tr

FOOD	PORTION	CALS	CHOL	FIBER
Flexible Serve Cornbread as prep w/ margarine	½ cup (3.3 oz)	160	0	1
Flexible Serve Homestyle Herb as prep w/ margarine	½ cup (3.3 oz)	170	0	1
For Beef as prep w/ margarine	½ cup (3.7 oz)	180	0	1
For Pork as prep w/ margarine	½ cup (3.6 oz)	170	0	1
For Turkey as prep w/ margarine	½ cup (3.6 oz)	170	0	tr
Long Grain & Wild Rice as prep w/ margarine	½ cup (3.7 oz)	180	0	tr
Lower Sodium Chicken as prep w/ margarine	½ cup (3.6 oz)	180	0	tr
Microwave Chicken as prep w/ margarine	½ cup (3.5 oz)	160	0	tr
Microwave Homestyle Cornbread as prep w/ margarine	½ cup (3 oz)	160	0	tr
Mushroom & Onion as prep w/ margarine	½ cup (3.6 oz)	180	0	tr
San Francisco Style as prep w/ margarine	½ cup (3.6 oz)	170	0	1
Savory Herb as prep w/ margarine	½ cup (3.6 oz)	170	0	1
Traditional Sage as prep w/ margarine	½ cup (3.6 oz)	180	0	1
TAKE-OUT				
bread	½ cup (3½ oz)	195	0	3
sausage	½ cup	292	12	1
SUCKER				
white baked	3 oz	101	45	–
SUGAR				
brown packed	1 cup (7.7 oz)	828	0	–
brown unpacked	1 cup (5.1 oz)	546	0	–
maple	1 piece (1 oz)	100	0	–

FOOD	PORTION	CALS	CHOL	FIBER
powdered	1 tbsp (0.3 oz)	31	0	—
powdered unsifted	1 cup (4.2 oz)	467	0	—
sugarcane stem	3 oz	54	0	3
white	1 cup (7 oz)	773	0	—
white	1 tbsp	45	0	—
white	1 packet (6 g)	25	0	—
white	1 tsp (4 g)	15	0	—
Domino				
Dark Brown	1 tsp	15	0	—
Light Brown	1 tsp	15	0	—
White	1 tsp	16	0	—
Maui Brand				
Raw Sugar	1 tsp	15	0	—

SUGAR SUBSTITUTES
Equal

FOOD	PORTION	CALS	CHOL	FIBER
Packet	1 pkg	4	0	—
Mrs. Bateman's				
Sugarlike	1 tsp (4 g)	4	0	0
NatraTaste				
Packet	1 pkg (1 g)	0	0	—
Sweet One				
Packet	1 pkg (1 g)	4	0	—
Sweet'N Low				
Granulated	1 pkg (1g)	4	0	—
Weight Watchers				
Sweetener	1 serv (1 g)	5	0	0

SUGAR-APPLE

FOOD	PORTION	CALS	CHOL	FIBER
fresh	1	146	0	—
fresh cut up	1 cup	236	0	—

SUNCHOKE

FOOD	PORTION	CALS	CHOL	FIBER
fresh raw sliced	½ cup	57	0	—

SUNFISH

FOOD	PORTION	CALS	CHOL	FIBER
pumpkinseed baked	3 oz	97	73	—

SUNFLOWER

FOOD	PORTION	CALS	CHOL	FIBER
seeds dried	1 oz	162	0	—
seeds dried	1 cup	821	0	—
seeds dry roasted	1 oz	165	0	—

FOOD	PORTION	CALS	CHOL	FIBER
seeds dry roasted	1 cup	745	0	—
seeds dry roasted salted	1 cup	745	0	—
seeds dry roasted salted	1 oz	165	0	—
seeds oil roasted	1 cup	830	0	—
seeds oil roasted salted	1 oz	175	0	—
seeds oil roasted salted	1 cup	830	0	—
seeds toasted	1 oz	176	0	—
seeds toasted	1 cup	826	0	—
seeds toasted salted	1 oz	176	0	—
seeds toasted salted	1 cup	826	0	—
sunflower butter	1 tbsp	93	0	—
sunflower butter w/o salt	1 tbsp	93	0	—
Dakota Gourmet				
Honey Roasted Kernels	1 pkg (1 oz)	158	0	1
Lightly Salted Kernels	1 pkg (1 oz)	168	0	2
Frito Lay				
Seeds	1 oz	180	0	2
Lance				
Seeds In Shell	⅔ cup (1.8 oz)	160	0	2
Seeds Roasted & Shelled	1 pkg (1⅛ oz)	190	0	2
Maranatha				
Tamari Seeds	¼ cup	160	0	2
Planters				
Kernels	1 pkg (2 oz)	340	0	8
Kernels	1 pkg (1.7 oz)	290	0	7
Kernels Barbecue	1 pkg (1.7 oz)	290	0	6
Kernels Honey Roasted	1 pkg (1.7 oz)	280	0	6
Kernels Salted	1 oz	170	0	4
Munch'N Go Singles Dry Roasted	1 pkg	120	0	1
Nuts Dry Roasted	¼ cup (1.1 oz)	190	0	4
Original With Shell Dry Roasted	¾ cup	160	0	2
Stone-Buhr				
Seeds Raw	4 tsp (1 oz)	170	0	6
SunGold				
SunButter	2 tbsp	200	0	4

FOOD	PORTION	CALS	CHOL	FIBER
SUSHI				
TAKE-OUT				
california roll	1 piece (0.8 oz)	28	1	–
sashimi	1 serv (6 oz)	198	63	–
tuna roll	1 piece (0.7 oz)	23	3	–
vegetable roll	1 piece (1.2 oz)	27	0	–
vinegared ginger	⅓ cup (1.6 oz)	48	0	–
wasabi	2 tsp (0.3 oz)	5	0	–
yellowtail roll	1 piece (0.6 oz)	25	0	–
SWAMP CABBAGE				
chopped cooked	½ cup	10	0	–
raw chopped	1 cup	11	0	–
SWEET POTATO (see also YAM)				
baked w/ skin	1 (3½ oz)	118	0	3
canned in syrup	½ cup	106	0	–
canned pieces	1 cup	183	0	–
frzn cooked	½ cup	88	0	–
leaves cooked	½ cup	11	0	–
mashed	½ cup	172	0	3
TAKE-OUT				
candied	3½ oz	144	0	–
SWEETBREADS				
lamb braised	3 oz	199	340	–
SWISS CHARD				
cooked	½ cup	18	0	–
raw chopped	½ cup	3	0	–
SWORDFISH				
cooked	3 oz	132	43	–
raw	3 oz	103	33	–
SYRUP				
corn	2 tbsp	122	0	–
corn dark	1 cup (11.5 oz)	925	0	–
corn dark	1 tbsp (0.7 oz)	56	0	–
corn light	1 cup (11.5 oz)	925	0	–
corn light	1 tbsp (0.7 oz)	56	0	–
malt	1 cup (13 oz)	1222	0	–
malt	1 tbsp (0.8 oz)	76	0	–

FOOD	PORTION	CALS	CHOL	FIBER
maple	1 cup (11.1 oz)	824	0	—
maple	1 tbsp (0.8 oz)	52	0	—
raspberry	1 oz	76	0	—
sorghum	1 tbsp (0.7 oz)	61	0	—
sorghum	1 cup (11.6 oz)	957	0	—
Eden				
Organic Barley Malt	1 tbsp	60	0	0
Estee				
Blueberry	¼ cup	80	0	0
Hershey				
Strawberry	2 tbsp (1.4 oz)	100	0	—
Karo				
Corn Syrup Light	2 tbsp (1 oz)	120	0	—
Quik				
Strawberry	2 tbsp (1.5 oz)	110	0	0
Red Wing				
Strawberry	2 tbsp (1.4 oz)	110	0	0
Smucker's				
Apricot	¼ cup	210	0	—
Blackberry	¼ cup	210	0	—
Plate Scapers Kiwi Lime	2 tbsp (1.3 oz)	100	0	—
Plate Scapers Mango Orange	2 tbsp	100	0	—
Plate Scapers Raspberry	2 tbsp (1.3 oz)	100	0	—
TAHINI (see SESAME)				
TAMARIND				
fresh	1	5	0	—
fresh cut up	1 cup	287	0	—
TANGERINE				
CANNED				
in light syrup	½ cup	76	0	—
juice pack	½ cup	46	0	—
FRESH				
sections	1 cup	86	0	—
tangerine	1	37	0	—
Chiquita				
Tangerine	1 med (3.5 oz)	50	0	2

FOOD	PORTION	CALS	CHOL	FIBER
TANGERINE JUICE				
canned sweetened	1 cup	125	0	—
fresh	1 cup	106	0	—
frzn sweetened as prep	1 cup	110	0	—
frzn sweetened not prep	6 oz	344	0	—
After The Fall				
Juice	1 can (12 oz)	170	0	0
Fresh Samantha				
Fresh Juice	1 cup (8 oz)	110	0	0
TAPIOCA				
pearl dry	½ cup (2.7 oz)	272	0	1
Minute				
Minute Tapioca	1½ tsp (6 g)	20	0	0
TARO				
chips	10 (0.8 oz)	115	0	—
chips	1 oz	141	0	—
leaves cooked	½ cup	18	0	—
raw sliced	½ cup	56	0	—
shoots sliced cooked	½ cup	10	0	—
sliced cooked	½ cup (2.3 oz)	94	0	—
tahitian sliced cooked	½ cup	30	0	—
TARRAGON				
ground	1 tsp	5	0	—
TEA/HERBAL TEA *(see also* ICED TEA)				
HERBAL				
chamomile brewed	1 cup	2	0	0
Celestial Seasonings				
Mandarin Orange Spice	1 tea bag	0	0	—
Eden				
Organic Genmaicha Tea	1 cup	0	0	0
Organic Kukicha Tea	1 cup	0	0	0
Lipton				
Bedtime Story	1 tea bag	0	0	—
Cinnamon Apple	1 tea bag	0	0	—
Ginger Twist	1 tea bag	0	0	0
Lemon	1 tea bag	0	0	—
Orange	1 tea bag	0	0	—

FOOD	PORTION	CALS	CHOL	FIBER
Peppermint	1 tea bag	0	0	–
Quietly Chamomile	1 tea bag	0	0	–
Silk				
Chai	1 cup	140	0	0
REGULAR				
brewed tea	6 oz	2	0	0
instant unsweetened as prep w/ water	8 oz	2	0	–
Activitea				
Green Tea	1 cup	36	0	–
General Foods				
International Instant Tea Decaffeinated English Breakfast Creme	1 serv (8 oz)	70	0	0
International Instant Tea Decaffeinated Viennese Cinnamon Creme	1 serv (8 oz)	70	0	0
International Instant Tea English Breakfast Creme as prep	1 serv (8 oz)	70	0	0
International Instant Tea English Raspberry Creme as prep	1 serv (8 oz)	70	0	0
International Instant Tea Island Orange Creme as prep	1 serv (8 oz)	70	0	0
International Instant Tea Viennese Cinnamon Creme as prep	1 serv (8 oz)	70	0	0
Lipton				
Brisk Tea as prep	1 serv	0	0	0
Decaffeinated Brisk Tea as prep	1 serv	0	0	0
English Blend as prep	1 cup	0	0	0
Flavored Decaffeinated Orange & Spice	1 tea bag	0	0	–
Green Tea	1 tea bag	0	0	–
Loose Tea	1 tsp (2 g)	0	0	0

FOOD	PORTION	CALS	CHOL	FIBER
Paradise				
Tropical Tea	8 fl oz	1	0	0
Tropical Tea Decafe	8 fl oz	1	0	0
Tropical Tea Passion Fruit	8 fl oz	1	0	0
Salada				
Green Tea	1 cup	0	0	0
Green Tea Decaffeinated	1 tea bag	0	0	–
Tetley				
British Blend Round Teabags	1 cup	0	0	0
Decaffeinated	1 tea bag	0	0	0
Tea Bag as prep	1	0	0	0
TAKE-OUT				
chai spiced latte decaf	1 cup	130	0	0
TEMPEH				
tempeh	½ cup	165	0	–
Lightlife				
Garden Vege	4 oz	200	0	6
Quinoa Sesame	4 oz	220	0	7
Smokey Strips	3 slices (2 oz)	80	0	1
Soy	4 oz	210	0	7
Three Grain	4 oz	200	0	6
Wild Rice	4 oz	190	0	6
Turtle Island				
Five Grain	3 oz	190	0	6
Low Fat Millet	3 oz	130	0	3
Soy	3 oz	160	0	7
Wild Rice Rhapsody	3 oz	160	0	7
White Wave				
Five Grain	⅓ block	140	0	4
Organic Original Soy	⅓ block	150	0	6
Organic Sea Veggie	⅓ block	120	0	8
Soy Rice	⅓ block	140	0	5
THYME				
ground	1 tsp	4	0	–
Watkins				
Thyme	¼ tsp (0.5 oz)	0	0	0

FOOD	PORTION	CALS	CHOL	FIBER
TOFU				
firm	¼ block (3 oz)	118	0	1
firm	½ cup	183	0	2
fresh fried	1 piece (0.5 oz)	35	0	tr
fuyu salted & fermented	1 block (⅓ oz)	13	0	tr
koyadofu dried frozen	1 piece (½ oz)	82	0	tr
okara	½ cup	47	0	1
regular	¼ block (4 oz)	88	0	1
regular	½ cup	94	0	1
Azumaya				
Baked Chili Picante	2 pieces	200	0	2
Baked Mesquite	2 pieces	100	0	2
Baked Spicy Thai Peanut	2 pieces	190	0	2
Baked Teriyaki	2 pieces	200	0	2
Extra Firm	1 serv (2.8 oz)	70	0	1
Firm	1 serv (2.8 oz)	70	0	0
Lite Extra Firm	1 serv (2.8 oz)	60	0	1
Lite Silken	1 serv (3.2 oz)	40	0	0
Silken	1 serv (3.2 oz)	40	0	—
Casbah				
Gyro as prep w/ tofu	1 patty (2 oz)	105	0	tr
Galaxy				
Slices Hickory Smoked	1 slice (1 oz)	50	0	0
Slices Italian Garlic Herb	1 slice (1 oz)	50	0	0
Slices Original	1 slice (1 oz)	50	0	0
Slices Savory	1 slice (1 oz)	50	0	0
Hinoichi				
Firm	1 inch slice (3 oz)	60	0	1
Long Life				
Tofu	3 oz	60	0	1
Mori-Nu				
Extra Firm	1 in slice (3 oz)	55	0	—
Firm	1 in slice (3 oz)	50	0	—
Lite Extra Firm	1 in slice (3 oz)	35	0	—
Lite Firm	1 in slice (3 oz)	35	0	—
Soft	1 in slice (3 oz)	45	0	—
Nasoya				
5 Spice	1 serv (3 oz)	70	0	0

FOOD	PORTION	CALS	CHOL	FIBER
Baked Mesquite Smoke	2 pieces	220	0	3
Baked Teriyaki	2 pieces	230	0	3
Baked TexMex	2 pieces	230	0	4
Baked Thai Peanut	2 pieces	240	0	3
Extra Firm	1 serv (3 oz)	90	0	0
Firm	1 serv (3 oz)	70	0	tr
Firm Enriched	1 serv (3 oz)	45	0	0
Garlic & Onion	1 serv (3 oz)	70	0	0
Silken	1 serv (3.2 oz)	45	0	0
Soft	1 serv (3 oz)	60	0	0
TofuMate Breakfast Scramble	¼ pkg	15	0	—
TofuMate Eggless Salad	¼ pkg	15	0	—
TofuMate Mandarin Stirfry	¼ pkg	30	0	—
TofuMate Mediterranean Herb	¼ pkg	15	0	—
TofuMate Szechwan StirFry	¼ pkg	25	0	—
TofuMate Texas Taco	¼ pkg	15	0	0
Pete's Tofu				
Dessert Peach Mango	1 serv (6 oz)	120	0	0
Dessert Very Berry	1 serv (6 oz)	120	0	0
Medium Firm	3 oz	70	0	0
Soft	3 oz	56	0	0
Super Firm Italian Herb	3 oz	120	0	tr
Super Frim	3 oz	130	0	0
Tofu 2 Go Lemon Pepper	2 pieces + sauce	160	0	2
Tofu 2 Go Santa Fe	2 pieces + sauce	150	0	2
Tofu 2 Go Sesame Ginger	2 pieces + sauce	160	0	2
Tofu 2 Go Thai Tango	2 pieces + sauce	165	0	2
Tree Of Life				
30% Reduced Fat Firm	⅕ block (3.2 oz)	90	0	2
Easymeal Pasta Primavera as prep	1 serv	460	10	3
Easymeal Southwest Medley as prep	1 serv	380	0	3

FOOD	PORTION	CALS	CHOL	FIBER
Easymeal Teriyaki Stir Fry as prep	1 serv	270	0	6
Easymeal Thai Stir Fry as prep	1 serv	270	0	6
Organic Baked	⅕ block (2.7 oz)	150	0	0
Organic Baked Island Spice	⅕ pkg (2.7 oz)	130	0	0
Organic Baked Oriental	⅓ pkg (2.7 oz)	130	0	0
Organic Baked Savory	⅕ block (2.7 oz)	140	0	0
Organic Firm	⅕ block (3.2 oz)	100	0	0
Raw Firm	⅕ block (3.2 oz)	100	0	0
White Wave				
Baked Garlic Herb Italian	1 piece	120	0	1
Baked Hickory Smoke BBQ	1 piece	75	0	1
Baked Roma Italian Basil	1 piece	100	0	2
Baked Teriyaki Oriental	1 piece	120	0	1
Baked Thai Style	1 piece	120	0	1
Baked Zesty Lemon Pepper	1 piece	120	0	1
Extra Firm	¼ block	80	0	1
Organic Extra Firm	⅕ block	90	0	1
Organic Soft	⅕ block	90	0	1
Reduced Fat	⅕ block	90	0	2

TOMATILLO
fresh	1 (1.2 oz)	11	0	—
fresh chopped	½ cup	21	0	—

TOMATO
CANNED
paste	½ cup	110	0	6
puree	1 cup	102	0	6
puree w/o salt	1 cup	102	0	6
red whole	½ cup	24	0	—
sauce	½ cup	37	0	2
sauce spanish style	½ cup	40	0	2
sauce w/ mushrooms	½ cup	42	0	—
sauce w/ onion	½ cup	52	0	—

FOOD	PORTION	CALS	CHOL	FIBER
stewed	½ cup	34	0	—
w/ green chiles	½ cup	18	0	—
wedges in tomato juice	½ cup	34	0	—
Amore				
Sun-Dried Tomato Paste	1 tsp (6 g)	15	0	0
Big R				
Cajun Stewed	½ cup (4.2 oz)	25	0	1
Diced w/ Chilies	½ cup (4.2 oz)	25	0	1
Mexican Stewed	½ cups (4.2 oz)	25	0	1
Stewed	½ cup (4.2 oz)	25	0	1
Whole	½ cup (4.2 oz)	25	0	1
Claussen				
Halves	1 serv (1 oz)	5	0	tr
Contadina				
Crushed	¼ cup	20	0	1
Italian Paste Roasted Garlic	2 tbsp	35	0	1
Italian Style Pear	½ cup	25	0	1
Italian Style Stewed	½ cup	40	0	1
Mexican Style Stewed	½ cup	40	0	1
Pasta Ready With Three Cheeses	½ cup	70	<5	tr
Paste	2 tbsp (1.2 oz)	30	0	1
Peeled Whole	½ cup	25	0	1
Puree	¼ cup (2.2 oz)	20	0	tr
Recipe Ready	½ cup	25	0	3
Recipe Ready Diced Roasted Garlic	½ cup (4.3 oz)	45	0	tr
Stewed	½ cup	40	0	1
Del Monte				
Chunky Chili Style	½ cup (4.5 oz)	30	0	2
Chunky Pasta Style	½ cup (4.5 oz)	45	0	2
Crushed Italian Recipe	½ cup (4.4 oz)	45	0	1
Crushed Original Recipe	½ cup (4.4 oz)	45	0	1
Crushed w/ Garlic	½ cup (4.4 oz)	50	0	1
Diced	½ cup (4.4 oz)	25	0	2
Diced No Salt Added	½ cup (4.4 oz)	25	0	2
Diced w/ Basil Garlic & Oregano	½ cup (4.4 oz)	50	0	1

FOOD	PORTION	CALS	CHOL	FIBER
Diced w/ Garlic & Onion	½ cup (4.4 oz)	40	0	1
Diced w/ Green Pepper & Onion	½ cup (4.4 oz)	40	0	2
Paste	2 tbsp (1.2 oz)	30	0	2
Sauce	¼ cup (2.1 oz)	20	0	1
Sauce No Salt Added	¼ cup (2.1 oz)	20	0	1
Stewed Cajun Recipe	½ cup (4.4 oz)	35	0	2
Stewed Italian Recipe	½ cup (4.4 oz)	30	0	2
Stewed Mexican Recipe	½ cup (4.4 oz)	35	0	2
Stewed Original	½ cup (4.4 oz)	35	0	2
Stewed Original No Salt Added	½ cup (4.4 oz)	35	0	2
Wedges	½ cup (4.4 oz)	35	0	2
Zesty Diced w/ Mild Green Chilies	½ cup (4.4 oz)	30	0	1
Eden				
Organic Diced	½ cup	30	0	2
Organic Diced w/ Green Chilies	½ cup	30	0	2
Hebrew National				
Pickled	⅓ tomato (1 oz)	4	0	–
Hunt's				
Angela Mia Puree	¼ cup (2.2 oz)	16	0	tr
Choice Cut	½ cup (4.2 oz)	23	0	1
Choice Cut Diced Tomatoes & Italian Herb	½ cup (4.2 oz)	24	0	1
Choice Cut Diced Tomatoes & Roasted Garlic	½ cup (4.2 oz)	24	0	1
Choice Cut Diced Tomatoes w/ Red Pepper & Basil	¼ cup (4.2 oz)	27	0	1
Crushed Pear Tomatoes	½ cup (4.2 oz)	29	0	2
Diced In Juice	½ cup (4.2 oz)	20	0	1
Diced In Puree	½ cup (4.3 oz)	23	0	1
Diced w/ Green Chilies	2 tbsp (0.4 oz)	1	0	tr
Paste	2 tbsp (1.2 oz)	30	0	2
Paste Italian	2 tbsp (1.2 oz)	27	0	2

FOOD	PORTION	CALS	CHOL	FIBER
Paste No Salt Added	2 tbsp (1.2 oz)	30	0	2
Paste With Garlic	2 tbsp (1.2 oz)	28	0	2
Petite Diced	½ cup	20	0	1
Puree	¼ cup (2.2 oz)	24	0	2
Ready Sauce Chunky Chili	¼ cup (2.2 oz)	22	0	1
Ready Sauce Chunky Italian	¼ cup (2.2 oz)	30	0	1
Ready Sauce Chunky Mexican	¼ cup (2.2 oz)	21	0	1
Ready Sauce Chunky Salsa	¼ cup (2.2 oz)	18	0	1
Ready Sauce Chunky Tomato	¼ cup (2.2 oz)	15	0	1
Ready Sauce Garlic & Herb	¼ cup (2.2 oz)	26	0	1
Sauce	¼ cup (2.2 oz)	16	0	1
Sauce Herb	¼ cup (2.2 oz)	32	0	1
Sauce Italian	¼ cup (2.2 oz)	32	0	1
Sauce Meatloaf Fixins	¼ cup (2.2 oz)	23	0	1
Sauce No Salt Added	¼ cup (2.2 oz)	16	0	1
Sauce Special	¼ cup (2.2 oz)	21	0	1
Stewed	½ cup (4.2 oz)	33	0	2
Stewed No Salt Added	½ cup (4.2 oz)	33	0	2
Whole Peeled	2 (5.2 oz)	24	0	1
Whole Peeled No Salt Added	2 (4.8 oz)	21	0	1
Muir Glen				
Diced Fire Roasted	¼ cup	30	0	1
Diced w/ Green Chilies	½ cup (4.5 oz)	25	0	1
Organic Chunky Sauce	¼ cup (2.3 oz)	20	0	1
Organic Crushed Fire Roasted	¼ cup	20	0	1
Organic Diced	½ cup (4.5 oz)	25	0	1
Organic Diced No Salt Added	½ cup (4.5 oz)	25	0	1
Organic Diced w/ Basil & Garlic	½ cup (4.5 oz)	25	0	1
Organic Diced w/ Italian Herbs	½ cup (4.4 oz)	25	0	1

FOOD	PORTION	CALS	CHOL	FIBER
Organic Ground Peeled	¼ cup (2.3 oz)	10	0	1
Organic Paste	2 tbsp (1.2 oz)	30	0	1
Organic Puree	¼ cup (2.2 oz)	20	0	1
Organic Sauce	¼ cup (2.2 oz)	20	0	1
Organic Sauce No Salt Added	¼ cup (2.2 oz)	20	0	1
Organic Stewed	½ cup (4.5 oz)	30	0	tr
Organic Whole Peeled	½ cup (4.6 oz)	30	0	1
Whole Peeled w/ Basil	½ cup (4.6 oz)	30	0	1
Old El Paso				
Tomatoes & Jalapenos	¼ cup (2 oz)	15	0	1
Tomatoes & Green Chilies	¼ cup (2 oz)	10	0	0
Progresso				
Crushed	¼ cup (2.1 oz)	20	0	1
Italian Style Peeled	½ cup (4.2 oz)	20	0	1
Paste	2 tbsp (1.2 oz)	30	0	1
Puree	¼ cup (2.2 oz)	25	0	1
Puree Thick Style	¼ cup (2.2 oz)	20	0	1
Sauce	¼ cup (2.1 oz)	20	0	1
Whole Peeled	½ cup (4.2 oz)	25	0	1
Red Pack				
Puree	¼ cup (2.2 oz)	25	0	1
Ro-Tel				
Diced Tomatoes & Green Chilies	½ cup (4.4 oz)	20	0	1
Rosoff's				
Pickled	⅓ tomato (1 oz)	5	0	—
Schorr's				
Pickled	⅓ tomato (1 oz)	4	0	—
Sonoma				
Dried Spice Medley oil drained	1 tbsp (0.5 oz)	50	0	1
Pesto	¼ cup (2 oz)	110	2	1
Tapenade	1 tbsp (0.7 oz)	70	0	1
DRIED				
sun dried	1 cup	140	0	—
sun dried	1 piece	5	0	—
sun dried in oil	1 cup (4 oz)	235	0	—

FOOD	PORTION	CALS	CHOL	FIBER
sun dried in oil	1 piece (3 g)	6	0	–
sun-dried	5 pieces (0.5 oz)	40	0	3
Sonoma				
Bits	2–3 tsp (5 g)	15	0	1
Dried	2–3 halves (5 g)	15	0	1
Julienne	7–9 pieces (5 g)	15	0	1
Pasta Toss	½ cup (0.7 oz)	70	0	3
Season It	2–3 tsp (5 g)	20	0	1
FRESH				
cooked	½ cup	32	0	–
green	1	30	0	–
red	1 (4.5 oz)	26	0	2
red chopped	1 cup	35	0	2
Chiquita				
Tomato	1 med (5.2 oz)	35	0	1
Eurofresh				
Tomatoes On The Vine	1 med (5.2 oz)	35	0	1
TAKE-OUT				
stewed	1 cup	80	0	–
TOMATO JUICE				
tomato juice	6 oz	32	0	–
tomato juice	½ cup	21	0	–
Del Monte				
Juice	8 fl oz	50	0	1
Snap-E-Tom Chile Cocktail	6 fl oz	40	0	1
Dole				
Juice	1 bottle (12 oz)	85	0	2
Hunt's				
Juice	1 can (6 oz)	22	0	1
No Salt Added	8 fl oz	34	0	2
Mott's				
Tomato Juice	8 fl oz	40	0	-
Muir Glen				
Organic	5.5 oz	40	0	4
TONGUE				
beef simmered	3 oz	241	91	–
lamb braised	3 oz	234	161	–
pork braised	3 oz	230	124	0

FOOD	PORTION	CALS	CHOL	FIBER
TORTILLA				
corn	1 (6-in diam)	56	0	1
corn w/o salt	1 6-in diam (.9 oz)	56	0	1
flour w/o salt	1 8-in diam (1.2 oz)	114	0	1
Alvarado St. Bakery				
Burrito Size	1 (2.2 oz)	170	0	1
Fajita Size	1 (1.6 oz)	130	0	1
La Mexicana				
Corn	1 (0.8 oz)	50	0	1
Flour	1 (0.8 oz)	80	0	1
Tortillas de Trigo	1 (1 oz)	140	0	1
Old El Paso				
Flour	1 (1.4 oz)	130	0	0
Soft Taco Tortilla	2 (1.8 oz)	180	0	0
Tyson				
Flour	1 (1.7 oz)	150	0	1
Flour Heat Pressed	2 (2 oz)	170	0	2
White Corn	2 (1.8 oz)	100	0	3
Whole Wheat Heat Pressed	1 (1.4 oz)	120	0	3
Yellow Corn	3 (1.9 oz)	140	0	3
TORTILLA CHIPS (see CHIPS)				
TREE FERN				
chopped cooked	½ cup	28	0	—
TRITICALE				
dry	1 cup (6.7 oz)	645	0	—
TROUT				
baked	3 oz	162	63	—
rainbow cooked	3 oz	129	62	—
seatrout baked	3 oz	113	90	—
Clear Springs				
Rainbow	3.5 oz	140	75	—
TRUFFLES				
fresh	0.5 oz	4	0	2
TUMERIC				
ground	1 tsp	8	0	—

FOOD	PORTION	CALS	CHOL	FIBER
TUNA				
CANNED				
light in oil	1 can (6 oz)	399	30	–
light in oil	3 oz	169	15	–
light in water	3 oz	99	25	–
light in water	1 can (5.8 oz)	192	49	–
white in oil	1 can (6.2 oz)	331	55	–
white in oil	3 oz	158	26	–
white in water	3 oz	116	35	–
white in water	1 can (6 oz)	234	72	–
Bumble Bee				
Chunk Light In Oil	2 oz	160	30	–
Chunk Light In Water Pouch	2 oz	60	30	0
Solid White in Oil	2 oz	130	30	–
Solid White In Water	2 oz	70	25	0
Progresso				
In Olive Oil drained	¼ cup (2 oz)	160	30	0
StarKist				
Chunk Light In Water	¼ cup (2 oz)	60	30	0
Chunk Light No Drain Package	¼ cup (2 oz)	60	30	0
Low Sodium Chunk White In Water	2 oz	60	25	0
Solid White Albacore In Spring Water	¼ cup (2 oz)	70	25	0
Tuna Fillet In Spring Water	¼ cup (2 oz)	60	30	0
FRESH				
bluefin cooked	3 oz	157	42	–
bluefin raw	3 oz	122	32	–
skipjack baked	3 oz	112	51	–
yellowfin baked	3 oz	118	49	–
TUNA DISHES				
MIX				
Tuna Helper				
AuGratin 50% Less Fat Recipe as prep	1 cup	240	15	1
AuGratin as prep	1 cup	300	20	1

FOOD	PORTION	CALS	CHOL	FIBER
Cheesy Broccoli 50% Less Fat Recipe as prep	1 cup	240	15	1
Cheesy Broccoli as prep	1 cup	290	20	1
Cheesy Pasta 50% Less Fat Recipe as prep	1 cup	230	15	tr
Cheesy Pasta as prep	1 cup	280	20	tr
Creamy Broccoli 50% Less Fat Recipe as prep	1 cup	240	15	1
Creamy Broccoli as prep	1 cup	310	20	1
Creamy Pasta 50% Less Fat Recipe as prep	1 cup	230	15	1
Creamy Pasta as prep	1 cup	300	20	1
Fettuccine Alfredo 50% Less Fat Recipe as prep	1 cup	240	15	1
Fettuccine Alfredo as prep	1 cup	310	15	1
Garden Cheddar 50% Less Fat Recipe as prep	1 cup	240	15	1
Garden Cheddar as prep	1 cup	290	20	1
Pasta Salad Low Fat Recipe as prep	⅔ cup	230	10	1
Pasta Salad as prep	⅔ cup	380	10	1
Tetrazzini 50% Less Fat Recipe as prep	1 cup	230	20	1
Tetrazzini as prep	1 cup	300	20	1
Tuna Melt Reduced Fat Recipe as prep	1 cup	240	15	1
Tuna Melt as prep	1 cup	300	20	1
Tuna Pot Pie as prep	1 cup	440	110	1
Tuna Romanoff 50% Less Fat Recipe as prep	1 cup	240	20	1
Tuna Romanoff as prep	1 cup	280	20	1
READY-TO-EAT				
Bumble Bee				
Tuna Salad Fat Free	1 pkg (3.5 oz)	190	15	0
Tuna Salad Kit	1 pkg (3.8 oz)	250	45	0
StarKist				
Lunch To-Go	1 pkg	310	40	tr

FOOD	PORTION	CALS	CHOL	FIBER
Ready-Mixed Tuna Salad Kit	1 pkg (3.5 oz)	190	5	2
Tuna Salad Lunch Kit	1 pkg (4.3 oz)	230	35	1
Wampler				
Salad	⅓ cup	180	20	—
Salad Chunky	⅓ cup	180	20	—
TAKE-OUT				
tuna salad	1 cup	383	27	—
tuna salad	3 oz	159	11	—

TURKEY *(see also* TURKEY DISHES, TURKEY SUBSTITUTES*)*
CANNED
Hormel

FOOD	PORTION	CALS	CHOL	FIBER
Chunk Turkey Ham	2 oz	70	40	0
Mary Kitchen				
Roast Turkey Hash	1 can (14.9 oz)	420	110	3
FRESH				
back w/ skin roasted	½ back (9 oz)	637	238	—
breast w/ skin roasted	4 oz	212	83	—
dark meat w/ skin roasted	3.6 oz	230	93	—
dark meat w/o skin roasted	3 oz	170	78	—
dark meat w/o skin roasted	1 cup (5 oz)	262	119	—
ground cooked	3 oz	188	57	—
leg w/ skin roasted	1 (1.2 lbs)	1133	466	—
leg w/ skin roasted	2.5 oz	147	61	—
light meat w/ skin roasted	4.7 oz	268	103	—
light meat w/ skin roasted	from ½ turkey (2.3 lbs)	2069	794	—
light meat w/o skin roasted	4 oz	183	81	—
neck simmered	1 (5.3 oz)	274	186	—
skin roasted	1 oz	141	36	—
skin roasted	from ½ turkey (9 oz)	1096	281	—
w/ skin roasted	½ turkey (4 lbs)	3857	1514	—
w/ skin roasted	8.4 oz	498	196	—

FOOD	PORTION	CALS	CHOL	FIBER
w/ skin neck & giblets roasted	½ turkey (8.8 lbs)	4123	1920	—
w/o skin roasted	1 cup (5 oz)	238	107	—
w/o skin roasted	7.3 oz	354	159	—
wing w/ skin roasted	1 (6.5 oz)	426	150	—
Butterball				
Ground All White Meat	3 oz	100	45	—
Louis Rich				
Ground	4 oz	190	90	0
Patties White	1 (4 oz)	170	65	0
Mr. Turkey				
Ground 85% Fat Free	3.5 oz	210	110	—
Ground 91% Fat Free	3.5 oz	170	95	—
Perdue				
Breast Tenderloins Butter Garlic	3 oz	100	45	—
Burger Cooked	1 (4 oz)	160	85	—
Dark Cooked	3 oz	180	85	—
Drumsticks Cooked	1 (2.2 oz)	110	80	—
Ground Cooked	3 oz	160	85	—
Tenderloins Black Pepper Cooked	3 oz	90	45	—
Thighs Cooked	1 (3.2 oz)	240	115	—
White Cooked	3 oz	150	65	—
Shady Brook				
Cutlets	4 oz	130	70	—
Drumstick	4 oz	170	70	—
Ground Breast	4 oz	120	70	—
Ground Lean	4 oz	170	90	—
Ground Turkey 85%	4 oz	220	75	—
Mesquite Seasoned Tenderloin	4 oz	110	50	—
OnlyOne Boneless Breast Roast	4 oz	130	70	—
Split Breast	4 oz	190	70	—
Tenderloin	4 oz	130	70	—
Teriyaki Seasoned Tenderloin	4 oz	120	50	—
Thigh	4 oz	220	75	—
Turkey Burgers	4 oz	170	90	—

FOOD	PORTION	CALS	CHOL	FIBER
Turkey Meatloaf Lean	4 oz	150	95	–
Whole Breast	4 oz	190	70	–
Whole Turkey	4 oz	180	75	–
Wing	4 oz	220	80	–
Zesty Lemon Seasoned Tenderlion	4 oz	120	50	–
Turkey Store				
Breakfast Sausage Patties Mild	2 patties (2.3 oz)	160	50	–
Lean Ground Italian Style	4 oz	190	80	–
Seasoned Cuts Turkey Breast Roast	4 oz	110	45	–
Wampler				
Boneless Breast Roast	4 oz	160	35	–
Breast Half	4 oz	160	35	–
Breast Steaks	4 oz	120	70	–
Drumsticks	4 oz	180	75	–
Ground	4 oz	210	100	–
Ground Breast	4 oz	130	70	–
Ground Lean	4 oz	160	90	–
Thighs	4 oz	170	80	–
Wings	4 oz	220	80	–
Woodfire Grill Burger	1 (3 oz)	180	65	
FROZEN				
roast boneless seasoned light & dark meat roasted	1 pkg (1.7 lbs)	1213	413	–
Empire				
Patties	1 (3.1 oz)	200	5	1
Wampler				
Burger BBQ	1 (4 oz)	240	140	–
Burgers Cracked Peppercorn & Garlic	1 (3 oz)	170	65	–
Seasoned Burgers Cracker Peppercorn & Garlic	1 (3 oz)	170	65	–
READY-TO-EAT				
bologna	1 oz	57	28	–
breast	1 slice (0.75 oz)	23	9	–

FOOD	PORTION	CALS	CHOL	FIBER
poultry salad sandwich spread	1 tbsp	109	4	–
poultry salad sandwich spread	1 oz	238	9	–
prebasted breast w/ skin roasted	1 breast (3.8 lbs)	2175	718	–
prebasted breast w/ skin roasted	½ breast (1.9 lbs)	1087	359	–
prebasted thigh w/ skin roasted	1 thigh (11 oz)	494	194	–
roll light & dark meat	1 oz	42	16	–
roll light meat	1 oz	42	12	–
salami cooked	2 oz	111	46	–
salami cooked	1 pkg (8 oz)	446	186	–
turkey loaf breast meat	1 pkg (6 oz)	187	69	–
turkey loaf breast meat	2 slices (1.5 oz)	47	17	–
Alpine Lace				
Breast Fat Free	2 oz	45	25	0
Boar's Head				
Breast Cracked Pepper Smoked	2 oz	60	30	0
Breast Golden Skin On	2 oz	60	25	0
Breast Golden Skinless	2 oz	60	25	0
Breast Hickory Smoked	2 oz	70	25	0
Breast Low Sodium Skinless	2 oz	60	25	0
Breast Lower Sodium Skin On	2 oz	60	25	0
Breast Maple Glazed Honey Coat	2 oz	70	30	0
Breast Ovengold Skin On	2 oz	60	35	0
Breast Ovengold Skinless	2 oz	60	20	0
Breast Roasted Mesquite Smoked Skinless	2 oz	60	25	0
Breast Roasted Salsalito	2 oz	60	25	0
Pastrami Seasoned	2 oz	60	25	0

FOOD	PORTION	CALS	CHOL	FIBER
Carl Buddig				
Honey Roasted Turkey Breast	1 pkg (2.5 oz)	120	40	—
Lean Slices Honey Roasted Breast	1 pkg (2.5 oz)	70	30	—
Lean Slices Oven Roasted Breast	1 pkg (2.5 oz)	70	30	—
Lean Slices Smoked Breast	1 pkg (2.5 oz)	70	30	—
Oven Roasted Breast	1 pkg (2.5 oz)	110	40	—
Smoked Breast	1 pkg (2.5 oz)	110	40	—
Turkey Ham	1 pkg (2.5 oz)	100	40	—
Empire				
Barbecue Whole	5 oz	250	100	0
Bologna	3 slices (1.8 oz)	90	30	0
Oven Prepared Breast Slices	3 slices (1.8 oz)	50	15	0
Pastrami	3 slices (1.8 oz)	60	30	1
Salami	3 slices (1.8 oz)	70	35	0
Smoked Breast Slices	3 slices (1.8 oz)	40	15	0
Falls				
BBQ	3 oz	140	55	—
Gourmet Breast	3 oz	80	35	—
Premium Cooked Breast	3 oz	100	40	—
Healthy Choice				
Deli-Thin Roasted Breast	6 slices (2 oz)	60	25	0
Deli-Thin Smoked Breast	6 slices (2 oz)	60	25	0
Deli-Thin Turkey Ham	6 slices (2 oz)	60	40	0
Fresh-Trak Honey Roast & Smoked Breast	1 slice (1 oz)	35	10	0
Fresh-Trak Oven Roasted Breast	1 slice (1 oz)	35	15	0
Honey Roasted & Smoked	1 slice (1 oz)	35	15	0
Oven Roasted Breast	1 slice (1 oz)	35	15	0

FOOD	PORTION	CALS	CHOL	FIBER
Smoked Breast	1 slice (1 oz)	30	10	0
Variety Pack Regular	3 slices (2.2 oz)	70	30	0
Hebrew National				
Deli Thin Hickory Smoked	1.8 oz	55	25	—
Deli Thin Lemon Garlic	1.8 oz	50	20	—
Deli Thin Oven Roasted	1.8 oz	80	20	—
Hormel				
Light & Lean 97 Breast Sliced	1 slice (1 oz)	30	15	0
Light & Lean 97 Mesquite Smoked Breast	1 slice (1 oz)	30	15	0
turkey pepperoni	17 slices (1 oz)	80	40	0
Jennie-O				
Turkey Breast Roast In Homestyle Gravy	1 serv (5 oz)	110	40	0
Jordan's				
Healthy Trim Fat Free Oven Roasted Breast	1 slice (1 oz)	20	15	0
Healthy Trim Fat Free Oven Roasted Smoked Breast	1 slice (1 oz)	20	15	0
Louis Rich				
Bologna	1 slice (28 g)	50	20	0
Breaded Nuggets	4 (3.2 oz)	260	35	0
Breaded Patties	1 (3 oz)	220	35	0
Breaded Sticks	3 (3 oz)	230	35	0
Breast Skinless Hickory Smoked	2 oz	50	25	0
Breast Skinless Honey Roasted	2 oz	60	20	0
Breast Skinless Oven Roasted	2 oz	50	20	0
Breast Skinless Rotisserie	2 oz	50	20	0
Breast Slices Hickory Smoked	1 slice (2 oz)	50	25	0
Breast Slices Honey Roasted	1 slice (2 oz)	60	20	0

FOOD	PORTION	CALS	CHOL	FIBER
Breast Slices Oven Roasted	1 slice (2 oz)	50	20	0
Breast Slices Rotisserie	1 slice (2 oz)	50	20	0
Carving Board Hickory Smoked	2 slices (1.6 oz)	40	20	0
Carving Board Oven Roasted Thin	6 slices (2.1 oz)	60	25	0
Carving Board Oven Roasted Traditional	2 slices (1.6 oz)	40	20	0
Carving Board Rotisserie	2 slices (1.6 oz)	40	20	0
Cotto Salami	1 slice (28 g)	40	25	0
Deli-Thin Oven Roasted	4 slices (1.8 oz)	50	20	0
Deli-Thin Smoked	4 slices (1.8 oz)	50	20	0
Fat Free Hickory Smoked Breast	1 slice (1 oz)	25	10	0
Fat Free Oven Roasted Breast	1 slice (1 oz)	25	10	0
Fat Free Oven Roasted Deli-Thin Breast	4 slices (1.8 oz)	45	15	0
Fat Free Turkey Ham Honey	2 slices (1.7 oz)	35	15	0
Fat Free Turkey Ham Smoked	2 slices (1.7 oz)	35	15	0
Hickory Smoked	1 slice (1 oz)	30	10	0
Oven Roasted	1 slice (1 oz)	30	10	0
Pastrami	1 slice (1 oz)	30	20	0
Salami	1 slice (28 g)	40	20	0
Smoked	1 slice (1 oz)	30	15	0
Turkey Ham	1 slice (1 oz)	30	20	0
Turkey Ham Chopped	1 slice (1 oz)	45	20	0
Turkey Ham Honey Cured	1 slice (1 oz)	30	20	0
Mr. Turkey				
Deli Cuts Hardwood Smoked Breast	3 slices	30	13	—
Deli Cuts Honey Roasted Breast	3 slices	30	15	—
Deli Cuts Oven Roasted Breast	3 slices	30	13	—

FOOD	PORTION	CALS	CHOL	FIBER
Deli Cuts Turkey Ham	3 slices	35	20	—
Deli Cuts Turkey Pastrami	3 slices	35	20	—
Hardwood Smoked Breast	1 slice	30	15	—
Hardwood Smoked Turkey Ham	1 slice	35	20	—
Honey Cured Turkey Ham	1 slice	30	20	—
Oven Roasted Breast	1 slice	30	15	—
Smoked Breakfast Turkey Ham	1 oz	30	18	—
Turkey Bologna	1 slice	70	25	—
Turkey Cotto Salami	1 slice	50	20	—
Turkey Ham	1 slice	35	20	—
Turkey Pastrami	1 slice	30	15	—
Oscar Mayer				
Free Oven Roasted Breast	4 slices (1.8 oz)	40	15	0
Free Smoked Breast	4 slices (1.8 oz)	40	15	0
Lunchables Fun Pack Turkey/Pacific Cooler	1 pkg (11.2 oz)	460	50	tr
Lunchables Fun Pack Turkey/Surger Cooler	1 pkg (11.2 oz)	440	45	0
Lunchables Turkey/Cheddar	1 pkg (4.5 oz)	360	70	1
Oven Roasted White	1 slice (1 oz)	30	10	0
Smoked White	1 slice (1 oz)	30	10	0
Perdue				
Breast Sliced Cajun Style	2 oz	50	20	—
Breast Sliced Honey Smoked	2 oz	50	20	—
Breast Sliced Pan Roasted	2 oz	70	30	—
Ham Hickory Smoked	2 oz	60	40	—
Healthsense Breast Sliced Oven Roasted	2 oz	60	20	—
Pastrami Hickory Smoked	2 oz	70	40	—

FOOD	PORTION	CALS	CHOL	FIBER
Sara Lee				
Hardwood Smoked Breast Of Turkey	2 oz	60	20	—
Hardwood Smoked Turkey Ham	2 oz	60	40	—
Honey Roasted Breast Of Turkey	2 oz	60	20	—
Honey Roasted Turkey Ham	2 oz	70	40	—
Mesquite Smoked Breast Of Turkey	2 oz	60	30	—
Oven Roasted Breast Of Turkey	2 oz	60	25	—
Peppered Breast Of Turkey	2 oz	50	20	—
Seasoned Breast Of Turkey Pastrami	2 oz	60	30	—
Shady Brook				
Black Forest Turkey Ham	2 oz	70	30	—
Browned Homestyle Oven Roasted Breast	2 oz	60	20	—
Browned Slow Roasted Breast	2 oz	60	20	—
Carved Breast Italian Seasoned	2 oz	60	20	—
Carved Breast Natural Roast	2 oz	60	20	—
Carved Breast Peppered	2 oz	60	20	—
Hickory Smoked Breast	2 oz	50	25	—
Honey Roasted Breast	2 oz	60	30	—
Honey Roasted Breast Covered w/ Cracked Pepper	2 oz	60	25	—
Meatballs Italian Style	3 (3 oz)	130	45	1
Smoked Drumstick	3 oz	180	70	—
Smoked Neck	3 oz	150	65	—
Smoked Whole Turkey	3 oz	150	60	—
Smoked Wing	3 oz	200	65	—

FOOD	PORTION	CALS	CHOL	FIBER
Wampler				
Bologna	2 oz	130	50	—
Dark Cured	2 oz	80	30	—
Deli Roast Breast	2 oz	50	25	—
Deli Roast Classic Spiced Breast	2 oz	70	25	—
Deli Roast Pan Roasted Breast	2 oz	70	20	—
Deli Roast Pan Roasted Skinless Breast	2 oz	50	20	—
Deli Roast Peppered Breast	21 oz	40	20	—
Deli Roast Rotisserie Breast	2 oz	50	20	—
Pastrami	2 oz	90	40	—
Salami	2 oz	90	55	—
Turkey Ham	2 oz	60	40	—

TURKEY DISHES
Banquet

FOOD	PORTION	CALS	CHOL	FIBER
Sandwich Toppers Gravy & Sliced Turkey	1 pkg (5 oz)	160	30	0
Dinty Moore				
Microwave Cup Stew	1 pkg (7.5 oz)	130	10	2
Stew	1 cup (8.5 oz)	140	20	2
Luigino's				
Gravy Dressing & Turkey	1 pkg (8 oz)	340	40	2
Mosey's				
Turkey Breast w/ Gravy	1 serv (5 oz)	140	90	0
Shady Brook				
Meatloaf	1 serv (16 oz)	470	175	—
Wampler				
Turkey Ham Salad	⅓ cup	150	30	—

TURKEY SUBSTITUTES
Lightlife

FOOD	PORTION	CALS	CHOL	FIBER
Smart Deli Turkey	3 slices (1.5 oz)	40	0	0
Soy Is Us				
Turkey Not!	½ cup (1.75 oz)	140	0	9

FOOD	PORTION	CALS	CHOL	FIBER
Tofurkey				
Deli Slices Hickory	1.5 oz	120	0	2
Deli Slices Original	1.5 oz	120	0	2
Deli Slices Peppered	1.5 oz	120	0	2
Drummettes	1 (3 oz)	105	0	4
Giblet Gravy	1 serv (3.5 oz)	42	0	1
Stuffed Tofu Roast	1 serv (4 oz)	193	0	2
Worthington				
Smoked Turkey Meatless	3 slices (2 oz)	140	0	2
Turkee Slices	3 slices (3.3 oz)	130	0	2
Yves				
Veggie Turkey Deli Slices	1 serv (2.2 oz)	85	0	1
TURNIPS				
canned greens	½ cup	17	0	—
cooked mashed	½ cup (4.2 oz)	47	0	—
cubed cooked	½ cup (3 oz)	33	0	—
frzn greens cooked	½ cup	24	0	2
greens chopped cooked	½ cup	15	0	2
greens raw chopped	½ cup	7	0	1
raw cubed	½ cup (2.4 oz)	25	0	—
Birds Eye				
Greens w/ Diced Turnip	1 cup	25	0	2
VANILLA				
Virginia Dare				
Vanilla Extract	1 tsp	10	0	—
VEAL *(see also* VEAL DISHES*)*				
cutlet lean only braised	3 oz	172	115	—
cutlet lean only fried	3 oz	156	91	—
ground broiled	3 oz	146	87	—
loin chop w/ bone lean & fat braised	1 chop (2.8 oz)	227	94	—
loin chop w/ bone lean only braised	1 chop (2.4 oz)	155	86	—
shoulder w/ bone lean only braised	3 oz	169	110	—

FOOD	PORTION	CALS	CHOL	FIBER
sirloin w/ bone lean & fat roasted	3 oz	171	87	—
sirloin w/ bone lean only roasted	3 oz	143	89	—

VEAL DISHES
TAKE-OUT

parmigiana	4.2 oz	279	136	2

VEGETABLE JUICE

vegetable juice cocktail	6 fl oz	34	0	—
vegetable juice cocktail	½ cup	22	0	—

Dole

Vegetable Blend	1 bottle (12 oz)	90	0	2

Hunt's

Cocktail	1 can (6 oz)	20	0	2

Muir Glen

Organic	5.5 oz	50	0	2

V8

Splash Tropical Blend	8 fl oz	120	0	—

VEGETABLES MIXED
CANNED

mixed vegetables	½ cup	39	0	—
peas & carrots	½ cup	48	0	—
peas & carrots low sodium	½ cup	48	0	—
peas & onions	½ cup	30	0	—
succotash	½ cup	102	0	—

Chi-Chi's

Diced Tomatoes & Green Chilies	¼ cup (2.5 oz)	20	0	0

Chun King

Chow Mein Vegetables	⅔ cup (3 oz)	14	0	1

Del Monte

Mixed	½ cup (4.4 oz)	40	0	2
Mixed No Salt Added	½ cup (4.4 oz)	40	0	2
Peas And Carrots	½ cup (4.5 oz)	60	0	2

FOOD	PORTION	CALS	CHOL	FIBER
Green Giant				
Garden Medley	½ cup (4.2 oz)	40	0	2
Mixed	½ cup (4.3 oz)	60	0	2
Sweet Peas & Carrots	½ cup (4.3 oz)	50	0	3
Sweet Peas & Tiny Pearl Onion	½ cup (4.4 oz)	60	0	4
House Of Tsang				
Vegetables & Sauce Cantonese Classic	½ cup (4.2 oz)	70	0	1
Vegetables & Sauce Hong Kong Sweet & Sour	½ cup (4.5 oz)	160	0	0
Vegetables & Sauce Szechuan Hot & Spicy	½ cup (4.2 oz)	70	0	1
Vegetables & Sauce Tokyo Teriyaki	½ cup (4.4 oz)	100	0	1
La Choy				
Chop Suey Vegetables	½ cup (2.2 oz)	10	0	1
LeSueur				
Early Peas w/ Mushrooms & Pearl Onions	½ cup (4.3 oz)	60	0	2
S&W				
Mixed	½ cup (4.4 oz)	35	0	2
Peas & Carrots	½ cup (4.5 oz)	60	0	2
Peas & Onions	½ cup (4.3 oz)	40	0	3
Veg-All				
Cajun Mixed	½ cup	50	0	3
FROZEN				
mixed vegetables cooked	½ cup	54	0	2
peas & carrots cooked	½ cup	38	0	—
peas & onions cooked	½ cup	40	0	—
succotash cooked	½ cup	79	0	—
Birds Eye				
Baby Sweet Peas & Pearl Onions	⅔ cup	60	0	4
Bavarian Vegetables	1 cup (5.5 oz)	150	30	3

FOOD	PORTION	CALS	CHOL	FIBER
Broccoli Cauliflower & Carrots	½ cup	25	0	2
Broccoli Cauliflower & Carrots In Cheese Sauce	½ cup	70	5	2
Broccoli Cauliflower & Red Peppers	½ cup	20	0	2
Broccoli & Cauliflower	½ cup	20	0	2
Broccoli Carrots & Water Chestnuts	½ cup	30	0	3
Broccoli Corn & Red Peppers	½ cup	50	0	3
Broccoli Red Peppers Onions & Mushrooms	½ cup	25	0	2
Brussels Sprouts Cauliflower & Carrots	½ cup	30	0	3
California Style Vegetables	½ cup	100	10	3
Cauliflower Nuggets Corn Carrots & Snow Peapods	½ cup	30	0	2
Gumbo Blend	¾ cup	40	0	2
Italian Style Vegetables & Bow Tie Pasta	1 cup	150	10	2
Mixed Vegetables	⅓ cup	50	0	3
New England Style Vegetables & Pasta Shells	1 pkg (9 oz)	260	15	3
Oriental Style Vegetables	½ cup	60	10	2
Peas & Pearl Onions	⅔ cup	90	0	5
Peas & Potatoes In Real Cream Sauce	½ cup	90	10	2
Radiatore Pasta & Vegetables	1 cup	200	5	1
Roasted Potatoes & Broccoli	⅔ cup (3.9 oz)	100	5	1
Roletti Pasta & Vegetables	1 cup (4.4 oz)	190	5	1
Stir Fry Asparagus	2 cups	90	0	3

FOOD	PORTION	CALS	CHOL	FIBER
Stir Fry Broccoli	1 cup	30	0	2
Stir Fry Pepper	1 cup	25	0	2
Stir Fry Sugar Snap	¾ cup	35	0	1
Stir Fry Whole Green Bean	1¾ cup	100	0	2
Stir Fry Style Vegetables	½ cup	60	10	1
Vegetables For Soup	⅔ cup	45	0	2
Vegetables For Stew	⅔ cup	40	0	1
Voila! Italian Pesto Chicken	2 cups	240	25	1
Voila! Three Cheese Chicken	1¾ cups	220	20	1
Budget Gourmet				
Mandarin Vegetables	1 pkg (5.25 oz)	160	10	—
New England Recipe Vegetables	1 pkg (5.5 oz)	230	25	—
Spring Vegetables In Cheese Sauce	1 pkg (5 oz)	130	20	—
Green Giant				
Alfredo Vegetables	¾ cup	70	5	3
American Mixtures Broccoli Carrots Cauliflower	¾ cup (2.6 oz)	25	0	2
American Mixtures Broccoli Carrots Waterchestnuts	¾ cup (3 oz)	30	0	3
American Mixtures Carrots Green Bean Cauliflower	¾ cup (2.7 oz)	25	0	2
American Mixtures Cauliflower Broccoli Sugar Snap & Sweet Pea	¾ cup (2.8 oz)	35	0	3
American Mixtures Corn Broccoli Red Pepper	¾ cup (3.1 oz)	60	0	2
American Mixtures Green Beans Potatoes Onions Red Peppers	¾ cup (2.8 oz)	45	0	2

FOOD	PORTION	CALS	CHOL	FIBER
American Mixtures Sweet Peas Potatoes Carrots	⅔ cup (3 oz)	70	0	3
Butter Sauce Broccoli Cauliflower Carrots Corn Sweet Peas	¾ cup (3.6 oz)	60	<5	2
Butter Sauce Broccoli Pasta Sweet Peas Corn Red Peppers	¾ cup (3.5 oz)	70	<5	2
Butter Sauce Mixed	¾ cup (3.6 oz)	70	<5	3
Cheese Sauce Broccoli Cauliflower Carrots	1 cup (4.1 oz)	60	5	2
Harvest Fresh Broccoli Cauliflower Carrots	1 cup (3.4 oz)	30	0	3
Harvest Fresh Mixed Vegetables	⅔ cup (3.1 oz)	50	0	3
Harvest Fresh Sweet Peas & Pearl Onions	½ cup (2.7 oz)	55	0	3
Mixed	¾ cup (2.9 oz)	50	0	3
Select Sweet Peas & Pearl Onions	⅔ cup (3.1 oz)	60	0	4
Health Is Wealth				
Veggie Munchees	2 (1 oz)	50	0	1
La Choy				
Fancy Chinese Mixed Vegetables	½ cup (2.9 oz)	9	0	1
McKenzie's				
Gumbo Mixture	1 serv (2.9 oz)	35	0	2
Ore Ida				
Stew Vegetables	⅔ cup (3 oz)	50	0	tr
Soglowek				
Golden Vegetarian Nuggets	4 pieces (2.5 oz)	190	0	1
Tree Of Life				
Mixed	½ cup (3 oz)	65	0	3
SHELF-STABLE				
TastyBite				
Curry Bangkok Red	½ pkg (5.3 oz)	88	0	1
Curry Patong Yellow	½ pkg (5.3 oz)	118	0	1
Curry Siam Green	½ pkg (5.3 oz)	63	0	1

FOOD	PORTION	CALS	CHOL	FIBER
Jaipur Vegetables	½ pkg (5 oz)	220	25	7
Malabar Mixed	½ pkg (5 oz)	67	0	1
TAKE-OUT				
buddha's delight	1 serv (16 oz)	174	35	3
caponata	¼ cup	28	0	–
gyoza potstickers vegetable	8 (4.9 oz)	210	0	5
ratatouille	1 serv (3.5 oz)	96	0	4
succotash	½ cup	111	0	–

VENISON

FOOD	PORTION	CALS	CHOL	FIBER
roasted	3 oz	134	95	–
Broken Arrow Ranch				
Antelope Chili Meat	3.5 oz	115	70	–
Antelope Ground Venison	3.5 oz	110	73	–
Antelope Stew Meat	3.5 oz	110	72	–
Nilgai Chili Meat	3.5 oz	115	70	–
Nilgai Leg	3.5 oz	100	65	–
Nilgai Stew Meat	3.5 oz	110	72	–

VINEGAR

FOOD	PORTION	CALS	CHOL	FIBER
balsamic	1 tbsp (0.5 oz)	5	0	–
cider	1 tbsp	tr	0	–
Eden				
Organic Brown Rice	1 tbsp	2	0	0
Ume Plum	1 tsp	2	0	0
Nakano				
Rice	1 tbsp	0	0	–
Progresso				
Balsamic	2 tbsp (0.5 oz)	10	0	0
Victoria				
Balsamic	1 tbsp (0.5 oz)	5	0	–
White House				
Apple Cider	1 tbsp (0.5 oz)	0	0	0
White	1 tbsp (0.5 oz)	0	0	–
Wild Thyme Farms				
Balsamic Red Raspberry	1 tbsp	13	0	–

FOOD	PORTION	CALS	CHOL	FIBER
WAFFLES				
FROZEN				
Aunt Jemima				
Blueberry	2 (2.5 oz)	190	10	1
Buttermilk	2 (2.5 oz)	170	10	1
Cinnamon	2 (2.5 oz)	180	10	1
Oatmeal	2 (2.5 oz)	170	0	3
Whole Grain	2 (2.5 oz)	170	0	2
Belgian Chef				
Belgian	2 (2.5 oz)	140	0	1
Eggo				
Apple Cinnamon	2 (2.7 oz)	220	20	1
Banana Bread	2 (2.7 oz)	200	0	2
Blueberry	2 (2.7 oz)	220	20	1
Buttermilk	2 (2.7 oz)	220	25	1
Golden Oat	2 (2.7 oz)	150	0	3
Homestyle	2 (2.7 oz)	220	25	1
Minis Cinnamon Toast	12 (3.2 oz)	290	25	2
Minis Cinnamon Toast	12 (3.2 oz)	280	25	0
Minis Homestyle	12 (3.3 oz)	260	25	2
Nut & Honey	2 (2.7 oz)	240	25	2
Nutri-Grain	2 (2.7 oz)	190	0	4
Nutri-Grain Multi-Bran	2 (2.7 oz)	180	0	6
Nutri-Grain Raisin & Bran	2 (2.9 oz)	210	0	5
Special K	2 (2 oz)	120	0	1
Strawberry	2 (2.7 oz)	220	20	1
Kellogg's				
Homestyle Low Fat	2 (2.7 oz)	180	20	1
Nutri-Grain Low Fat	2 (2.7 oz)	160	0	3
Nutri-Grain Low Fat Blueberry	2 (2.7 oz)	160	0	3
Kid Cuisine				
Wave Rider Waffle Sticks	1 meal (6.6 oz)	380	30	3
Van's				
7 Grain Belgain	2	152	0	8
Belgian Original	2	145	0	2
Belgian Original Toaster	2	145	0	2

FOOD	PORTION	CALS	CHOL	FIBER
Blueberry Toaster	2	157	0	2
Blueberry Wheat Free Toaster	2	225	0	5
Fat Free	2	155	0	7
Mini	4	107	0	6
Multigrain Toaster	2	160	0	6
Organic Whole Wheat	2	190	0	6
Organic Whole Wheat Blueberry	2	190	0	6
Wheat Free Cinnamon Apple Toaster	2	220	0	5
Wheat Free Toaster	2	220	0	5
MIX				
plain as prep	1 7 in diam (2.6 oz)	218	39	1
READY-TO-EAT				
Thomas'				
Buttermilk	1 (1.6 oz)	130	0	tr
TAKE-OUT				
plain	1 (7 in diam)	218	52	–
WALNUTS				
black dried chopped	1 cup	759	0	–
english dried	1 oz	182	0	1
english dried chopped	1 cup	770	0	6
halves	14 (1 oz)	190	0	2
Planters				
Black	1 pkg (2 oz)	340	0	3
Gold Measure Halves	1 pkg (2 oz)	380	0	2
Halves	⅓ cup (1.2 oz)	220	0	1
Pieces	¼ cup (1 oz)	190	0	1
WASABI (see HORSERADISH)				
WATER				
ice cubes	3	0	0	–
tap water	8 oz	0	0	–
Absopure				
Natural Spring	8 fl oz	0	0	–
Aquafina				
Essentials B-Power Wild Berry	8 fl oz	40	0	–

FOOD	PORTION	CALS	CHOL	FIBER
Essentials Calcium + Tangerine Pineapple	8 fl oz	40	0	–
Essentials Daily C Citrus	8 fl oz	40	0	–
Essentials Multi-V Watermelon	8 fl oz	40	0	–
Water	8 fl oz	0	0	–
Aquess				
Purified Water w/ Soluble Fiber	1 bottle (18 oz)	30	0	5
Canada Dry				
Sparkling Water	8 fl oz	0	0	0
Castellina				
Sparking Spring	8 fl oz	0	0	0
Crystal Geyser				
Sparking Natural Wild Cherry	1 bottle (12 fl oz)	0	0	–
Sparkling Lemon	1 bottle (12 fl oz)	0	0	–
Sparkling Mineral	1 bottle (12 fl oz)	0	0	–
Sparkling Natural Cola Berry	1 bottle (12 fl oz)	0	0	–
Sparkling Orange	1 bottle (12 fl oz)	0	0	–
Spring Water	8 fl oz	0	0	0
Dasani				
Purfied Water	8 oz	0	0	–
Diamond Spring				
Water	1 qt	0	0	–
Evian				
Spring Water	1 bottle (11.5 oz)	0	0	0
Ferrarelle				
Sparkling	8 fl oz	0	0	1
Gerolsteiner				
Sparling Mineral	8 fl oz	0	0	0
Glaceau				
Smartwater	8 oz	0	0	0
Vitamin Water Tropical Citrus	1 cup (8 oz)	40	0	–
Glacier Springs				
Drinking Water	8 fl oz	0	0	0

FOOD	PORTION	CALS	CHOL	FIBER
Glennpatrick				
Irish Spring Pure	8 oz	0	0	—
Hansen's				
Energy Water Lemon	8 oz	10	0	—
LaCroix				
Sparkling Berry	12 fl oz	0	0	—
Sparkling Lemon	12 fl oz	0	0	—
Sparkling Lime	12 fl oz	0	0	—
Sparkling Orange	12 fl oz	0	0	—
Sparkling Regular	12 fl oz	0	0	—
Spring	1 bottle (12 oz)	0	0	0
Meridian				
Clear All Flavors	8 oz	100	0	—
Mountain Valley				
Mineral Water	1 qt	0	0	—
Mt Shasta				
Natural Spring	1 bottle (20 oz)	0	0	0
Propel				
Fitness Water Berry	8 fl oz	10	0	—
Fitness Water Black Cherry	8 fl oz	10	0	—
Reebok				
Fitness Water Berry	1 bottle (24 oz)	30	0	0
Fitness Water Natural	1 bottle (24 oz)	0	0	0
Replenish				
Elements Enhanced Water Orange	8 oz	40	0	—
San Pellegrino				
Acqua Panna	8 fl oz	0	0	0
Saratoga				
Spring	8 oz	0	0	—
Snapple				
Natural Spring	8 fl oz	0	0	0
Veryfine				
Fruit₂O Lemon	8 oz	0	0	—
Fruit₂O Lemon Lime	8 fl oz	0	0	—
Fruit₂O Orange	8 fl oz	0	0	—
Fruit₂O Raspberry	8 fl oz	0	0	—
Volvic				
Spring Water	8 oz	0	0	0

FOOD	PORTION	CALS	CHOL	FIBER
Water Joe				
Caffeine Enhanced	8 fl oz	0	0	—
WATER CHESTNUTS				
chinese sliced canned	½ cup	35	0	—
fresh sliced	½ cup	66	0	—
Chun King				
Sliced	2 tbsp (0.8 oz)	11	0	1
Whole	2 (0.7 oz)	10	0	1
La Choy				
Chopped	2 tbsp (0.6 oz)	9	0	1
Sliced	2 tbsp (0.8 oz)	11	0	1
Whole	2 (0.7 oz)	10	0	1
WATERCRESS				
fresh chopped	½ cup	2	0	tr
garden fresh	½ cup	8	0	—
garden fresh cooked	½ cup	16	0	—
WATERMELON				
cut up	1 cup	50	0	1
seeds dried	1 oz	158	0	—
seeds dried	1 cup	602	0	—
wedge	⅟₁₆	152	0	2
WATERMELON JUICE				
Kool-Aid				
Splash Drink	1 serv (8 oz)	110	0	0
WAX BEANS				
CANNED				
Del Monte				
Cut Golden	½ cup (4.2 oz)	20	0	2
Owatonna				
Cut	½ cup	20	0	—
S&W				
Cut	½ cup (4.2 oz)	20	0	2
WHEAT				
sprouted	1 cup (3.8 oz)	214	0	1
Lightlife				
Savory Seitan Barbecue	4 oz	160	0	0
Savory Seitan Teriyaki	4 oz	160	0	0

FOOD	PORTION	CALS	CHOL	FIBER
Near East				
Taboule Salad Mix as prep	⅔ cup	120	0	3
Wheat Pilaf as prep	1 cup	220	0	5
Sonoma				
Wheat Nuts Salted	2 tbsp (0.5 oz)	60	0	1
WHEAT GERM				
plain toasted	¼ cup (1 oz)	108	0	4
plain toasted	1 cup	431	0	—
Kretschmer				
Original Toasted	2 tbsp (0.5 oz)	50	0	2
Stone-Buhr				
Untoasted	2 tbsp (0.5 oz)	58	0	2
WHIPPED TOPPINGS				
cream pressurized	1 cup (2.1 oz)	154	46	—
cream pressurized	1 tbsp (3 g)	8	2	—
nondairy frzn	1 tbsp	13	0	—
nondairy powdered as prep w/ whole milk	1 cup	151	8	—
nondairy powdered as prep w/ whole milk	1 tbsp (4 g)	8	tr	—
nondairy pressurized	1 tbsp (4 g)	11	0	—
nondairy pressurized	1 cup	184	0	—
Cool Whip				
Extra Creamy	2 tbsp (0.3 oz)	25	0	0
Free	2 tbsp (0.3 oz)	15	0	0
Lite	2 tbsp (0.3 oz)	20	0	0
Original	2 tbsp (0.3 oz)	25	0	0
Dream Whip				
Mix as prep	2 tbsp (0.3 oz)	20	0	0
Estee				
Whipped Topping	1 serv	10	0	0
Hood				
Instant	2 tbsp	20	<5	0
Light Instant	2 tbsp	15	<5	0
Kraft				
Dairy Whip Light Cream	2 tbsp (0.2 oz)	10	<5	0
Fat Free	1 tbsp (0.3 oz)	15	0	0

FOOD	PORTION	CALS	CHOL	FIBER
Reddiwip				
Lite	2 tbsp (8 g)	15	0	—
Non-Dairy	2 tbsp (8 g)	20	0	—
Real Whipped Heavy Cream	2 tbsp (8 g)	30	10	—
Real Whipped Light Cream	2 tbsp (8 g)	20	<5	—
WHITE BEANS				
canned	1 cup	306	0	—
dried regular cooked	1 cup	249	0	—
dried small cooked	1 cup	253	0	—
Progresso				
Cannellini	½ cup (4.6 oz)	100	0	5
WHITEFISH				
baked	3 oz	146	65	—
smoked	1 oz	39	9	—
smoked	3 oz	92	28	—
WHITING				
cooked	3 oz	98	71	—
raw	3 oz	77	57	—
WILD RICE				
cooked	1 cup (5.7 oz)	166	0	3
Haddon House				
Extra Fancy	¼ cup (1.6 oz)	170	0	2
WINE				
japanese plum	3 oz	139	0	0
japanese sake	1 oz	33	0	0
red	3½ oz	74	0	—
rose	3½ oz	73	0	—
sherry	2 oz	84	0	—
sweet dessert	2 oz	90	0	—
vermouth dry	3½ oz	105	0	—
vermouth sweet	3½ oz	167	0	—
white	3½ oz	70	0	—
Boone's				
Country Kwencher	4 fl oz	96	0	—
Delicious Apple	4 fl oz	84	0	—

FOOD	PORTION	CALS	CHOL	FIBER
Sangria	4 fl oz	88	0	–
Snow Creek Berry	4 fl oz	72	0	–
Strawberry Hill	4 fl oz	88	0	–
Sun Peak Peach	4 fl oz	72	0	–
Wild Island	4 fl oz	72	0	–
Carlo Rossi				
Blush	4 fl oz	84	0	–
Burgundy	4 fl oz	88	0	–
Chablis	4 fl oz	84	0	–
Paisano	4 fl oz	92	0	–
Red Sangria	4 fl oz	92	0	–
Rhine	4 fl oz	84	0	–
Vin Rosé	4 fl oz	84	0	–
White Grenache	4 fl oz	80	0	–
Eden				
Mirin Rice Cooking Wine	1 tbsp	25	0	0
Fairbanks				
Cream Sherry	4 fl oz	168	0	–
Port	4 fl oz	176	0	–
Sherry	4 fl oz	136	0	–
White Port	4 fl oz	136	0	–
Gallo				
Blush Chablis	4 fl oz	88	0	–
Burgundy	4 fl oz	88	0	–
Cabernet Sauvignon	4 fl oz	88	0	–
Chablis Blanc	4 fl oz	80	0	–
Chardonnay	4 fl oz	92	0	–
Classic Burgundy	4 fl oz	84	0	–
French Colombard	4 fl oz	84	0	–
Hearty Burgundy	4 fl oz	88	0	–
Johannisberg Riesling '88	4 fl oz	80	0	–
Pink Chablis	4 fl oz	80	0	–
Red Rosé	4 fl oz	92	0	–
Rhine	4 fl oz	88	0	–
Sauvignon Blanc '90	1 fl oz	20	0	–
White Grenache '92	1 fl oz	20	0	–
White Grenache New Vintage	1 fl oz	20	0	–
White Zinfandel '91	1 fl oz	18	0	–

FOOD	PORTION	CALS	CHOL	FIBER
White Zinfandel New Vintage	1 fl oz	18	0	–
Zinfandel '87	1 fl oz	23	0	–
Sheffield Cellars				
Sherry	4 fl oz	136	0	–
Tawny Port	4 fl oz	180	0	–
Vermouth Extra Dry	1 fl oz	28	0	–
Vermouth Sweet	1 fl oz	43	0	–
Very Dry Sherry	4 fl oz	128	0	–

WINE COOLERS
Bartles & Jaymes

FOOD	PORTION	CALS	CHOL	FIBER
Berry	12 fl oz	210	0	–
Margarita	12 fl oz	260	0	–
Original	12 fl oz	190	0	–
Peach	12 fl oz	210	0	–
Pina Colada	12 fl oz	280	0	–
Planter's Punch	12 fl oz	230	0	–
Strawberry	12 fl oz	210	0	–
Strawberry Daquiri	12 fl oz	230	0	–
Tropical	12 fl oz	230	0	–

WINGED BEANS

FOOD	PORTION	CALS	CHOL	FIBER
dried cooked	1 cup	252	0	–

WOLFFISH

FOOD	PORTION	CALS	CHOL	FIBER
atlantic baked	3 oz	105	50	–

WRAPS *(see BREAD)*

YAM *(see also SWEET POTATO)*
CANNED
S&W

FOOD	PORTION	CALS	CHOL	FIBER
Candied	½ cup (4.9 oz)	170	0	4
FRESH				
mountain yam hawaii cooked	½ cup	59	0	–
yam cubed cooked	½ cup	79	0	–

YAMBEAN

FOOD	PORTION	CALS	CHOL	FIBER
cooked	¾ cup	38	0	–

FOOD	PORTION	CALS	CHOL	FIBER
YARDLONG BEANS				
dried cooked	1 cup	202	0	–
YAUTIA (TANNIER)				
fresh sliced	1 cup (4.7 oz)	132	0	2
root raw	1 (10.7 oz)	299	0	5
YEAST				
baker's compressed	1 cake (0.6 oz)	18	0	2
baker's dry	1 pkg (¼ oz)	21	0	–
baker's dry	1 tbsp	35	0	3
brewer's dry	1 tbsp	25	0	–
Hodgson Mill				
Fast Rise	1 tsp (9 g)	25	0	1
Red Star				
Yeast	4 tbsp (0.5 oz)	47	0	4
Yeast Flakes	3 tbsp (0.5 oz)	47	0	4
YELLOW BEANS				
canned	½ cup	13	0	1
canned low sodium	½ cup	13	0	1
dried cooked	1 cup	254	0	–
fresh cooked	½ cup	22	0	–
fresh raw	½ cup	17	0	–
frozen cooked	½ cup	18	0	–
YELLOWEYE BEANS				
CANNED				
B&M				
Baked	½ cup (4.6 oz)	170	<5	7
YOGURT *(see also* YOGURT FROZEN*)*				
coffee lowfat	8 oz	194	11	–
fruit lowfat	8 oz	225	10	–
fruit lowfat	4 oz	113	5	–
plain	8 oz	139	29	–
plain lowfat	8 oz	144	14	–
plain no fat	8 oz	127	4	–
vanilla lowfat	8 oz	194	11	–
Breyers				
Blended Blueberry	4.4 oz	130	10	0
Blended Peach	4.4 oz	130	10	0

FOOD	PORTION	CALS	CHOL	FIBER
Blended Strawberry	4.4 oz	130	10	0
Light Nonfat Apple Pie A La Mode	8 oz	120	10	0
Light Nonfat Berry Banana Split	8 oz	120	10	0
Light Nonfat Black Cherry Jubilee	8 oz	120	10	0
Light Nonfat Blueberries N' Cream	8 oz	120	10	0
Light Nonfat Cherry Bon-Bon	8 oz	120	10	0
Light Nonfat Cherry Vanilla Cream	8 oz	120	10	0
Light Nonfat Classic Strawberry	8 oz	120	10	0
Light Nonfat Key Lime Pie	8 oz	120	10	0
Light Nonfat Lemon Chiffon	8 oz	120	10	0
Light Nonfat Peaches N' Cream	8 oz	120	10	0
Light Nonfat Raspberries N' Cream	8 oz	120	10	0
Light Nonfat Strawberry Cheesecake	8 oz	120	10	tr
Lowfat Black Cherry	8 oz	240	15	0
Lowfat Blueberry	8 oz	230	15	0
Lowfat Mixed Berry	8 oz	320	15	0
Lowfat Peach	8 oz	240	15	0
Lowfat Pineapple	8 oz	240	15	0
Lowfat Red Raspberry	8 oz	230	15	2
Lowfat Strawberry	8 oz	230	15	0
Lowfat Strawberry Banana	8 oz	240	15	tr
Lowfat Vanilla	8 oz	220	20	0
Smooth & Creamy Apple Cobbler	8 oz	230	20	0
Smooth & Creamy Black Cherry Parfait	8 oz	240	20	0

FOOD	PORTION	CALS	CHOL	FIBER
Smooth & Creamy Black Cherry Parfait	4.4 oz	130	10	0
Smooth & Creamy Blueberries 'N Cream	8 oz	240	20	0
Smooth & Creamy Blueberries 'N Cream	4.4 oz	130	10	0
Smooth & Creamy Classic Strawberry	8 oz	230	20	0
Smooth & Creamy Classic Strawberry	4.4 oz	130	10	0
Smooth & Creamy Orange Vanilla Cream	8 oz	230	20	0
Smooth & Creamy Peaches 'N Cream	4.4 oz	130	10	0
Smooth & Creamy Peaches 'N Cream	8 oz	230	20	0
Smooth & Creamy Raspberries 'N Cream	8 oz	230	20	0
Smooth & Creamy Strawberry Banana Split	8 oz	240	10	tr
Smooth & Creamy Strawberry Cheesecake	8 oz	240	20	0
Colombo				
99% Fat Free Peach	4 oz	110	5	0
99% Fat Free Strawberry	4 oz	110	5	0
Banana Strawberry	8 oz	210	15	0
Black Cherry	8 oz	200	15	0
Blueberry	8 oz	200	15	0
Fat Free Apples 'n Spice	8 oz	190	5	0
Fat Free Apricot	8 oz	190	5	0
Fat Free Blueberry	8 oz	190	5	0
Fat Free Cappuccino	8 oz	180	<5	0
Fat Free Cherry	8 oz	190	5	0
Fat Free Cranberry Strawberry	8 oz	200	5	0
Fat Free French Roast	8 oz	180	<5	0
Fat Free Fruit Cocktail	8 oz	190	5	0

FOOD	PORTION	CALS	CHOL	FIBER
Fat Free Lemon	8 oz	170	<5	0
Fat Free Peach	8 oz	190	5	0
Fat Free Plain	8 oz	110	5	0
Fat Free Raspberry	8 oz	190	5	0
Fat Free Strawberry Pineapple Orange	8 oz	190	5	0
Fat Free Vanilla	8 oz	170	5	0
French Vanilla	8 oz	180	20	0
Light 100 Blueberry	8 oz	100	<5	0
Light 100 Cherry Vanilla	8 oz	100	<5	0
Light 100 Coffee & Cream	8 oz	100	<5	0
Light 100 Creamy Vanilla	8 oz	100	<5	0
Light 100 Juicy Peach	8 oz	100	<5	0
Light 100 Lemon Creme	8 oz	100	<5	0
Light 100 Mandarin Orange	8 oz	100	<5	0
Light 100 Mixed Berries	8 oz	100	<5	0
Light 100 Raspberry	8 oz	100	<5	0
Light 100 Strawberry	8 oz	100	<5	0
Peach Melba	8 oz	200	15	0
Plain	8 oz	120	20	0
Raspberry	8 oz	200	15	0
Strawberry	8 oz	200	15	0
Dannon				
Chunky Fruit Nonfat Apple Cinnamon	6 oz	160	5	0
Chunky Fruit Nonfat Blueberry	6 oz	160	5	0
Chunky Fruit Nonfat Cherry Vanilla	6 oz	160	5	0
Chunky Fruit Nonfat Peach	6 oz	160	5	0
Chunky Fruit Nonfat Strawberry	6 oz	160	5	0
Chunky Fruit Nonfat Strawberry Banana	6 oz	160	5	0
Danimals Lowfat Tropical Punch	4.4 oz	130	5	0

FOOD	PORTION	CALS	CHOL	FIBER
Danimals Lowfat Blueberry	4.4 oz	130	5	0
Danimals Lowfat Grape Lemonade	4.4 oz	120	5	0
Danimals Lowfat Lemon Ice	4.4 oz	120	5	0
Danimals Lowfat Orange Banana	4.4 oz	130	5	0
Danimals Lowfat Strawberry	4.4 oz	130	5	0
Danimals Lowfat Vanilla	4.4 oz	120	5	0
Danimals Lowfat Wild Raspberry	4.4 oz	120	5	0
Double Delights Banana Creme Strawberry	6 oz	160	10	0
Double Delights Bavarian Creme Raspberry	6 oz	170	10	0
Double Delights Cheesecake Cherry	6 oz	170	10	0
Double Delights Cheesecake Strawberry	6 oz	170	10	0
Double Delights Chocolate Cheesecake	6 oz	220	10	0
Double Delights Chocolate Dipped Strawberry	6 oz	210	10	0
Double Delights Chocolate Eclair	6 oz	220	10	0
Double Delights Vanilla Strawberry	6 oz	170	10	0
Double Delights Vanilla Peach & Apricot	6 oz	170	10	0
Fruit On The Bottom Lowfat Apple Cinnamon	8 oz	240	15	1

FOOD	PORTION	CALS	CHOL	FIBER
Fruit On The Bottom Lowfat Blueberry	8 oz	240	15	1
Fruit On The Bottom Lowfat Boysenberry	8 oz	240	15	1
Fruit On The Bottom Lowfat Cherry	8 oz	240	15	1
Fruit On The Bottom Lowfat Minipack Mixed Berry	4.4 oz	130	10	tr
Fruit On The Bottom Lowfat Minipack Strawberry	4.4 oz	130	10	tr
Fruit On The Bottom Lowfat Mixed Berries	8 oz	240	15	1
Fruit On The Bottom Lowfat Orange	8 oz	240	15	0
Fruit On The Bottom Lowfat Peach	8 oz	240	15	1
Fruit On The Bottom Lowfat Raspberry	8 oz	240	15	1
Fruit On The Bottom Lowfat Strawberry	8 oz	240	15	1
Fruit On The Bottom Lowfat Strawberry Banana	8 oz	240	15	1
LaCreme Vanilla	1 pkg (4.4 oz)	140	20	—
Light 'N Crunchy Mint Chocolate Chip	8 oz	140	5	0
Light 'N Crunchy Nonfat Caramel Apple Crunch	8 oz	140	<5	0
Light 'N Crunchy Nonfat Lemon Blueberry Cobbler	8 oz	140	<5	0
Light 'N Crunchy Nonfat Mocha Cappuccino	8 oz	140	<5	0
Light 'N Crunchy Nonfat Raspberry w/ Granola	8 oz	140	<5	2

FOOD	PORTION	CALS	CHOL	FIBER
Light 'N Crunchy Nonfat Vanilla Chocolate Crunch	8 oz	130	<5	0
Light Duets Cherry Cheesecake	6 oz	90	0	0
Light Duets Peaches N' Cream	6 oz	90	0	0
Light Duets Raspberry Royale	6 oz	90	0	0
Light Duets Strawberry Cheesecake	6 oz	90	0	0
Light Nonfat Banana Cream Pie	8 oz	100	<5	0
Light Nonfat Blueberry	8 oz	100	<5	0
Light Nonfat Cappuccino	8 oz	100	5	0
Light Nonfat Cherry Vanilla	8 oz	100	<5	0
Light Nonfat Coconut Cream Pie	8 oz	100	5	0
Light Nonfat Creme Caramel	8 oz	100	<5	0
Light Nonfat Lemon Chiffon	8 oz	100	5	0
Light Nonfat Mint Chocolate Cream Pie	8 oz	100	<5	0
Light Nonfat Peach	8 oz	100	<5	0
Light Nonfat Raspberry	8 oz	100	<5	0
Light Nonfat Strawberry	8 oz	100	<5	0
Light Nonfat Strawberry Banana	8 oz	100	<5	0
Light Nonfat Strawberry Kiwi	8 oz	100	5	0
Light Nonfat Tangerine Chiffon	8 oz	100	5	0
Light Nonfat Vanilla	8 oz	100	<5	0
Lowfat Coffee	8 oz	210	15	0
Lowfat Cranberry Raspberry	8 oz	210	15	0
Lowfat Lemon	8 oz	210	15	0

FOOD	PORTION	CALS	CHOL	FIBER
Lowfat Vanilla	8 oz	210	15	0
Minipack Blended Nonfat Blueberry	4.4 oz	120	5	0
Minipack Blended Nonfat Cherry	4.4 oz	110	5	0
Minipack Blended Nonfat Peach	4.4 oz	120	5	0
Minipack Blended Nonfat Raspberry	4.4 oz	120	5	0
Minipack Blended Nonfat Strawberry	4.4 oz	120	5	0
Minipack Blended Nonfat Strawberry Banana	4.4 oz	120	5	0
Sprinkl'ins Cherry Vanilla	1 (4.1 oz)	130	5	0
Sprinkl'ins Strawberry	1 (4.1 oz)	130	5	0
Sprinkl'ins Strawberry Banana	1 (4.1 oz)	130	5	0
Sprinkl'ins Vanilla w/ Cherry Crystals	1 (4.1 oz)	110	5	0
Sprinkl'ins Vanilla w/ Orange Crystals	1 (4.1 oz)	110	5	0
Friendship				
Coffee	8 oz	210	20	0
Fruit Crunch Peach	6 oz	190	10	0
Fruit Crunch Strawberry	6 oz	190	10	0
Fruit Crunch Strawberry Banana	6 oz	190	10	0
Plain	8 oz	150	20	0
Hood				
Fat Free Blueberry	1 (8 oz)	190	5	1
Fat Free Cherry	1 (8 oz)	190	5	1
Fat Free Peach	1 (8 oz)	190	5	1
Fat Free Plain	1 (8 oz)	130	5	0
Fat Free Raspberry	1 (8 oz)	190	5	1
Fat Free Strawberry	1 (8 oz)	190	5	1
Fat Free Strawberry Banana	1 (8 oz)	190	5	1
Fat Free Vanilla	1 (8 oz)	190	5	1

FOOD	PORTION	CALS	CHOL	FIBER
Fat Free Swiss Blueberry	1 (8 oz)	210	5	0
Fat Free Swiss Lemon	1 (8 oz)	210	5	0
Fat Free Swiss Raspberry	1 (8 oz)	210	5	0
Fat Free Swiss Strawberry	1 (8 oz)	210	5	0
Fat Free Swiss Strawberry Banana	1 (8 oz)	210	5	0
Fat Free Swiss Vanilla	1 (8 oz)	210	5	0
Horizon Organic				
Fat Free Apricot Mango	¾ cup (6 oz)	120	<5	0
Fat Free Honey	1 cup (8 oz)	160	<5	0
Jell-O				
Lowfat Cherry	4.4 oz	130	10	0
Lowfat Grape	4.4 oz	130	10	0
Lowfat Raspberry	4.4 oz	130	10	0
Lowfat Tropical Berry Twist	4.4 oz	130	10	0
Lowfat Tropical Punch	4.4 oz	130	10	0
Lowfat Watermelon	4.4 oz	130	10	0
Lowfat Wild Berry	4.4 oz	130	10	0
Lowfat Wild Strawberry	4.4 oz	130	10	0
La Yogurt				
French Style Banana	6 oz	180	10	0
French Style Blueberry	6 oz	180	10	1
French Style Cherry	6 oz	180	10	0
French Style Cherry Vanilla	6 oz	190	10	0
French Style Guava	6 oz	180	10	1
French Style Key Lime	6 oz	180	10	0
French Style Mango	6 oz	180	10	0
French Style Mixed Berry	6 oz	180	10	0
French Style Nonfat Blueberry	6 oz	70	5	0
French Style Nonfat Cherry	6 oz	75	5	0
French Style Nonfat Raspberry	6 oz	70	5	0

FOOD	PORTION	CALS	CHOL	FIBER
French Style Nonfat Strawberry	6 oz	70	5	0
French Style Nonfat Strawberry Banana	6 oz	70	5	0
French Style Peach	6 oz	180	10	0
French Style Pina Colada	6 oz	180	10	0
French Style Raspberry	6 oz	180	10	1
French Style Strawberry	6 oz	180	10	0
French Style Strawberry Banana	6 oz	180	10	0
French Style Strawberry Fruit Cup	6 oz	180	10	0
French Style Tropical Orange	6 oz	180	10	0
French Style Vanilla	6 oz	170	15	0
Latin Style Banana	6 oz	190	10	0
Latin Style Guava	6 oz	190	10	0
Latin Style Mango	6 oz	190	10	0
Latin Style Papaya	6 oz	190	10	0
Latin Style Passion Fruit	6 oz	190	10	0
Latin Style Strawberry Kiwi	6 oz	180	10	0
Light N'Lively				
Free Blueberry	4.4 oz	70	5	0
Free Peach	4.4 oz	70	5	0
Free Strawberry	4.4 oz	70	5	0
Free Strawberry Banana Cream	4.4 oz	70	5	0
Free Strawberry Fruit Cup	4.4 oz	70	5	0
Lowfat Blueberry	4.4 oz	130	10	0
Lowfat Peach	4.4 oz	130	10	0
Lowfat Pineapple	4.4 oz	130	10	0
Lowfat Red Raspberry	4.4 oz	120	10	0
Lowfat Strawberry	4.4 oz	130	10	0
Lowfat Strawberry Banana Cream	4.4 oz	130	10	0
Lowfat Strawberry Fruit Cup	4.4 oz	130	10	0

FOOD	PORTION	CALS	CHOL	FIBER
Oberweis				
Peach	1 pkg (8 oz)	210	15	0
Pascual				
Nonfat Cherries & Berries	1 pkg (4.4 oz)	100	0	5
Nonfat Peach	1 pkg (4.4 oz)	100	0	5
Silk				
Organic Soy Strawberry	1 pkg (6 oz)	160	0	1
Soy Apricot Mango	1 pkg	160	0	1
Soy Banana Strawberry	1 pkg	160	0	1
Soy Black Cherry	1 pkg	160	0	1
Soy Blueberry	1 pkg	160	0	1
Soy Key Lime	1 pkg	170	0	1
Soy Lemon	1 pkg	160	0	1
Soy Lemon Kiwi	1 pkg	150	0	1
Soy Peach	1 pkg	170	0	1
Soy Plain	8 oz	120	0	1
Soy Raspberry	1 pkg	160	0	1
Soy Vanilla	1 pkg (8 oz)	120	0	1
Stonyfield Farm				
Creamy Maple	1 pkg	160	25	0
Mocho-Ccino	1 pkg	170	20	0
Nonfat Apricot Mango	1 pkg (8 oz)	160	0	tr
Nonfat Black Cherry	1 pkg (8 oz)	160	0	tr
Nonfat Cappuccino	1 pkg (8 oz)	160	0	0
Nonfat Cherry Vanilla	1 pkg (8 oz)	190	0	tr
Nonfat Chocolate Underground	1 pkg (8 oz)	200	0	tr
Nonfat French Vanilla	1 pkg (8 oz)	180	0	0
Nonfat Lotsa Lemon	1 pkg (8 oz)	160	0	0
Nonfat Peach	1 pkg (8 oz)	150	0	tr
Nonfat Plain	1 pkg (8 oz)	100	<5	0
Nonfat Raspberry	1 pkg (8 oz)	160	0	tr
Nonfat Strawberry	1 pkg (8 oz)	180	0	tr
Organic French Vanilla	1 pkg	170	20	0
Organic Wild Blueberry	1 pkg	160	20	tr
Organic Lowfat Blueberry	1 pkg (6 oz)	130	5	1

FOOD	PORTION	CALS	CHOL	FIBER
Organic Lowfat Luscious Lemon	1 pkg (6 oz)	130	5	1
Organic Lowfat Maple Vanilla	1 pkg (6 oz)	120	6	0
Organic Lowfat Mocha Latte	1 pkg (6 oz)	120	5	0
Organic Lowfat Plain	1 cup (8 oz)	110	10	0
Organic Lowfat Raspberry	1 pkg (6 oz)	130	5	1
Organic Lowfat Strawberry	1 pkg (6 oz)	130	5	1
Organic Lowfat Vanilla	1 pkg (6 oz)	120	5	0
Strawberries & Cream	1 pkg	160	20	tr
Vanilla Truffle	1 pkg	220	20	tr
YoSelf Organic Chocolate	1 (4 oz)	110	0	2
YoSelf Organic Creme Carmel	1 (4 oz)	110	5	2
Yosqueeze Strawberry	1 tube (2 oz)	60	5	1
Total				
Greek Yogurt	1 pkg (5 oz)	180	25	0
Greek Yogurt 0% Fat	1 pkg (5 oz)	80	0	0
Greek Yogurt 1% Fat	1 pkg (5 oz)	120	25	0
Yoplait				
99% Fat Free Blueberry	6 oz	180	10	0
99% Fat Free Boysenberry	6 oz	180	10	0
99% Fat Free Cherry	6 oz	180	10	0
99% Fat Free Harvest Peach	6 oz	120	5	0
99% Fat Free Harvest Peach	6 oz	180	10	0
99% Fat Free Key Lime Pie	6 oz	180	10	0
99% Fat Free Lemon	6 oz	180	10	0
99% Fat Free Mixed Berry	6 oz	120	5	0
99% Fat Free Mixed Berry	6 oz	180	10	0
99% Fat Free Orange	6 oz	180	10	0

FOOD	PORTION	CALS	CHOL	FIBER
99% Fat Free Pina Colada	6 oz	180	10	0
99% Fat Free Pineapple	6 oz	180	10	0
99% Fat Free Raspberry	6 oz	180	10	0
99% Fat Free Strawberry	6 oz	180	10	0
99% Fat Free Strawberry	6 oz	120	5	0
99% Fat Free Strawberry Banana	6 oz	180	10	0
99% Fat Free Strawberry Banana	6 oz	120	5	0
99% Fat Free Strawberry Cheesecake	6 oz	180	10	0
Custard Style Banana	6 oz	190	15	0
Custard Style Blueberry	6 oz	190	15	0
Custard Style Cherry Vanilla	6 oz	190	15	0
Custard Style Key Lime Pie	6 oz	190	15	0
Custard Style Lemon	6 oz	190	15	0
Custard Style Peaches'n Cream	6 oz	190	15	0
Custard Style Raspberry	6 oz	190	15	0
Custard Style Raspberry Cheesecake	6 oz	190	15	0
Custard Style Strawberry	6 oz	190	15	0
Custard Style Strawberry Banana	6 oz	190	15	0
Custard Style Strawberry Vanilla	4 oz	120	10	0
Custard Style Vanilla	6 oz	190	15	0
Go-Gurt Strawberry Banana Burst	1 pkg (2.25 oz)	80	5	0
Go-Gurt Watermelon Meltdown	1 pkg (2.25 oz)	80	5	0
Light Amaretto Cheesecake	6 oz	90	5	0

FOOD	PORTION	CALS	CHOL	FIBER
Light Apricot Mango	6 oz	90	5	0
Light Banana Cream	6 oz	90	5	0
Light Blueberry	6 oz	90	5	0
Light Boston Cream Pie	6 oz	90	5	0
Light Caramel Apple	6 oz	90	5	0
Light Cherry	6 oz	90	5	0
Light Key Lime Pie	6 oz	90	5	0
Light Lemon Cream Pie	6 oz	90	5	0
Light Peach	6 oz	90	5	0
Light Raspberry	6 oz	90	5	0
Light Strawberry	6 oz	90	5	0
Light Strawberry Banana	6 oz	90	5	0
Light White Chocolate Strawberry	6 oz	90	5	0
Original Cafe Au Lait	6 oz	170	10	0
Original Coconut Cream Pie	6 oz	200	10	0
Original French Vanilla	6 oz	180	10	0
Trix Rainbow Punch	6 oz	190	10	0
Trix Raspberry Rainbow	6 oz	190	10	0
Trix Strawberry Banana Bash	6 oz	190	10	0
Trix Strawberry Punch	4 oz	130	5	0
Trix Triple Cherry	6 oz	190	10	0
Trix Watermelon Burst	4 oz	130	5	0
Trix Wild Berry Blue	4 oz	130	5	0
Whips! Orange Creme	1 pkg (4 oz)	140	10	—
Whips! Raspberry Mousse	1 pkg (4 oz)	140	10	—
YOGURT FROZEN				
chocolate soft serve	½ cup (4 fl oz)	115	3	—
vanilla soft serve	½ cup (4 fl oz)	114	2	—
Ben & Jerry's				
Cherry Garcia	½ cup	170	20	0
Chocolate Cherry Garcia	½ cup	190	15	1

FOOD	PORTION	CALS	CHOL	FIBER
Chocolate Chip Cookie Dough	½ cup	200	10	0
Chocolate Fudge Brownie	½ cup	190	5	1
Chocolate Heath Bar Crunch	½ cup	210	10	1
Chunky Monkey Pop	½ cup	200	5	tr
Cherry Garcia	1	260	15	2
Breyers				
Chocolate	½ cup (2.6 oz)	130	10	tr
Fat Free Chocolate	½ cup (2.6 oz)	100	<5	0
Fat Free Cookies N Cream	½ cup (2.6 oz)	110	0	tr
Fat Free Peach	½ cup (2.6 oz)	90	0	0
Fat Free Strawberry	½ cup (2.6 oz)	100	0	0
Fat Free Take Two Vanilla Chocolate	½ cup (2.6 oz)	100	0	tr
Fat Free Vanilla	½ cup (2.6 oz)	100	0	tr
Fat Free Vanilla Fudge Twirl	½ cup (2.6 oz)	110	0	0
Vanilla	½ cup (2.6 oz)	120	10	0
Vanilla Chocolate Strawberry	½ cup (2.6 oz)	120	10	0
Dannon				
Light Cappuccino	½ cup (2.8 oz)	80	0	0
Light Cherry Vanilla Swirl	½ cup (2.8 oz)	90	0	0
Light Chocolate	½ cup (2.7 oz)	80	0	tr
Light Mint Chocolate Fudge	½ cup (2.8 oz)	90	0	0
Light Peach Raspberry Melba	½ cup (2.8 oz)	90	0	0
Light Strawberry Cheesecake	½ cup (2.8 oz)	90	0	0
Light Vanilla	½ cup (2.8 oz)	80	0	0
Light Duets Strawberry Sundae	6 oz	90	0	0
Light Nonfat Cappuccino	8 oz	100	<5	0

FOOD	PORTION	CALS	CHOL	FIBER
Light'N Crunchy Banana Cream Pie	½ cup (2.8 oz)	110	0	0
Light'N Crunchy Carmel Toffee Crunch	½ cup (2.8 oz)	110	0	0
Light'N Crunchy Mocha Chocolate Chunk	½ cup (2.8 oz)	110	0	0
Light'N Crunchy Peanut Chocolate Crunch	½ cup (2.8 oz)	110	0	0
Light'N Crunchy Rocky Road	½ cup (2.8 oz)	110	0	tr
Light'N Crunchy Triple Chocolate	½ cup (2.8 oz)	110	0	tr
Light'N Crunchy Vanilla Streusel	½ cup (2.8 oz)	110	0	0
Edy's				
Black Cherry Vanilla Swirl	½ cup	90	0	—
Caramel Fudge Cosmo	½ cup	140	10	—
Caramel Praline Crunch	½ cup	100	0	—
Chocolate Decadence	½ cup	120	10	—
Chocolate Fudge	½ cup	100	0	—
Coffee Fudge Sundae	½ cup	100	0	—
Cookies'N Cream	½ cup	120	10	—
Heath Toffee Crunch	½ cup	120	10	—
Raspberry	½ cup	90	10	—
Ultimate Tin Roof Sundae	½ cup	130	5	—
Vanilla	½ cup	90	0	—
Vanilla Chocolate Swirl	½ cup	90	0	—
Friendly's				
Apple Bettie	½ cup (2.6 oz)	140	10	0
Fabulous Fudge Swirl	½ cup (2.6 oz)	140	10	0
Fudge Berry Swirl	½ cup (2.6 oz)	150	10	0
Lowfat Perfectly Peach	½ cup (2.6 oz)	110	10	0
Lowfat Purely Chocolate	½ cup (2.6 oz)	120	10	0
Lowfat Raspberry Delight	½ cup (2.6 oz)	120	10	0
Lowfat Simply Vanilla	½ cup (2.6 oz)	120	10	0

FOOD	PORTION	CALS	CHOL	FIBER
Lowfat Strawberry Patch	½ cup (2.6 oz)	110	10	0
Mint Chocolate Chip	½ cup (2.6 oz)	130	10	0
Strawberry Cheesecake Blast	½ cup (2.6 oz)	140	15	0
Toffee Almond Crunch	½ cup (2.6 oz)	160	15	tr
Good Humor				
Creamsicle Raspberry	1 (2.8 oz)	100	<5	0
Frista Cup	1 (6.2 oz)	220	15	1
Häagen-Dazs				
Lowfat Dulce De Leche	½ cup	190	5	0
Nonfat Chocolate	½ cup	140	<5	tr
Nonfat Coffee	½ cup	140	<5	0
Nonfat Strawberry	½ cup	140	<5	0
Nonfat Vanilla	½ cup	140	<5	0
Nonfat Vanilla Raspberry Swirl	½ cup	130	<5	tr
Nonfat Vanilla Fudge	½ cup	160	<5	0
Hood				
Bavarian Truffle & Twist	½ cup (2.6 oz)	150	10	0
Coffee Toffee Chunk Sundae	½ cup (2.6 oz)	150	10	0
Combo Bars	1 (2.2 oz)	90	5	0
Cookies & Cream	½ cup (2.6 oz)	140	10	0
Grandma's Raisin Oatmeal Cookie Dough	½ cup (2.6 oz)	140	10	0
Mixed Berry Swirl	½ cup (2.6 oz)	120	10	0
Natural Strawberry	½ cup (2.6 oz)	110	10	0
Natural Strawberry Banana	½ cup (2.6 oz)	110	10	0
Natural Vanilla	½ cup (2.6 oz)	120	10	0
Nonfat Caramel & Brownie Sundae	½ cup (2.6 oz)	120	0	0
Nonfat Chocolate Marshmallow	½ cup (2.6 oz)	110	0	0
Nonfat Double Raspberry	½ cup (2.6 oz)	120	0	0
Nonfat Mocha Fudge	½ cup (2.6 oz)	120	0	0

FOOD	PORTION	CALS	CHOL	FIBER
Nonfat Olde Fashioned Vanilla	½ cup (2.6 oz)	110	0	0
Nonfat Peach Cobbler A La Mode	½ cup (2.6 oz)	110	0	0
Nonfat Strawberry	½ cup (2.6 oz)	100	0	0
Nonfat Vanilla Fudge	½ cup (2.6 oz)	120	0	0
Raspberry Swirl	½ cup (2.6 oz)	130	10	0
Sundae Cups Chocolate & Strawberry	1 (2.2 oz)	110	5	1
Vanilla Chocolate Strawberry	½ cup (2.6 oz)	120	10	0
Vanilla Swiss Almond Sundae	½ cup (2.6 oz)	150	10	0
Sealtest				
Chocolate	½ cup (2.7 oz)	120	5	tr
Mocha Fudge	½ cup (2.6 oz)	130	10	tr
Vanilla	½ cup (2.6 oz)	120	10	0
Tofutti				
Better Than Yogurt Chocolate Fudge	4 fl oz	120	0	0
Better Than Yogurt Coffee Mashmallow Swirl	4 fl oz	100	0	0
Better Than Yogurt Passion Island Fruit	4 fl oz	100	0	0
Better Than Yogurt Peach Mango	4 fl oz	100	0	0
Better Than Yogurt Strawberry Banana	4 fl oz	100	0	0
Better Than Yogurt Vanilla Fudge	4 fl oz	120	0	0
Turkey Hill				
Black Raspberry	½ cup	110	10	—
Caramel Cashew Crunch	½ cup	160	25	—
Chocolate Chip Cookie Dough	½ cup	140	10	0
Chocolate Chip Cookie Dough	½ cup	190	30	—
Clark Bar	½ cup	140	10	—

FOOD	PORTION	CALS	CHOL	FIBER
Fat Free Chocolate Cherry Cordial	½ cup	100	0	0
Fat Free Chocolate Marshmallow	½ cup	130	0	0
Fat Free Mint Cookie 'N Cream	½ cup	110	0	0
Fat Free Neapolitan	½ cup	100	0	0
Fat Free Orange Swirl	½ cup	100	0	—
Fat Free Vanilla Fudge	½ cup	110	0	0
Peach Raspberry	½ cup	110	10	0
Tin Roof Sundae	½ cup	140	10	0
Vanilla & Chocolate	½ cup	110	10	0
Vanilla Bean	½ cup	110	10	0

ZUCCHINI

FOOD	PORTION	CALS	CHOL	FIBER
baby raw	1 (0.5 oz)	3	0	tr
canned italian style	½ cup	33	0	—
frzn cooked	½ cup	19	0	—
raw sliced	½ cup	9	0	1
sliced cooked	½ cup	14	0	1
Empire				
Breaded	1 (2.9 oz)	100	0	1
Progresso				
Italian Style	½ cup (4.2 oz)	50	0	2
TAKE-OUT				
indian paalkora	1 serv	46	1	2

PART TWO

Restaurant Chains

Americans spend 48% of every food dollar
on foods eaten away from home.

FOOD	PORTION	CALS	CHOL	FIBER
APPLEBEE'S				
DESSERTS				
Apple Betty Cobbler Ala Mode	1 serv	598	31	2
Fudge Brownie Sundae	1 serv	739	66	6
Low Fat Bikini Banana Strawberry Shortcake	1 serv	248	8	2
Low Fat Brownie Sundae	1 serv	415	3	3
Low Fat Marble Cheesecake	1 serv	261	10	4
MAIN MENU SELECTIONS				
Applebee's Burger w/ Fries	1 serv	1274	263	7
Basic Hamburger w/ Fries	1 serv	980	118	6
Beef Fajita Quesadilla	1 serv	1205	159	6
Bourbon Street Steak w/ Fried New Potatoes	1 serv	1115	168	—
Low Fat Asian Chicken Salad	1 med serv (2.5 oz)	370	40	7
Low Fat Asian Chicken Salad	1 serv (5 oz)	623	76	14
Low Fat Blackened Chicken Salad	1 med serv (2.5 oz)	287	43	6
Low Fat Blackened Chicken Salad	1 serv (5 oz)	411	82	11
Low Fat Garlic Chicken Pasta	1 serv	587	39	9
Low Fat Lemon Chicken Pasta	1 serv	528	50	8
Low Fat Quesadilla Chicken Fajita	1 serv	518	35	2
Low Fat Quesadilla Veggie	1 serv	344	8	3
Mozzarella Stix	8 pieces	963	64	1
Quesadillas	1 serv	684	99	4

FOOD	PORTION	CALS	CHOL	FIBER
Riblet Basket w/ Fries	1 serv	1317	219	7
Salad Dinner w/o Dressing	1 serv	303	277	3
Salad Santa Fe Chicken	1 med	724	96	7
Sandwich Bacon Cheese Chicken Grill w/o Fries	1	746	133	1
Sandwich Gyro	1	880	15	3
Stir Fry Chicken	1 serv	566	76	5

ARBY'S
BEVERAGES

FOOD	PORTION	CALS	CHOL	FIBER
Chocolate Shake	1 (14 oz)	480	45	0
Hot Chocolate	1 serv (8.6 oz)	110	0	0
Jamocha Shake	1 (14 oz)	470	45	0
Milk	1 serv (8 oz)	120	20	0
Orange Juice	1 serv (10 oz)	140	0	0
Strawberry Shake	1 (14 oz)	500	15	0
Vanilla Shake	1 (14 oz)	470	45	0

BREAKFAST SELECTIONS

FOOD	PORTION	CALS	CHOL	FIBER
Add Egg To Breakfast	1 serv (2 oz)	110	175	0
Add Swiss Cheese Slice	1 slice (0.5 oz)	45	10	0
Biscuit w/ Bacon	1 (3.4 oz)	360	10	1
Biscuit w/ Butter	1 (2.9 oz)	280	0	1
Biscuit w/ Ham	1 (4.3 oz)	330	30	1
Biscuit w/ Sausage	1 (4.2)	460	25	1
Croissant w/ Bacon	1 (2.7 oz)	340	30	1
Croissant w/ Ham	1 (3.7 oz)	310	11	0
Croissant w/ Sausage	1 (3.6 oz)	440	45	0
Maple Syrup	1 serv (0.5 oz)	130	0	0
Sourdough w/ Bacon	1 (5.1 oz)	420	10	3
Sourdough w/ Ham	1 (6.1 oz)	390	30	2
Sourdough w/ Sausage	1 (5.9 oz)	520	25	2
Toastix w/o Syrup	6 pieces (4.4 oz)	370	0	4

DESSERTS

FOOD	PORTION	CALS	CHOL	FIBER
Apple Turnover Iced	1 (4.5 oz)	420	0	2
Cherry Turnover Iced	1 (4.5 oz)	410	0	1

MAIN MENU SELECTIONS

FOOD	PORTION	CALS	CHOL	FIBER
Arby's Sauce	1 serv (0.5 oz)	15	0	0
Au Jus Sauce	1 serv (3 oz)	5	0	tr

FOOD	PORTION	CALS	CHOL	FIBER
BBQ Dipping Sauce	1 serv (1 oz)	40	0	0
Baked Potato Broccoli'N Cheddar	1 (14 oz)	540	50	7
Baked Potato Deluxe	1 (13 oz)	650	90	6
Baked Potato w/ Butter & Sour Cream	1 (11.2 oz)	500	55	6
Bronco Berry Sauce	1 serv (1.5 oz)	90	0	0
Caesar Salad w/o Dressing	1 serv (8 oz)	90	10	3
Cheddar Curly Fries	1 serv (6 oz)	460	5	4
Chicken Finger 4-Pak	1 serv (6.77 oz)	640	70	0
Chicken Finger Salad w/o Dressing	1 serv (13 oz)	570	65	3
Chicken Finger Snack	1 serv (6.4 oz)	580	35	3
Curly Fries	1 lg (7 oz)	620	0	7
Curly Fries	1 med (4.5 oz)	400	0	4
Curly Fries	1 sm (3.8 oz)	310	0	3
German Mustard	1 pkg (0.25 oz)	5	0	0
Grilled Chicken Caesar Salad w/o Dressing	1 serv (12 oz)	230	80	3
Homestyle Fries	1 lg (7.5 oz)	560	0	6
Homestyle Fries	1 med (5 oz)	370	0	4
Homestyle Fries	1 sm (4 oz)	300	0	3
Homestyle Fries Child-Size	1 serv (3 oz)	220	0	3
Honey Mustard	1 serv (1 oz)	130	10	0
Horsey Sauce	1 pkg (0.5 oz)	60	0	0
Jalapeno Bites	1 serv (4 oz)	330	40	2
Ketchup	1 pkg (0.3 oz)	10	0	0
Light Grilled Chicken Salad	1 (16.3 oz)	210	65	6
Marinara Sauce	1 serv (1.5 oz)	35	0	0
Mayonnaise	1 pkg (0.4 oz)	90	10	0
Mayonnaise Light Cholesterol Free	1 pkg (0.4 oz)	20	0	0
Mozzarella Sticks	1 serv (4.8 oz)	470	60	2
Onion Petals	1 serv (4 oz)	410	0	2
Potato Cakes	2 (3.5 oz)	250	0	3

FOOD	PORTION	CALS	CHOL	FIBER
Roast Beef Sandwich Arby's Melt w/ Cheddar	1 (5.2 oz)	320	45	2
Roast Beef Sandwich Arby-Q	1 (6.4 oz)	360	70	2
Roast Beef Sandwich Beef'N Cheddar	1 (6.9 oz)	460	50	2
Roast Beef Sandwich Big Montana	1 (11 oz)	560	50	3
Roast Beef Sandwich Giant	1 (7.9 oz)	440	45	3
Roast Beef Sandwich Junior	1 (4.4 oz)	290	40	2
Roast Beef Sandwich Regular	1 (5.4 oz)	330	45	2
Roast Beef Sandwich Super	1 (8.5 oz)	450	45	3
Sandwich Chicken Bacon'N Swiss	1 (7.4 oz)	610	110	2
Sandwich Chicken Breast Fillet	1 (7.2 oz)	550	90	2
Sandwich Chicken Cordon Bleu	1 (8.4 oz)	630	120	2
Sandwich Grilled Chicken Deluxe	1 (8.7 oz)	450	110	2
Sandwich Hot Ham 'N Swiss	1 (5.9 oz)	340	90	1
Sandwich Light Roast Chicken Deluxe	1 (7.2 oz)	260	40	3
Sandwich Light Roast Turkey Deluxe	1 (7.2 oz)	260	40	3
Sandwich Market Fresh Roast Beef & Swiss	1 (12.5 oz)	780	80	6
Sandwich Market Fresh Roast Chicken Caesar	1 (12.7 oz)	820	140	5
Sandwich Market Fresh Roast Ham & Swiss	1 (12.5 oz)	730	125	5

FOOD	PORTION	CALS	CHOL	FIBER
Sandwich Market Fresh Roast Turkey & Swiss	1 (12.5 oz)	760	135	5
Sandwich Roast Chicken Club	1 (8.4 oz)	520	115	2
Sub Sandwich French Dip	1 (10 oz)	410	45	2
Sub Sandwich Hot Ham'N Swiss	1 (9.7 oz)	530	110	3
Sub Sandwich Italian	1 (11 oz)	780	120	3
Sub Sandwich Pilly Beef'N Swiss	1 (10.8 oz)	670	75	4
Sub Sandwich Roast Beef	1 (11.6 oz)	730	76	3
Sub Sandwich Turkey	1 (10.6 oz)	630	100	2
Tangy Southwest Sauce	1 serv (1.5 oz)	250	30	0
SALAD DRESSINGS				
Bleu Cheese	1 serv (2 oz)	300	45	0
Buttermilk Ranch	1 serv (2 oz)	360	5	0
Buttermilk Ranch Reduced Calorie	1 serv (2 oz)	60	0	1
Caesar	1 serv (2 oz)	310	60	0
Honey French	1 serv (2 oz)	290	0	tr
Italian Reduced Calorie	1 serv (2 oz)	25	0	tr
Thousand Island	1 serv (2 oz)	290	35	0
SALADS AND SALAD BARS				
Croutons Seasoned	1 serv (0.25 oz)	30	0	1
Garden Salad	1 (12.3 oz)	70	0	6
Light Grilled Chicken Sandwich	1 (7.5 oz)	280	55	3
Light Roast Chicken Salad	1 (14.8 oz)	160	40	6
Side Salad	1 (6.1 oz)	30	0	3
Turkey Club Salad w/o Dressing	1 serv (12 oz)	350	90	3

FOOD	PORTION	CALS	CHOL	FIBER
AU BON PAIN				
BAKED SELECTIONS				
Apple Coffee Cake	1 piece (4.6 oz)	480	96	2
Bagel Chocolate Chip	1 (5 oz)	380	5	3
Bagel Dutch Apple w/ Walnut Streussel	1 (5 oz)	360	0	4
Baguette Loaf	1 slice (1.8 oz)	140	0	1
Biscotti	1 (1.5 oz)	200	35	1
Biscotti Chocolate	1 (1.7 oz)	240	35	2
Braided Roll	1 (1.8 oz)	170	0	1
Cinnamon Roll	1 (7 oz)	710	100	3
Cookie Chocolate Chip	1 (2.1 oz)	280	40	2
Cookie Oatmeal Raisin	1 (2.1 oz)	250	30	2
Cookie Peanut Butter	1 (2.1 oz)	280	30	1
Cookie Shortbread	1 (2.4 oz)	390	65	1
Croissant Almond	1 (4.3 oz)	560	105	4
Croissant Apple	1 (3.4 oz)	280	25	1
Croissant Chocolate	1 (3.4 oz)	440	30	4
Croissant Cinnamon Raisin	1 (3.7 oz)	380	35	2
Croissant Plain	1 (2.1 oz)	270	40	1
Croissant Raspberry Cheese	1 (3.5 oz)	380	60	1
Croissant Sweet Cheese	1 (3.6 oz)	390	75	1
Danish Cheese Swirl	1 (3.8 oz)	450	95	1
Danish Lemon Swirl	1 (4 oz)	450	80	1
Danish Raspberry	1 (3.6 oz)	370	65	2
Danish Sweet Cheese	1 (3.6 oz)	420	90	1
Four Grain Loaf	1 slice (1.8 oz)	130	0	1
French Sandwich Roll	1 (1.8 oz)	120	0	1
Hazelnut Fudge Brownie	1 (4 oz)	380	100	4
Holiday Cookie Cranberry Almond Macaroon	1 (1.5 oz)	160	0	2

FOOD	PORTION	CALS	CHOL	FIBER
Holiday Cookie Cranberry Almond Macaroon w/ Chocolate	1 (1.9 oz)	210	0	2
Holiday Cookie English Toffee	1 (1.8 oz)	220	45	0
Holiday Cookie Ginger Pecan	1 (2 oz)	260	40	1
Mochaccino Bar	1 (4 oz)	404	37	1
Muffin Blueberry	1 (4.5 oz)	410	85	1
Muffin Carrot	1 (5 oz)	480	55	3
Muffin Chocolate Chip	1 (4.5 oz)	490	35	2
Muffin Corn	1 (4.6 oz)	470	65	2
Muffin Pumpkin w/ Streusel Topping	1 (5.5 oz)	470	60	2
Muffin Low Fat Chocolate Cake	1 (4 oz)	290	20	3
Muffin Low Fat Triple Berry	1 (4.2 oz)	270	25	2
Multigrain Loaf	1 slice (1.8 oz)	130	0	1
Parisienne Loaf	1 slice (1.8 oz)	120	0	1
Pear Ginger Tea Cake	1 piece (4 oz)	380	0	1
Pecan Roll	1 (6.8 oz)	900	50	4
Roll 3 Seed Pecan Raisin	1 (2.7 oz)	250	0	3
Roll Hearth Sandwich	1 (2.8 oz)	220	0	2
Roll Petit Pan	1 (2.5 oz)	200	0	1
Rye Loaf	1 slice (1.8 oz)	110	0	2
Scone Cinnamon	1 (4.1 oz)	520	145	1
Scone Current	1 (3.7 oz)	430	155	2
Scone Orange	1 (4.1 oz)	440	155	2
Sourdough Bagel Asiago Cheese	1 (4.2 oz)	380	15	3
Sourdough Bagel Cinnamon Raisin	1 (4.5 oz)	390	0	4
Sourdough Bagel Cranberry Walnut	1 (5 oz)	460	0	7
Sourdough Bagel Everything	1 (4.2 oz)	360	0	3

FOOD	PORTION	CALS	CHOL	FIBER
Sourdough Bagel Honey 8 Grain	1 (4.2 oz)	360	0	6
Sourdough Bagel Mocha Chip Swirl	1 (5 oz)	370	0	3
Sourdough Bagel Plain	1 (4 oz)	350	0	3
Sourdough Bagel Sesame	1 (4.2 oz)	380	0	3
Sourdough Bagel Wild Blueberry	1 (4.5 oz)	380	0	4
Valentine Cookie Chocolate Dipped Shortbread	1 (2.8 oz)	410	55	2
Valentine Cookie Red Sugar Shortbread Heart	1 (2.4 oz)	350	60	1
Valentine Cookie Shortbread	1 (2.4 oz)	340	60	1
BEVERAGES				
Frozen Java Blast	1 serv (16 oz)	220	10	0
Frozen Mocha Blast	1 serv (16 oz)	320	10	2
Hot Apple Cider	1 med (16 oz)	310	0	0
Hot Apple Cider	1 sm (10 oz)	190	0	0
Hot Apple Cider	1 lg (20 oz)	350	0	0
Hot Hazelnut Blast	1 serv (16 oz)	310	25	0
Hot Mocha Blast	1 lg (17 oz)	310	30	0
Hot Mocha Blast	1 med (13 oz)	260	25	0
Hot Mocha Blast	1 sm (9 oz)	160	15	0
Hot Raspberry Mocha Blast	1 serv (16 oz)	300	25	0
Hot Raspberry Mocha Blast	1 serv (10 oz)	180	15	0
Hot Raspberry Mocha Blast	1 serv (20 oz)	350	30	0
Hot Strawberry Chocolate Blast	1 serv (16 oz)	330	25	0
Hot Vanilla Chocolate Blast	1 serv (16 oz)	310	25	0
Iced Caffee Latte	1 lg (20.5 oz)	270	40	0
Iced Caffee Latte	1 sm (9 oz)	130	20	0
Iced Caffee Latte	1 med (12 oz)	150	25	0

FOOD	PORTION	CALS	CHOL	FIBER
Iced Cappuccino	1 sm (9 oz)	110	15	0
Iced Cappuccino	1 lg (20.5 oz)	270	40	0
Iced Cappuccino	1 med (12 oz)	150	25	0
Iced Cocoa	1 lg (20.5 oz)	440	40	0
Iced Cocoa	1 sm (9 oz)	200	20	0
Iced Cocoa	1 med (12 oz)	280	25	0
Iced Hazelnut Blast	1 serv (16 oz)	310	25	0
Iced Mocha Blast	1 med (12 oz)	260	25	0
Iced Mocha Blast	1 lg (20.5 oz)	360	40	0
Iced Mocha Blast	1 sm (9 oz)	180	20	0
Iced Raspberry Mocha Blast	1 serv (24 oz)	330	25	0
Iced Raspberry Mocha Blast	1 serv (16 oz)	310	25	0
Iced Raspberry Mocha Blast	1 serv (12 oz)	160	15	0
Iced Strawberry Chocolate Blast	1 serv (16 oz)	310	25	0
Iced Vanilla Chocolate Blast	1 serv (16 oz)	310	25	0
Iced Tea Peach	1 med (12 oz)	130	0	0
Iced Tea Peach	1 sm (8 oz)	90	0	0
Iced Tea Peach	1 lg (16 oz)	170	0	0
Iced Tea Raspberry	1 lg (16 oz)	150	0	0
Iced Tea Raspberry	1 med (12 oz)	110	0	0
Iced Tea Raspberry	1 sm (8 oz)	80	0	0
Whipped Cream	1 serv (1.2 oz)	160	55	0
SALAD DRESSINGS				
Bleu Cheese	1 serv (3 oz)	370	40	0
Buttermilk Ranch	1 serv (3 oz)	310	35	0
Caesar	1 serv (3 oz)	380	25	0
Fat Free Tomato Basil	1 serv (3 oz)	70	0	1
Greek	1 serv (3 oz)	440	0	0
Lemon Basil Vinaigrette	1 serv (3 oz)	330	0	0
Lite Honey Mustard	1 serv (3 oz)	280	40	1
Lite Italian	1 serv (3 oz)	230	0	0
Sesame French	1 serv (3 oz)	370	0	1
SALADS AND SALAD BARS				
Caesar	1 serv (8.9 oz)	270	20	5
Chicken Caesar	1 serv (11.4 oz)	360	65	5

FOOD	PORTION	CALS	CHOL	FIBER
Garden	1 lg (10.6 oz)	160	0	6
Garden	1 sm (7.5 oz)	100	0	4
Mozzarella & Roasted Pepper Salad	1 serv (13.7 oz)	340	60	10
Pesto Chicken Salad	1 serv (10.7 oz)	230	45	4
Tuna	1 serv (15 oz)	490	45	7
SANDWICHES AND FILLINGS				
Bagel Spreads Lite Strawberry	1 serv (2 oz)	150	35	1
Bagel Spreads Lite Vanilla Hazelnut	1 serv (2 oz)	150	35	1
Cheddar	½ serv (1.5 oz)	170	45	0
Chicken Tarragon	1 serv (4 oz)	240	65	0
Club Sandwich Hot Roasted Turkey	1 (14.9 oz)	950	135	4
Country Ham	1 serv (3.7 oz)	150	55	0
Cracked Pepper Chicken	1 serv (3.9 oz)	140	72	0
Cream Cheese Lite	1 serv (2 oz)	130	35	1
Cream Cheese Lite Honey Walnut	1 serv (2 oz)	260	20	—
Cream Cheese Lite Raspberry	1 serv (2 oz)	200	20	—
Cream Cheese Lite Sun-Dried Tomato	1 serv (2 oz)	130	35	1
Cream Cheese Plain	1 serv (2 oz)	190	55	—
Cream Cheese Veggie Lite	1 serv (2 oz)	100	20	—
Grilled Chicken	1 serv (3.9 oz)	140	72	0
Hot Croissant Ham & Cheese	1 (4.2 oz)	380	70	1
Hot Croissant Spinach & Cheese	1 (3.6 oz)	270	40	2
Provolone	½ serv (1.5 oz)	150	30	0
Roast Beef	1 serv (3.7 oz)	140	50	0
Sandwich Arizona Chicken	1 (12.7 oz)	720	125	4
Sandwich Buffalo Chicken	1 (13.7 oz)	640	85	3

FOOD	PORTION	CALS	CHOL	FIBER
Sandwich California Chicken	1 (13.2 oz)	820	135	4
Sandwich Fresh Mozzarella Tomato & Pesto	1 (10.5 oz)	650	55	4
Sandwich Honey Dijon Chicken	1 (15.3 oz)	730	135	4
Sandwich Parmesan Chicken	1 (11.1 oz)	740	70	5
Sandwich Steak & Cheese Melt	1 (11.7 oz)	750	90	2
Sandwich Thai Chicken	1 (8.3 oz)	420	20	3
Swiss	½ serv (1.5 oz)	160	40	0
Tuna Salad	1 serv (4.5 oz)	360	50	1
Turkey Breast	1 serv (3.7 oz)	120	20	0
Wraps Chicken Caesar	1 (9.9 oz)	630	80	2
Wraps Southwestern Tuna	1 (14.4 oz)	950	110	4
Wraps Summer Turkey	1 (11.7 oz)	340	35	9
SOUPS				
Beef Barley	1 serv (12 oz)	112	18	3
Beef Barley	1 serv (16 oz)	150	25	5
Beef Barley	1 serv (8 oz)	75	15	2
Beef Stew	1 serv (8 oz)	140	25	2
Bohemian Cabbage	1 serv (8 oz)	70	0	2
Bohemian Cabbage	1 serv (12 oz)	110	0	4
Bohemian Cabbage	1 serv (16 oz)	140	0	5
Bread Bowl	1 (9 oz)	640	0	5
Broccoli & Cheddar	1 serv (8 oz)	260	50	1
Broccoli & Cheddar	1 serv (16 oz)	520	100	2
Broccoli & Cheddar	1 serv (12 oz)	390	75	2
Caribbean Black Bean	1 serv (16 oz)	250	10	16
Caribbean Black Bean	1 serv (12 oz)	180	10	12
Caribbean Black Bean	1 serv (8 oz)	120	5	8
Chicken Chili	1 serv (12 oz)	350	65	5
Chicken Chili	1 serv (8 oz)	240	45	4
Chicken Chili	1 serv (16 oz)	470	90	8
Chicken Noodle	1 serv (16 oz)	170	35	2
Chicken Noodle	1 serv (8 oz)	80	15	1

FOOD	PORTION	CALS	CHOL	FIBER
Chicken Noodle	1 serv (12 oz)	120	25	2
Chili	1 serv (12 oz)	340	50	7
Chili	1 serv (16 oz)	460	70	9
Chili	1 serv (8 oz)	230	35	5
Clam Chowder	1 serv (12 oz)	400	95	1
Clam Chowder	1 serv (16 oz)	540	125	1
Clam Chowder	1 serv (8 oz)	270	65	0
Corn Chowder	1 serv (16 oz)	530	95	3
Corn Chowder	1 serv (12 oz)	390	70	2
Corn Chowder	1 serv (8 oz)	260	50	1
Cream Of Broccoli	1 serv (16 oz)	440	80	3
Cream Of Broccoli	1 serv (12 oz)	330	60	2
Cream Of Broccoli	1 serv (8 oz)	220	40	1
Cream Of Chicken With Wild Rice	1 serv (16 oz)	330	90	1
French Onion	1 serv (12 oz)	120	0	3
French Onion	1 serv (16 oz)	170	0	4
French Onion	1 serv (8 oz)	80	0	2
In A Bread Bowl Beef Barley	1 serv (21 oz)	760	20	8
In A Bread Bowl Carribean Black Bean	1 serv (21 oz)	830	10	17
In A Bread Bowl Chicken Chili	1 serv (21 oz)	990	65	12
In A Bread Bowl Chicken Noodle	1 serv (21 oz)	760	20	7
In A Bread Bowl Clam Chowder	1 serv (21 oz)	1050	100	5
In A Bread Bowl Cream of Broccoli	1 serv (21 oz)	970	60	7
In A Bread Bowl French Onion	1 serv (21 oz)	760	0	8
In A Bread Bowl New England Potato & Cheese w/ Ham	1 serv (21 oz)	860	40	9
In A Bread Bowl Tomato Florentine	1 serv (21 oz)	760	10	8
In A Bread Bowl Vegetarian Chili	1 serv (21 oz)	870	0	8

FOOD	PORTION	CALS	CHOL	FIBER
Louisiana Beans & Rice	1 serv (16 oz)	360	20	3
Louisiana Beans & Rice	1 serv (8 oz)	180	10	1
Louisiana Beans & Rice	1 serv (12 oz)	280	15	2
New England Potato & Cheese w/ Ham	1 serv (8 oz)	150	25	3
New England Potato & Cheese w/ Ham	1 serv (12 oz)	220	40	4
New England Potato & Cheese w/ Ham	1 serv (16 oz)	290	55	5
Potato Leek	1 serv (12 oz)	320	70	2
Potato Leek	1 serv (8 oz)	200	45	2
Potato Leek	1 serv (16 oz)	400	85	3
Sante Fe Chicken Tortilla	1 serv (16 oz)	300	30	4
Sante Fe Chicken Tortilla	1 serv (8 oz)	150	15	2
Sante Fe Chicken Tortilla	1 serv (12 oz)	230	25	3
Seafood Gumbo	1 serv (8 oz)	130	20	1
Seafood Gumbo	1 serv (12 oz)	190	25	2
Seafood Gumbo	1 serv (16 oz)	260	35	3
Tomato Florentine	1 serv (8 oz)	61	5	2
Tomato Florentine	1 serv (12 oz)	90	5	2
Tomato Florentine	1 serv (16 oz)	122	5	3
Tomato Tortellini	1 serv (12 oz)	90	5	2
Tomato Tortellini	1 serv (8 oz)	60	5	2
Tomato Tortellini	1 serv (16 oz)	110	10	3
Vegetable Stew	1 serv (8 oz)	60	5	2
Vegetable Stew	1 serv (12 oz)	100	5	4
Vegetable Stew	1 serv (16 oz)	130	5	5
Vegetarian Lentil	1 serv (16 oz)	270	0	5
Vegetarian Lentil	1 serv (8 oz)	130	0	2
Vegetarian Lentil	1 serv (12 oz)	200	0	4
Vegetarian Chili	1 serv (12 oz)	210	0	3
Vegetarian Chili	1 serv (8 oz)	139	0	2
Vegetarian Chili	1 serv (16 oz)	278	0	4
Vegetarian Corn & Green Chili Bisque	1 serv (8 oz)	190	30	3
Vegetarian Corn & Green Chili Bisque	1 serv (16 oz)	380	60	5

FOOD	PORTION	CALS	CHOL	FIBER
Vegetarian Corn & Green Chili Bisque	1 serv (12 oz)	300	45	4

AUNTIE ANNE'S

FOOD	PORTION	CALS	CHOL	FIBER
Caramel Dip	1 serv (1.5 oz)	135	5	0
Cheese Sauce	1 serv (1 oz)	70	15	0
Chocolate Dip	1 serv (1.25 oz)	130	2	1
Cream Cheese Light	1 serv (075 oz)	45	15	0
Cream Cheese Pineapple	1 serv (.75 oz)	70	20	0
Cream Cheese Strawberry	1 serv (.75 oz)	70	20	0
Dutch Ice Kiwi Banana	1 (18 oz)	250	0	0
Dutch Ice Kiwi Banana	1 (12 oz)	160	0	0
Dutch Ice Lemonade	1 (12 oz)	270	0	0
Dutch Ice Lemonade	1 (18 oz)	405	0	1
Dutch Ice Mocha	1 (18 oz)	500	0	0
Dutch Ice Mocha	1 (12 oz)	340	0	0
Dutch Ice Orange Creme	1 (12 oz)	240	0	0
Dutch Ice Orange Creme	1 (18 oz)	360	0	0
Dutch Ice Raspberry	1 (18 oz)	220	0	1
Dutch Ice Raspberry	1 (12 oz)	150	0	1
Dutch Ice Strawberry	1 (12 oz)	190	0	0
Dutch Ice Strawberry	1 (18 oz)	280	0	1
Marinara Sauce	1 serv (1 oz)	10	0	0
Pretzel Almond w/ Butter	1	400	20	2
Pretzel Almond w/o Butter	1	350	0	2
Pretzel Cinnamon Raisin w/o Butter	1	350	0	2
Pretzel Cinnamon Sugar w/ Butter	1	450	25	3
Pretzel Garlic w/ Butter	1	350	10	2
Pretzel Garlic w/o Butter	1	320	0	2

FOOD	PORTION	CALS	CHOL	FIBER
Pretzel Glazin' Raisin w/ Butter	1	510	10	4
Pretzel Glazin' Raisin w/o Butter	1	470	0	3
Pretzel Jalapeno w/ Butter	1	310	10	2
Pretzel Jalapeno w/o Butter	1	270	0	2
Pretzel Original w/ Butter	1	370	10	2
Pretzel Original w/o Butter	1	340	0	3
Pretzel Sesame w/ Butter	1	410	15	7
Pretzel Sesame w/o Butter	1	350	0	3
Pretzel Sour Cream & Onion w/ Butter	1	340	10	2
Pretzel Sour Cream & Onion w/o Butter	1	310	0	2
Pretzel Whole Wheat w/ Butter	1	370	10	7
Pretzel Whole Wheat w/o Butter	1	350	0	7
Sweet Mustard	1 serv (1 oz)	60	40	0

BASKIN-ROBBINS
FROZEN YOGURT

FOOD	PORTION	CALS	CHOL	FIBER
Maui Brownie Madness	½ cup	140	5	1
Perils Of Pauline	½ cup	140	5	0

ICE CREAM

FOOD	PORTION	CALS	CHOL	FIBER
Banana Strawberry	½ cup	130	25	0
Baseball Nut	½ cup	160	30	0
Black Walnut	½ cup	160	30	1
Cherries Jubilee	½ cup	140	30	0
Chocolate	½ cup	150	30	0
Chocolate Almond	½ cup	180	30	1
Chocolate Chip	½ cup	150	35	0
Chocolate Chip Cookie Dough	½ cup	170	35	0

FOOD	PORTION	CALS	CHOL	FIBER
Chocolate Fudge	½ cup	160	30	0
Chocolate Mousse Royale	½ cup	170	25	1
Chocolate Raspberry Truffle	½ cup	180	30	0
Chunky Heath Bar	½ cup	170	30	0
Cookies N Cream	½ cup	170	30	0
Dirt'N Worms	½ cup	160	25	0
Egg Nog	½ cup	150	40	0
Everybody's Favorite Candy Bar	½ cup	170	30	2
French Vanilla	½ cup	160	70	0
Fudge Brownie	½ cup	170	25	1
German Chocolate Cake	½ cup	180	25	0
Gold Medal Ribbon	½ cup	150	30	0
Jamoca	½ cup	140	35	0
Jamoca Almond Fudge	½ cup	140	25	0
Lemon Custard	½ cup	150	45	0
Lowfat Carmel Apple AlaMod	½ cup	100	5	0
Lowfat Espresso'N Cream	½ cup	100	5	1
Mint Chocolate Chip	½ cup	150	35	0
No Sugar Added Call Me Nuts	½ cup	110	5	1
No Sugar Added Cherry Cordial	½ cup	100	5	0
No Sugar Added Mad About Chocolate	½ cup	100	5	0
No Sugar Added Pineapple Coconut	½ cup	90	5	0
No Sugar Added Thin Mint	½ cup	100	5	0
Nonfat Berry Innocent Cheese	½ cup	110	0	0
Nonfat Check-It-Out Cherry	½ cup	100	0	0
Nonfat Jamoca Swirl	½ cup	110	5	0
Ocean Commotion	½ cup	150	25	0

FOOD	PORTION	CALS	CHOL	FIBER
Old Fashion Butter Pecan	½ cup	160	35	0
Oregon Blueberry	½ cup	140	30	0
Peanut Butter N Chocolate	½ cup	180	30	1
Pink Bubblegum	½ cup	150	30	0
Pistachio Almond	½ cup	170	30	1
Pralines N Cream	½ cup	160	30	0
Pumpkin Pie	½ cup	130	30	0
Quarterback Crunch	½ cup	160	30	0
Reeses Peanut Butter	½ cup	180	30	0
Rocky Road	½ cup	170	30	0
Rum Raisin	½ cup	140	30	0
Strawberry Cheesecake	½ cup	150	35	0
Triple Chocolate Passion	½ cup	180	35	0
Vanilla	½ cup	140	40	0
Very Berry Strawberry	½ cup	130	25	0
Winter White Chocolate	½ cup	150	25	0
World Class Chocolate	½ cup	160	30	0
ICES AND ICE POPS				
Daiquiri Ice	½ cup	110	0	0
Sherbet Blue Raspberry	½ cup	120	5	0
Sherbet Orange	½ cup	120	5	0
Sherbet Rainbow	½ cup	120	5	0
Sorbet Pink Raspberry Lemon	½ cup	120	0	0
The Mask Ice	½ cup	120	0	0
Watermelon Ice	½ cup	110	0	0
BEN & JERRY'S				
Sugar Cone	1	48	0	tr
FROZEN YOGURT				
Cherry Garcia	½ cup (3.3 oz)	150	15	tr
Chocolate Cherry Garcia	½ cup (3.3 oz)	170	5	1
Chocolate Fudge Brownie	½ cup (3.3 oz)	180	15	1
No Fat Black Raspberry	½ cup (3.4 oz)	140	5	0

FOOD	PORTION	CALS	CHOL	FIBER
No Fat Coffee Fudge	½ cup (3.4 oz)	140	0	0
No Fat Vanilla	½ cup (3.4 oz)	140	5	0
No Fat Vanilla Fudge Swirl	½ cup (3.4 oz)	130	0	0
ICE CREAM				
Bovinity Divinity	½ cup (3.1 oz)	240	30	1
Butter Pecan	½ cup (3.1 oz)	270	60	tr
Cherry Garcia	½ cup (3.1 oz)	210	55	tr
Chocolate Chip Cookie Dough	½ cup (3.1 oz)	180	55	0
Chocolate Fudge Brownie	½ cup (3.1 oz)	230	35	2
Chubby Hubby	½ cup (3.1 oz)	280	50	1
Chunky Monkey	½ cup (3.1 oz)	220	50	0
Coconut Almond Fudge Chip	½ cup (3.1 oz)	250	30	2
Coffee Coffee Buzz Buzz	½ cup (3.1 oz)	240	55	tr
Coffee Ole	½ cup (3.1 oz)	200	65	0
Coffee w/ Heath Bar Crunch	½ cup (3.1 oz)	250	30	0
Deep Dark Chocolate	½ cup (3.1 oz)	210	40	2
Dilbert's World Totally Nuts	½ cup (3.1 oz)	260	30	tr
Low Fat Blackberry Cobbler	½ cup (3.2 oz)	160	10	0
Low Fat Chocolate Comfort	½ cup (3.2 oz)	150	10	–
Low Fat Coconut Creme Pie	½ cup (3.2 oz)	160	15	0
Low Fat Mocha Latte	½ cup (3.2 oz)	150	10	–
Low Fat Rockin Road	½ cup (3.2 oz)	180	5	2
Low Fat S'mores	½ cup (3.2 oz)	180	5	1
Low Fat Vanilla & Chocolate Mint Patty	½ cup (3.2 oz)	170	20	tr
Maple Walnut	½ cup (3.1 oz)	240	55	0
Mint Chocolate Chunk	½ cup (3.1 oz)	240	60	0
Mint Chocolate Cookie	½ cup (3.1 oz)	230	60	tr

FOOD	PORTION	CALS	CHOL	FIBER
New York Super Fudge Chunk	½ cup (3.1 oz)	250	35	0
Peanut Butter Cup	½ cup (3.1 oz)	270	55	1
Phish Food	½ cup (3.1 oz)	230	30	1
Pistachio Pistachio	½ cup (3.1 oz)	190	35	0
Praline Pecan	½ cup (3.1 oz)	230	30	0
Southern Pecan Pie	½ cup (3.1 oz)	240	35	0
Strawberry	½ cup (3.1 oz)	180	50	tr
Sweet Cream Cookie	½ cup (3.1 oz)	230	60	tr
Triple Caramel Chunk	½ cup (3.1 oz)	240	30	0
Vanilla Caramel Fudge	½ cup (3.1 oz)	230	60	0
Vanilla Chocolate Chunk	½ cup (3.1 oz)	240	60	0
Vanilla World's Best	½ cup (3.1 oz)	200	65	0
Vanilla w/ Heath Toffee Crunch	½ cup (3.1 oz)	250	35	0
Wavy Gravy	½ cup (3.1 oz)	260	50	1
White Russian	½ cup (3.1 oz)	200	65	0
SORBETS				
Doonesberry	½ cup (3.2 oz)	100	0	0
Lemon Swirl	½ cup (3.2 oz)	100	0	0
Purple Passion Fruit	½ cup (3.2 oz)	100	0	0
Strawberry Kiwi	½ cup (3.2 oz)	110	0	tr

BIG BOY

DESSERTS

FOOD	PORTION	CALS	CHOL	FIBER
Frozen Yogurt Fat Free	1 serv	118	0	—
Frozen Yogurt Shake	1	156	2	—
MAIN MENU SELECTIONS				
Baked Cod w/ Salad Baked Potato Roll & Margarine	1 meal	744	76	—
Baked Potato	1	163	0	—
Breast of Chicken Pita w/ Mozzarella & Ranch Dressing	1	361	84	—
Breast of Chicken w/ Mozzarella Salad Baked Potato Roll & Margarine	1 meal	697	76	—
Cabbage Soup	1 bowl	40	0	—

FOOD	PORTION	CALS	CHOL	FIBER
Cabbage Soup	1 cup	34	0	–
Cajun Cod w/ Salad Baked Potato Roll & Margarine	1 meal	736	76	–
Chicken & Pasta Primavera w/ Salad Roll & Margarine	1 meal	676	65	–
Chicken 'n Vegetable Stir Fry w/ Salad Baked Potato Roll & Margarine	1 meal	795	65	–
Dinner Roll	1	210	0	–
Plain Egg Beaters Omelette w/ Whole Wheat Bread & Margarine	1 meal	305	0	–
Promise Margarine	1 pat	25	0	–
Rice Pilaf	1 serv	153	10	–
Scrambled Egg Beaters w/ Whole Wheat Bread & Margarine	1 meal	305	0	–
Southwest Chicken w/ Salad Baked Potato Roll & Margarine	1 meal	702	76	–
Spaghetti Marinara w/ Salad Roll & Margarine	1 meal	754	8	–
Turkey Pita w/ Ranch Dressing	1	245	83	–
Vegetable Stir Fry w/ Salad Baked Potato Roll & Margarine	1 meal	616	0	–
Vegetarian Egg Beaters Omelette w/ Whole Wheat Bread & Margarine	1 meal	330	0	–
SALAD DRESSINGS				
Italian Fat Free	1 oz	11	0	–
Lo Cal Oriental	1 oz	20	0	–
Lo Cal Ranch	1 oz	41	8	–

FOOD	PORTION	CALS	CHOL	FIBER
SALADS AND SALAD BARS				
Chicken Breast Salad w/ Roll & Margarine	1 serv	523	73	—
Oriental Chicken Breast Salad w/ Dinner Roll & Margarine	1 serv	660	65	—
Tossed Salad	1	35	0	—
BLIMPIE				
6 INCH SUB				
5 Meatball	1 (7.8 oz)	500	25	2
Blimpie Best	1 (8.5 oz)	410	50	4
Cheese Trio	1 (8.2 oz)	510	60	2
Club	1 (9.8 oz)	450	40	3
Grilled Chicken	1 (9.1 oz)	400	30	2
Ham & Swiss	1 (8.2 oz)	400	35	5
Ham Salami Provolone	1 (9.8 oz)	590	70	3
Roast Beef	1 (8.5 oz)	340	20	2
Steak & Cheese	1 (7.1 oz)	550	70	2
Tuna	1 (10.2 oz)	570	50	2
Turkey	1 (8.2 oz)	320	10	3
SALADS AND SALAD BARS				
Grilled Chicken Salad	1 serv (16.2 oz)	350	140	0
BOJANGLES				
BAKED SELECTIONS				
Biscuit	1	243	2	2
Multi-Grain Roll	1	150	0	3
Sweet Biscuit Apple Cinnamon	1	330	tr	1
Sweet Biscuit Bo*Berry	1	220	tr	1
Sweet Biscuit Cinnamon	1	320	tr	1
MAIN MENU SELECTIONS				
Biscuit Sandwich Bacon	1	290	10	1
Biscuit Sandwich Bacon Egg & Cheese	1	550	160	1
Biscuit Sandwich Cajun Filet	1	454	41	1

FOOD	PORTION	CALS	CHOL	FIBER
Biscuit Sandwich Country Ham	1	270	20	1
Biscuit Sandwich Egg	1	400	120	1
Biscuit Sandwich Sausage	1	350	20	1
Biscuit Sandwich Smoked Sausage	1	380	20	1
Biscuit Sandwich Steak	1	649	34	1
Bo Rounds	1 serv	235	13	3
Buffalo Bites	1 serv	180	105	0
Cajun Pintos	1 serv	110	0	6
Cajun Roast Skinfree Breast	1 serv	143	84	tr
Cajun Roast Skinfree Leg	1 serv	161	125	tr
Cajun Roast Skinfree Thigh	1 serv	215	95	tr
Cajun Roast Wing	1 serv	231	117	tr
Cajun Spiced Breast	1 serv	278	75	tr
Cajun Spiced Leg	1 serv	310	67	tr
Cajun Spiced Thigh	1 serv	264	96	tr
Cajun Spiced Wing	1 serv	355	94	tr
Chicken Supremes	1 serv	337	58	1
Corn On The Cob	1 serv	140	0	2
Dirty Rice	1 serv	166	10	1
Green Beans	1 serv	25	0	2
Macaroni & Cheese	1 serv	198	26	tr
Marinated Cole Slaw	1 serv	136	0	3
Potatoes w/o Gravy	1 serv	80	0	1
Sandwich Cajun Filet w/ Mayonnaise	1	437	55	3
Sandwich Cajun Filet w/o Mayonnaise	1	337	45	3
Sandwich Cajun Steak w/ Horseradish Sauce & Pickles	1	434	55	2
Sandwich Grilled Filet w/ Mayonnaise	1	335	61	2
Sandwich Grilled Filet w/o Mayonnaise	1 serv (5.2 oz)	329	59	–

FOOD	PORTION	CALS	CHOL	FIBER
Seasoned Fries	1 serv	344	13	4
Southern Style Breast	1 serv	261	76	tr
Southern Style Leg	1 serv	254	94	tr
Southern Style Thigh	1 serv	308	78	tr
Southern Style Wing	1 serv	337	86	tr

BOSTON MARKET
BAKED SELECTIONS

Brownie	1 (3.3 oz)	450	80	3
Cinnamon Apple Pie	⅛ pie (4.8 oz)	390	0	2
Cookie Chocolate Chip	1 (2.8 oz)	340	25	1

MAIN MENU SELECTIONS

½ Chicken w/ Skin	1 serv (9.7 oz)	590	280	0
¼ Dark Meat Chicken No Skin	1 serv (3.3 oz)	190	115	0
¼ Dark Meat Chicken w/ Skin	1 serv (4.4 oz)	320	155	0
¼ White Meat Chicken No Skin Or Wing	1 serv (4.9 oz)	170	85	0
¼ White Meat Chicken w/ Skin And Wing	1 serv (5.3 oz)	280	135	0
BBQ Baked Beans	¾ cup (7.1 oz)	270	0	12
BBQ Chicken Sandwich	1 (9.9 oz)	540	75	3
Baked Sweet Potato Low Fat	1 (12.5 oz)	460	0	10
Black Beans & Rice	1 cup (8 oz)	300	0	5
Boston Hearth Ham Lean	1 serv (5 oz)	210	75	0
Broccoli Cauliflower Au Gratin	¾ cup (6.1 oz)	200	20	3
Broccoli Rice Casserole	¾ cup (6 oz)	240	40	2
Broccoli w/ Red Peppers	¾ cup (3.4 oz)	60	0	3
Butternut Squash Low Fat	¾ cup (6.8 oz)	160	15	3
Chicken Gravy	1 serv (1 oz)	15	0	0
Chicken Salad Sandwich	1 (11.5 oz)	680	120	4

FOOD	PORTION	CALS	CHOL	FIBER
Chicken Sandwich w/ Cheese & Sauce	1 (12.4 oz)	750	135	5
Chicken Sandwich w/o Cheese & Sauce Low Fat	1 (10 oz)	430	65	4
Chunky Chicken Salad	¾ cup (5.5 oz)	370	120	1
Chunky Cinnamon Apple Sauce No Fat	¾ cup (6.4 oz)	250	0	2
Cole Slaw	¾ cup (6.5 oz)	300	20	3
Corn Bread	1 (2.4 oz)	200	25	1
Coyote Bean Salad	¾ cup (5.3 oz)	190	0	9
Cranberry Relish Low Fat	¾ cup (7.9 oz)	370	0	5
Creamed Spinach	¾ cup (6.4 oz)	260	55	2
Fruit Salad Low Fat	¾ cup (5.5 oz)	70	0	1
Green Bean Casserole	¾ cup (6 oz)	130	20	2
Green Beans	¾ cup (3 oz)	80	0	3
Ham Sandwich w/ Cheese & Sauce	1 (11.8 oz)	760	100	5
Ham Sandwich w/o Cheese & Sauce	1 (9.3 oz)	440	45	4
Homestyle Mashed Potatoes & Gravy	¾ cup (6.6 oz)	210	25	1
Honey Glazed Carrots	¾ cup (5.4 oz)	280	0	4
Hot Cinnamon Apples	¾ cup (6.4 oz)	250	0	3
Macaroni & Cheese	¾ cup (6.7 oz)	280	30	1
Mashed Potatoes	⅔ cup (5.6 oz)	190	25	1
Meat Loaf & Brown Gravy	1 serv (7 oz)	390	120	1
Meat Loaf & Chunky Tomato Sauce	1 serv (8 oz)	370	120	2
Meat Loaf Sandwich w/ Cheese	1 (13.8 oz)	860	165	6
Meat Loaf Sandwich w/o Cheese	1 (12.3 oz)	690	120	6
New Potatoes Low Fat	¾ cup (4.6 oz)	130	0	2
Old Fashioned Potato Salad	¾ cup (6.2 oz)	340	30	2

FOOD	PORTION	CALS	CHOL	FIBER
Open Face Turkey Sandwich	1 (13.4 oz)	500	80	3
Original Chicken Pot Pie	1 pie (14.9 oz)	780	135	4
Oven Roasted Potato Planks Low Fat	5 pieces (5.8 oz)	180	0	3
Pastry Sandwich BBQ Chicken	1 (7.2 oz)	640	60	1
Pastry Sandwich Broccoli Chicken Cheddar	1 (7.2 oz)	690	85	2
Pastry Sandwich Ham & Cheddar	1 (6.6 oz)	640	60	1
Pastry Sandwich Italian Chicken	1 (7.2 oz)	630	60	2
Red Beans And Rice Low Fat	1 cup (8 oz)	260	5	4
Rice Pilaf	⅔ cup (5.1 oz)	180	0	2
Rotisserie Turkey Breast Skinless Low Fat	1 serv (5 oz)	170	100	0
Savory Stuffing	¾ cup (6.1 oz)	310	0	3
Southwest Savory Chicken	1 serv (9.6 oz)	400	100	4
Squash Casserole	¾ cup (6.6 oz)	330	70	3
Steamed Vegetables Low Fat	⅔ cup (3.7 oz)	35	0	3
Sweet Potato Casserole	¾ cup (6.4 oz)	280	10	2
Tabasco BBQ Drumstick	1 (2.4 oz)	130	50	0
Tabasco BBQ Wing	1 (1.8 oz)	110	30	0
Teriyaki Chicken ¼ White w/ Skin	1 serv (6.8 oz)	340	135	0
Teriyaki Chicken ¼ w/ Skin	1 serv (5.9 oz)	380	155	0
Triple Topped Chicken	1 serv (9.2 oz)	470	155	1
Turkey Club Sandwich	1 (11.1 oz)	650	105	4
Turkey Sandwich w/ Cheese & Sauce	1 (11.8 oz)	710	110	4
Turkey Sandwich w/o Cheese & Sauce	1 (9.3 oz)	400	60	4
Whole Kernel Corn	¾ cup (5.8 oz)	180	0	2

FOOD	PORTION	CALS	CHOL	FIBER
Zucchini Marinara Low Fat	¾ cup (6.6 oz)	60	0	2
SALADS AND SALAD BARS				
Caesar Salad Entree	1 serv (10 oz)	510	35	3
Caesar Salad w/o Dressing	1 serv (8 oz)	230	20	3
Caesar Side Salad	1 (4 oz)	200	15	1
Chicken Caesar Salad	1 serv (13 oz)	650	105	3
Tossed Salad w/ Caesar Dressing	1 serv (8 oz)	380	15	3
Tossed Salad w/ Fat Free Ranch	1 serv (8 oz)	160	0	4
Tossed Salad w/ Old Venice Dressing	1 serv (8 oz)	340	0	3
SOUPS				
Chicken Chili	1 cup (8.7 oz)	220	40	6
Chicken Noodle	1 cup (8.4 oz)	130	40	2
Chicken Tortilla	1 cup (8.4 oz)	220	35	2
Potato	1 cup (8 oz)	270	40	2
Tomato Bisque	1 cup (8 oz)	280	50	2
BROWN'S CHICKEN				
Breadsticks w/ Garlic Butter	1	199	tr	–
Breast	3.5 oz	284	67	–
Coleslaw	3.5 oz	131	6	–
Corn Fritters	3.5 oz	415	4	–
Corn On Cob	1 ear (3 inch)	126	1	–
Fettucini Alfredo	1 serv (12 oz)	1507	51	–
French Fries	3.5 oz	503	1	–
Gizzard	3.5 oz	387	88	–
Leg	3.5 oz	287	52	–
Liver	3.5 oz	341	147	–
Mostaccioli w/ Meat	1 serv (12 oz)	835	17	–
Mostaccioli w/o Meat	1 serv (12 oz)	792	0	–
Mushrooms	3.5 oz	289	1	–
Potato Salad	3.5 oz	94	11	–
Ravioli w/ Meat	1 serv (12 oz)	865	17	–
Ravioli w/o Meat	1 serv (12 oz)	822	0	–
Shrimp	3.5 oz	277	31	–

FOOD	PORTION	CALS	CHOL	FIBER
Thigh	3.5 oz	355	63	—
Wing	3.5 oz	385	81	—

BRUEGGER'S BAGELS

Blueberry	1	300	0	2
Cinnamon Raisin	1	290	0	3
Egg	1	280	25	3
Everything	1	290	0	2
Garlic	1	280	0	2
Honey Grain	1	300	0	3
Onion	1	280	0	2
Orange Cranberry	1	290	0	2
Pesto	1	280	0	2
Plain	1	280	0	2
Poppy Seed	1	280	0	2
Pumpernickel	1	280	0	4
Salt	1	270	0	2
Sesame	1	290	0	2
Spinach	1	280	0	3
Sun Dried Tomato	1	280	0	3
Wheat Bran	1	280	0	5

BURGER KING
BEVERAGES

Coca Cola Classic	1 med (22 fl oz)	280	0	0
Coffee	1 serv (12 oz)	5	0	0
Diet Coke	1 med (22 fl oz)	1	0	0
Milk 2%	1 (8 oz)	130	20	0
Shake Chocolate	1 med (13.9 oz)	440	30	4
Shake Chocolate	1 sm (10.7 oz)	330	25	3
Shake Chocolate Syrup Added	1 med (15.9 oz)	570	30	3
Shake Chocolate Syrup Added	1 sm (11.7 oz)	390	20	2
Shake Strawberry Syrup Added	1 med (15.9 oz)	550	30	2
Shake Strawberry Syrup Added	1 sm (11.7 oz)	390	20	1
Shake Vanilla	1 med (13.9 oz)	430	50	2
Shake Vanilla	1 sm (10.7 oz)	330	20	1
Sprite	1 med (22 fl oz)	260	0	0

FOOD	PORTION	CALS	CHOL	FIBER
Tropicana Orange Juice	1 serv (10 oz)	140	0	0
BREAKFAST SELECTIONS				
AM Express Dip	1 serv (1 oz)	80	0	—
AM Express Grape Jam	1 serv (0.4 oz)	30	0	—
AM Express Strawberry Jam	1 serv (0.4 oz)	30	0	—
Bacon	3 strips (0.3 oz)	40	10	—
Biscuit	1 (3.3 oz)	300	0	1
Biscuit w/ Bacon Egg & Cheese	1 (6.6 oz)	620	185	1
Biscuit w/ Egg	1 (4.6 oz)	380	140	tr
Biscuit w/ Sausage	1 (4.6 oz)	490	35	1
Cini-minis w/o Icing	4 (3.8 oz)	440	25	1
Croissan'wich Sausage Egg & Cheese	1 (5.3 oz)	530	185	1
Croissan'wich w/ Sausage & Cheese	1 (3.7 oz)	450	45	1
French Toast Sticks	5 sticks (4 oz)	440	2	3
Ham	1 serv (1.2 oz)	35	15	—
Hash Browns	1 sm (2.6 oz)	240	0	2
Land O'Lakes Whipped Classic Blend	1 serv (0.4 oz)	65	0	—
Vanilla Icing Cini-Minis	1 serv (1 oz)	110	0	—
MAIN MENU SELECTIONS				
American Cheese	2 slices (0.9 oz)	90	25	—
BK Big Fish Sandwich	1 (8.8 oz)	720	80	3
BK Broiler Chicken Breast Patty	1 (3.5 oz)	140	90	—
BK Broiler Chicken Sandwich	1 (8.7 oz)	530	105	2
BK Broiler Chicken Sandwich w/o Mayo	1 (8.7 oz)	370	105	2
Bacon Cheeseburger	1 (4.9 oz)	400	70	1
Bacon Double Cheeseburger	1 (7.2 oz)	630	125	1
Big King Sandwich	1 (7.6 oz)	640	125	1
Bull's Eye Barbecue Sauce	1 serv (0.5 oz)	20	0	—
Cheeseburger	1 (4.7 oz)	360	60	1
Chick'N Crisp Sandwich	1 (4.9 oz)	460	35	3

FOOD	PORTION	CALS	CHOL	FIBER
Chick'N Crisp Sandwich w/o Mayo	1 (4.9 oz)	360	35	3
Chicken Sandwich	1 (8 oz)	710	60	2
Chicken Sandwich w/o Mayo	1 (8 oz)	500	60	2
Chicken Tenders	4 (2.2 oz)	180	30	0
Chicken Tenders	8 (4.3 oz)	350	65	1
Chicken Tenders	5 (2.7 oz)	230	40	tr
Dipping Sauce Barbecue	1 serv (1 oz)	35	0	—
Dipping Sauce Honey	1 serv (1 oz)	90	0	—
Dipping Sauce Honey Mustard	1 serv (1 oz)	90	10	—
Dipping Sauce Ranch	1 serv (1 oz)	170	0	—
Dipping Sauce Sweet & Sour	1 serv (1 oz)	45	0	—
Double Cheeseburger	1 (6.9 oz)	580	120	1
Double Whopper	1 (12.2 oz)	920	155	3
Double Whopper w/ Cheese	1 (13.1 oz)	1010	180	3
Double Whopper w/ Mayo	1 (13.1 oz)	850	180	3
Double Whopper w/o Mayo	1 (12.2 oz)	760	155	3
Dutch Apple Pie	1 serv (4 oz)	300	0	2
French Fries No Salt	1 king size (6 oz)	590	0	5
French Fries No Salt	1 med (4.1 g)	400	0	4
French Fries No Salt	1 sm (2.6 oz)	250	0	2
French Fries Salted	1 med (4.1 oz)	400	0	4
French Fries Salted	1 sm (2.6 oz)	250	0	2
French Fries Salted	1 king size (6 oz)	590	0	5
Hamburger	1 (4.2 oz)	320	50	1
Hamburger Bun	1 (4.6 oz)	130	0	—
Hamburger Patty	1 (1.9 oz)	170	50	—
Hash Browns	1 lg (4.5 oz)	410	0	4
Ketchup	1 serv (0.5 oz)	15	0	—
King Sauce	1 serv (0.5 oz)	70	4	—
Lettuce	1 leaf (0.7 oz)	0	0	—
Mustard	1 serv (3 g)	0	0	—
Onion	1 serv (0.5 oz)	5	0	—

FOOD	PORTION	CALS	CHOL	FIBER
Onion Rings	1 med serv (3.3 oz)	380	2	4
Onion Rings	1 king serv (5.3 oz)	600	4	6
Pickles	4 slices (0.5 oz)	0	0	—
Tartar Sauce	1 serv (1.5 oz)	260	20	—
Tomato	2 slices (1 oz)	5	0	—
Whopper	1 (9.5 oz)	660	85	3
Whopper Bun	1 (2.7 oz)	220	0	—
Whopper Jr.	1 (5.5 oz)	400	55	2
Whopper Jr. w/ Cheese	1 (6 oz)	450	65	2
Whopper Jr. w/ Cheese w/o Mayo	1 (6 oz)	370	65	2
Whopper Jr. w/o Mayo	1 (5.5 oz)	320	55	2
Whopper Patty	1 (2.8 oz)	250	70	—
Whopper w/ Cheese	1 (10.4 oz)	760	110	3
Whopper w/ Cheese w/o Mayo	1 (10.4 oz)	600	110	3
Whopper w/o Mayo	1 (9.5 oz)	510	85	3

CARL'S JR.
BAKED SELECTIONS

FOOD	PORTION	CALS	CHOL	FIBER
Cheese Danish	1 (4.1 oz)	400	15	1
Cheesecake Strawberry Swirl	1 serv (3.5 oz)	300	55	0
Chocolate Cake	1 serv (3 oz)	300	13	4
Chocolate Chip Cookie	1 (2.5 oz)	370	25	1
Cinnamon Roll	1 (4.2 oz)	420	15	4
Muffin Blueberry	1 (4.2 oz)	340	40	1
Muffin Bran	1 (4.7 oz)	370	45	6
BEVERAGES				
Coca-Cola Classic	1 reg (16 fl oz)	190	0	0
Coffee	1 reg (12 oz)	10	0	0
Diet 7UP	1 reg (16 oz)	0	0	0
Diet Coke	1 reg (16 oz)	0	0	0
Dr. Pepper	1 reg (16 oz)	200	0	0
Hot Chocolate	1 reg (12 oz)	110	<5	tr
Iced Tea	1 reg (14 fl oz)	5	0	—
Milk 1%	1 (10 fl oz)	150	15	0
Minute Maid Orange Soda	1 reg (16 oz)	230	0	0
Orange Juice	1 (6 fl oz)	90	0	0

FOOD	PORTION	CALS	CHOL	FIBER
Ramblin' Root Beer	1 reg (16 oz)	230	0	0
Shake Chocolate	1 sm (13.5 oz)	390	30	0
Shake Strawberry	1 sm (13.5 oz)	400	30	0
Shake Vanilla	1 sm (13.5 fl oz)	330	35	0
Sprite	1 reg (16 fl oz)	190	0	0
BREAKFAST SELECTIONS				
Breakfast Burrito	1 (5.3 oz)	430	460	tr
Breakfast Quesadilla Cheese	1 (5.2 oz)	300	225	1
English Muffin w/ Margarine	1 (2.6 oz)	230	0	2
French Toast Dips w/o Syrup	1 serv (3.7 oz)	410	0	3
Grape Jelly	1 serv (0.5 oz)	35	0	0
Hash Brown Nuggets	1 serv (3.3 oz)	270	0	2
Sausage	1 patty (1.8 oz)	200	35	0
Scrambed Eggs	1 serv (3.5 oz)	160	425	0
Strawberry Jam	1 serv (0.5 oz)	35	0	0
Sunrise Sandwich	1 (4.6 oz)	370	225	2
Table Syrup	1 serv (1 oz)	90	0	0
MAIN MENU SELECTIONS				
American Cheese	1 slice (0.5 oz)	60	15	0
BBQ Chicken Sandwich	1 (6.7 oz)	310	55	3
BBQ Sauce	1 serv (1.1 oz)	50	0	0
Big Burger	1 (6.8 oz)	470	55	2
Breadstick	1 (0.3 oz)	35	0	1
Carl's Catch Fish Sandwich	1 (7.5 oz)	560	60	5
Chicken Club Sandwich	1 (8.8 oz)	550	85	3
Chicken Stars	6 pieces (3 oz)	230	85	0
CrissCut Fries	1 lg (5.7 oz)	550	0	3
Croutons	1 serv (7 g)	35	0	0
Double Western Bacon Cheeseburger	1 (11.5 oz)	970	145	2
Famous Big Star Hamburger	1 (8.6 oz)	610	70	2
French Fries	1 reg (4.4 oz)	370	0	3
Great Stuff Potato Bacon & Cheese	1 (14.2 oz)	630	40	6

FOOD	PORTION	CALS	CHOL	FIBER
Great Stuff Potato Broccoli & Cheese	1 (14.2 oz)	530	15	8
Great Stuff Potato Plain	1 (9.4 oz)	290	0	6
Great Stuff Potato Sour Cream & Chive	1 (10.9 oz)	430	10	6
Hamburger	1 (3.1 oz)	200	25	1
Honey Sauce	1 serv (1 oz)	90	0	0
Hot & Crispy Sandwich	1 (5 oz)	400	45	2
Mustard Sauce	1 serv (1 oz)	45	0	0
Onion Rings	1 serv (5.3 oz)	520	0	3
Salsa	1 serv (0.9 oz)	10	0	0
Sante Fe Chicken Sandwich	1 (7.9 oz)	530	85	3
Super Star Hamburger	1 (11.2 oz)	820	120	2
Sweet N'Sour Sauce	1 serv (1 oz)	50	0	0
Swiss Cheese	1 slice (0.5 oz)	45	10	0
Western Bacon Cheeseburger	1 (8.1 oz)	870	90	2
Zucchini	1 serv (5.9 oz)	380	0	3
SALAD DRESSINGS				
1000 Island	2 fl oz	250	20	0
Blue Cheese	2 fl oz	310	25	0
French Fat Free	2 fl oz	70	0	1
House	2 fl oz	220	20	0
Italian Fat Free	2 fl oz	15	0	0
SALADS AND SALAD BARS				
Salad-To-Go Charbroiled Chicken	1 serv (12 oz)	260	70	4
Salad-To-Go Garden	1 (4.8 oz)	50	5	2
CARVEL				
ICE CREAM				
Brown Bonnet Cone	1 (4.7 oz)	380	40	1
Cake	1 pkg (7 oz)	450	45	1
Cake	1 pkg (4 oz)	270	30	tr
Cake Cheesecake	1 serv (4 oz)	280	30	—
Cake Chocolate Vanilla Chocolate Crunchies	1/15 cake (3.4 oz)	230	35	1

FOOD	PORTION	CALS	CHOL	FIBER
Cake Cookies & Cream	1 serv (4 oz)	270	35	1
Cake Fudge Drizzle	⅛ cake (4 oz)	310	30	1
Cake Fudgie The Whale	¼ cake (3.6 oz)	290	30	1
Cake Holiday	¹⁄₁₅ cake (3.4 oz)	240	30	1
Cake S'mores	1 serv (4 oz)	270	25	1
Cake Sinfully Chocolate	1 serv (4 oz)	280	25	1
Cake Strawberries & Cream	⅛ cake (3.8 oz)	240	35	1
Chocolate	4 fl oz	190	25	0
Chocolate No Fat	4 fl oz	120	0	0
Flying Saucer Chocolate	1 (4 oz)	230	30	2
Flying Saucer Chocolate w/ Sprinkles	1 (4 oz)	330	30	2
Flying Saucer Low Fat Chocolate	1 (4 oz)	190	0	1
Flying Saucer Low Fat Vanilla	1 (4 oz)	180	0	1
Flying Saucer Vanilla	1 (4 oz)	240	40	1
Flying Saucer Vanilla w/ Sprinkles	1 (4 oz)	340	40	1
Lil'Love Cake All Vanilla	1 piece (4.4 oz)	330	35	tr
Lil'Love Cake Chocolate & Vanilla	1 piece (4 oz)	260	30	tr
Nature's Crunch	1 (4.2 g)	450	20	2
Olde Fashion Sundae Butterscotch	1 (8 oz)	500	60	1
Olde Fashion Sundae Chocolate	1 (8 oz)	470	55	1
Olde Fashion Sundae Strawberry	1 (8 oz)	420	55	2
Sheet Cake Chocolate Vanilla Chocolate Crunchies	½6 cake (3.3 oz)	230	35	1
Sinful Love Bar	1 (4.2 oz)	460	20	3
Thick Shake Chocolate	1 (16 oz)	719	116	tr
Thick Shake Low Fat Chocolate	1 (16 oz)	490	15	1

FOOD	PORTION	CALS	CHOL	FIBER
Thick Shake Low Fat Strawberry	1 (16 oz)	460	15	1
Thick Shake Low Fat Vanilla	1 (16 oz)	460	15	1
Thick Shake No Fat Chocolate	1 (16 oz)	524	36	1
Thick Shake No Fat Strawberry	1 (16 oz)	453	36	1
Thick Shake No Fat Vanilla	1 (16 oz)	462	36	1
Thick Shake Strawberry	1 (16 oz)	648	116	tr
Thick Shake Vanilla	1 (16 oz)	657	116	tr
Vanilla	4 fl oz	200	40	0
Vanilla No Fat	4 fl oz	120	0	0
SHERBET				
Black Raspberry	½ cup (3.4 oz)	150	5	0
Blueberry	½ cup (3.4 oz)	150	5	0
Lemon	½ cup (3.5 oz)	150	5	0
Lime	½ cup (3.5 oz)	150	5	0
Mango	½ cup (3.5 oz)	140	5	0
Orange	½ cup (3.5 oz)	150	5	0
Peach	½ cup (3.4 oz)	150	5	0
Pineapple	½ cup (3.5 oz)	150	5	0
Strawberry	½ cup (3.5 oz)	150	5	0

CHICK-FIL-A
BEVERAGES

FOOD	PORTION	CALS	CHOL	FIBER
Coca-Cola Classic	1 sm	110	0	0
Diet Coke	1 sm	0	0	0
Diet Lemonade	1 sm	25	0	0
Ice Tea Sweetened	1 sm	80	0	0
Iced Tea Unsweetened	1 serv	0	0	0
Lemonade	1 sm	170	0	0
DESSERTS				
Cheesecake w/ Blueberry Topping	1 slice	370	90	2
Cheesecake w/ Strawberry Topping	1 slice	360	90	2
Fudge Nut Brownie	1	330	20	2
IceDream Cup	1 sm	230	25	0

FOOD	PORTION	CALS	CHOL	FIBER
IceDream Cone	1 sm	160	15	0
Lemon Pie	1 slice	320	110	3
MAIN MENU SELECTIONS				
Barbecue Sauce	1 pkg	45	0	0
Carrot & Raisin Salad	1 sm	130	0	2
Chargrilled Chicken Caesar Salad	1 serv	240	85	2
Chargrilled Chicken Club Sandwich w/o Sauce	1	360	80	2
Chargrilled Chicken Deluxe Sandwich	1	280	60	2
Chargrilled Chicken Filet	1	100	60	0
Chargrilled Chicken Sandwich	1	280	60	1
Chargrilled Chicken Sandwich w/o Butter	1	240	60	1
Chick-N-Strips	4	250	70	0
Chicken Deluxe Sandwich	1	420	60	2
Chicken Sandwich	1	410	60	1
Chicken Sandwich w/o Butter	1	380	60	1
Chicken Filet	1	230	60	0
Chicken Salad Sandwich On Whole Wheat	1	350	65	5
Cole Slaw	1 sm	210	20	2
Cool Wrap Chargrilled Chicken	1	390	70	3
Cool Wrap Chicken Caesar	1	460	85	3
Cool Wrap Spicy Chicken	1	390	70	3
Dijon Honey Mustard Sauce	1 pkg	50	5	0
Hearty Breast of Chicken Soup	1 cup	100	50	1
Honey Mustard Sauce	1 pkg	45	0	0

FOOD	PORTION	CALS	CHOL	FIBER
Nuggets	8	260	70	tr
Polynesian Sauce	1 pkg	110	0	0
Waffle Fries w/o Salt	1 sm	280	15	4
Waffle Potato Fries	1 sm	280	15	5
SALAD DRESSINGS				
Basil Vinaigrette	1 pkg	210	0	0
Blue Cheese	1 pkg	190	20	0
Buttermilk Ranch	1 pkg	190	10	0
Caesar	1 pkg	200	45	0
Fat Free Dijon Honey Mustard	1 pkg	60	0	0
Light Italian	1 pkg	20	0	0
Spicy	1 pkg	210	10	0
Thousand Island	1 pkg	170	10	0
SALADS AND SALAD BARS				
Chargrilled Chicken Garden Salad	1 serv	180	70	3
Chick-N-Strips Salad	1 serv	340	85	3
Croutons Garlic & Butter	1 pkg	90	0	0
Roasted Sunflower Kernels Unsalted	1 pkg	80	0	tr
Side Salad	1 serv	80	15	2

CHILI'S
DESSERTS

FOOD	PORTION	CALS	CHOL	FIBER
Diet By Chocolate Cake	1 serv	370	0	8
Diet By Chocolate Cake w/ Yogurt	1 serv	465	3	8
Diet By Chocolate Cake w/ Yogurt & Fudge Topping	1 serv	534	3	8
MAIN MENU SELECTIONS				
Guiltless Grill Chicken Fijitas	1 serv	726	44	24
Guiltless Grill Chicken Platter	1 serv	563	58	12
Guiltless Grill Chicken Salad w/ Dressing	1 serv	254	47	6

FOOD	PORTION	CALS	CHOL	FIBER
Guiltless Grill Chicken Sandwich	1	527	43	18
Guiltless Grill Veggie Pasta	1 serv	590	55	16
Guiltless Grill Veggie Pasta w/ Chicken	1 serv	696	97	17

CHURCH'S CHICKEN

FOOD	PORTION	CALS	CHOL	FIBER
Apple Pie	1 serv (3.1 oz)	280	<5	1
Biscuit	1 (2.1 oz)	250	<5	1
Breast	1 serv (2.8 oz)	200	65	0
Cajun Rice	1 serv (3.1 oz)	130	5	tr
Cole Slaw	1 serv (3 oz)	92	0	2
Corn On The Cob	1 serv (5.7 oz)	139	0	9
French Fries	1 serv (2.7 oz)	210	0	2
Leg	1 serv (2 oz)	140	45	0
Okra	1 serv (2.8 oz)	210	0	4
Potatoes & Gravy	1 serv (3.7 oz)	90	0	1
Tender Strip	1 (1.1 oz)	80	15	1
Thigh	1 serv (2.8 oz)	230	80	0
Wing	1 serv (3.1 oz)	250	60	0

D'ANGELO'S SANDWICH SHOP
SALADS AND SALAD BARS

FOOD	PORTION	CALS	CHOL	FIBER
Antipasto Salad w/o Dressing	1	420	40	—
Caesar Salad w/ Dressing	1	740	70	—
Caesar Salad w/o Dressing	1	490	15	—
Chicken Caesar Salad w/ Dressing	1	860	130	—
Chicken Caesar Salad w/o Dressing	1	600	70	—
Chicken Salad D'Lite	1	325	49	—
Chicken Salad w/o Dressing	1	390	60	—
D'Lite Turkey	1 serv	355	79	—
Greek Salad w/ Dressing	1	940	50	—
Greek Salad w/ Tuna & Dressing	1	1010	65	—

FOOD	PORTION	CALS	CHOL	FIBER
Greek Salad w/ Tuna w/o Dressing	1	490	65	—
Greek Salad w/o Dressing	1	420	50	—
Roast Beef Salad D'Lite	1	350	63	—
Roast Beef Salad w/o Dressing	1	400	50	—
Tossed Garden Salad w/o Dressing	1	270	0	—
Tuna Salad D'Lite	1	305	32	—
Tuna Salad w/o Dressing	1	330	15	—
Turkey Salad w/o Dressing	1	400	80	—
SANDWICHES				
BLT w/ Cheese	1	1170	165	—
BLT w/ Cheese Medium Sub	1	870	125	—
BLT w/ Cheese Pokket	1	570	90	—
BLT w/ Cheese Small Sub	1	600	90	—
Barbecue Curls	1	480	70	—
Buffalo Chicken Wrap w/ Blue Cheese Dressing	1	621	93	—
Buffalo Chicken Wrap w/o Dressing	1	417	78	—
Caesar Salad w/ Dressing Pokket	1	590	40	—
Caesar Salad w/o Dressing Pokket	1	460	10	—
Caesar Salad w/ Chicken w/ Dressing Pokket	1	700	100	—
Caesar Salad w/ Chicken w/ Dressing Pokket	1	570	70	—
Caesar Wrap w/ Dressing	1	484	10	—

FOOD	PORTION	CALS	CHOL	FIBER
Caesar Wrap w/ Fat Free Dressing	1	484	10	—
Capicola Ham & Cheese Large Sub	1	740	85	—
Capicola Ham & Cheese Medium Sub	1	550	65	—
Capicola Ham & Cheese Pokket	1	350	45	—
Capicola Ham & Cheese Small Sub	1	390	45	—
Cheeseburger Large Sub	1	1060	165	—
Cheeseburger Medium Sub	1	780	125	—
Cheeseburger Pokket	1	490	80	—
Cheeseburger Small Sub	1	530	80	—
Chicken Salad Large Sub	1	1370	155	—
Chicken Salad Medium Sub	1	970	110	—
Chicken Salad Pokket	1	650	80	—
Chicken Salad Small Sub	1	690	80	—
Chicken Stir Fry D'Lite Pokket	1	360	70	—
Chicken Stir Fry D'Lite Sub	1	280	70	—
Chicken Stir Fry Large Sub	1	800	160	—
Chicken Stir Fry Medium Sub	1	560	110	—
Chicken Stir Fry Pokket	1	360	70	—
Chicken Stir Fry Small Sub	1	380	70	—
Classic Vegetable D'Lite Pokket	1	340	23	—
Classic Vegetable Large Sub	1	860	80	—

FOOD	PORTION	CALS	CHOL	FIBER
Classic Vegetable Medium Sub	1	610	55	—
Classic Vegetable Pokket	1	400	40	—
Classic Vegetable Small Sub	1	430	40	—
Crunchy Vegetable D'Lite Pokket	1	350	23	—
Crunchy Vegetable D'Lite Small Sub	1	385	23	—
Crunchy Vegetable Large Sub	1	880	80	—
Crunchy Vegetable Pokket	1	410	40	—
Crunchy Vegetables Medium Sub	1	620	55	—
Crunchy Vegetables Small Sub	1	440	40	—
Ginger Chicken Stir Fry D'Lite Pokket	1	400	72	—
Greek Pokket	1	910	50	—
Grilled Spicy Steak D'Lite Pokket	1	425	41	—
Grilled Steak Cheese Large Sub	1	1160	195	—
Grilled Steak Cheese Medium Sub	1	820	135	—
Grilled Steak Cheese Pokket	1	550	100	—
Grilled Steak Cheese Small Sub	1	580	100	—
Grilled Steak Combo Large Sub	1	1170	195	—
Grilled Steak Combo Medium Sub	1	830	135	—
Grilled Steak Combo Pokket	1	550	100	—
Grilled Steak Combo Small Sub	1	590	100	—

FOOD	PORTION	CALS	CHOL	FIBER
Grilled Steak D'Lite Pokket	1	390	41	—
Grilled Steak Large Sub	1	990	155	—
Grilled Steak Medium Sub	1	680	105	—
Grilled Steak Mushrooms Large Sub	1	1000	155	—
Grilled Steak Mushrooms Medium Sub	1	690	105	—
Grilled Steak Mushrooms Pokket	1	450	70	—
Grilled Steak Mushrooms Small Sub	1	480	70	—
Grilled Steak Onion Large Sub	1	1000	155	—
Grilled Steak Onion Medium Sub	1	700	105	—
Grilled Steak Onion Small Sub	1	480	70	—
Grilled Steak Onions Pokket	1	450	70	—
Grilled Steak Peppers	1	690	105	—
Grilled Steak Peppers Large Sub	1	1000	155	—
Grilled Steak Peppers Pokket	1	540	70	—
Grilled Steak Pokket	1	440	70	—
Grilled Steak Small Sub	1	470	70	—
Ham & Cheese Large Sub	1	760	105	—
Ham & Cheese Medium Sub	1	550	75	—
Ham & Cheese Pokket	1	370	55	—
Ham & Cheese Small Sub	1	400	55	—
Ham Salami & Cheese Large Sub	1	870	110	—

FOOD	PORTION	CALS	CHOL	FIBER
Ham Salami & Cheese Medium Sub	1	630	80	—
Ham Salami & Cheese Pokket	1	420	60	—
Ham Salami & Cheese Small Sub	1	450	60	—
Hamburger Large Sub	1	920	130	—
Hamburger Medium Sub	1	680	95	—
Hamburger Pokket	1	430	65	—
Hamburger Small Sub	1	460	65	—
Italian Cold Cut Large Sub	1	1130	155	—
Italian Cold Cut Medium Sub	1	820	110	—
Italian Cold Cut Pokket	1	550	80	—
Italian Cold Cut Small Sub	1	580	80	—
Meatball Large Sub	1	1010	135	—
Meatball Medium Sub	1	750	100	—
Meatball Pokket	1	480	65	—
Meatball Small Sub	1	520	65	—
Meatball w/ Cheese Large Sub	1	1170	165	—
Meatball w/ Cheese Medium Sub	1	880	125	—
Meatball w/ Cheese Pokket	1	580	85	—
Meatball w/ Cheese Small Sub	1	620	85	—
Pastrami Large Sub	1	1250	175	—
Pastrami Medium Sub	1	860	115	—
Pastrami Pokket	1	550	75	—
Pastrami Small Sub	1	580	75	—
Pastrami w/ Cheese Large Sub	1	1640	270	—
Pastrami w/ Cheese Medium Sub	1	1170	195	—

FOOD	PORTION	CALS	CHOL	FIBER
Pastrami w/ Cheese Pokket	1	780	135	—
Pastrami w/ Cheese Small Sub	1	820	135	—
Roast Beef D'Lite Pokket	1	330	48	—
Roast Beef D'Lite Small Sub	1	365	48	—
Roast Beef Large Sub	1	710	95	—
Roast Beef Medium Sub	1	520	70	—
Seafood Salad Large Sub	1	1210	50	—
Seafood Salad Medium Sub	1	860	35	—
Seafood Salad Pokket	1	570	25	—
Seafood Salad Small Sub	1	610	25	—
Stuffed Turkey D'Lite Pokket	1	510	82	—
Stuffed Turkey D'Lite Small Sub	1	545	82	—
Stuffed Turkey Large Sub	1	1070	165	—
Stuffed Turkey Medium Sub	1	790	120	—
Tuna Salad Large Sub	1	1510	120	—
Tuna Salad Medium Sub	1	1070	85	—
Tuna Salad Pokket	1	720	60	—
Turkey D'Lite Pokket	1	330	79	—
Turkey D'Lite Small Sub	1	365	79	—
Turkey Large Sub	1	710	160	—
Turkey Medium Sub	1	520	115	—
Turkey Club Large Sub	1	860	180	—
Turkey Club Medium Sub	1	630	130	—
Turkey Club Pokket	1	400	90	—
Turkey Club Small Sub	1	430	90	—

FOOD	PORTION	CALS	CHOL	FIBER
DAIRY QUEEN				
FOOD SELECTIONS				
Chicken Breast Fillet Sandwich	1 (6.7 oz)	430	55	2
Chicken Strip Basket	1 serv (14.5 oz)	1000	55	5
Chili 'n' Cheese Dog	1 (5 oz)	330	45	2
DQ Homestyle Bacon Double Cheeseburger	1 (8.9 oz)	610	130	2
DQ Homestyle Cheeseburger	1 (5.3 oz)	340	55	2
DQ Homestyle Double Cheeseburger	1 (7.7 oz)	540	115	2
DQ Homestyle Hamburger	1 (4.8 oz)	290	45	2
DQ Ultimate Burger	1 (9.4 oz)	670	135	2
French Fries	1 sm (4 oz)	350	0	3
French Fries	1 med (3.9 oz)	440	0	4
Grilled Chicken Sandwich	1 (6.5 oz)	310	50	3
Hot Dog	1 (3.5 oz)	240	25	1
Onion Rings	1 serv (4 oz)	320	0	3
The Great Steakmelt Basket	1 serv (13.2 oz)	770	75	5
ICE CREAM				
Banana Split	1 (12.9 oz)	510	30	3
Blizzard Chocolate Sandwich Cookie	1 med (11.4 oz)	640	45	1
Blizzard Chocolate Sandwich Cookie	1 sm (12 oz)	520	40	1
Blizzard Chocolate Chip Cookie Dough	1 med (15.4 oz)	950	75	2
Blizzard Chocolate Chip Cookie Dough	1 sm (12 oz)	660	55	1
Breeze Heath	1 med (14.2 oz)	710	20	1
Breeze Heath	1 sm (10.2 oz)	470	10	1
Breeze Strawberry	1 sm (12 oz)	320	5	1
Breeze Strawberry	1 med (13.4 oz)	460	10	1

FOOD	PORTION	CALS	CHOL	FIBER
Buster Bar	1 (5.2 oz)	450	15	2
Chocolate Malt	1 sm (14.7 oz)	650	55	0
Chocolate Malt	1 med (19.9 oz)	880	70	0
Cone Chocolate	1 med (6.9 oz)	340	30	0
Cone Chocolate	1 sm (5 oz)	240	20	0
Cone Vanilla	1 sm (5 oz)	230	20	0
Cone Vanilla	1 med (6.9 oz)	330	30	0
Cone Vanilla	1 lg (8.9 oz)	410	40	0
Cone Yogurt	1 med (6.9 oz)	260	5	0
Cone Dipped	1 med (7.7 oz)	490	30	1
Cone Dipped	1 sm (5.5 oz)	340	20	1
Cup Of Yogurt	1 med (6.7 oz)	230	5	0
DQ 8 Inch Round Cake Undecorated	⅛ of cake (6.2 oz)	340	25	1
DQ Fudge Bar No Sugar Added	1 (2.3 oz)	50	0	0
DQ Lemon Freez'r	½ cup (3.2 oz)	80	0	0
DQ Nonfat Frozen Yogurt	½ cup (3 oz)	100	<5	0
DQ Sandwich	1 (2.1 oz)	200	10	1
DQ Soft Serve Chocolate	½ cup (3.3 oz)	150	15	0
DQ Soft Serve Vanilla	½ cup (3.3 oz)	140	15	0
DQ Treatzza Pizza Heath	⅛ of pie (2.3 oz)	180	5	1
DQ Treatzza Pizza M&M	⅛ of pie (2.4 oz)	190	5	1
DQ Vanilla Orange Bar No Sugar Added	1 (2.3 oz)	60	0	0
Dilly Bar Chocolate	1 (3 oz)	210	10	0
Frozen Hot Chocolate	1 (20.9 oz)	860	50	3
Misty Slush	1 sm (15.9 oz)	220	0	0
Misty Slush	1 med (20.9 oz)	290	0	0
Peanut Buster Parfait	1 (10.7 oz)	730	35	2
Pecan Mudslide Treat	1 (4.6 oz)	650	35	2
S'more Galore Parfait	1 (10.7 oz)	730	30	3
Shake Chocolate	1 sm (13.9 oz)	560	50	0
Shake Chocolate	1 med (18.9 oz)	770	70	0
Starkiss	1 (3 oz)	80	0	0
Strawberry Shortcake	1 (8.5 oz)	430	60	1
Sundae Chocolate	1 med (8.2 oz)	400	30	0

FOOD	PORTION	CALS	CHOL	FIBER
Sundae Chocolate	1 sm (5.7 oz)	280	20	0
Yogurt Sundae Strawberry	1 med (8.2 oz)	280	5	1

DELTACO
BEVERAGES

FOOD	PORTION	CALS	CHOL	FIBER
Coffee	1 serv (8 oz)	0	0	0
Coke Classic	1 sm (10 oz)	120	0	0
Coke Classic	1 med (12 oz)	150	0	0
Coke Classic	1 lg (20 oz)	230	0	0
Coke Classic Best Value	1 serv (27 oz)	320	0	0
Diet Coke	1 lg (20 oz)	5	0	0
Diet Coke	1 med (12 oz)	0	0	0
Diet Coke	1 sm (10 oz)	0	0	0
Diet Coke Best Value	1 serv (27 oz)	10	0	0
Iced Tea	1 sm (10 oz)	0	0	0
Iced Tea	1 lg (20 oz)	5	0	0
Iced Tea	1 med (12 oz)	0	0	0
Iced Tea Best Value	1 serv (27 oz)	10	0	0
Milk 1% Lowfat	1 serv (11 oz)	130	10	0
Mr Pibb	1 lg (20 oz)	230	0	0
Mr Pibb	1 sm (10 oz)	120	0	0
Mr Pibb	1 med (12 oz)	150	0	0
Mr Pibb Best Value	1 serv (27 oz)	320	0	0
Orange Juice	1 serv (11 oz)	140	0	1
Shake Chocolate	1 lg (15 oz)	680	45	1
Shake Chocolate	1 sm (11.4 oz)	520	35	1
Shake Strawberry	1 lg (15 oz)	540	40	1
Shake Strawberry	1 sm (11.4 oz)	410	30	1
Shake Vanilla	1 lg (15 oz)	550	50	0
Shake Vanilla	1 sm (11.4 oz)	420	35	0
Sprite	1 med (12 oz)	140	0	0
Sprite	1 lg (20 oz)	230	0	0
Sprite	1 sm (10 oz)	110	0	0
Sprite Best Value	1 serv (27 oz)	310	0	0

BREAKFAST SELECTIONS

FOOD	PORTION	CALS	CHOL	FIBER
Burrito Breakfast	1 (3.8 oz)	250	160	1
Burrito Egg & Cheese	1 (7.5 oz)	450	530	3
Burrito Macho Bacon & Egg	1 (15.9 oz)	1030	790	6

FOOD	PORTION	CALS	CHOL	FIBER
Burrito Steak & Egg	1 (9 oz)	580	560	3
Quesadilla Bacon & Egg	1 (6.1 oz)	450	260	2
Side of Bacon	2 strips (0.3 oz)	50	10	0
MAIN MENU SELECTIONS				
Beans 'n Cheese Cup	1 serv (7.7 oz)	260	5	16
Burrito Combo	1 (8.2 oz)	490	55	8
Burrito Del Beef	1 (8 oz)	550	90	3
Burrito Del Classic Chicken	1 (8.5 oz)	580	70	3
Burrito Deluxe Combo	1 (10.7 oz)	530	60	9
Burrito Deluxe Del Beef	1 (10.5 oz)	590	95	4
Burrito Green	1 (5 oz)	280	15	6
Burrito Macho Beef	1 (18.9 oz)	1170	190	7
Burrito Macho Combo	1 (19.4 oz)	1050	115	17
Burrito Red	1 (5 oz)	270	15	6
Burrito Red Regular	1 (7.5 oz)	390	20	11
Burrito Regular Green	1 (7.5 oz)	400	10	10
Burrito Spicy Chicken	1 (8.7 oz)	480	40	8
Burrito The Works	1 (10.2 oz)	480	25	9
Cheeseburger	1 (4.6 oz)	330	35	3
Del Cheeseburger	1 (5.6 oz)	430	45	4
Double Del Cheeseburger	1 (7.1 oz)	560	85	4
Fries	1 sm (3 oz)	210	0	2
Fries	1 reg (5 oz)	350	0	3
Fries Best Value	1 serv (7 oz)	490	0	5
Fries Chili Cheese	1 serv (10.5 oz)	670	45	5
Fries Deluxe Chili Cheese	1 serv (11.9 oz)	710	50	6
Get A Lot Meals #1 Combo Burrito Fries Drink	1 meal	980	55	11
Get A Lot Meals #2 Del Classic Chicken Burrito Fries Drink	1 meal	1080	70	7
Get A Lot Meals #3 Regular Red Burrito Fries Drink	1 meal	890	20	14

FOOD	PORTION	CALS	CHOL	FIBER
Get A Lot Meals #4 Two Chicken Soft Tacos Fries Drink	1 meal	910	60	5
Get A Lot Meals #5 Taco Combo Burrito Drink	1 meal	790	75	9
Get A Lot Meals #6 Two Tacos Quesadilla Drink	1 meal	960	115	3
Get A Lot Meals #7 Macho Combo Burrito Fries Drink	1 meal	1530	115	20
Get A Lot Meals #8 Two Big Fat Tacos Fries Drink	1 meal	802	70	10
Get A Lot Meals #9 Double Del Cheeseburger Fries Drink	1 meal	1050	85	7
Nachos	1 serv (4 oz)	380	5	2
Nachos Macho	1 serv (17 oz)	1200	55	16
Quesadilla Chicken	1 (6.8 oz)	580	104	2
Quesadilla Regular	1 (5.3 oz)	500	75	2
Quesadilla Spicy Jack Chicken	1 (6.8 oz)	570	105	2
Quesadilla Spicy Jack Regular	1 (5.3 oz)	490	75	2
Rice Cup	1 serv (4 oz)	150	2	1
Soft Taco	1 (2.8 oz)	160	20	1
Soft Taco Chicken	1 (3.3 oz)	210	30	1
Taco	1 (2.2 oz)	160	20	1
Taco Big Fat	1 (5.4 oz)	320	35	3
Taco Big Fat Chicken	1 (5.4 oz)	340	45	3
TacoBig Fat Steak	1 (5.4 oz)	390	45	3
Taco Salad Deluxe	1 (18.8 oz)	760	70	14
Tostada Salad	1 (4.5 oz)	210	15	6

FOOD	PORTION	CALS	CHOL	FIBER
DENNY'S				
BEVERAGES				
2% Milk	1 serv (10 oz)	151	22	0
Chocolate Milk	1 serv (10 oz)	235	37	0
Coffee French Vanilla	1 serv (8 oz)	76	2	0
Coffee Hazelnut	1 serv (8 oz)	66	2	0
Coffee Irish Cream	1 serv (8 oz)	73	2	0
Grapefruit Juice	1 serv (10 oz)	115	0	0
Hot Chocolate	1 serv (8 oz)	90	0	0
Lemonade	1 serv (16 oz)	150	0	0
Orange Juice	1 serv (10 oz)	126	0	0
Raspberry Ice Tea	1 serv (16 oz)	78	0	0
Tomato Juice	1 serv (10 oz)	56	0	2
BREAKFAST SELECTIONS				
All American Slam	1 serv (15 oz)	1028	724	2
Applesauce	1 serv (3 oz)	60	0	1
Bacon	4 strips (1 oz)	162	36	0
Bagel Dry	1 (3 oz)	235	0	0
Banana	1 (4 oz)	110	0	4
Banana Strawberry Medley	1 serv (4 oz)	108	0	2
Biscuit Plain	1 (3 oz)	375	0	0
Biscuit w/ Sausage Gravy	1 serv (7 oz)	570	24	0
Blueberry Topping	1 serv (3 oz)	106	0	0
Canadian Bacon	1 serv (3 oz)	110	43	0
Cantaloup	1 serv (3 oz)	32	0	1
Cheddar Cheese Omelette	1 serv (13 oz)	770	675	2
Cherry Topping	1 serv (3 oz)	86	0	0
Chicken Fried Steak & Eggs	1 serv (14 oz)	723	452	8
Country Scramble	1 serv (16 oz)	795	409	2
Cream Cheese	1 oz	100	31	0
Egg	1 (2 oz)	134	205	0
Egg Beaters	1 serv (2.3 oz)	71	1	0
Eggs Benedict	1 serv (19 oz)	860	525	3
English Muffin Dry	1 (4 oz)	125	0	1
Farmer's Omelette	1 serv (18 oz)	912	633	3
French Slam	1 serv (14 oz)	1029	777	2

FOOD	PORTION	CALS	CHOL	FIBER
French Toast	2 pieces (8 oz)	510	317	2
Fresh Fruit Mix	1 serv (3 oz)	36	0	1
Grapefruit	½ (5 oz)	60	0	6
Grapes	1 serv (3 oz)	55	0	1
Grits	1 serv (4 oz)	80	0	0
Ham	1 serv (3 oz)	94	23	0
Ham'n'Cheddar Omelette	1 serv (14 oz)	743	657	2
Hashed Browns	1 serv (4 oz)	218	0	2
Hashed Browns Covered	1 serv (6 oz)	318	30	2
Hashed Browns Covered & Smothered	1 serv (8 oz)	359	30	2
Honeydew	1 serv (3 oz)	31	0	1
Junior Meals Basic Breakfast	1 serv (9 oz)	558	230	3
Junior Meals Junior French Slam	1 serv (7 oz)	461	386	1
Junior Meals Junior Grand Slam	1 serv (5 oz)	397	230	1
Junior Meals Junior Waffle Supreme	1 serv (4 oz)	190	73	0
Meat Lover's Sampler	1 serv (14 oz)	806	481	2
Moon Over My Hammy	1 serv (12 oz)	807	430	2
Muffin Blueberry	1 (3 oz)	309	0	0
Oatmeal	1 serv (4 oz)	100	0	3
Original Grand Slam	1 serv (10 oz)	795	460	2
Pancakes	3 (5 oz)	491	0	3
Pork Chop & Eggs	1 serv (12 oz)	555	469	2
Porterhouse Steak & Eggs	1 serv (18 oz)	1223	570	2
Ready To Eat Cereal	1 serv (1 oz)	100	0	1
Sausage	4 links (3 oz)	354	64	0
Sausage Cheddar Omelette	1 serv (16 oz)	1036	721	2
Scram Slam	1 serv (18 oz)	974	694	4
Senior Belgian Waffle Slam	1 serv (6 oz)	399	302	0
Senior Omelette	1 serv (12 oz)	623	439	3
Senior Starter	1 serv (7 oz)	336	205	2

FOOD	PORTION	CALS	CHOL	FIBER
Senior Triple Play	1 serv (8 oz)	537	409	2
Sirloin Steak & Eggs	1 serv (13 oz)	808	474	2
Slim Slam	1 serv (14 oz)	638	34	1
Southern Slam	1 serv (13 oz)	1065	484	0
Strawberries w/ Sugar	1 serv (3 oz)	115	0	1
Strawberry Topping	1 serv (3 oz)	115	0	1
Sunshine Slam	1 serv (8 oz)	537	409	2
Super Play It Again Slam	1 serv (15 oz)	1192	690	3
Syrup	3 tbsp (1.5 oz)	143	0	0
Syrup Reduced Calorie	1 serv (1.5 oz)	25	0	0
T-Bone Steak & Eggs	1 serv (16 oz)	1045	530	2
Toast Dry	1 slice (1 oz)	92	0	1
Ultimate Omelette	1 serv (17 oz)	780	639	4
Veggie Cheese Omelette	1 serv (16 oz)	714	644	4
Waffle	1 (6 oz)	304	146	0
Whipped Cream	1 serv (2 oz)	23	7	0
Whipped Margarine	1 serv (0.5 oz)	87	0	0
DESSERTS				
Apple Pie	1 serv (7 oz)	430	<5	1
Apple Pie w/ Equal	1 serv (7 oz)	370	<5	2
Banana Split	1 serv (19 oz)	894	78	6
Blueberry Topping	1 serv (3 oz)	106	0	0
Cheesecake Pie	1 serv (4 oz)	470	90	0
Cherry Topping	1 serv (3 oz)	86	0	0
Cherry Pie	1 serv (7 oz)	540	<5	2
Chocolate Topping	1 serv (2 oz)	317	0	0
Chocolate Cake	1 serv (4 oz)	370	29	2
Chocolate Pecan Pie	1 serv (6 oz)	790	70	3
Chocolate Shake	1 serv (10 oz)	579	108	0
Coconut Cream Pie	1 serv (7 oz)	480	15	1
Double Scoop Sundae	1 serv (6 oz)	375	74	0
Dutch Apple Pie	1 serv (7 oz)	440	0	1
French Silk Pie	1 serv (6 oz)	650	165	2
Fudge Topping	1 serv (2 oz)	201	3	1
German Chocolate Pie	1 serv (7 oz)	580	15	2
Hot Fudge Cake Sundae	1 serv (8 oz)	687	62	3

FOOD	PORTION	CALS	CHOL	FIBER
Ice Cream Float	1 serv (12 oz)	280	39	0
Key Lime Pie	1 serv (6 oz)	600	35	0
Lemon Meringue Pie	1 serv (7 oz)	460	95	1
Pecan Pie	1 serv (6 oz)	600	50	2
Single Scoop Sundae	1 serv (3 oz)	188	37	0
Strawberry Topping	1 serv (3 oz)	115	0	1
Vanilla Shake	1 serv (11 oz)	581	108	0
MAIN MENU SELECTIONS				
BBQ Sauce	1 serv (1.5 oz)	47	0	0
Bacon Cheddar Burger	1 (14 oz)	935	164	3
Bacon Lettuce & Tomato Sandwich	1 (6 oz)	634	54	3
Baked Potato Plain	1 (6 oz)	186	0	4
Battered Cod Dinner w/ Tartar Sauce	1 serv (9 oz)	732	105	3
Broccoli In Butter Sauce	2 serv (4 oz)	50	5	3
Brown Gravy	1 serv (1 oz)	13	0	0
Buffalo Chicken Strips	1 serv (10 oz)	734	96	0
Buffalo Wings	12 pieces (15 oz)	856	500	1
Carrots In Honey Glaze	2 serv (4 oz)	80	0	3
Charleston Chicken Sandwich	1 (11 oz)	632	81	4
Chicken Fried Chicken	1 serv (6 oz)	327	65	1
Chicken Fried Steak w/ Gravy	1 serv (4 oz)	265	27	1
Chicken Gravy	1 serv (1 oz)	14	2	0
Chicken Melt Sandwich	1 (7 oz)	520	39	2
Chicken Quesadilla	1 serv (16 oz)	827	181	2
Chicken Strip w/ Dressing	1 serv (10 oz)	635	95	0
Chicken Strips	5 pieces (10 oz)	720	95	0
Classic Burger	1 (11 oz)	673	106	3
Classic Burger w/ Cheese	1 (13 oz)	836	137	3
Club Sandwich	1	485	90	–
Corn In Butter Sauce	2 serv (4 oz)	120	5	5
Cornbread Stuffing Plain	1 serv (2 oz)	182	0	0

FOOD	PORTION	CALS	CHOL	FIBER
Cottage Cheese	1 serv (3 oz)	72	10	0
Country Gravy	1 serv (1 oz)	17	0	0
Delidinger Sandwich	1 (14 oz)	852	80	3
Deluxe Grilled Cheese Sandwich	1 (7 oz)	482	1	2
Dinner Roll	1 (1.5 oz)	132	0	1
French Fries Unsalted	1 serv (4 oz)	323	0	0
Fried Fish Sandwich	1 (11 oz)	905	69	4
Gardenburger Patty	1 patty (3.4 oz)	160	10	3
Gardenburger Patty w/ Bun & Fat Free Honey Mustard Dressing	1 serv (11.1 oz)	653	26	6
Green Beans w/ Bacon	2 serv (4 oz)	60	5	3
Green Peas In Butter Sauce	2 serv (4 oz)	100	5	4
Grilled Alaskan Salmon	1 serv (7 oz)	296	102	0
Grilled Chicken Breast	1 serv (4 oz)	130	67	0
Grilled Chicken Dinner	1 serv (4 oz)	130	67	0
Grilled Chicken Sandwich	1 (11 oz)	509	83	3
Grilled Chopped Steak w/ Gravy	1 serv (10 oz)	400	91	2
Grilled Mushrooms	1 serv (2 oz)	14	0	1
Ham & Swiss On Rye	1 (9 oz)	533	36	5
Hashed Browns	1 serv (4 oz)	218	0	2
Herb Toast	1 serv (2 oz)	200	0	1
Horseradish Sauce	1 serv (1.5 oz)	170	43	0
Junior Meals Junior Burger	1 serv (3 oz)	261	41	0
Junior Meals Junior Chicken Strips	1 serv (5 oz)	318	48	0
Junior Meals Junior Fried Fish	1 serv (5 oz)	465	68	1
Junior Meals Junior Grilled Cheese	1 serv (4 oz)	375	1	1

FOOD	PORTION	CALS	CHOL	FIBER
Junior Meals Junior Shrimp Basket	1 serv (4 oz)	291	60	2
Lunch Basket Charleston Chicken Ranch Melt	1 serv (14 oz)	975	96	4
Lunch Basket Chicken Strips	1 serv (8 oz)	568	70	0
Lunch Basket Classic Burger	1 serv (12 oz)	674	121	3
Lunch Basket Delidinger	1 serv (14 oz)	852	80	3
Lunch Basket Five Star Philly	1 serv (10 oz)	657	97	4
Lunch Basket Patty Melt	1 serv (8 oz)	696	129	2
Mashed Potatoes Plain	1 serv (6 oz)	105	0	2
Mayonnaise	2 tbsp (1 oz)	200	16	0
Mozzarella Sticks w/ Sauce	8 pieces (10 oz)	756	48	7
Onion Ring Basket	1 serv (5 oz)	439	7	1
Onion Rings	1 serv (3 oz)	264	4	0
Patty Melt Sandwich	1 (8 oz)	695	114	2
Pork Chop Dinner w/ Gravy	1 serv (8 oz)	386	121	0
Porterhouse Steak	1 (14 oz)	708	161	0
Pot Roast Dinner w/ Gravy	1 serv (7 oz)	260	140	0
Rice Pilaf	1 serv (3 oz)	112	0	0
Roast Turkey & Stuffing	1 serv (12 oz)	701	100	0
Sampler	1 serv (15 oz)	1120	69	5
Seasoned Fries	1 serv (4 oz)	261	0	0
Senior Battered Cod	1 serv (5 oz)	465	68	1
Senior Chicken Fried Steak	1 serv (8 oz)	341	27	2
Senior Grilled Cheese Sandwich	1 serv	360	50	–
Senior Grilled Chicken Breast	1 serv (6 oz)	219	67	0
Senior Liver w/ Bacon & Onions	1 serv (8 oz)	322	270	2
Senior Pork Chop	1 serv (4 oz)	193	60	0

FOOD	PORTION	CALS	CHOL	FIBER
Senior Pot Roast	1 serv (5 oz)	149	71	0
Senior Roast Turkey & Stuffing	1 serv (8 oz)	596	51	0
Senior Turkey Sandwich	1	340	75	—
Senior Sandwich Ham & Swiss	1 serv (9 oz)	497	36	4
Shrimp Dinner	1 serv (8 oz)	558	135	3
Sirloin Steak Dinner	1 serv (5.5 oz)	271	62	0
Sliced Tomatoes	3 slices (2 oz)	13	0	1
Sour Cream	1 serv (1.5 oz)	91	19	0
Steak & Shrimp Dinner w/ Gravy	1 serv (9 oz)	645	150	2
Super Bird Sandwich	1 (9 oz)	620	60	2
T-Bone Steak Dinner	1 serv (10 oz)	530	121	0
Turkey Breast On Multigrain	1 (9 oz)	476	57	5
SALAD DRESSINGS				
Bleu Cheese	1 oz	124	18	0
Caesar	1 oz	142	2	0
Creamy Italian	1 oz	106	0	0
Fat Free Honey Mustard	1 oz	38	0	0
French	1 oz	106	7	0
Oriental Peanut Dressing	1 serv (1 oz)	106	0	0
Ranch	1 oz	101	8	0
Reduced Calorie French	1 oz	76	0	0
Reduced Calorie Italian	1 oz	32	0	0
Thousand Island	1 oz	104	21	0
SALADS AND SALAD BARS				
Buffalo Chicken Salad	1 serv (17 oz)	615	88	3
Fried Chicken Salad	1 serv (13 oz)	506	94	3
Garden Chicken Delight Salad	1 serv (16 oz)	277	67	6
Grilled Chicken Caesar Salad w/ Dressing	1 serv (13 oz)	655	86	4

FOOD	PORTION	CALS	CHOL	FIBER
Oriental Chicken Salad w/ Dressing	1 serv (20 oz)	568	67	7
Side Caesar w/ Dressing	1 serv (6 oz)	338	7	3
Side Garden Salad w/ Dressing	1 serv (7 oz)	113	0	3
SOUPS				
Cheese	1 serv (8 oz)	293	19	4
Chicken Noodle	1 serv (8 oz)	60	10	0
Clam Chowder	1 serv (8 oz)	214	5	1
Cream Of Broccoli	1 serv (8 oz)	193	0	2
Cream of Potato	1 serv (8 oz)	222	0	2
Split Pea	1 serv (8 oz)	146	5	2
Vegetable Beef	1 serv (8 oz)	79	5	2

DOMINO'S PIZZA
12 INCH MEDIUM PIZZAS

FOOD	PORTION	CALS	CHOL	FIBER
Add A Topping Anchovies	1 topping serv	23	9	0
Add A Topping Bacon	1 topping serv	81	12	0
Add A Topping Canned Mushrooms	1 topping serv	4	0	tr
Add A Topping Cheddar Cheese	1 topping serv	57	15	0
Add A Topping Cooked Beef	1 topping serv	56	11	tr
Add A Topping Extra Cheese	1 topping serv	48	7	tr
Add A Topping Fresh Mushrooms	1 topping serv	4	0	tr
Add A Topping Green Olives	1 topping serv	12	0	tr
Add A Topping Green Peppers	1 topping serv	3	0	tr
Add A Topping Ham	1 topping serv	18	7	0
Add A Topping Italian Sausage	1 topping serv	55	11	tr
Add A Topping Onion	1 topping serv	4	0	tr

FOOD	PORTION	CALS	CHOL	FIBER
Add A Topping Pepperoni	1 topping serv	62	13	tr
Add A Topping Pineapple Tidbits	1 topping serv	10	0	tr
Add A Topping Ripe Olives	1 topping serv	14	0	tr
Deep Dish Cheese	2 slices (6.3 oz)	477	19	3
Hand Tossed Cheese	2 slices (5.2 oz)	347	15	3
Thin Crust Cheese	¼ pie (3.7 oz)	271	15	2
14 INCH LARGE PIZZAS				
Add A Topping Anchovies	1 topping serv	23	tr	0
Add A Topping Anchovies	1 topping serv	23	9	0
Add A Topping Bacon	1 topping serv	75	11	0
Add A Topping Canned Mushrooms	1 topping serv	3	0	tr
Add A Topping Cheddar Cheese	1 topping serv	48	12	0
Add A Topping Cooked Beef	1 topping serv	44	8	tr
Add A Topping Extra Cheese	1 topping serv	45	7	tr
Add A Topping Fresh Mushrooms	1 topping serv	3	0	tr
Add A Topping Green Olives	1 topping serv	11	0	tr
Add A Topping Green Peppers	1 topping serv	2	0	tr
Add A Topping Ham	1 topping serv	17	7	0
Add A Topping Italian Sausage	1 topping serv	44	9	tr
Add A Topping Onion	1 topping serv	3	0	tr
Add A Topping Pepperoni	1 topping serv	55	12	tr
Add A Topping Pineapple Tidbits	1 topping serv	8	0	tr

FOOD	PORTION	CALS	CHOL	FIBER
Add A Topping Ripe Olives	1 topping serv	12	0	tr
Deep Dish Cheese	2 slices (6.1 oz)	455	18	3
Hand-Tossed Cheese	2 slices (4.8 oz)	317	14	3
Thin Crust Cheese	⅛ pie (3.5 oz)	253	14	2
6 INCH DEEP DISH PIZZAS				
Add A Topping Anchovies	1 topping serv	45	18	0
Add A Topping Bacon	1 topping serv	82	12	0
Add A Topping Canned Mushrooms	1 topping serv	2	0	tr
Add A Topping Cheddar Cheese	1 topping serv	86	22	0
Add A Topping Cooked Beef	1 topping serv	44	8	tr
Add A Topping Extra Cheese	1 topping serv	57	9	tr
Add A Topping Fresh Mushrooms	1 topping serv	2	0	tr
Add A Topping Green Olives	1 topping serv	10	0	tr
Add A Topping Green Peppers	1 topping serv	2	0	tr
Add A Topping Ham	1 topping serv	17	7	0
Add A Topping Italian Sausage	1 topping serv	44	9	tr
Add A Topping Onion	1 topping serv	3	0	tr
Add A Topping Pepperoni	1 topping serv	50	10	tr
Add A Topping Pineapple Tidbits	1 topping serv	5	0	tr
Add A Topping Ripe Olives	1 topping serv	11	0	tr
Cheese	1 pie (7.6 oz)	595	23	4
MAIN MENU SELECTIONS				
Breadstick	1 (0.8 oz)	78	0	tr
Buffalo Wings Barbeque	1 piece (0.9 oz)	50	26	tr
Buffalo Wings Hot	1 piece (0.9 oz)	45	26	tr
Cheesy Bread	1 piece (1 oz)	103	5	tr
Garden Salad	1 lg (7.7 oz)	39	0	3

FOOD	PORTION	CALS	CHOL	FIBER
Garden Salad	1 sm (4.3 oz)	22	0	2
SALAD DRESSINGS				
Marzetti Blue Cheese	1 serv (1.5 oz)	220	40	0
Marzetti Creamy Caesar	1 serv (1.5 oz)	200	10	0
Marzetti Fat Free Ranch	1 serv (1.5 oz)	40	0	1
Marzetti Honey French	1 serv (1.5 oz)	210	0	0
Marzetti House Italian	1 serv (1.5 oz)	220	0	0
Marzetti Light Italian	1 serv (1.5 oz)	20	0	0
Marzetti Ranch	1 serv (1.5 oz)	260	5	0
Marzetti Thousand Island	1 serv (1.5 oz)	200	25	0

DUNKIN' DONUTS

BAGELS AND CREAM CHEESE

FOOD	PORTION	CALS	CHOL	FIBER
Bagel Blueberry	1	340	0	tr
Bagel Cinnamon Raisin	1	340	0	1
Bagel Egg	1	350	25	0
Bagel Everything	1	360	0	0
Bagel Garlic	1	360	0	0
Bagel Onion	1	330	0	0
Bagel Plain	1	340	0	0
Bagel Poppyseed	1	360	0	tr
Bagel Pumpernickel	1	350	0	2
Bagel Salt	1	340	0	0
Bagel Sesame	1	380	0	0
Bagel Wheat	1	330	0	4
Cream Cheese Chive	1 pkg	190	55	tr
Cream Cheese Garden Vegetable	1 pkg	180	45	tr
Cream Cheese Lite	1 pkg	130	30	0
Cream Cheese Plain	1 pkg	200	60	0
Cream Cheese Salmon	1 pkg	180	50	0
BAKED SELECTIONS				
Bow Tie Donut	1	300	0	tr
Cake Donut Blueberry	1	290	10	tr
Cake Donut Butternut	1	300	0	tr
Cake Donut Chocolate Coconut	1	300	0	1
Cake Donut Chocolate Frosted	1	300	0	tr

FOOD	PORTION	CALS	CHOL	FIBER
Cake Donut Chocolate Glazed	1	290	0	1
Cake Donut Cinnamon	1	270	0	tr
Cake Donut Coconut	1	290	0	tr
Cake Donut Double Chocolate	1	310	0	2
Cake Donut Glazed	1	270	0	tr
Cake Donut Old Fashioned	1	250	0	tr
Cake Donut Powdered	1	270	0	tr
Cake Donut Toasted Coconut	1	300	0	tr
Cake Donut Whole Wheat Glazed	1	310	0	2
Chocolate Frosted Donut	1	200	0	tr
Chocolate Kreme Filled Donut	1	270	0	tr
Cinnamon Bun	1	510	10	0
Coffee Roll	1	270	0	1
Coffee Roll Chocolate Frosted	1	290	0	1
Coffee Roll Maple Frosted	1	290	0	1
Coffee Roll Vanilla Frosted	1	290	0	1
Cookie Chocolate Chocolate Chunk	1	210	35	2
Cookie Chocolate Chunk	1	220	35	1
Cookie Chocolate Chunk w/ Nut	1	230	35	1
Cookie Chocolate White Chocolate Chunk	1	230	35	1
Cookie Oatmeal Raisin Pecan	1	220	30	1
Cookie Peanut Butter Chocolate Chunk w/ Nuts	1	240	25	2

FOOD	PORTION	CALS	CHOL	FIBER
Cookie Peanut Butter w/ Nuts	1	240	30	1
Croissant Almond	1	350	5	2
Croissant Chocolate	1	400	5	2
Croissant Plain	1	290	5	tr
Cruller Glazed	1	290	0	tr
Cruller Glazed Chocolate	1	280	0	1
Cruller Plain	1	240	0	tr
Cruller Powdered	1	270	0	tr
Cruller Sugar	1	250	0	tr
Donut Apple Crumb	1	230	0	tr
Donut Apple N' Spice	1	200	0	tr
Donut Bavarian Kreme	1	210	0	tr
Donut Black Raspberry	1	210	0	tr
Donut Blueberry Crumb	1	240	0	tr
Donut Boston Kreme	1	240	0	tr
Donut Chocolate Iced Bismark	1	340	0	tr
Dunkin' Donut	1	240	0	tr
Eclair Donut	1	270	0	tr
Fritter Glazed	1	260	0	1
Glazed Donut	1	180	0	tr
Jelly Filled Donut	1	210	0	tr
Jelly Stick	1	290	0	tr
Lemon Donut	1	200	0	tr
Maple Frosted Donut	1	210	0	tr
Marble Frosted Donut	1	200	0	tr
Muffin Apple Cinnamon Pecan	1	510	70	1
Muffin Apple N'Spice	1	350	35	2
Muffin Banana Nut	1	360	35	3
Muffin Blueberry	1 (4 oz)	320	35	3
Muffin Blueberry	1 (6 oz)	490	75	2
Muffin Bran	1	390	20	3
Muffin Cherry	1	340	40	2

FOOD	PORTION	CALS	CHOL	FIBER
Muffin Chocolate Hazelnut	1	610	70	3
Muffin Chocolate Chip	1 (6 oz)	590	75	3
Muffin Chocolate Chip	1 (4 oz)	400	35	4
Muffin Corn	1 (4 oz)	390	55	2
Muffin Corn	1 (6 oz)	500	80	1
Muffin Cranberry Orange	1	470	75	2
Muffin Cranberry Orange Nut	1	350	35	3
Muffin Honey Raisin Bran	1 (3.3 oz)	330	15	4
Muffin Lemon Poppyseed	1	360	35	1
Muffin Oat Bran	1	370	20	3
Muffin Lowfat Apple & Spice	1	240	0	tr
Muffin Lowfat Banana	1	250	0	tr
Muffin Lowfat Blueberry	1	250	0	1
Muffin Lowfat Bran	1	240	0	4
Muffin Lowfat Cherry	1	250	0	tr
Muffin Lowfat Chocolate	1	250	0	2
Muffin Lowfat Corn	1	240	45	0
Muffin Lowfat Cranberry Orange	1	240	0	1
Muffin Reduced Fat Blueberry	1	450	65	2
Muffin Reduced Fat Corn	1	460	75	1
Munchkins Chocolate Cake Glazed	3	200	0	tr
Munchkins Cake Butternut	3	200	0	tr
Munchkins Cake Cinnamon	4	250	0	tr
Munchkins Cake Coconut	3	200	0	tr
Munchkins Cake Glazed	3	200	0	0

FOOD	PORTION	CALS	CHOL	FIBER
Munchkins Cake Plain	4	220	0	tr
Munchkins Cake Powdered	4	250	0	tr
Munchkins Cake Sugared	4	240	0	tr
Munchkins Cake Toasted Coconut	3	200	0	tr
Munchkins Yeast Glazed	5	200	0	tr
Munchkins Yeast Jelly Filled	5	210	0	tr
Munchkins Yeast Lemon Filled	4	170	0	0
Munchkins Yeast Sugar Raised	7	220	0	tr
Strawberry Frosted Donut	1	210	0	tr
Strawberry Donut	1	210	0	tr
Sugar Raised Donut	1	170	0	tr
Sugared Cake Donut	1	250	0	tr
Vanilla Frosted Donut	1	210	0	tr
Vanilla Kreme Filled Donut	1	270	0	tr
BEVERAGES				
Coffee Coolatta w/ 2% Milk	1 (16 oz)	240	10	0
Coffee Coolatta w/ Cream	1 (16 oz)	410	75	0
Coffee Coolatta w/ Milk	1 (16 oz)	260	15	0
Coffee Coolatta w/ Skim Milk	1 (16 oz)	230	<5	0
Coolatta Orange Mango Fruit	1 (16 oz)	290	0	tr
Coolatta Pink Lemonade Fruit	1 (16 oz)	350	0	0
Coolatta Raspberry Lemonade	1 (16 oz)	280	0	0

FOOD	PORTION	CALS	CHOL	FIBER
Coolatta Strawberry Fruit	1 (16 oz)	280	0	1
Coolatta Vanilla	1 (16 oz)	450	0	0
Cream	1 serv (1 oz)	60	20	0
Dark Roast Coffee	1 serv (10 oz)	5	0	0
Decaf Coffee	1 serv (10 oz)	0	0	0
Dunkaccino	1 (10 oz)	250	10	tr
Dunkaccino	1 (20 oz)	510	20	1
Dunkaccino	1 (18.75 oz)	480	20	1
Dunkaccino	1 (14 oz)	360	15	1
French Vanilla Coffee	1 serv (10 oz)	5	0	0
Hazelnut Coffee	1 serv (10 oz)	5	0	0
Hot Cocoa	1 (20 oz)	470	0	3
Hot Cocoa	1 (10 oz)	230	0	2
Hot Cocoa	1 (18.75 oz)	440	0	3
Hot Cocoa	1 (14 oz)	330	0	2
Regular Coffee	1 serv (10 oz)	5	0	0
SANDWICHES				
Breakfast Sandwich Ham Egg Cheese	1	320	195	2
Omwich Bagel Bacon Cheddar	1	600	295	tr
Omwich Bagel Spanish Cheese	1	570	280	tr
Omwich Bagel Three Cheese	1	610	305	tr
Omwich Croissant Spanish Cheese	1	530	285	1
Omwich Croissant Bacon Cheddar	1	560	295	1
Omwich Croissant Three Cheese	1	560	305	1
Omwich English Muffin Bacon Cheddar	1	400	295	2
Omwich English Muffin Spanish Cheese	1	370	280	2
Omwich English Muffin Three Cheese	1	400	305	2

FOOD	PORTION	CALS	CHOL	FIBER
EINSTEIN BROS BAGELS				
BAGELS				
Bagel Chips Cinnamon Raisin Swirl	1 serv (1 oz)	90	0	1
Bagel Chips Plain	1 serv (1 oz)	90	0	1
Bagel Chips Sourdough Dill	1 serv (1 oz)	90	0	1
Bagel Chips Sun Dried Tomato	1 serv (1 oz)	90	0	1
Bagel Chips Sunflower	1 serv (1 oz)	100	0	1
Bagel Chips Wild Blueberry	1 serv (1 oz)	90	0	1
Chocolate Chip	1 (4 oz)	380	0	2
Chopped Garlic	1 (4.2 oz)	377	0	5
Chopped Onion	1 (4 oz)	340	0	2
Cinnamon Raisin Swirl	1 (4 oz)	360	0	2
Cinnamon Sugar	1	330	0	2
Dark Pumpernickel	1 (3.8 oz)	330	0	5
Everything	1 (4 oz)	342	0	2
Honey 8 Grain	1 (4 oz)	320	0	4
Nutty Banana	1 (4 oz)	370	0	2
Plain	1 (3.7 oz)	330	0	2
Poppy Dip'd	1 (3.9 oz)	346	0	2
Salt	1 (3.9 oz)	330	0	2
Sesame Dip'd	1 (4.1 oz)	381	0	3
Spinach Herb	1 (3.8 oz)	320	0	3
Sun Dried Tomato	1 (3.8 oz)	320	0	3
Veggie Confetti	1 (3.8 oz)	330	0	3
Wild Blueberry	1 (4 oz)	360	0	3
SANDWICHES AND FILLINGS				
Butter & Margarine Blend	1 serv (0.4 oz)	60	0	0
Capers	1 tbsp	0	0	0
Cheddar Cheese	1 serv (0.75 oz)	110	30	0
Classic New York Lox & Bagel	1 (11.4 oz)	560	75	3
Cream Cheese Cheddarpeno	1 serv (1 oz)	90	30	0
Cream Cheese Chive	1 serv (1 oz)	90	35	0

FOOD	PORTION	CALS	CHOL	FIBER
Cream Cheese Maple Walnut Raisin	1 serv (1 oz)	100	25	0
Cream Cheese Plain	1 serv (1 oz)	100	35	0
Cream Cheese Smoked Salmon	1 serv (1 oz)	90	35	0
Cream Cheese Strawberry	1 serv (1 oz)	90	30	0
Cream Cheese Sun Dried Tomato	1 serv (1 oz)	90	35	0
Cucumbers	1 serv (1 oz)	0	0	0
Fruit Spreads	1 tbsp	40	0	0
Ham	1 serv (2.5 oz)	75	20	0
Ham & Cheese Sandwich	1 (9.9 oz)	520	70	3
Honey	1 tbsp	64	0	0
Hummus	2 tbsp	60	0	1
Hummus Sandwich	1 (6 oz)	440	0	4
Lettuce	1 leaf	0	0	0
Lite Cream Cheese Plain	1 serv (1 oz)	60	20	0
Lite Cream Cheese Spinach Dill	1 serv (1 oz)	60	20	0
Lite Cream Cheese Veggie	1 serv (1 oz)	60	20	0
Lite Cream Cheese Wildberry	1 serv (1 oz)	70	15	0
Lowfat Chicken Salad Sandwich	1 (11.6 oz)	440	45	3
Lowfat Tuna Salad Sandwich	1 (11.6 oz)	440	30	3
Marshall's Lox	1 serv (2 oz)	90	10	0
Mayonnaise Lite Reduced Calorie	1 serv (0.5 oz)	50	5	0
Peanut Butter	1 serv (1.1 oz)	190	0	2
Peanut Butter & Jelly Sandwich	1 (6 oz)	595	0	4
Scrambled Egg Sandwich	1 (7.7 oz)	480	385	2
Scrambled Egg Sandwich w/ Meat & Cheese	1 (8.9 oz)	520	8	2

FOOD	PORTION	CALS	CHOL	FIBER
Smoked Turkey	1 serv (2.5 oz)	75	20	0
Smoked Turkey Sandwich	1 (9.9 oz)	480	45	3
Spouts Alfalfa	1 serv (0.5 oz)	0	0	1
Sweet Onions	1 serv (1 oz)	0	0	0
Swiss Cheese	1 serv (0.75 oz)	100	25	0
Tasty Turkey Sandwich	1 (10 oz)	530	90	2
Tomato	1 serv (1.5 oz)	0	0	1
Turkey Pastrami 99% Fat Free	1 serv (2.5 oz)	75	0	0
Turkey Pastrami Sandwich	1 (9.7 oz)	460	20	3
Veg Out Sandwich	1 (8.9 oz)	350	3	3
Whitefish Salad Sandwich	1 (9.2 oz)	630	45	3

EL POLLO LOCO
MAIN MENU SELECTIONS

FOOD	PORTION	CALS	CHOL	FIBER
Broccoli Slaw	1 serv (5 oz)	203	0	3
Burrito BRC	1 (9.3 oz)	482	15	9
Burrito Classic Chicken	1 (9.3 oz)	556	117	8
Burrito Grilled Steak	1 (11.3 oz)	705	77	10
Burrito Loco Grande	1 (13.1 oz)	632	129	8
Burrito Smokey Black Bean	1 (9.3 oz)	566	22	9
Burrito Spicy Hot Chicken	1 (9.8 oz)	559	117	8
Burrito Whole Wheat Chicken	1 (10.8 oz)	592	146	8
Chicken Breast	1 piece (3 oz)	160	110	0
Chicken Leg	1 piece (1.75 oz)	90	75	0
Chicken Soft Taco	1 (4 oz)	224	66	0
Chicken Thigh	1 piece (2 oz)	180	130	0
Chicken Wing	1 (1.5 oz)	110	80	0
Chicken Tamale	1 (3.5 oz)	190	10	2
Cole Slaw	1 serv (5 oz)	206	11	2
Corn-On-Cob	1 ear (5.5 oz)	146	0	2
Cornbread Stuffing	1 serv (6 oz)	281	0	6
Crispy Green Beans	1 serv (5 oz)	41	0	3
Cucumber Salad	1 serv (4.2 oz)	34	0	1

FOOD	PORTION	CALS	CHOL	FIBER
Fiesta Corn	1 serv (5 oz)	152	0	6
Flame Broiled Chicken Salad	1 serv (14.9 oz)	167	56	4
French Fries	1 serv (4.4 oz)	323	0	0
Garden Salad	1 serv (6.4 oz)	29	0	2
Gravy	1 serv (1 oz)	14	2	0
Honey Glazed Carrots	1 serv (5 oz)	104	0	3
Lime Parfait	1 serv (5 oz)	125	0	0
Macaroni & Cheese	1 serv (6 oz)	238	31	1
Mashed Potatoes	1 serv (5 oz)	97	0	2
Pinto Beans	1 serv (6 oz)	185	0	8
Polo Bowl	1 serv (19 oz)	504	56	9
Potato Salad	1 serv (6 oz)	256	15	3
Rainbow Pasta Salad	1 serv (5 oz)	157	0	2
Salad Shell	1 (5.6 oz)	440	0	0
Smokey Black Beans	1 serv (5 oz)	255	11	4
Southwest Cole Slaw	1 serv (5 oz)	178	8	3
Spanish Rice	1 serv (4 oz)	130	0	1
Spiced Apples	1 serv (5 oz)	146	0	0
Steak Bowl	1 serv (15.2 oz)	616	68	8
Taco Al Carbon Chicken	1 serv (4.4 oz)	265	28	3
Taco Al Carbon Steak	1 (4.4 oz)	394	46	3
Taquito	1 serv (5 oz)	370	25	3
Tortilla Corn	1 (1.1 oz)	70	0	1
Tortilla Flour	1 (1 oz)	90	0	0
Tortilla Wrap Chicken Caesar	1 (10.47 oz)	518	48	3
Tortilla Wrap Southwest	1 (11.97 oz)	632	61	5
Tostada Salad Chicken	1 serv (14.7 oz)	332	80	4
Tostado Salad Steak	1 serv (13.2 oz)	525	100	4
SALAD DRESSINGS				
Blue Cheese	1 serv (2 oz)	300	50	0
Light Italian	1 serv (2 oz)	25	0	0
Ranch	1 serv (2 oz)	350	5	0
Thousand Island	1 serv (2 oz)	270	30	0

FAZOLI'S

DESSERTS

FOOD	PORTION	CALS	CHOL	FIBER
Cheesecake	1 slice	290	950	0
Cheesecake Turtle	1 slice	420	100	2

FOOD	PORTION	CALS	CHOL	FIBER
Cookie Milk Chocolate Chunk	1	360	30	0
Lemon Ice	1 serv	190	0	0
Specialty Cheesecake	1 serv	300	85	1
Strawberry Topping	1 serv	35	0	0
MAIN MENU SELECTIONS				
Baked Chicken Parmesan	1 serv	740	65	6
Baked Spaghetti Parmesan	1 serv	700	60	5
Baked Ziti	1 reg	750	55	6
Baked Ziti	1 sm	490	35	4
Breadstick	1	140	0	1
Breadstick Dry	1	90	0	1
Broccoli Fettuccine Alfredo	1 sm	560	15	6
Broccoli Fettuccine Alfredo	1 reg	830	20	6
Cheese Ravioli w/ Marinara Sauce	1 serv	480	65	4
Cheese Ravioli w/ Meat Sauce	1 serv	510	70	4
Classic Sampler	1 serv	710	85	6
Fettuccine Alfredo	1 reg	800	20	5
Fettuccine Alfredo	1 sm	530	15	3
Fettuccine w/ Shrimp & Scallop	1 serv	590	95	3
Homestyle Lasagna	1 serv	440	145	4
Homestyle Lasagna w/ Broccoli	1 serv	420	140	5
Minestrone Soup	1 serv	120	0	8
Peppery Chicken Alfredo	1 serv	610	50	3
Pizza Cheese	1 serv	460	40	2
Pizza Combination Double Slice	1 serv	570	60	3
Pizza Pepperoni	1 serv	530	53	2
Pizza Baked Spaghetti	1 serv	750	75	5
Spaghetti w/ Marinara Sauce	1 sm	420	0	5

FOOD	PORTION	CALS	CHOL	FIBER
Spaghetti w/ Marinara Sauce	1 reg	620	0	7
Spaghetti w/ Meat Sauce	1 reg	670	10	8
Spaghetti w/ Meat Sauce	1 sm	450	10	5
Spaghetti w/ Meatballs	1 reg	1020	80	8
Spaghetti w/ Meatballs	1 sm	730	60	6
SALAD DRESSINGS				
Honey French	1 serv	150	0	0
House Italian	1 serv	110	0	0
Ranch	1 serv	150	3	0
Reduced Calorie Italian	1 serv	50	0	0
Thousand Island	1 serv	130	15	0
SALADS AND SALAD BARS				
Caesar Side Salad	1	220	5	3
Chicken & Pasta Caesar Salad	1	500	55	4
Chicken Caesar Salad	1	420	45	4
Chicken Finger Salad	1	190	45	2
Chicken Finger Salad w/ Bacon & Honey Mustard	1	400	50	2
Garden Salad	1	25	0	1
Garden Salad w/ Balsamic Vinaigrette	1	120	0	1
Italian Chef Salad	1	260	45	3
Pasta Salad	1 serv	590	20	5
SANDWICHES				
Panini Chicken Caesar Club	1	660	110	3
Panini Chicken Pesto	1	510	60	3
Panini Four Cheese & Tomato	1	720	75	3
Panini Ham & Swiss	1	600	70	2
Panini Italian Club	1	670	85	3

FOOD	PORTION	CALS	CHOL	FIBER
Panini Italian Deli	1	660	90	4
Panini Smoked Turkey	1	710	110	3
Submarinos Club	half	1100	120	7
Submarinos Ham & Swiss	1	1000	75	7
Submarinos Meatball	half	1260	125	8
Submarinos Orignal	half	1160	105	8
Submarinos Pepperoni Pizza	half	1060	95	6
Submarinos Turkey	half	990	90	7

FOSTERS FREEZE

FOOD	PORTION	CALS	CHOL	FIBER
Soft Serve Vanilla	1 serv (4 oz)	152	9	–

FRULLATI CAFE
BAKED SELECTIONS

FOOD	PORTION	CALS	CHOL	FIBER
Muffin Banana Nut	1 (4 oz)	394	31	1
Muffin Cranberry Orange	1 (4 oz)	357	31	1
Muffin Fat Free Apple Streusel	1 (4 oz)	260	0	2
Muffin Fat Free Chocolate	1 (4 oz)	260	0	2
Muffin Fat Free Very Berry	1 (4 oz)	260	0	2
Muffin Sugar Free Blueberry	1 (4 oz)	308	12	1
Muffin Wild Blueberry	1 (4 oz)	344	31	1

BEVERAGES

FOOD	PORTION	CALS	CHOL	FIBER
Apple Juice	1 serv (12 oz)	131	0	0
Carrot Juice	1 serv (12 oz)	111	0	2
Celery Juice	1 serv (12 oz)	22	0	2
Lemondae	1 serv	209	0	2
Lemondae Apple	1 serv	245	0	3
Lemondae Cherry	1 serv	237	0	2
Lemondae Orange	1 serv	270	0	5
Lemondae Strawberry	1 serv	234	0	2
Orange Banana Juice	1 serv (12 oz)	150	0	2
Orange Juice	1 serv (12 oz)	126	0	1

FOOD	PORTION	CALS	CHOL	FIBER
Smoothie A La Frullati	1 sm	275	10	3
Smoothie A La Frullati	1 lg	426	20	3
Smoothie Affinity	1 lg	378	20	2
Smoothie Affinity	1 sm	226	10	2
Smoothie Fiesta	1 lg	257	0	6
Smoothie Fiesta	1 sm	234	0	6
Smoothie Peach Banana	1 sm	266	0	5
Smoothie Peach Banana	1 lg	289	0	5
Smoothie Pina Colada	1 sm	236	10	2
Smoothie Pina Colada	1 lg	387	82	2
Smoothie Strawberry Banana	1 sm	165	0	4
Smoothie Strawberry Banana	1 lg	188	0	4
Smoothie Strawberry Blueberry	1 sm	90	0	3
Smoothie Strawberry Blueberry	1 lg	113	0	3
Smoothie Strawberry Fruit	1 lg	101	0	3
Smoothie Strawberry Fruit	1 sm	79	0	3
Smoothie Strawberry Watermelon	1 lg	123	0	2
Smoothie Strawberry Watermelon	1 sm	100	0	2
DESSERTS				
Frozen Yogurt	1 reg	205	3	0
Frozen Yogurt	1 lg	263	3	0
Frozen Yogurt	1 sm	146	2	0
Yogurt Smoothie Cappuccino	1 serv	472	17	0
Yogurt Smoothie Chocolate Fudge	1 serv	555	17	1
Yogurt Smoothie Fiesta	1 serv	432	17	3

FOOD	PORTION	CALS	CHOL	FIBER
Yogurt Smoothie Oreo Cookie	1 serv	566	19	2
Yogurt Smoothie Peach	1 serv	486	17	1
Yogurt Smoothie Peach Banana	1 serv	519	17	2
Yogurt Smoothie Peanut Butter	1 serv	630	17	2
Yogurt Smoothie Pina Colada	1 serv	519	5	1
Yogurt Smoothie Strawberry Banana	1 serv	514	17	2
Yogurt Smoothie Strawberry Fruit	1 serv	487	17	2
Yogurt Smoothie Strawberry Vanilla	1 serv	462	17	0
Yogurt Smoothie Strawberry Watermelon	1 serv	503	17	2
SALADS AND SALAD BARS				
Fruit Salad	1 lg	148	0	3
Fruit Salad	1 sm	99	0	2
Garden Salad	1 sm	56	0	2
Garden Salad w/ Italian Fat Free Dressing	1 lg	72	8	3
Pasta Salad	1 lg	256	0	0
Pasta Salad	1 sm	179	0	0
SANDWICHES				
Chicken On Croissant	1	481	109	4
Chicken On Honey Wheat	1	297	34	6
Chicken On Jewish Rye	1	261	34	5
Chicken On Pita	1	281	34	4
Chicken On White	1	291	35	4
Ham & Cheese On Croissant	1	797	192	3
Ham & Cheese On Honey Wheat	1	613	117	5

FOOD	PORTION	CALS	CHOL	FIBER
Ham & Cheese On Jewish Rye	1	577	117	4
Ham & Cheese On Pita	1	597	117	3
Ham & Cheese On White	1	607	118	3
Roast Beef On Croissant	1	631	155	3
Roast Beef On Honey Wheat	1	348	72	5
Roast Beef On Jewish Rye	1	312	72	4
Roast Beef On Pita	1	332	72	3
Roast Beef On White	1	342	72	3
Tuna On Croissant	1	480	90	4
Tuna On Honey Wheat	1	295	16	7
Tuna On Jewish Rye	1	259	16	5
Tuna On Pita	1	280	16	4
Tuna On White	1	289	16	4
Turkey On Croissant	1	566	122	3
Turkey On Honey Wheat	1	342	56	5
Turkey On Jewish Rye	1	306	56	4
Turkey On Pita	1	326	56	3
Turkey On White	1	338	57	3
Veggie On Croissant	1	510	83	4
Veggie On Honey Wheat	1	227	0	6
Veggie On Jewish Rye	1	191	0	5
Veggie On Pita	1	211	0	4
Veggie On White	1	221	0	4

GODFATHER'S PIZZA

FOOD	PORTION	CALS	CHOL	FIBER
Golden Crust Cheese	1/10 lg (3.5 oz)	242	14	—
Golden Crust Cheese	1/8 med (3.1 oz)	212	12	—
Golden Crust Combo	1/8 med (4.4 oz)	271	22	—
Golden Crust Combo	1/10 lg (4.9 oz)	305	25	—
Original Crust Cheese	1/10 jumbo (5.8 oz)	382	27	—
Original Crust Cheese	1/4 mini (1.9 oz)	131	8	—
Original Crust Cheese	1/8 med (3.5 oz)	231	14	—

FOOD	PORTION	CALS	CHOL	FIBER
Original Crust Cheese	⅒ lg (4 oz)	258	18	—
Original Crust Combo	¼ mini (2.9 oz)	176	16	—
Original Crust Combo	⅒ lg (5.6 oz)	338	31	—
Original Crust Combo	⅛ med (5.1 oz)	306	27	—
Original Crust Combo	⅒ jumbo (8.3 oz)	503	47	—

GODIVA

FOOD	PORTION	CALS	CHOL	FIBER
Chocolatier Dark Chocolate w/ Raspberry	1 bar (1.5 oz)	220	3	0
Chocolatier Milk Chocolate	1 bar (1.5 oz)	230	10	0
Mochaccino Mousse	2 pieces (1.25 oz)	210	4	0
Nut Croquant	3 pieces	140	<5	2
Truffle Assorted	2 pieces (1.5 oz)	220	10	0

HAAGEN-DAZS
FROZEN YOGURT

FOOD	PORTION	CALS	CHOL	FIBER
Pinapple Coconut	½ cup	230	90	0
Soft Serve Nonfat Chocolate	½ cup	110	0	0
Soft Serve Nonfat Chocolate Mousse	½ cup	80	0	1
Soft Serve Nonfat Coffee	½ cup	110	<5	0
Soft Serve Nonfat Strawberry	½ cup	110	0	0
Soft Serve Nonfat Vanilla	½ cup	110	<5	0
Soft Serve Nonfat Vanilla Mousse	½ cup	70	<5	0
Soft Serve Nonfat White Chocolate	½ cup	110	<5	0
Vanilla Fudge	½ cup	160	<5	0
Vanilla Raspberry Swirl	½ cup	130	<5	tr

ICE CREAM

FOOD	PORTION	CALS	CHOL	FIBER
Bailey's Irish Cream	½ cup	270	115	0
Bar Chocolate	1 (2.7 oz)	200	85	tr

FOOD	PORTION	CALS	CHOL	FIBER
Bar Chocolate & Dark Chocolate	1 (3.6 oz)	350	85	2
Bar Coffee	1 (2.7 oz)	190	85	0
Bar Coffee & Almond Crunch	1 (3.7 oz)	370	90	tr
Bar Vanilla	1 (2.7 oz)	190	85	0
Bar Vanilla & Almonds	1 (3.7 oz)	380	90	1
Bar Vanilla & Milk Chocolate	1 (3.5 oz)	340	90	tr
Belgian Chocolate Chocolate	½ cup	330	85	2
Brownies A La Mode	½ cup	280	90	tr
Butter Pecan	½ cup	300	105	tr
Cappuccino Commotion	½ cup	310	100	1
Chocolate	½ cup	269	110	1
Chocolate Chocolate Chip	½ cup	300	100	2
Chocolate Chocolate Mint	½ cup	300	95	1
Chocolate Swiss Almond	½ cup	300	100	2
Coffee	½ cup	250	115	0
Coffee Mocha Chip	½ cup	270	105	tr
Cookie Dough Dynamo	½ cup	310	95	0
Cookies & Cream	½ cup	270	105	0
Cookies & Fudge	½ cup	180	15	tr
Deep Chocolate Peanut Butter	½ cup	350	80	4
Dulce De Leche Caramel	½ cup	270	95	0
Lowfat Coffee Fudge	½ cup	170	25	0
Macadamia Brittle	½ cup	280	105	0
Macadamia Nut	½ cup	320	110	0
Mint Chip	½ cup	280	105	tr
Pistachio	½ cup	280	110	tr
Pralines & Cream	½ cup	280	95	0
Rum Raisin	½ cup	260	105	0
Strawberry	½ cup	250	90	tr

FOOD	PORTION	CALS	CHOL	FIBER
Vanilla	½ cup	250	115	0
Vanilla Chocolate Chip	½ cup	290	100	tr
Vanilla Swiss Almond	½ cup	290	100	tr
SORBET				
Bar Raspberry & Vanilla	1 (2.5 oz)	90	0	tr
Mango	½ cup	120	0	tr
Orange	½ cup	120	0	tr
Raspberry	½ cup	120	0	2
Soft Serve Raspberry	½ cup	110	0	2
Strawberry	½ cup	120	0	1
Zesty Lemon	½ cup	120	0	tr
HARDEE'S				
BEVERAGES				
Orange Juice	1 serv (11 oz)	140	0	—
Shake Chocolate	1 (12.2 oz)	370	30	—
Shake Peach	1 (12.1 oz)	390	25	—
Shake Strawberry	1 (12.7 oz)	420	20	—
Shake Vanilla	1 (12.2 oz)	350	20	—
BREAKFAST SELECTIONS				
Apple Cinnamon 'N' Raisin Biscuit	1 (2.18 oz)	200	0	—
Bacon & Egg Biscuit	1 (5.5 oz)	570	275	—
Bacon Egg & Cheese Biscuit	1 (5.9 oz)	610	280	—
Big Country Breakfast Bacon	1 serv (9.4 oz)	820	535	—
Big Country Breakfast Sausage	1 serv (11.4 oz)	1000	570	—
Biscuit 'N' Gravy	1 (7.8 oz)	510	15	—
Country Ham Biscuit	1 (3.8 oz)	430	25	—
Frisco Breakfast Sandwich Ham	1 (7.4 oz)	500	290	—
Ham Biscuit	1 (4 oz)	400	15	—
Ham Egg & Cheese Biscuit	1 (6.5 oz)	540	285	—
Hash Rounds	1 serv (2.8 oz)	230	0	—
Jelly Biscuit	1 (3.5 oz)	440	0	—
Rise 'N' Shine Biscuit	1 (2.9 oz)	390	0	—

FOOD	PORTION	CALS	CHOL	FIBER
Sausage Biscuit	1 (4.1 oz)	510	25	—
Sausage & Egg Biscuit	1 (6.3 oz)	630	285	—
Three Pancakes	1 serv (4.8 oz)	280	15	—
Ultimate Omelet Biscuit	1 (5.8 oz)	570	120	—
DESSERTS				
Big Cookie	1 (2.0 oz)	280	15	—
Cone Chocolate	1 (4.1 oz)	180	15	—
Cone Vanilla	1 (4.1 oz)	170	10	—
Cool Twist Cone Vanilla/Chocolate	1 (4.1 oz)	180	10	—
Peach Cobbler	1 serv (6 oz)	310	0	—
Sundae Hot Fudge	1 (5.5 oz)	290	20	—
Sundae Strawberry	1 (5.8 oz)	210	10	—
MAIN MENU SELECTIONS				
Baked Beans	1 serv (5 oz)	170	0	—
Big Roast Beef Sandwich	1 (6.5 oz)	460	70	—
Cheeseburger	1 (4.3 oz)	310	40	—
Chicken Fillet Sandwich	1 (7.5 oz)	480	55	—
Cole Slaw	1 serv (4 oz)	240	10	—
Cravin' Bacon Cheeseburger	1 (8.1 oz)	690	95	—
Fisherman's Fillet	1 (8.3 oz)	560	65	—
French Fries	1 lg (6 oz)	430	0	—
French Fries	1 sm (3.4 oz)	240	0	—
French Fries	1 med (5 oz)	350	0	—
Fried Chicken Breast	1 piece (5.2 oz)	370	75	—
Fried Chicken Leg	1 piece (2.4 oz)	170	45	—
Fried Chicken Thigh	1 piece (4.2 oz)	330	60	—
Fried Chicken Wing	1 piece (2.3 oz)	200	30	—
Frisco Burger	1 (8.1 oz)	720	95	—
Gravy	1 serv (1.5 oz)	20	0	—
Grilled Chicken Sandwich	1 (7.1 oz)	350	65	—
Hamburger	1 (3.9 oz)	270	35	—
Hot Ham 'N' Cheese	1 (5.1 oz)	310	50	—
Mashed Potatoes	1 serv (4 oz)	70	0	—

FOOD	PORTION	CALS	CHOL	FIBER
Mesquite Bacon Cheeseburger	1 (4.5 oz)	370	45	—
Mushroom 'N' Swiss Burger	1 (6.8 oz)	490	80	—
Quarter Pound Double Cheeseburger	1 (6 oz)	470	80	—
Regular Roast Beef	1 (4.3 oz)	320	43	—
The Boss	1 (7 oz)	570	85	—
The Works Burger	1 (8.1 oz)	530	80	—
SALAD DRESSINGS				
French Fat Free	1 serv (2 oz)	70	0	0
Ranch	1 serv (2 oz)	290	25	—
Thousand Island	1 serv (2 oz)	250	35	—
SALADS AND SALAD BARS				
Garden Salad	1 (10.2 oz)	220	40	—
Grilled Chicken Salad	1 (11.5 oz)	150	60	—
Side Salad	1 (4.6 oz)	25	0	—

HOT SAM'S PRETZELS

FOOD	PORTION	CALS	CHOL	FIBER
Bavarian	1 lg (5.1 oz)	390	0	4
Bavarian	1 reg (2.5 oz)	200	0	2
Bavarian Stix	10 (5 oz)	390	0	4
Sweet Dough	1 (4.5 oz)	360	0	4
Sweet Dough Blueberry	1 (4.5 oz)	400	0	2

HUNGRY HOWIE'S
MAIN MENU SELECTIONS

FOOD	PORTION	CALS	CHOL	FIBER
Howie Wings	6 (3 oz)	180	70	0
Three Cheeser Bread	1 serv	370	17	1
PIZZA				
Large Cheese	1 slice	175	11	1
Large Cheese + Bacon	1 slice	208	13	1
Large Cheese + Beef	1 slice	197	16	1
Large Cheese + Black Olives	1 slice	181	12	1
Large Cheese + Green Olives	1 slice	181	12	1
Large Cheese + Green Peppers	1 slice	175	11	1
Large Cheese + Ham	1 slice	179	14	1

FOOD	PORTION	CALS	CHOL	FIBER
Large Cheese + Mushrooms	1 slice	175	11	1
Large Cheese + Onions	1 slice	175	12	1
Large Cheese + Pepperoni	1 slice	191	16	1
Large Cheese + Pineapple	1 slice	388	12	1
Large Cheese + Sausage	1 slice	195	14	1
Medium Cheese	1 slice	153	9	1
Medium Cheese + Bacon	1 slice	179	10	1
Medium Cheese + Beef	1 slice	177	14	1
Medium Cheese + Black Olives	1 slice	159	11	1
Medium Cheese + Green Olives	1 slice	159	11	1
Medium Cheese + Green Peppers	1 slice	155	10	1
Medium Cheese + Ham	1 slice	159	12	1
Medium Cheese + Mushrooms	1 slice	155	9	1
Medium Cheese + Onions	1 slice	155	10	1
Medium Cheese + Pepperoni	1 slice	171	14	1
Medium Cheese + Pineapple	1 slice	158	10	1
Medium Cheese + Sausage	1 slice	175	12	1
Small Cheese	1 slice	121	8	1
Small Cheese + Bacon	1 slice	138	9	1
Small Cheese + Beef	1 slice	137	12	1
Small Cheese + Black Olives	1 slice	125	9	1
Small Cheese + Green Olives	1 slice	125	9	1
Small Cheese + Green Peppers	1 slice	122	8	1

FOOD	PORTION	CALS	CHOL	FIBER
Small Cheese + Ham	1 slice	126	11	1
Small Cheese + Mushrooms	1 slice	123	8	1
Small Cheese + Onions	1 slice	122	8	1
Small Cheese + Pepperoni	1 slice	136	12	1
Small Cheese + Pineapple	1 slice	124	8	1
Small Cheese + Sausage	1 slice	136	11	1
SALADS AND SALAD BARS				
Antipasto Salad w/o Dressing	1 lg	101	24	1
Chef Salad w/o Dressing	1 lg	99	24	2
Garden Salad w/o Dressing	1 lg	17	0	2
Greek Salad w/o Dressing	1 lg	109	25	2
SANDWICHES				
Sub Deluxe Italian	½ sub	506	44	2
Sub Ham & Cheese	½ sub	475	44	2
Sub Pizza	½ sub	689	86	3
Sub Pizza Special	½ sub	606	65	3
Sub Steak Cheese Mushroom	½ sub	491	47	2
Sub Turkey	½ sub	466	38	2
Sub Turkey Club	½ sub	556	44	2
Sub Vegetarian	½ sub	530	39	3
IHOP				
Pancake Buckwheat	1 (2.5 oz)	134	61	1
Pancake Buttermilk	1 (2 oz)	108	31	tr
Pancake Country Griddle	1 (2.25 oz)	134	38	1
Pancake Egg	1 (2 oz)	102	66	tr
Pancake Harvest Grain 'N Nut	1 (2.25 oz)	160	38	1
Waffle	1 (4 oz)	305	70	1

FOOD	PORTION	CALS	CHOL	FIBER
Waffle Belgian	1 (6 oz)	408	146	1
Waffle Belgian Harvest Grain 'N Nut	1 (6 oz)	445	147	3

JACK IN THE BOX
BEVERAGES
2% Milk	1 serv (8 fl oz)	130	20	0
Barq's Root Beer	1 reg (20 fl oz)	180	0	0
Classic Ice Cream Shake Chocolate	1 reg (11 fl oz)	630	85	tr
Classic Ice Cream Shake Oreo Cookie	1 reg (12 oz)	740	95	tr
Classic Ice Cream Shake Strawberry	1 reg (10 fl oz)	640	85	0
Classic Ice Cream Shake Vanilla	1 reg (11 oz)	610	95	0
Classice Ice Cream Shake Cappuccino	1 reg (11 oz)	630	90	0
Coca-Cola Classic	1 reg (20 fl oz)	170	0	0
Coffee	1 reg (12 fl oz)	5	0	0
Diet Coke	1 reg (20 fl oz)	0	0	0
Dr Pepper	1 reg (20 fl oz)	190	0	0
Iced Tea	1 reg (20 fl oz)	0	0	0
Minute Maid Lemonade	1 reg (20 fl oz)	190	0	0
Orange Juice	1 serv (10 oz)	150	0	1
Sprite	1 reg (20 fl oz)	160	0	0
BREAKFAST SELECTIONS
Breakfast Jack	1 (4.2 oz)	300	185	0
Country Crock Spread	1 pat (5 g)	25	0	0
Grape Jelly	1 serv (0.5 oz)	40	0	0
Pancake Syrup	1 serv (1.5 oz)	120	0	0
Pancakes w/ Bacon	1 serv (5.6 oz)	400	30	3
Sausage Croissant	1 (6.4 oz)	670	250	2
Sourdough Breakfast Sandwich	1 (5.2 oz)	380	355	0
Supreme Croissant	1 (6 oz)	570	235	2
Ultimate Breakfast Sandwich	1 (8.5 oz)	620	245	tr

FOOD	PORTION	CALS	CHOL	FIBER
DESSERTS				
Carrot Cake	1 serv (3.5 oz)	370	35	2
Cheesecake	1 serv (3.5 oz)	310	65	2
Double Fudge Cake	1 serv (3 oz)	300	50	1
Hot Apple Turnover	1 (3.8 oz)	340	0	2
MAIN MENU SELECTIONS				
¼ lb Burger	1 (6 oz)	510	65	0
American Cheese	1 slice (0.4 oz)	45	10	0
Bacon & Cheddar Potato Wedges	1 serv (9.3 oz)	800	55	4
Bacon Ultimate Cheeseburger	1 (10.4 oz)	1150	230	0
Barbeque Dipping Sauce	1 serv (1 fl oz)	45	0	0
Cheeseburger	1 (4 oz)	330	60	2
Chicken & Fries	1 serv (9.3 oz)	730	65	5
Chicken Caesar Sandwich	1 (8.3 oz)	520	55	4
Chicken Fajita Pita	1 (6.6 oz)	280	75	3
Chicken Sandwich	1 (5.9 oz)	450	45	2
Chicken Strips Breaded	5 pieces (5.3 oz)	360	80	1
Chicken Supreme Sandwich	1 (8.2 oz)	680	85	4
Chili Cheese Curly Fries	1 serv (8.1 oz)	650	25	13
Double Cheeseburger	1 (5.3 oz)	450	75	0
Egg Rolls	3 pieces (6 oz)	440	35	4
Egg Rolls	5 pieces (10 oz)	730	60	7
Fish & Chips	1 serv (9 oz)	720	35	6
French Fries	1 reg (4.1 oz)	360	0	3
Grilled Chicken Fillet Sandwich	1 (8.1 oz)	520	140	4
Hamburger	1 (3.6 oz)	280	45	2
Jumbo Fries	1 serv (5 oz)	430	0	4
Jumbo Jack	1 (7.8 oz)	560	80	4
Jumbo Jack w/ Cheese	1 (8.6 oz)	650	105	4
Ketchup	1 pkg (0.3 oz)	10	0	0
Monster Taco	1 (4 oz)	290	40	3
Onion Rings	1 serv (4.2 oz)	460	0	3
Pilly Cheesesteak Sandwich	1 (7.6 oz)	520	155	4

FOOD	PORTION	CALS	CHOL	FIBER
Salsa	1 serv (1 oz)	10	0	0
Seasoned Curly Fries	1 serv (4.5 oz)	420	0	4
Sour Cream	1 serv (1 oz)	60	20	0
Sourdough Jack	1 (7.8 oz)	670	110	0
Soy Sauce	1 serv (0.3 oz)	5	0	0
Spicy Crispy Chicken Sandwich	1 (7.9 oz)	560	50	0
Stuffed Jalapenos	10 pieces (7.6 oz)	680	75	5
Stuffed Jalapenos	7 pieces (5.3 oz)	470	50	3
Super Scoop French Fries	1 serv (7 oz)	610	0	5
Sweet & Sour Dipping Sauce	1 serv (1 oz)	40	0	0
Swiss-Style Cheese	1 slice (0.4 oz)	40	10	0
Taco	1 (2.7 oz)	190	20	2
Tartar Dipping Sauce	1 pkg (1.5 oz)	220	20	0
Teriyaki Bowl Chicken	1 serv (17.6 oz)	670	15	5
Ultimate Cheeseburger	1 (9.8 oz)	1030	205	0
SALAD DRESSINGS				
Blue Cheese	1 serv (2 fl oz)	210	15	0
Buttermilk House	1 serv (2 fl oz)	290	20	0
Buttermilk House Dipping Sauce	1 serv (0.9 oz)	130	10	tr
Low Calorie Italian	1 serv (2 fl oz)	25	0	0
Thousand Island	1 serv (2 fl oz)	250	20	0
SALADS AND SALAD BARS				
Croutons	1 serv (0.4 oz)	50	0	0
Garden Chicken Salad	1 serv (8.9 oz)	200	65	3
Side Salad	1 (3 oz)	50	10	1

KENNY ROGERS ROASTERS
MAIN MENU SELECTIONS

FOOD	PORTION	CALS	CHOL	FIBER
½ Chicken w/ Skin	1 serv (9.06 oz)	515	301	–
½ Chicken w/o Skin & Wing	1 serv (7.03 oz)	313	221	–
¼ Chicken Dark Meat w/ Skin	1 serv (4.35 oz)	271	165	–
¼ Chicken Dark Meat w/o Skin & Wing	1 serv (3.29 oz)	169	130	–

FOOD	PORTION	CALS	CHOL	FIBER
¼ Chicken White Meat w/ Skin	1 serv (4.71 oz)	244	136	—
¼ Chicken White Meat w/o Skin & Wing	1 serv (3.74 oz)	144	92	—
Baked Sweet Potato	1 (9 oz)	263	0	1
Chicken Caesar Salad	1 serv (9.4 oz)	285	122	1
Cinnamon Apples	1 serv (5.27 oz)	199	13	3
Cole Slaw	1 serv (5.05 oz)	225	13	2
Corn Muffin	1 (2 oz)	175	0	1
Corn On The Cob	1 (2.25 oz)	68	0	2
Corn Stuffing	1 serv (7.1 oz)	326	5	tr
Creamy Parmesan Spinach	1 serv (5.3 oz)	119	12	tr
Garlic Parsley Potatoes	1 serv (6.5 oz)	259	16	3
Honey Baked Beans	1 serv (5 oz)	148	0	tr
Italian Green Beans	1 serv (6.1 oz)	116	0	tr
Macaroni & Cheese	1 serv (5.51 oz)	197	26	1
Pasta Salad	1 serv (5 oz)	236	40	1
Pita BBQ Chicken	1 (7.33 oz)	401	112	—
Pita Chicken Caesar	1 (9.2 oz)	606	122	1
Pita Roasted Chicken	1 (10.8 oz)	685	159	tr
Pot Pie Chicken	1 (12 oz)	708	69	tr
Potato Salad	1 serv (7.01 oz)	390	0	2
Real Mashed Potatoes	1 serv (8 oz)	295	2	1
Rice Pilaf	1 serv (5 oz)	173	0	0
Roasted Chicken Salad	1 serv (16.9 oz)	292	218	6
Sandwich Turkey	1 (9.2 oz)	385	88	1
Side Salad	1 serv (4.73 oz)	23	0	2
Sour Cream & Dill Pasta Salad	1 serv (5 oz)	233	16	1
Steamed Vegetables	1 serv (4.25 oz)	48	0	4
Sweet Corn Niblets	1 serv (5 oz)	112	0	1
Tomato Cucumber Salad	1 serv (6 oz)	123	0	1
Turkey Sliced Breast	1 serv (4.5 oz)	158	78	—
Zucchini & Squash Santa Fe	1 serv (5 oz)	70	0	1

FOOD	PORTION	CALS	CHOL	FIBER
SALAD DRESSINGS				
Blue Cheese	1 serv (2.47 oz)	370	65	0
Buttermilk Ranch	1 serv (2.47 oz)	430	10	0
Caesar	1 serv (2.47 oz)	340	15	0
Honey French	1 serv (2.47 oz)	350	0	0
Honey Mustard	1 serv (2.47 oz)	320	40	1
Italian Fat Free	1 serv (2.47 oz)	35	0	0
Thousand Island	1 serv (2.47 oz)	330	40	0
SOUPS				
Chicken Noodle	1 cup (6 oz)	55	13	1
Chicken Noodle	1 bowl (10 oz)	91	22	tr
KFC				
BBQ Baked Beans	1 serv (5.5 oz)	190	5	6
Biscuit	1 (2 oz)	180	0	tr
Chicken Pot Pie	1 (13 oz)	770	70	5
Chicken Twister	1 (8.7 oz)	550	85	1
Cole Slaw	1 serv (5 oz)	180	5	3
Corn On The Cob	1 ear (5.7 oz)	150	0	2
Cornbread	1 (2 oz)	228	42	1
Crispy Strips Colonel's	3 (3.25 oz)	261	40	3
Crispy Strips Spicy Buffalo	3 (4.2 oz)	350	35	2
Extra Tasty Crispy Breast	1 (5.9 oz)	470	80	1
Extra Tasty Crispy Drumstick	1 (2.4 oz)	190	60	tr
Extra Tasty Crispy Thigh	1 (4.2 oz)	370	70	2
Extra Tasty Crispy Whole Wing	1 (1.9 oz)	200	45	tr
Green Beans	1 serv (4.7 oz)	45	5	3
Hot & Spicy Breast	1 (6.5 oz)	530	110	2
Hot & Spicy Drumstick	1 (2.3 oz)	190	50	tr
Hot & Spicy Thigh	1 (3.8 oz)	370	90	1
Hot & Spicy Whole Wing	1 (1.9 oz)	210	50	tr
Hot Wings	6 (4.8 oz)	471	150	2
Macaroni & Cheese	1 serv (5.4 oz)	180	10	2
Mashed Potatoes With Gravy	1 serv (4.8 oz)	120	tr	2

FOOD	PORTION	CALS	CHOL	FIBER
Mean Greens	1 serv (5.4 oz)	70	10	5
Original Recipe Breast	1 (5.4 oz)	400	135	1
Original Recipe Chicken Sandwich	1 (7.3 oz)	497	52	3
Original Recipe Drumstick	1 (2.2 oz)	140	75	0
Original Recipe Thigh	1 (3.2 oz)	250	95	1
Original Recipe Whole Wing	1 (1.6 oz)	140	55	0
Potato Salad	1 serv (5.6 oz)	230	15	3
Potato Wedges	1 serv (4.8 oz)	280	5	5
Tender Roast Breast w/ Skin	1 (4.9 oz)	251	151	0
Tender Roast Breast w/o Skin	1 (4.2 oz)	169	112	0
Tender Roast Drumstick w/ Skin	1 (1.9 oz)	97	85	0
Tender Roast Drumstick w/o Skin	1 (1.2 oz)	67	63	0
Tender Roast Thigh w/ Skin	1 (3.2 oz)	207	120	0
Tender Roast Thigh w/o Skin	1 (2.1 oz)	106	84	0
Tender Roast Wing w/ Skin	1 (1.8 oz)	121	74	0
Value BBQ Chicken Sandwich	1 (5.3 oz)	256	57	2

KRISPY KREME

FOOD	PORTION	CALS	CHOL	FIBER
Chocolate Iced	1 (2 oz)	260	<5	1
Chocolate Iced Cake	1 (2 oz)	230	15	tr
Chocolate Iced Creme Filled	1 (2.3 oz)	270	<5	2
Chocolate Iced Cruller	1 (1.7 oz)	240	10	tr
Chocolate Iced Custard Filled	1 (2.7 oz)	250	5	3
Chocolated Iced w/ Sprinkles	1 (2 oz)	220	<5	tr
Cinnamon Apple Filled	1 (2.3 oz)	210	<5	3

FOOD	PORTION	CALS	CHOL	FIBER
Cinnamon Bun	1 (2.1 oz)	220	0	4
Glazed Blueberry	1 (2.4 oz)	300	5	1
Glazed Creme Filled	1 (2.3 oz)	270	<5	2
Glazed Cruller	1 (1.5 oz)	220	10	0
Glazed Devil's Food	1 (1.9 oz)	240	10	3
Lemon Filled	1 (2.2 oz)	210	5	tr
Maple Iced	1 (1.8 oz)	200	0	2
Original Glazed	1 (1.3 oz)	180	<5	tr
Powdered Blueberry Filled	1 (2.1 oz)	200	5	2
Powdered Cake	1 (1.8 oz)	220	15	0
Raspberry Filled	1 (2 oz)	210	<5	3
Traditional Cake	1 (1.7 oz)	200	15	tr

KRYSTAL
BEVERAGES

Chocolate Shake	1 (16 fl oz)	275	32	—

BREAKFAST SELECTIONS

Biscuit	1 (2.5 oz)	244	2	—
Biscuit Bacon	1 (2.9 oz)	306	14	—
Biscuit Bacon, Egg & Cheese	1 (4.7 oz)	421	153	—
Biscuit Country Ham	1 (3.7 oz)	334	23	—
Biscuit Egg	1 (4 oz)	327	134	—
Biscuit Gravy	1 (7.5 oz)	419	23	—
Biscuit Sausage	1 (4.1 oz)	437	49	—
Sunriser	1 (3.8 oz)	259	162	—

DESSERTS

Apple Pie	1 serv (4.5 oz)	300	0	—
Donut Plain	1 (1.3 oz)	150	5	—
Donut w/ Chocolate Icing	1 (1.8 oz)	212	5	—
Donut w/ Vanilla Icing	1 (1.8 oz)	198	5	—
Lemon Meringue Pie	1 serv (4 oz)	340	50	—
Pecan Pie	1 serv (4 oz)	450	55	—

MAIN MENU SELECTIONS

Big K	1 (8 oz)	540	93	—
Burger Plus	1 (6.5 oz)	415	63	—
Burger Plus w/ Cheese	1 (7.1 oz)	473	77	—
Cheese Krystal	1 (2.5 oz)	187	29	—

FOOD	PORTION	CALS	CHOL	FIBER
Chili	1 reg (8 oz)	218	19	—
Chili	1 lg (12 oz)	327	28	—
Chili Cheese Pup	1 (2.7 oz)	211	31	—
Chili Pup	1 (2.5 oz)	182	24	—
Corn Pup	1 (2.3 oz)	214	24	—
Crispy Crunchy Chicken Sandwich	1 (5.75 oz)	467	56	—
Double Cheese Krystal	1 (4.5 oz)	337	57	—
Double Krystal	1 (4 oz)	277	43	—
Fries	1 lg (5.3 oz)	463	16	—
Fries	1 sm (3 oz)	262	9	—
Fries	1 reg (4.1 oz)	358	12	—
Krys Kross Fries	1 serv (4.3 oz)	486	31	—
Krys Kross Fries Chili Cheese	1 serv (6.8 oz)	625	61	—
Krys Kross Fries w/ Cheese	1 serv (5.3 oz)	515	31	—
Krystal	1 (2.2 oz)	158	22	—
Plain Pup	1 (1.9 oz)	160	20	—

LITTLE CAESARS
MAIN MENU SELECTIONS

FOOD	PORTION	CALS	CHOL	FIBER
Crazy Bread	1 piece (1.4 oz)	106	0	1
Crazy Sauce	1 serv (6 oz)	170	0	5
Deli-Style Sandwich Ham & Cheese	1 (11.6 oz)	728	54	3
Deli-Style Sandwich Italian	1 (11.9 oz)	740	62	3
Deli-Style Sandwich Veggie	1 (11.9 oz)	647	29	4
Hot Oven-Baked Sandwich Cheeser	1 (12.1 oz)	822	580	5
Hot Oven-Baked Sandwich Meatsa	1 (15 oz)	1036	130	5
Hot Oven-Baked Sandwich Pepperoni	1 (11.2 oz)	899	58	4
Hot Oven-Baked Sandwich Supreme	1 (13.1 oz)	894	700	5

FOOD	PORTION	CALS	CHOL	FIBER
Hot Oven-Baked Sandwich Veggie	1 (13.7 oz)	669	58	6
PIZZA				
Baby Pan!Pan!	1 serv (8.4 oz)	616	47	4
Pan!Pan! Cheese	1 med slice (2.9 oz)	181	15	1
Pan!Pan! Pepperoni	1 med slice (3 oz)	199	15	1
Pizza!Pizza! Cheese	1 med slice (3.2 oz)	201	17	1
Pizza!Pizza! Pepperoni	1 med slice (3.3 oz)	220	17	1
SALAD DRESSINGS				
1000 Island	1 serv (1.5 oz)	183	30	—
Blue Cheese	1 serv (1.5 oz)	160	17	—
Caesar	1 serv (1.5 oz)	255	13	—
French	1 serv (1.5 oz)	166	0	—
Greek	1 serv (1.5 oz)	268	9	—
Italian	1 serv (1.5 oz)	200	12	—
Italian Fat Free	1 serv (1.5 oz)	15	0	—
Ranch	1 serv (1.5 oz)	221	18	—
SALADS AND SALAD BARS				
Antipasto Salad	1 serv (8.4 oz)	176	19	2
Caesar Salad	1 serv (5 oz)	140	11	2
Greek Salad	1 serv (10.3 oz)	168	37	3
Tossed Salad	1 serv (8.5 oz)	116	0	3

LONG JOHN SILVER'S
MAIN MENU SELECTIONS

FOOD	PORTION	CALS	CHOL	FIBER
Breaded Chicken Strips	1 piece (1.15 oz)	100	10	0
Breaded Clams	1 serv (3 oz)	300	40	5
Breaded Fish	1 piece (1.6 oz)	110	20	0
Cheese Sticks	1 serv (1.6 oz)	160	10	tr
Chicken Salsa	1 reg (11 oz)	690	20	5
Corn Cobbette w/ Butter	1 piece (3.3 oz)	140	0	0
Corn Cobbette w/o Butter	1 (3.1 oz)	80	0	0
Fish Cajun	1 lg (23 oz)	1450	60	10
Flavorbaked Chicken	1 piece (2.6 oz)	110	55	tr
Flavorbaked Fish	1 piece (2.3 oz)	90	35	0
Fries	1 reg (3 oz)	250	0	3
Fries	1 lg (5 oz)	420	0	4
Honey Mustard Sauce	1 serv (0.4 oz)	20	0	0

FOOD	PORTION	CALS	CHOL	FIBER
Hushpuppy	1 (0.8 oz)	60	0	0
Ketchup	1 serv (.32 oz)	10	0	0
Popcorn Chicken Munchers	1 serv (4 oz)	380	35	2
Popcorn Fish Munchers	1 serv (4 oz)	300	50	tr
Popcorn Shrimp Munchers	1 serv (4 oz)	320	85	1
Rice	1 serv (3 oz)	140	0	tr
Sandwich Batter Dipped Fish No Sauce	1 (5.4 oz)	320	30	6
Sandwich Flavorbaked Chicken	1 (5.8 oz)	290	60	2
Sandwich Flavorbaked Fish	1 (6 oz)	320	55	2
Sandwich Ultimate Fish	1 (6.4 oz)	430	35	3
Shrimp Sauce	1 serv (0.4 oz)	15	0	0
Side Salad	1 (4.3 oz)	25	0	tr
Slaw	1 serv (3.4 oz)	140	0	3
Sweet'N'Sour Sauce	1 serv (0.4 oz)	20	0	0
Tartar Sauce	1 serv (0.4 oz)	35	0	0
Wraps Chicken Cajun	1 reg (11 oz)	720	25	5
Wraps Chicken Cajun	1 lg (22 oz)	1440	50	11
Wraps Chicken Ranch	1 reg (11 oz)	730	25	5
Wraps Chicken Ranch	1 lg (22 oz)	1450	50	10
Wraps Chicken Salsa	1 lg (22 oz)	1370	35	10
Wraps Chicken Tartar	1 lg (22 oz)	1450	45	11
Wraps Chicken Tartar	1 reg (11 oz)	730	25	6
Wraps Fish Cajun	1 reg (11.5 oz)	730	30	5
Wraps Fish Ranch	1 reg (11.5 oz)	730	30	5
Wraps Fish Ranch	1 lg (23 oz)	1460	60	10
Wraps Fish Salsa	1 reg (11.5 oz)	690	25	5
Wraps Fish Salsa	1 lg (23 oz)	1380	45	10
Wraps Fish Tartar	1 reg (11.5 oz)	730	25	5
Wraps Fish Tartar	1 lg (23 oz)	1470	55	10
Wraps Popcorn Shrimp Cajun	1 reg (11 oz)	720	50	5
Wraps Popcorn Shrimp Cajun	1 lg (22 oz)	1450	95	10

FOOD	PORTION	CALS	CHOL	FIBER
Wraps Popcorn Shrimp Ranch	1 lg (22 oz)	1460	100	10
Wraps Popcorn Shrimp Ranch	1 reg (11 oz)	720	50	5
Wraps Popcorn Shrimp Salsa	1 reg (11 oz)	690	40	5
Wraps Popcorn Shrimp Salsa	1 lg (22 oz)	1380	85	9
Wraps Popcorn Shrimp Tartar	1 reg (11 oz)	730	45	5
Wraps Popcorn Shrimp Tartar	1 lg (22 oz)	1460	95	10
SALAD DRESSINGS				
Fat-Free French	1 serv (1.5 oz)	50	0	–
Fat-Free Ranch	1 serv (1.5 oz)	50	0	–
Italian	1 serv (1 oz)	130	0	–
Malt Vinegar	1 serv (0.3 oz)	0	0	0
Ranch Dressing	1 serv (1 oz)	170	5	–
Thousand Island	1 serv (1 oz)	110	15	–

MACHEEZMO MOUSE
CHILDREN'S MENU SELECTIONS

FOOD	PORTION	CALS	CHOL	FIBER
Quesadilla Kid Cheese	1 serv (5 oz)	360	40	–
Quesadilla Kid Chicken	1 serv (7 oz)	430	100	–
MAIN MENU SELECTIONS				
Broccoli	1 oz	4	0	–
Burrito Vegetarian	1 (14 oz)	655	20	–
Dinner Rice, Beans, Broccoli	1 serv (10 oz)	328	0	–
Dinner Rice, Beans, Salad	1 serv (12 oz)	344	0	–
Green Sauce	1 oz	5	0	–
Snack Famouse #5	1 serv (14 oz)	585	20	–
Snack Tacos Chicken	1 serv (6 oz)	290	82	–
Snack Tacos Veggie	1 serv (6 oz)	290	22	–

MANHATTAN BAGEL

FOOD	PORTION	CALS	CHOL	FIBER
Blueberry	1	260	0	2
Cheddar Cheese	1	270	10	2
Chocolate Chip	1	290	0	2
Cinnamon Raisin	1	280	0	3

FOOD	PORTION	CALS	CHOL	FIBER
Egg	1	270	0	2
Everything	1	290	0	3
Jalapeno Cheddar	1	260	0	2
Marble	1	260	0	3
Oat Bran	1	260	0	3
Oat Bran Raisin Walnut	1	270	0	3
Onion	1	270	0	2
Plain	1	260	0	2
Poppy	1	300	0	5
Pumpernickel	1	250	0	3
Rye	1	260	0	3
Salt	1	260	0	2
Sesame	1	310	0	3
Spinach	1	270	0	3
Sun-Dried Tomato	1	260	0	3
Whole Wheat	1	260	0	3

MAX & ERMA'S

FOOD	PORTION	CALS	CHOL	FIBER
Black Bean Roll Up	1 serv	401	13	8
Black Bean Salsa	½ cup	215	0	5
Fruit Smoothie	1 serv	124	0	1
Garden Grill Sandwich w/ Tex Mex Dressing	1	569	19	14
Garlic Breadstick	1	156	0	0
Hula Bowl w/ Fat Free Honey Mustard Dressing w/o Breadsticks	1 serv	583	111	5
Salad Dressing Fat Free French	2 tbsp	126	0	2
Salad Dressing Fat Free Honey Mustard	2 tbsp	60	0	0
Salad Dressing Tex Mex	2 tbsp	33	5	tr
Sugar Snap Peas w/ Lemon Pepper Butter	1 serv (4 oz)	106	15	3

MCDONALD'S
BAKED SELECTIONS

FOOD	PORTION	CALS	CHOL	FIBER
Apple Pie Baked	1 (2.7 oz)	260	0	tr
Chocolate Chip Cookie	1 (1.2 oz)	170	20	1

FOOD	PORTION	CALS	CHOL	FIBER
Cinnamon Roll	1	390	65	—
Danish Apple	1	340	20	—
Danish Cheese	1	400	40	—
Lowfat Muffin Apple Bran	1 (4 oz)	300	0	3
McDonaldland Cookies	1 pkg (1.5 oz)	180	0	1
BEVERAGES				
Coca-Cola Classic	1 sm (16 oz)	150	0	—
Cocoa-Cola Classic	1 lg (32 oz)	310	0	—
Cocoa-Cola Classic	1 child serv (12 oz)	110	0	—
Cocoa-Cola Classic	1 med (21 oz)	210	0	—
Diet Coke	1 sm (16 oz)	1	0	—
Diet Coke	1 med (21 oz)	0	0	—
Diet Coke	1 child serv (12 oz)	0	0	—
Diet Coke	1 lg (32 oz)	0	0	—
Hi-C Orange	1 sm (16 oz)	160	0	—
Hi-C Orange	1 lg (32 oz)	350	0	—
Hi-C Orange	1 med (21 oz)	240	0	—
Hi-C Orange	1 child serv (12 oz)	120	0	—
Milk 1%	1 serv (8 oz)	100	10	0
Orange Juice	1 serv (6 oz)	80	0	0
Shake Chocolate	1 sm (14.5 oz)	360	40	1
Shake Strawberry	1 sm (14.5 oz)	360	40	0
Shake Vanilla	1 sm (14.5 oz)	360	40	0
Sprite	1 sm (16 fl oz)	150	0	—
Sprite	1 med (21 oz)	210	0	—
Sprite	1 child serv (12 oz)	110	0	—
Sprite	1 lg (32 oz)	310	0	—
BREAKFAST SELECTIONS				
Bacon Egg & Cheese Biscuit	1	540	250	—
Bagel Ham & Egg Cheese	1	550	255	—
Bagel Spanish Omelet	1	690	275	—
Bagel Steak & Egg Cheese	1	660	285	—
Biscuit	1 (2.9 oz)	290	0	1
Breakfast Burrito	1 (4.1 oz)	320	195	—
Egg McMuffin	1 (4.8 oz)	290	235	1

FOOD	PORTION	CALS	CHOL	FIBER
English Muffin	1 (1.9 oz)	140	0	1
Hash Browns	1 serv (1.9 oz)	130	0	1
Hotcakes Margarine & Syrup	1 serv	600	20	—
Hotcakes Plain	1 serv	340	20	—
Sausage	1 (1.5 oz)	170	35	0
Sausage Biscuit	1 (4.5 oz)	470	35	1
Sausage Biscuit w/ Egg	1 (6.2 oz)	550	245	1
Sausage McMuffin	1 (3.9 oz)	360	45	1
Sausage McMuffin w/ Egg	1 (5.7 oz)	440	255	1
Scrambled Eggs	2 (3.6 oz)	160	425	0
DESSERTS				
McFlurry Butterfinger	1	620	70	—
McFlurry M&M	1	630	75	—
McFlurry Nestle Crunch	1	630	75	—
McFlurry Oreo	1	570	70	—
Nuts For Sundaes	1 serv (7 g)	40	0	0
Reduced Fat Ice Cream Cone Vanilla	1 (3.2 oz)	150	20	0
Sundae Hot Caramel	1 (6.4 oz)	360	35	0
Sundae Hot Fudge	1 (6.3 oz)	340	30	1
Sundae Strawberry	1 (6.2 oz)	290	30	tr
MAIN MENU SELECTIONS				
Barbeque Sauce	1 pkg (1 oz)	45	0	0
Big Mac	1	570	85	3
Big Xtra!	1	710	95	—
Big Xtra! w/ Cheese	1	810	120	—
Cheeseburger	1 (4.2 oz)	320	40	2
Chicken McNuggets	6 pieces (3.7 oz)	290	55	—
Chicken McNuggets	4 pieces (2.5 oz)	190	35	—
Chicken McNuggets	9 pieces	430	80	—
Crispy Chicken Deluxe	1 (7.8 oz)	500	55	3
Filet-O-Fish	1	470	50	—
French Fries	1 sm (2.4 oz)	210	0	2
French Fries	1 lg	540	0	—
French Fries	1 med	450	0	—
French Fries	1 super	610	0	—

FOOD	PORTION	CALS	CHOL	FIBER
Grilled Chicken Deluxe	1 (7.8 oz)	440	60	3
Grilled Chicken Deluxe Plain w/o Mayonnaise	1 (7.2 oz)	300	50	3
Grilled Chicken Salad Deluxe	1 serv (9 oz)	120	45	2
Hamburger	1	270	30	–
Honey	1 pkg (0.5 oz)	45	0	0
Honey Mustard	1 pkg (0.5 oz)	50	10	0
Hot Mustard	1 pkg (1 oz)	60	5	tr
Light Mayonnaise	1 pkg (0.4 oz)	40	5	0
Quarter Pounder	1	430	70	2
Quarter Pounder w/ Cheese	1 (7 oz)	530	95	2
Sweet 'N Sour Sauce	1 pkg (1 oz)	50	0	0
SALAD DRESSINGS				
Caesar	1 pkg (2.1 oz)	160	20	0
Fat Free Herb Vinaigrette	1 pkg (2.1 oz)	50	0	0
Ranch	1 pkg (2.1 oz)	230	20	0
Reduced Calorie Red French	1 pkg (2.1 oz)	160	0	0
SALADS AND SALAD BARS				
Croutons	1 pkg	50	0	–
Garden Salad	1 serv (6.2 oz)	35	0	2
MRS. FIELDS				
Brownie Double Fudge	1 (3.1 oz)	420	35	3
Brownie Fudge Walnut	1 (3.4 oz)	500	40	4
Brownie Pecan Fudge	1 (2.8 oz)	390	40	2
Brownie Pecan Pie	1 (3 oz)	400	55	4
Cookie Chewy Fudge	1 (1.7 oz)	230	25	1
Cookie Coconut Macadamia	1 (1.7 oz)	250	35	1
Cookie Milk Chocolate Chip	1 (1.7 oz)	240	35	1
Cookie Milk Chocolate Macadamia	1 (1.7 oz)	250	30	1

FOOD	PORTION	CALS	CHOL	FIBER
Cookie Milk Chocolate w/ Walnuts	1 (1.7 oz)	250	30	1
Cookie Oatmeal Raisin	1 (1.7 oz)	220	30	2
Cookie Peanut Butter	1 (1.7 oz)	240	40	1
Cookie Semi-Sweet Chocolate	1 (1.7 oz)	230	30	1
Cookie Semi-Sweet Chocolate w/ Walnuts	1 (1.8 oz)	240	30	2
Cookie Triple Chocolate	1 (1.7 oz)	230	30	1
Cookie White Chunk Macadamia	1 (1.7 oz)	260	30	tr
Muffin Banana Walnut	1 (3.9 oz)	460	45	5
Muffin Blueberry	1 (4 oz)	390	45	2
Muffin Chocolate Chip	1 (4 oz)	450	40	5
Muffin Mandarin Orange	1 (4 oz)	420	45	1
Peanut Butter Dream Bar	1 (5 oz)	750	40	8
Stokabunga Energy Cookie	1 (5 oz)	750	60	5
MY FAVORITE MUFFIN				
Basic Muffin	⅓ muffin	220	0	0
Double Chocolate	⅓ muffin	190	0	2
Fat Free Bavarian	⅓ muffin	100	0	1
Fat Free Bavarian Chocolate	⅓ muffin	130	0	3
NEWPORT CREAMERY				
BEVERAGES				
Skim Milk	1 serv (16 oz)	206	20	–
ICE CREAM				
Reduced Fat No Sugar Added Chocolate	½ cup (2.6 oz)	110	0	1
Reduced Fat No Sugar Added Coffee	½ cup (2.6 oz)	100	15	0

FOOD	PORTION	CALS	CHOL	FIBER
Soft Serve Nonfat Frozen Yogurt Cone or Dish	1 reg (5 oz)	125	0	–
SALAD DRESSINGS				
Corn Oil & Vinegar	1 tbsp	45	0	–
Fat Free Ranch	1½ oz	48	0	–
Low-Cal French	1½ oz	48	0	–
SALADS AND SALAD BARS				
Chef's Salad	1 serv	215	50	–
Chicken Fajita	1 serv	295	44	–
Grilled Chicken	1 serv	247	48	–
SANDWICHES				
Lite Chicken Salad	1	379	63	–
Lite Grilled Cheese	1	274	30	–
Lite Grilled Chicken Breast Pocket	1	327	74	–
Lite Sliced Turkey	1	288	32	–
Lite Tuna Salad	1	358	23	–
Lite Vegetarian Pocket Broccoli Mushrooms Onions Peppers Cheese	1	211	15	–
Lite Vegetarian Pocket Broccoli Cheese	1	214	15	–
Lite Vegetarian Pocket Peppers Onions Mushrooms Cheese	1	230	15	–
Low Fat Cheese	1 slice	73	15	–
Mayonnaise	2 tsp	71	5	–
Smart Sides Broccoli	1 serv	23	0	–
Smart Sides Cottage Cheese	1 serv	90	13	–
Smart Sides Side Salad	1 serv	30	0	–
OLIVE GARDEN				
Garden Fare Apple Carmellina	1 serv (12.2 oz)	560	5	–
Garden Fare Dinner Capellini Pomodoro	1 serv (21.1 oz)	610	5	–

FOOD	PORTION	CALS	CHOL	FIBER
Garden Fare Dinner Capellini Primavera	1 serv (20.1 oz)	400	15	—
Garden Fare Dinner Capellini Primavera w/ Chicken	1 serv (23.8 oz)	560	95	—
Garden Fare Dinner Chicken Giardino	1 serv (20.6 oz)	550	85	—
Garden Fare Dinner Linguine Alla Marinara	1 serv (16.3 oz)	500	0	—
Garden Fare Dinner Penne Fra Diavolo	1 serv (14.3 oz)	420	10	—
Garden Fare Dinner Shrimp Primavera	1 serv (28.4 oz)	740	290	—
Garden Fare Lunch Capellini Pamodoro	1 serv (11.7 oz)	360	5	—
Garden Fare Lunch Capellini Primavera	1 serv (11.2 oz)	260	15	—
Garden Fare Lunch Capellini Primavera w/ Chicken	1 serv (14.9 oz)	420	90	—
Garden Fare Lunch Chicken Giardino	1 serv (12.8 oz)	360	50	—
Garden Fare Lunch Linguine Alla Marinara	1 serv (10.2 oz)	310	0	—
Garden Fare Lunch Penne Fra Diavolo	1 serv (10.2 oz)	300	10	—
Garden Fare Lunch Shrimp Primavera	1 serv (15.2 oz)	410	145	—
Minestrone Soup	1 serv (6 oz)	80	0	—

PANDA EXPRESS

Mixed Vegetables	1 serv (5 oz)	80	0	—
Steamed Rice	1 serv (8 oz)	220	0	—
Sweet & Sour Sauce	1 serv (2 oz)	60	0	—

PICCADILLY CAFETERIA
BAKED SELECTIONS

Corn Sticks	1 (2 oz)	165	26	tr
French Bread	1 slice	132	6	4

FOOD	PORTION	CALS	CHOL	FIBER
Garlic Bread	1 serv (15.8 oz)	1154	48	34
Mexican Corn Bread	1 piece	220	31	1
Roll	1 (2 oz)	130	0	4
Roll Whole Wheat	1 (1.7 oz)	117	19	3
Texas Toast	1 serv (15.5 oz)	1088	48	34
BEVERAGES				
Iced Tea	1 serv (6.5 oz)	2	0	0
Punch	1 serv (9 oz)	133	0	0
DESSERTS				
Apple Pie	1 slice (7.2 oz)	439	0	3
Cantaloupe	1 serv (9 oz)	89	0	3
Cantaloupe	1 serv (5.5 oz)	55	0	2
Chocolate Cream Pie	1 slice (7.5 oz)	512	66	tr
Custard	1 cup (5.4 oz)	183	25	0
Custard Pie	1 slice (6.2 oz)	412	18	tr
Dole Whip Topping	1 serv (3 oz)	68	0	0
Fresh Fruit Plate	1 serv (21.1 oz)	389	11	9
Gelatin	1 serv (4.75 oz)	128	14	0
Honeydew Melon	1 serv (5.5 oz)	55	0	1
Honeydew Melon	1 serv (9 oz)	89	0	2
Lemon Chiffon Pie	1 slice (6.3 oz)	481	32	tr
Pound Cake	1 slice (3.8 oz)	371	76	0
Watermelon	1 serv (11 oz)	100	0	1
MAIN MENU SELECTIONS				
Au Jus	1 serv (3 oz)	5	0	0
Baby Lima Beans	1 serv (4.5 oz)	151	0	4
Baked Potato	1	218	0	4
Baked Potato w/ Topping	1	350	33	4
Beef Chopped Steak Fried	1 serv (4 oz)	311	59	0
Beef Leg Roast	1 serv (4 oz)	311	92	tr
Beef Liver Fried	1 serv (4.5 oz)	430	418	2
Beef Tips Braised	1 serv (10 oz)	470	56	3
Black-eyed Peas w/ Pork Jowls	1 serv (4 oz)	108	7	0
Broccoli Buttered	1 serv (4 oz)	77	0	3
Broccoli & Rice Au Gratin	½ cup	184	18	1
Carrots Young Buttered	½ cup	90	0	1

FOOD	PORTION	CALS	CHOL	FIBER
Cauliflower Buttered	1 serv	80	0	2
Chicken Baked w/o Skin	¼ chicken	352	168	0
Chicken Teriyaki	1 serv (4 oz)	445	124	tr
Chicken Teriyaki Polynesian	1 serv (4 oz)	537	104	1
Corn	1 serv (4.5 oz)	128	0	0
Cornbread Stuffing	1 serv (4.5 oz)	164	26	tr
Cranberry Sauce	1 serv (1.5 oz)	64	0	tr
Eggplant Escalloped	½ cup	180	15	1
Fish Baked	1 serv (7 oz)	195	54	tr
Green Beans	1 serv (4.5 oz)	77	7	1
Ham Baked	1 serv (4 oz)	224	67	0
Macaroni & Cheese	½ cup	317	22	2
Mashed Potatoes	1 serv (4.8 oz)	120	0	0
Meatballs Baked & Spaghetti	1 serv (11.5 oz)	108	23	tr
New Potatoes Boiled	½ cup	148	0	tr
Okra Smothered	1 serv (4 oz)	121	0	1
Onion Sauce	1 serv (4 oz)	152	0	1
Rice	½ cup	99	0	tr
Rice Polynesian	1 serv (4 oz)	140	0	tr
Spaghetti Baked	1 serv (9.5 oz)	256	13	2
Squash Baked Italian	1 serv (4.75 oz)	73	8	1
Squash Mixed Yellow & Zucchini	1 serv (4 oz)	72	0	1
Squash Yellow Baked French Style	⅓ cup	86	5	1
Vegetables Unseasoned	1 serv (5 oz)	29	0	2
SALADS AND SALAD BARS				
Broccoli Salad	1 serv (4 oz)	202	13	2
Cabbage Combination Salad	1 serv (4.5 oz)	50	0	1
Carrot & Raisin Salad	1 serv (4.5 oz)	321	10	2
Cole Slaw w/ Cream	1 serv (4 oz)	182	9	1
Cucumber & Celery Salad	1 serv (4 oz)	82	0	1
Fruit Salad	1 serv (6 oz)	59	0	2
Neptune Salad	1 serv	361	25	1

FOOD	PORTION	CALS	CHOL	FIBER
Spinach Tossed Salad	1 serv (4 oz)	88	44	2
Spring Salad Bowl	1 serv (4 oz)	22	0	1
SOUPS				
Gumbo Chicken	1 serv (8 oz)	92	22	1
Gumbo Seafood	1 serv (8 oz)	98	45	1
Vegetable	1 serv (8 oz)	49	0	tr

PIZZA HUT
DESSERTS

FOOD	PORTION	CALS	CHOL	FIBER
Apple Pizza	1 slice (2.8 oz)	250	0	2
Cherry Pizza	1 slice (2.8 oz)	250	0	3
MAIN MENU SELECTIONS				
Bread Stick	1 (1.3 oz)	130	0	1
Bread Stick Dipping Sauce	1 serv (1.2 oz)	30	0	tr
Buffalo Wings Hot	4 pieces (2.1 oz)	210	130	tr
Buffalo Wings Mild	5 pieces (2.9 oz)	200	150	0
Cavatini Pasta	1 serv (12.5 oz)	480	8	9
Cavatini Supreme Pasta	1 serv (13.9 oz)	560	10	10
Garlic Bread	1 slice (1.3 oz)	150	0	1
Ham & Cheese Sandwich	1 (9.7 oz)	550	22	4
Spaghetti Marinara	1 serv (16.6 oz)	490	0	8
Spaghetti Meat Sauce	1 serv (16.4 oz)	600	25	9
Spaghetti Meatballs	1 serv (18.8 oz)	850	17	10
Supreme Sandwich	1 (10.2 oz)	640	28	4
PIZZA				
Edge Chicken Supreme	1 sq (2.5 oz)	90	15	tr
Edge Meat Lover's	1 sq (2 oz)	160	20	tr
Edge The Works	1 sq (2.2 oz)	110	10	tr
Edge Veggie Lover's	1 sq (1.9 oz)	70	<5	tr
Hand Tossed Beef Topping	1 slice	330	25	3
Hand Tossed Cheese	1 slice	240	10	2
Hand Tossed Chicken Supreme	1 slice	230	15	2
Hand Tossed Ham	1 slice	260	20	2
Hand Tossed Italian Sausage	1 slice	340	30	2

FOOD	PORTION	CALS	CHOL	FIBER
Hand Tossed Meat Lover's	1 slice	320	30	2
Hand Tossed Pepperoni	1 slice	280	20	2
Hand Tossed Pepperoni Lover's	1 slice	250	15	2
Hand Tossed Pork Topping	1 slice	320	25	3
Hand Tossed Super Supreme	1 slice	290	25	2
Hand Tossed Supreme	1 slice	270	20	3
Hand Tossed Veggie Lover's	1 slice	220	5	2
Insider Cheese	1 med slice (4.9 oz)	370	30	3
Pan Beef Topping	1 med slice (4.3 oz)	330	20	3
Pan Cheese	1 med slice (3.9 oz)	290	10	2
Pan Chicken Supreme	1 med slice (4.5 oz)	270	15	2
Pan Ham	1 med slice (3.8 oz)	260	15	2
Pan Italian Sausage	1 med slice (4.3 oz)	340	25	2
Pan Meat Lover's	1 med slice (4.7 oz)	360	30	3
Pan Pepperoni	1 med slice (3.7 oz)	280	15	2
Pan Pepperoni Lover's	1 med slice (4.3 oz)	330	20	2
Pan Pork Topping	1 med slice (3.7 oz)	320	20	3
Pan Super Supreme	1 med slice (5 oz)	340	25	3
Pan Supreme	1 med slice (4.7 oz)	320	20	3
Pan Veggie Lover's	1 med slice (4.6 oz)	270	5	3
Personal Pan Beef Topping	1 pie (10.2 oz)	710	45	6
Personal Pan Cheese	1 pie (9.2 oz)	630	25	6
Personal Pan Ham	1 pie (9.1 oz)	580	35	5
Personal Pan Italian Sausage	1 pie (10.2 oz)	740	55	6
Personal Pan Pepperoni	1 pie (9 oz)	620	30	5
Personal Pan Pork Topping	1 pie (10.2 oz)	700	40	6
Sicilian Beef Topping	1 slice (4 oz)	260	15	2
Sicilian Cheese	1 slice (4 oz)	290	10	2
Sicilian Chicken Supreme	1 slice (4.6 oz)	270	15	2

FOOD	PORTION	CALS	CHOL	FIBER
Sicilian Ham	1 slice (3.8 oz)	257	14	3
Sicilian Italian Sausage	1 slice (4.4 oz)	333	24	3
Sicilian Meat Lover's	1 slice (4.7 oz)	350	25	2
Sicilian Pepperoni	1 slice (3.9 oz)	280	15	2
Sicilian Pepperoni Lover's	1 slice (4.4 oz)	320	20	2
Sicilian Pork Topping	1 slice (4.4 oz)	320	20	2
Sicilian Super Supreme	1 slice (5 oz)	340	20	2
Sicilian Supreme	1 slice (4.7 oz)	310	15	2
Sicilian Veggies Lover's	1 slice (4.6 oz)	270	15	2
Stuffed Crust Beef Topping	1 lg slice (5.8 oz)	390	30	3
Stuffed Crust Cheese	1 lg slice (5.5 oz)	360	25	3
Stuffed Crust Chicken Supreme	1 lg slice (6.5 oz)	350	35	3
Stuffed Crust Ham	1 lg slice (5.5 oz)	330	30	3
Stuffed Crust Italian Sausage	1 lg slice (5.8 oz)	400	35	3
Stuffed Crust Meat Lover's	1 lg slice (6.7 oz)	470	50	3
Stuffed Crust Pepperoni	1 lg slice (5.4 oz)	360	30	3
Stuffed Crust Pepperoni Lover's	1 lg slice (6.2 oz)	420	40	3
Stuffed Crust Pork Topping	1 lg slice (5.7 oz)	380	30	3
Stuffed Crust Super Supreme	1 lg slice (7.2 oz)	430	40	3
Stuffed Crust Supreme	1 lg slice (6.7 oz)	410	35	3
Stuffed Crust Veggie Lover's	1 lg slice (6.6 oz)	340	20	3
The Big New Yorker Beef Topping	1 slice (7.2 oz)	480	40	8
The Big New Yorker Cheese	1 slice (6.1 oz)	380	20	7
The Big New Yorker Ham	1 slice (5.9 oz)	340	25	7

FOOD	PORTION	CALS	CHOL	FIBER
The Big New Yorker Pepperoni	1 slice (5.6 oz)	370	20	7
The Big New Yorker Pork Topping	1 slice (7.2 oz)	470	35	8
The Big New Yorker Sausage	1 slice (8 oz)	570	55	8
The Big New Yorker Supreme	1 slice (7.8 oz)	450	35	8
The Big New Yorker Veggie Lover's	1 slice (12 oz)	450	10	9
Thin'N Crispy Cheese	1 med slice (3 oz)	200	10	2
Thin'N Crispy Chicken Supreme	1 med slice (4 oz)	200	20	2
Thin'N Crispy Ham	1 med slice (2.9 oz)	170	15	2
Thin'N Crispy Italian Sausage	1 med slice (3.7 oz)	290	30	2
Thin'N Crispy Meat Lovers	1 med slice (4.1 oz)	310	35	2
Thin'N Crispy Pepperoni	1 med slice (2.8 oz)	190	15	2
Thin'N Crispy Pepperoni Lover's	1 med slice (3.4 oz)	250	20	2
Thin'N Crispy Pork Topping	1 med slice (3.7 oz)	270	25	2
Thin'N Crispy Super Supreme	1 med slice (4.6 oz)	280	25	2
Thin'N Crispy Supreme	1 med slice (4.1 oz)	250	20	2
Thin'N Crispy Veggie Lover's	1 med slice (4 oz)	190	5	2
Thin'n Crispy Beef Topping	1 med slice (3.7 oz)	270	25	2
Twist Crust Cheese	1 lg slice (6.7 oz)	450	15	3
Twist Crust Marinara Sauce	1 serv (3 oz)	60	0	2
Twist Crust Ranch Sauce	1 serv (3 oz)	440	20	0
Twist Crust Supreme	1 lg slice (7.5 oz)	470	25	3

FOOD	PORTION	CALS	CHOL	FIBER
POPEYE'S				
Apple Pie	1 serv (3.1 oz)	290	10	2
Biscuit	1 serv (2.3 oz)	250	<5	1
Breast Mild	1 (3.7 oz)	270	60	2
Breast Spicy	1 (3.7 oz)	270	60	2
Cajun Rice	1 serv (3.9 oz)	150	25	3
Cole Slaw	1 serv (4 oz)	149	3	3
Corn On The Cob	1 serv (5.2 oz)	127	0	9
French Fries	1 serv (3 oz)	240	10	3
Leg Mild	1 (1.7 oz)	120	40	0
Leg Spicy	1 (1.7 oz)	120	40	0
Nuggets	1 serv (4.2 oz)	410	55	3
Nuggets Mild Tender	1 (1.2 oz)	110	15	1
Nuggets Spicy Tender	1 (1.2 oz)	110	15	1
Onion Rings	1 serv (3.1 oz)	310	25	2
Potatoes & Gravy	1 serv (3.8 oz)	100	<5	3
Red Beans & Rice	1 serv (5.9 oz)	270	10	7
Shrimp	1 serv (2.8 oz)	250	110	3
Thigh Mild	1 (3.1 oz)	300	70	tr
Thigh Spicy	1 (3.1 oz)	300	70	tr
Wing Mild	1 (1.6 oz)	160	40	0
Wing Spicy	1 (1.6 oz)	160	40	0
QUINCY'S				
BAKED SELECTIONS				
Banana Nut Bread	1 serv (2 oz)	165	5	–
Biscuit	1 (2.5 oz)	270	11	–
Cornbread	1 serv (2 oz)	140	0	–
Yeast Roll	1 (2 oz)	160	0	–
BREAKFAST SELECTIONS				
Bacon	1 serv (0.25 oz)	35	5	–
Corned Beef Hash	1 serv (4.5 oz)	210	45	–
Country Ham	1 serv (1.5 oz)	90	35	–
Escalloped Apples	1 serv (3.5 oz)	120	0	–
Oatmeal	1 serv (1 oz)	175	0	–
Pancakes	1 (1.5 oz)	95	30	–
Sausage Gravy	1 serv (4 oz)	70	10	–
Sausage Links	1 (2 oz)	225	20	–
Sausage Patties	1 (2 oz)	230	45	–
Scrambled Eggs	1 serv (2 oz)	95	215	–

FOOD	PORTION	CALS	CHOL	FIBER
Steak Fingers	1 serv (3.5 oz)	360	50	—
Syrup	1 oz	75	0	—
DESSERTS				
Banana Pudding	1 serv (5 oz)	240	10	—
Brownie Pudding Cake	1 serv (4 oz)	310	0	—
Caramel Topping	1 serv (1 oz)	105	0	—
Chocolate Chip Cookies	1 (0.5 oz)	60	5	—
Cobbler Apple	1 serv (6 oz)	255	5	—
Cobbler Cherry	1 serv (6 oz)	410	5	—
Cobbler Peach	1 serv (6 oz)	305	5	—
Frozen Yogurt	1 serv (4 oz)	135	5	—
Fudge Topping	1 serv (1 oz)	105	0	—
Sugar Cookie	1 (0.5 oz)	60	5	—
MAIN MENU SELECTIONS				
⅓ Pound Hamburger	1 serv (8 oz)	565	66	—
BBQ Beans	1 serv (4 oz)	114	0	—
Bacon Cheese Burger	1 (9 oz)	663	87	—
Baked Potato	1 (6 oz)	115	0	—
Broccoli	1 serv (4 oz)	34	0	—
Cheese Sauce	1 serv (1 oz)	58	11	—
Chopped Steak Steak	1 serv (8 oz)	499	89	—
Cinnamon Apples	1 serv (4 oz)	172	0	—
Corn	1 serv (4 oz)	96	0	—
Country Steak w/ Gravy	1 serv (8 oz)	530	54	—
Cowboy Steak	1 serv (14 oz)	580	176	—
Filet w/ Bacon	1 serv (8 oz)	340	124	—
Green Beans	1 serv (4 oz)	61	0	—
Grilled Chicken	1 reg serv (5 oz)	120	55	—
Grilled Chicken Sandwich	1 (9 oz)	324	55	—
Grilled Salmon	1 serv (7 oz)	228	109	—
Homestyle Chicken Fillet	1 serv (3 oz)	217	25	—
Junior Sirloin Steak	1 serv (5.5 oz)	194	69	—
Large Sirloin Steak	1 serv (10 oz)	368	119	—
Mashed Potatoes	1 serv (4 oz)	54	0	—
NY Strip Steak	1 serv (10 oz)	450	148	—
Philly Cheese Steak	1 serv (11 oz)	588	87	—
Porterhouse Steak	1 serv (17 oz)	683	154	—

FOOD	PORTION	CALS	CHOL	FIBER
Regular Sirloin Steak	1 serv (8 oz)	285	71	—
Ribeye Steak	1 serv (10 oz)	452	116	—
Rice Pilaf	1 serv (4 oz)	119	0	1
Roasted BBQ Chicken	1 serv (14 oz)	941	340	—
Roasted Herb Chicken	1 serv (14 oz)	875	340	—
Sirloin Tips w/ Mushroom Gravy	1 serv (6 oz)	196	64	—
Sirloin Tips w/ Peppers & Onions	1 serv (5 oz)	203	63	—
Smothered Steak Sandwich	1 (9 oz)	429	69	—
Smothered Strip Steak	1 serv (10 oz)	622	148	—
Southern Breaded Shrimp	1 serv (7 oz)	546	135	—
Spicy BBQ Chicken Sandwich	1 (10 oz)	368	55	—
Steak & Shrimp	1 serv (9 oz)	677	170	—
Steak Fries	1 serv (4 oz)	358	0	—
T-Bone Steak	1 serv (13 oz)	521	118	—
SALAD DRESSINGS				
Blue Cheese	1 serv (1 oz)	155	10	—
French	1 serv (1 oz)	125	0	—
Honey Mustard	1 serv (1 oz)	100	0	—
Italian	1 serv (1 oz)	135	0	—
Light Creamy Italian	1 serv (1 oz)	65	0	—
Light French	1 serv (1 oz)	85	0	—
Light Italian	1 serv (1 oz)	20	0	—
Light Thousand Island	1 serv (1 oz)	65	20	—
Parmesan Peppercorn	1 serv (1 oz)	150	0	—
Ranch	1 serv (1 oz)	110	10	—
SOUPS				
Chili With Beans	1 serv (6 oz)	235	15	—
Clam Chowder	1 serv (6 oz)	180	0	—
Cream Of Broccoli	1 serv (6 oz)	170	0	—
Vegetable Beef	1 serv (6 oz)	90	0	—
QUIZNO'S				
Sub Honey Bourbon Chicken	1 sm	329	38	3
Sub Turkey Lite	1 sm	334	19	3

FOOD	PORTION	CALS	CHOL	FIBER
Sub Tuscan Chicken Salad	1 sm	326	35	4

RALLY'S
BEVERAGES

FOOD	PORTION	CALS	CHOL	FIBER
Coke	1 serv (20 oz)	177	0	—
Coke	1 serv (16 oz)	132	0	—
Coke	1 serv (32 oz)	264	0	—
Coke	1 serv (42 oz)	372	0	—
Diet Coke	1 serv (42 oz)	2	0	—
Diet Coke	1 serv (32 oz)	1	0	—
Diet Coke	1 serv (20 oz)	1	0	—
Fanta Orange	1 serv (20 oz)	202	0	—
Fanta Orange	1 serv (32 oz)	301	0	—
Fanta Orange	1 serv (16 oz)	150	0	—
Fanta Orange	1 serv (42 oz)	424	0	—
Mr. Pibb	1 serv (32 oz)	237	0	—
Mr. Pibb	1 serv (42 oz)	334	0	—
Mr. Pibb	1 serv (20 oz)	159	0	—
Mr. Pibb	1 serv (16 oz)	113	0	—
Root Beer	1 serv (20 oz)	197	0	—
Root Beer	1 serv (16 oz)	146	0	—
Root Beer	1 serv (32 oz)	294	0	—
Root Beer	1 serv (42 oz)	414	0	—
Shake Banana	1 serv	399	38	—
Shake Chocolate	1 serv	411	38	—
Shake Strawberry	1 serv	399	38	—
Shake Vanilla	1 serv	320	38	—
Sprite	1 serv (20 oz)	161	0	—
Sprite	1 serv (32 oz)	264	0	—
Sprite	1 serv (16 oz)	132	0	—
Sprite	1 serv (42 oz)	338	0	—

MAIN MENU SELECTIONS

FOOD	PORTION	CALS	CHOL	FIBER
Big Buford	1	743	151	—
Chicken Fillet Sandwich	1	399	42	—
Chili w/ Cheese & Onion	1 serv (13 oz)	669	137	—
Chili w/ Cheese & Onion	1 serv (7 oz)	360	74	—
French Fries	1 extra lg (8 oz)	423	13	—
French Fries	1 reg (4 oz)	211	7	—
French Fries	1 lg (6 oz)	317	10	—

FOOD	PORTION	CALS	CHOL	FIBER
Onion Rings	1 serv	210	0	—
Rallyburger	1	433	63	—
Rallyburger w/ Cheese	1	488	27	—
Spicy Chicken Sandwich	1	437	40	—
Super Barbecue Bacon	1	593	88	—
Super Double Cheeseburger	1	762	154	—

RED LOBSTER
CHILDREN'S MENU SELECTIONS

Cheeseburger	1 serv	1040	130	—
Fried Chicken Fingers	1 serv	680	35	—
Fried Shrimp	1 serv	650	80	—
Grilled Chicken Tenders	1 serv	580	55	—
Hamburger	1 serv	920	100	—
Popcorn Shrimp	1 serv	650	120	—
Popcorn Shrimp & Cheesesticks	1 serv	750	125	—
Spaghetti & Cheesesticks	1 serv	830	5	—

DESSERTS

Fudge Overboard	1 serv	620	105	—
Ice Cream	1 serv (4.5 oz)	140	30	—
Sensational 7	1 serv	790	140	—

MAIN MENU SELECTIONS

Admiral's Feast	1 serv	1060	265	—
Appetizer Calamari	1 serv	350	190	—
Appetizer Chicken Fingers	1 serv	390	65	—
Appetizer Chilled Shrimp In The Shell	1 serv (6 oz)	110	235	—
Appetizer Crab & Shrimp Cakes	1 serv	480	80	—
Appetizer Crab Add-On	1 serv	60	55	—
Appetizer Fresh Fried Mushrooms	1 serv	790	<5	—
Appetizer Lobster Quesadilla	1 serv	760	160	—

FOOD	PORTION	CALS	CHOL	FIBER
Appetizer Lobster Stuffed Mushroom	1 serv	400	100	—
Appetizer Mozzarella Cheesesticks	1 serv	730	50	—
Appetizer Parmesan Zucchini	1 serv	620	10	—
Appetizer Shrimp Cocktail	1 serv	50	105	—
Appetizer Stuffed Mushrooms	1 serv	420	90	—
Applesauce	1 serv (4 oz)	90	0	—
Atlantic Cod	1 serv (8 oz)	200	105	—
Atlantic Cod	1 lunch serv (5 oz)	110	60	—
Atlantic Salmon	1 lunch serv (5 oz)	200	80	—
Atlantic Salmon	1 serv (8 oz)	340	135	—
Baked Atlantic Cod	1 serv	220	100	—
Baked Atlantic Haddock	1 serv	220	100	—
Baked Flounder	1 lunch serv	190	90	—
Baked Potato	1 (8 oz)	130	0	—
Broccoli	1 serv (3 oz)	25	0	—
Broiled Fisherman's Platter	1 serv	600	250	—
Broiled Rock Lobster Tail	1 tail	190	110	—
Broiled Seafarer's Platter	1 serv	450	190	—
Caesar Salad w/ Dressing	1 serv	240	15	—
Catfish	1 serv (8 oz)	220	130	—
Catfish	1 lunch serv (5 oz)	130	75	—
Catfish Santa Fe	1 serv	340	165	—
Catfish Sante Fe	1 lunch serv	180	85	—
Chicken Fingers	1 lunch serv	390	64	—
Chicken Fresco	1 serv	1320	240	—
Chicken Fresco	1 lunch serv	660	120	—
Clam Strips	1 serv	720	35	—
Clam Strips	1 lunch serv	360	15	—
Cocktail Sauce	1 oz	30	0	—
Cole Slaw	1 serv (4 oz)	190	25	—

FOOD	PORTION	CALS	CHOL	FIBER
Crab Alfredo	1 serv	1170	270	–
Crab Alfredo	1 lunch serv	590	135	–
Fish & Shrimp Combo	1 serv	730	230	–
Fish Nuggets	1 lunch serv	320	95	–
Fish Seasoning Add On For Blackened Dinner	1 serv	70	0	–
Fish Seasoning Add On For Blackened Lunch	1 serv	50	0	–
Fish Seasoning Add On For Broiled Dinner	1 serv	45	0	–
Fish Seasoning Add On For Broiled Lunch	1 serv	35	0	–
Fish Seasoning Add On For Grilled Dinner	1 serv	35	0	–
Fish Seasoning Add On For Grilled Lunch	1 serv	25	0	–
Fish Seasoning Add On For Lemon Pepper Dinner	1 serv	35	0	–
Fish Seasoning Add On For Lemon Pepper Lunch	1 serv	30	0	–
Fish Seasoning Add On For Santa Fe Style Dinner	1 serv	60	0	–
Fish Seasoning Add On For Santa Fe Style Lunch	1 serv	40	0	–
Flounder	1 lunch serv (5 oz)	130	75	–
Flounder	1 serv (8 oz)	220	130	–
French Fries	1 serv (4 oz)	350	0	–
Fried Flounder	1 lunch serv	230	60	–

FOOD	PORTION	CALS	CHOL	FIBER
Fried Shrimp	1 lunch serv	270	115	—
Fried Shrimp	12 lg	500	290	—
Garden Salad w/o Dressing	1 serv	50	0	—
Garlic Cheese Biscuit	1	140	5	—
Grilled Cheeseburger	1	580	130	—
Grilled Chicken Breasts	1 serv	230	105	—
Grilled Chicken Salad w/o Dressing	1 serv	320	70	—
Grouper	1 lunch serv (5 oz)	130	50	—
Grouper	1 serv (8 oz)	220	90	—
Haddock	1 serv (8 oz)	210	140	—
Haddock	1 lunch serv (5 oz)	120	80	—
Halibut	1 lunch serv (5 oz)	150	45	—
Halibut	1 serv (8 oz)	260	75	—
King Salmon	1 lunch serv (5 oz)	250	95	—
King Salmon	1 serv (8 oz)	420	160	—
Lake Trout	1 lunch serv (5 oz)	200	80	—
Lake Trout	1 serv (8 oz)	340	140	—
Lemon Pepper Grilled Mahi Mahi	1 serv	240	130	—
Lobster Shrimp & Scallop Scampi	1 lunch serv	430	80	—
Lobster Shrimp & Scallop Scampi	1 serv	870	135	—
Mahi Mahi	1 lunch serv (5 oz)	130	75	—
Mahi Mahi	1 serv (8 oz)	220	130	—
Maine Lobster Steamed	1 serv (1.25 lb)	160	125	—
Maine Lobster Stuffed	1 serv (2 lb)	430	210	—
Marinara Sauce	1 serv	50	0	—
Melted Butter	1 oz	200	60	—
Neptune's Feast	1 serv	1210	290	—
New York Strip Steak	1 serv	560	180	—
Perch	1 serv (8 oz)	220	130	—
Perch	1 lunch serv (5 oz)	130	75	—
Pollack	1 lunch serv (5 oz)	120	100	—
Pollock	1 serv (8 oz)	120	100	—
Popcorn Shrimp	1 lunch serv	380	235	—

FOOD	PORTION	CALS	CHOL	FIBER
Popcorn Shrimp	1 serv	580	360	–
Red Rockfish	1 lunch serv (5 oz)	130	50	–
Red Rockfish	1 serv (8 oz)	230	85	–
Red Snapper	1 lunch serv (5 oz)	140	50	–
Red Snapper	1 serv (8 oz)	240	90	–
Rice Pilaf	1 serv (4 oz)	180	0	–
Roasted Vegetables	1 serv (6 oz)	120	0	–
Roasted Vegetables	1 lunch serv (4 oz)	80	0	–
Sailor's Platter	1 lunch serv	250	170	–
Sandwich Blackened Catfish	1	340	85	–
Sandwich Broiled Fish	1	300	80	–
Sandwich Cajun Grilled Chicken	1	370	55	–
Sandwich Classic Fish	1	520	90	–
Sandwich Grilled Chicken	1	290	50	–
Sassy Sauce	1 oz	80	5	–
Seafood Broil	1 lunch serv	310	110	–
Shrimp & Chicken	1 serv	340	225	–
Shrimp Caesar Salad w/o Dressing	1 serv	240	110	–
Shrimp Carbonara	1 serv	1290	310	–
Shrimp Carbonara	1 lunch serv	650	155	–
Shrimp Combo	1 serv	380	210	–
Shrimp Feast	1 serv	470	390	–
Shrimp Milano	1 serv	1190	340	–
Shrimp Milano	1 lunch serv	590	170	–
Shrimp Scampi	1 lunch serv	110	100	–
Smothered Chicken	1 serv	530	170	–
Snow Crab Legs	1 serv	110	115	–
Sockeye Salmon	1 lunch serv (5 oz)	240	95	–
Sockeye Salmon	1 serv (8 oz)	410	165	–
Sole	1 serv (8 oz)	220	130	–
Sole	1 lunch serv (5 oz)	130	75	–
Soup Bread Salad w/o Dressing	1 lunch serv	430	40	–
Steak & Fried Shrimp	1 serv	780	340	–
Steak & Rock Lobster Tail	1 serv	570	220	–

FOOD	PORTION	CALS	CHOL	FIBER
Swordfish	1 serv (8 oz)	290	115	–
Swordfish	1 lunch serv (5 oz)	170	70	–
Tartar Sauce	1 oz	160	15	–
Teriyaki Grilled Chicken Breast	1 serv	240	105	–
Twice Baked Potato	1	430	60	–
Walleye	1 serv (8 oz)	210	205	–
Walleye	1 lunch serv (5 oz)	120	120	–
Yellow Lake Perch	1 serv (8 oz)	220	130	–
Yellow Lake Perch	1 lunch serv (5 oz)	130	75	–
SALAD DRESSINGS				
Blue Cheese	1 serv	170	30	–
Buttermilk Ranch	1 serv	110	15	–
Caesar	1 serv	170	10	–
Dijon Honey Mustard	1 serv	140	20	–
Fat Free Ranch	1 serv	50	0	–
Lite Red Wine Vinaigrette	1 serv	50	0	–
SOUPS				
Bayou Style Gumbo	1 serv (6 oz)	120	65	–
Broccoli Cheese	1 serv	160	25	–
Clam Chowder	1 serv (6 oz)	130	20	–
SBARRO				
Pizza Veggie Slice	1 serv (10 oz)	490	15	1
SEE'S CANDIES				
Bridge Mix	14 pieces (1.4 oz)	200	10	1
Dark Chocolate Bordeaux	2 (1.4 oz)	170	25	1
Dark Chocolates	2 (1.2 oz)	160	10	2
Lollypop Butterscotch	1	90	10	0
Lollypop Cafe Latte	1	90	10	0
Lollypop Chocolate	1	90	5	tr
Lollypop Peanut Butter	1	90	0	0
Marshmints	3 (1.4 oz)	140	0	tr
Milk Chocolate Bordeaux	2 (1.4 oz)	170	15	tr
Milk Chocolate Butter	2 (1.4 oz)	190	15	tr
Milk Chocolate Buttercreams	2 (1.4 oz)	180	15	0

FOOD	PORTION	CALS	CHOL	FIBER
Milk Chocolate California Brittle	2 (1.3 oz)	220	25	0
Milk Chocolate Nuts & Chews	3 (1.7 oz)	250	15	2
Milk Chocolate Peanuts	3 (1.5 oz)	230	5	2
Milk Chocolate Soft Centers	2 (1.4 oz)	170	15	tr
Milk Chocolates	2 (1.2 oz)	160	10	tr
Nuts & Chews	3 (1.6 oz)	240	10	2
P-Nut Crunch	2 (1.4 oz)	220	10	1
Peanut Brittle	1.5 oz	230	25	0
Pecan Buds	3 (1.7 oz)	270	10	tr
Red Hot Swamp Goo	3 pieces (1.4 oz)	140	0	tr
Soft Centers	2 (1.4 oz)	170	10	tr
Truffles Black or Gold	2 (1.4 oz)	180	10	1
Truffles Mint	3 (1.6 oz)	200	15	tr
Victoria Toffee	1.5 oz	250	20	1

SIZZLER
DESSERTS

FOOD	PORTION	CALS	CHOL	FIBER
Chocolate & Vanilla Soft Serve	4 oz	136	0	0
Chocolate Syrup	1 oz	90	0	0
Strawberry Topping	1 oz	70	0	0
Whipped Topping	1 tbsp	12	0	0

HOT BUFFET

FOOD	PORTION	CALS	CHOL	FIBER
Broccoli Cheese Soup	1 serv (4 oz)	139	8	0
Chicken Noodle Soup	1 serv (4 oz)	31	7	0
Chicken Wings	1 oz	73	20	0
Clam Chowder	1 serv (4 oz)	118	6	0
Fettucine	2 oz	80	5	0
Focaccia Bread	2 pieces	108	1	0
Marinara Sauce	1 oz	13	0	0
Meatballs	4	157	30	1
Minestrone Soup	1 serv (4 oz)	36	1	2
Nacho Cheese Soup	1 serv (4 oz)	120	30	0
Potato Skins	2 oz	160	0	3
Refried Beans	¼ cup	62	5	3
Saltine Crackers	2	25	2	0

FOOD	PORTION	CALS	CHOL	FIBER
Spaghetti	2 oz	80	0	1
Taco Filling	2 oz	103	16	1
Taco Shells	1	50	0	1
Vegetable Sirloin Soup	1 serv (4 oz)	60	10	0
MAIN MENU SELECTIONS				
Buttery Dipping Sauce	1 serv (1.5 oz)	330	0	0
Cheese Toast	1 piece	273	5	1
Cocktail Sauce	1 serv (1.5 oz)	40	0	0
Dakota Ranch Steak	1 (6 oz)	316	101	—
Dakota Ranch Steak	1 (9.5 oz)	500	160	—
Dakota Ranch Steak	1 (8 oz)	421	135	—
French Fries	1 serv (4 oz)	358	0	4
Hamburger	1	626	142	1
Hibachi Chicken Breast w/ Pineapple	5 oz	193	65	1
Hibachi Sauce	1 serv (1.5 oz)	57	0	0
Lemon Herb Chicken Breast	5 oz	140	65	0
Malibu Chicken Patty	1	310	75	0
Malibu Sauce	1 serv (1.5 oz)	283	28	0
Margarine Whipped	1½ tbsp	105	0	0
Potato Baked Plain	1 (4 oz)	105	0	2
Rice Pilaf	1 serv (6 oz)	256	0	1
Salmon	8 oz	110	41	0
Sante Fe Chicken Breast	5 oz	150	65	0
Shrimp Broiled	5 oz	150	218	0
Shrimp Fried	4 pieces	223	118	2
Shrimp Mini	4 oz	152	80	1
Shrimp Scampi	5 oz	143	150	0
Sour Dressing	2 tbsp	60	0	0
Swordfish	8 oz	315	89	0
Tartar Sauce	1 serv (1.5 oz)	170	14	0
SALAD DRESSINGS				
Blue Cheese	1 oz	111	8	0
Honey Mustard	1 oz	160	10	0
Italian Lite	1 oz	14	0	0
Japanese Rice Vinegar Fat Free	1 oz	10	0	0

FOOD	PORTION	CALS	CHOL	FIBER
Parmesan Italian	1 oz	100	0	0
Ranch	1 oz	120	10	0
Ranch Reduced Calorie	1 oz	90	10	0
Thousand Island	1 oz	143	11	0
SALADS AND SALAD BARS				
Alfafa Sprouts	¼ cup	2	0	0
Avocado	½	153	0	3
Bean Sprouts	¼ cup	8	0	0
Beets	¼ cup	13	0	1
Bell Peppers	2 oz	8	0	1
Broccoli	½ cup	12	0	1
Cabbage Red	¼ cup	5	0	0
Cantoupe	½ cup	28	0	1
Carrot & Raisin Salad	2 oz	130	10	1
Carrots	¼ cup	12	0	1
Chinese Chicken Salad	2 oz	54	10	1
Chives	1 oz	62	0	1
Cottage Cheese	2 oz	51	5	0
Cucumber	2 oz	7	0	1
Eggs	1 oz	44	122	0
Garbanzo Beans	¼ cup	63	0	3
Grapes	½ cup	29	0	1
Guacamole	1 oz	42	0	0
Honeydew Melon	½ cup	30	0	1
Iceberg Lettuce	1 cup	7	0	1
Jicama	2 oz	13	0	0
Kidney Beans	¼ cup	52	0	4
Kiwifruit	2 oz	35	0	2
Mediterranean Minted Fruit Salad	2 oz	29	0	0
Mexican Fiesta Salad	2 oz	54	0	1
Mushrooms	¼ cup	4	0	0
Old Fashioned Potato Salad	2 oz	84	6	1
Onions Red	2 tbsp	8	0	0
Peaches	¼ cup	34	0	1
Peas	¼ cup	31	0	2
Pineapple	½ cup	38	0	1
Real Bacon Bits	1 tbsp	27	0	1
Red Herb Potato Salad	2 oz	121	9	1

FOOD	PORTION	CALS	CHOL	FIBER
Romaine Lettuce	1 cup	9	0	1
Salsa	1 oz	7	0	0
Seafood Louis Pasta Salad	2 oz	64	17	1
Seafood Salad	2 oz	56	7	0
Spicy Jicama Salad	2 oz	16	0	0
Spinach	½ cup	6	0	1
Strawberries	½ cup	22	0	2
Teriyaki Beef Salad	2 oz	49	7	1
Tomatoes Cherry	¼ cup	12	0	1
Tuna Pasta Salad	2 oz	133	10	0
Turkey Ham	1 oz	62	19	0
Watermelon	½ cup	26	0	0
Zucchini	¼ cup	5	0	1

SMOOTHIE KING

FOOD	PORTION	CALS	CHOL	FIBER
Activator Banana	1 (20 oz)	429	2	4
Activator Chocolate	1 (20 oz)	429	2	4
Activator Strawberry	1 (20 oz)	559	2	5
Activator Vanilla	1 (20 oz)	429	2	4
Angel Food	1 (20 oz)	330	2	4
Blackberry Dream	1 (20 oz)	343	0	3
Caribbean Way	1 (20 oz)	392	0	5
Celestial Cherry High	1 (20 oz)	285	0	4
Coconut Surprise	1 (20 oz)	457	3	5
Cranberry Supreme	1 (20 oz)	577	24	3
Cranberry Cooler	1 (20 oz)	538	0	3
GoGuava	1 (20 oz)	300	0	2
Grape Expectations	1 (20 oz)	399	0	2
Grape Expectations II	1 (20 oz)	529	0	4
Hawaiian Cafe Au Lei	1 (20 oz)	286	5	tr
High Protein Almond Mocha	1 (20 oz)	402	17	4
High Protein Banana	1 (20 oz)	412	14	6
High Protein Chocolate	1 (20 oz)	401	17	4
High Protein Lemon	1 (20 oz)	390	12	3
High Protein Pineapple	1 (20 oz)	380	12	7
Hulk Chocolate	1 (20 oz)	846	102	6
Hulk Strawberry	1 (20 oz)	953	102	6
Hulk Vanilla	1 (20 oz)	846	102	5

FOOD	PORTION	CALS	CHOL	FIBER
Immune Builder	1 (20 oz)	333	24	4
Instant Vigor	1 (20 oz)	359	0	2
Island Treat	1 (20 oz)	334	0	5
Lemon Twist Banana	1 (20 oz)	339	0	2
Lemon Twist Strawberry	1 (20 oz)	399	0	2
Light & Fluffy	1 (20 oz)	389	0	4
Malt	1 (20 oz)	887	166	tr
Mangofest	1 (20 oz)	320	0	2
Mo'cuccino	1 (20 oz)	440	75	1
Muscle Punch	1 (20 oz)	339	2	4
Muscle Punch Plus	1 (20 oz)	340	2	5
Peach Slice	1 (20 oz)	341	2	3
Peach Slice Plus	1 (20 oz)	471	2	5
Peanut Power	1 (20 oz)	502	2	4
Peanut Power Plus Grape	1 (20 oz)	703	2	4
Peanut Power Plus Strawberry	1 (20 oz)	632	2	5
Pep Upper	1 (20 oz)	334	0	5
Pineapple Pleasure	1 (20 oz)	313	0	4
Power Punch	1 (20 oz)	430	2	4
Power Punch Plus	1 (20 oz)	499	2	4
Raspberry Sunrise	1 (20 oz)	335	0	4
Shake	1 (20 oz)	875	166	0
Slim & Trim Chocolate	1 (20 oz)	270	4	3
Slim & Trim Strawberry	1 (20 oz)	357	2	3
Slim & Trim Vanilla	1 (20 oz)	227	2	2
Super Punch	1 (20 oz)	425	0	6
Super Punch Plus	1 (20 oz)	516	0	6
Yogurt D'Lite	1 (20 oz)	341	14	2
Youth Fountain	1 (20 oz)	267	0	5

STARBUCKS
ICE CREAM

FOOD	PORTION	CALS	CHOL	FIBER
Biscotte Bliss	½ cup	240	55	—
Caffe Almond Fudge	½ cup	260	55	—
Caffe Almond Roast	1 bar	280	25	—
Dark Roast Expresso Swirl	½ cup	220	55	—
Frappuccino Coffee	1 bar	110	10	—

FOOD	PORTION	CALS	CHOL	FIBER
Italian Roast Coffee	½ cup	230	65	—
Javachip	½ cup	250	60	—
Low Fat Latte	½ cup	170	10	—
Low Fat Mocha Mambo	½ cup	170	10	—
Vanilla Mochachip	½ cup	270	75	—
SNACKS				
Crunchy Honey Bar	1 (1.06 oz)	150	0	1
Lively Lemon Bar	1 (1.23 oz)	140	0	1
Tangy Apple Bar	1 (1.23 oz)	140	0	1

STUFF'N TURKEY

FOOD	PORTION	CALS	CHOL	FIBER
Chef's Salad	1 serv	288	58	3
Grilled Turkey Breast	1 serv	244	23	5
Homemade Turkey Salad	1 serv	651	110	9
Real Fresh Roasted Turkey Breast	1 serv	384	29	8
Rotisserie Turkey Breast	1 serv	251	48	4
Thanksgiving Dinner On A Sandwich	1 serv	605	33	10
Turkey Barbecue	1 serv	478	48	8
Turkey Powerhouse	1 serv	482	50	10

SUBWAY

FOOD	PORTION	CALS	CHOL	FIBER
BEVERAGES				
Fruizle Smoothie Berry Lishus	1 sm (13 oz)	113	15	1
Fruizle Smoothie Berry Lishus w/ Banana	1 sm (17 oz)	221	15	4
Fruizle Smoothie Peach Pizazz	1 sm (12 oz)	103	0	0
Fruizle Smoothie Pineapple Delight w/ Banana	1 sm (17 oz)	241	0	4
Fruizle Smoothie Pineapple Delite	1 sm (13 oz)	133	0	1
Fruizle Smoothie Sunrise Refresher	1 sm (12 oz)	119	0	1

FOOD	PORTION	CALS	CHOL	FIBER
COOKIES				
Chocolate Chip	1	215	13	1
Chocolate Chunk	1	217	12	1
Double Chocolate	1	209	15	1
M&M	1	215	13	1
Oatmeal Raisin	1	210	14	2
Peanut Butter	1	221	12	1
Sugar	1	227	17	0
White Macadamia Nut	1	221	15	1
SALAD DRESSINGS				
Fat Free French	1 serv (2 oz)	70	0	0
Fat Free Italian	1 serv (2 oz)	20	0	0
Fat Free Ranch	1 serv (2 oz)	60	0	0
SALADS AND SALAD BARS				
BMT	1 serv	275	55	3
Cold Cut Trio	1 serv	234	57	3
Ham	1 serv	112	25	3
Meatball	1 serv	320	56	4
Roast Beef	1 serv	117	25	3
Roasted Chicken Breast	1 serv	130	50	3
Seafood & Crab	1 serv	197	24	4
Steak & Cheese	1 serv	181	37	4
Subway Club	1 serv	146	33	3
Subway Melt	1 serv	203	44	3
Tuna	1 serv	238	42	3
Turkey Breast	1 serv	105	20	3
Turkey Breast & Ham	1 serv	117	26	3
Veggie Delight	1 serv	50	0	3
SANDWICHES				
6 Inch Steak & Cheese	1	362	37	4
6 Inch Subway Melt	1	384	44	3
6 Inch Sub BMT	1	456	55	3
6 Inch Sub Cold Cut Trio	1	415	57	3
6 Inch Sub Ham	1	261	25	3
6 Inch Sub Meatball	1	501	56	4
6 Inch Sub Roast Beef	1	267	20	3
6 Inch Sub Roasted Chicken Breast	1	291	46	3

FOOD	PORTION	CALS	CHOL	FIBER
6 Inch Sub Seafood & Crab	1	378	24	3
6 Inch Sub Subway Club	1	296	33	3
6 Inch Sub Tuna	1	419	42	3
6 Inch Sub Turkey Breast	1	254	20	3
6 Inch Sub Turkey Breast & Ham	1	267	26	3
6 Inch Sub Veggie Delight	1	200	0	3
American Cheese Triangles	2	41	10	0
Asiago Caesar Sauce	1.5 tbsp	110	10	0
Bacon Strips	2	45	8	0
Breakfast Bacon & Egg	1	321	184	3
Breakfast Cheese & Egg	1	317	187	3
Breakfast Ham & Egg	1	338	201	3
Breakfast Western Egg	1	300	182	3
Cheddar Triangles	2	59	15	0
Cucumber Slices	3	2	0	0
Deli Ham	1	210	12	3
Deli Roast Beef	1	223	13	3
Deli Tuna	1	325	26	3
Deli Turkey Breast	1	215	13	3
Deli Style Roll	1	165	0	3
Dijon Horseradish	1.5 tbsp	91	8	0
Dijon Horseradish Melt	6 inch	465	52	4
Fat Free Red Wine Vinaigrette	1.5 tbsp	29	1	0
Fat Free Sweet Onion	1.5 tbsp	38	0	0
Green Pepper Strips	3 (0.2 oz)	2	0	0
Hearty Italian Bread	6 inch	207	0	3
Honey Mustard	1.5 tbsp	28	0	0
Honey Mustard Ham	6 inch	311	25	4
Honey Oat Bread	6 inch	249	0	4
Italian Bread	6 inch	178	0	2
Lettuce	1 serv (0.7 oz)	3	0	0

FOOD	PORTION	CALS	CHOL	FIBER
Mayonnaise	1 tbsp	111	9	0
Mayonnaise Light	1 tbsp	46	6	0
Moneterey Cheddar Bread	6 inch	235	10	3
Mustard	2 tsp	7	0	0
Olive Oil Blend	1 tsp	45	0	0
Olive Rings	3 (3 g)	3	0	0
Onions	1 serv (0.5 oz)	5	0	0
Parmesan Oregano Bread	6 inch	211	0	3
Pepperjack Cheese Triangles	2	40	11	0
Pickle Chips	3 pieces (0.3 oz)	1	0	0
Provolone Circles	2 havles	51	11	0
Red Wine Vinaigrette Club	6 inch	350	33	4
Roasted Garlic Bread	6 inch	225	0	4
Sourdough Bread	6 inch	208	0	3
Southwest Sauce	1.5 tbsp	86	7	0
Southwest Turkey Bacon	6 inch	407	35	4
Sweet Onion Chicken Teriyaki	6 inch	374	50	4
Swiss Triangles	2	53	13	0
Tomato Slices	3 (1.2 oz)	7	0	0
Vinegar	1 tsp	1	0	0
Wheat Sub	6 inch	186	0	3
SOUPS				
Black Bean	1 cup	180	5	15
Brown & Wild Rice w/ Chicken	1 cup	190	20	2
Cheese w/ Ham & Bacon	1 cup	230	20	2
Chicken & Dumplings	1 cup	130	30	1
Cream Of Broccoli	1 cup	130	15	1
Cream Of Potato w/ Bacon	1 cup	210	20	4
Golden Broccoli Cheese	1 cup	180	10	9
Hearty Chili Beef	1 cup	250	20	9

FOOD	PORTION	CALS	CHOL	FIBER
Minestrone	1 cup	70	5	0
New England Clam Chowder	1 cup	140	15	1
Potato Cheese Chowder	1 cup	210	25	2
Roasted Chicken Noodle	1 cup	90	20	1
Tomato Bisque	1 cup	90	0	3
Vegetable Beef	1 cup	90	5	2
TACO BELL				
BEVERAGES				
2% Lowfat Milk	1 serv (8 oz)	110	15	0
Coffee Black	1 serv (12 oz)	5	0	0
Diet Pepsi	1 serv (16 oz)	0	0	0
Dr. Pepper	1 serv (16 oz)	208	0	0
Lipton Iced Tea Sweetened	1 serv (16 oz)	140	0	0
Lipton Iced Tea Unsweetened	1 serv (16 oz)	0	0	0
Mountain Dew	1 serv (16 oz)	227	0	0
Orange Juice	1 serv (6 oz)	80	0	0
Pepsi Cola	1 serv (16 oz)	200	0	0
Slice	1 serv (16 oz)	200	0	0
BREAKFAST SELECTIONS				
Breakfast Quesadilla Cheese	1 (5.5 oz)	380	280	1
Breakfast Quesadilla w/ Bacon	1 (6 oz)	450	290	2
Breakfast Quesadilla w/ Sausage	1 (6 oz)	430	285	1
Country Breakfast Burrito	1 (4 oz)	270	195	2
Double Bacon & Egg Burrito	1 (6.25 oz)	480	405	2
Fiesta Breakfast Burrito	1 (3.5 oz)	280	25	2
Grande Breakfast Burrito	1 (6.25 oz)	420	205	3
Hash Brown Nuggets	1 serv (3.5 oz)	280	0	1

FOOD	PORTION	CALS	CHOL	FIBER
MAIN MENU SELECTIONS				
7-Layer Burrito	1 (10 oz)	530	25	13
BLT Soft Taco	1 (4.5 oz)	340	40	7
Bacon Cheeseburger Burrito	1 (8.5 oz)	570	70	6
Bean Burrito	1 (7 oz)	380	10	13
Big Beef Burrito Supreme	1 (10.5 oz)	520	55	11
Big Beef MexiMelt	1 (4.75 oz)	290	45	4
Big Chicken Burrito Supreme	1 (9 oz)	510	95	4
Border Sauce Fire	1 serv (0.3 oz)	0	0	0
Border Sauce Hot	1 serv (0.3 oz)	0	0	0
Border Sauce Mild	1 serv (0.3 oz)	0	0	0
Burger Sauce	1 serv (0.5 oz)	60	5	0
Burrito Supreme	1 (9 oz)	440	35	10
Cheddar Cheese	1 serv (0.25 oz)	30	5	0
Cheese Quesadilla	1 (4.25 oz)	350	50	2
Chicken Fajita Wrap	1 (8 oz)	470	60	4
Chicken Fajita Wrap Supreme	1 (9 oz)	520	70	4
Chicken Quesadilla	1 (6 oz)	410	90	3
Chicken Club Burrito	1 (8 oz)	540	80	4
Chili Cheese Burrito	1 (5 oz)	330	35	5
Choco Taco Ice Cream Dessert	1 serv (4 oz)	310	20	1
Cinnamon Twists	1 serv (1 oz)	140	0	0
Club Sauce	1 serv (0.5 oz)	80	10	0
Double Decker Taco	1 (5.75 oz)	340	25	9
Double Decker Taco Supreme	1 (7 oz)	390	35	9
Fajita Sauce	1 serv (0.5 oz)	70	5	0
Green Sauce	1 serv (1 oz)	5	0	0
Grilled Chicken Burrito	1 (7 oz)	410	55	4
Grilled Chicken Soft Taco	1 (4.5 oz)	240	45	3
Grilled Steak Soft Taco	1 (4.5 oz)	230	25	2
Grilled Steak Soft Taco Supreme	1 (5.75 oz)	290	35	3

FOOD	PORTION	CALS	CHOL	FIBER
Guacamole	1 serv (0.75 oz)	35	0	1
Mexican Pizza	1 serv (7.75 oz)	570	45	8
Mexican Rice	1 serv (4.75 oz)	190	15	1
Nacho Cheese Sauce	2 serv (2 oz)	120	5	0
Nachos	1 serv (3.5 oz)	320	5	3
Nachos Beef Beef Supreme	1 serv (7 oz)	450	30	9
Nachos Bellgrande	1 serv (11 oz)	770	35	17
Picante Sauce	1 serv (0.3 oz)	0	0	0
Pico De Gallo	1 serv (0.75 oz)	5	0	0
Pintos 'n Cheese	1 serv (4.5 oz)	190	15	10
Red Sauce	1 serv (1 oz)	10	0	0
Soft Taco	1 (3.5 oz)	220	25	3
Soft Taco Supreme	1 (5 oz)	260	35	3
Sour Cream	1 serv (0.75 oz)	40	10	0
Steak Fajita Wrap	1 (8 oz)	470	40	3
Steak Fajita Wrap Supreme	1 (9 oz)	510	50	3
Taco	1 (2.75 oz)	180	25	3
Taco Supreme	1 (4 oz)	220	35	3
Taco Salad w/ Salsa	1 (19 oz)	850	60	16
Taco Salad w/ Salsa w/o Shell	1 (16.5 oz)	420	60	15
Three Cheese Blend	1 serv (0.25 oz)	25	5	0
Tostada	1 (6.25 oz)	300	15	12
Veggie Fajita Wrap	1 (8 oz)	420	20	3
Veggie Fajita Wrap Supreme	1 (9 oz)	470	30	3

TACO JOHN'S
CHILDREN'S MENU SELECTIONS

FOOD	PORTION	CALS	CHOL	FIBER
Kid's Meal Crispy Taco	1 serv (8 oz)	579	35	—
Kid's Meal Softshell Taco	1 serv (8.5 oz)	617	35	—

DESSERTS

FOOD	PORTION	CALS	CHOL	FIBER
Choco Taco	1 serv (3.5 oz)	320	20	—
Churro	1 serv (1.5 oz)	147	4	—
Flauta Apple	1 serv (2 oz)	84	0	—
Flauta Cherry	1 serv (2 oz)	143	0	—

FOOD	PORTION	CALS	CHOL	FIBER
Flauta Cream Cheese	1 serv (2 oz)	181	10	–
Italian Ice	1 serv (4 oz)	80	0	–
MAIN MENU SELECTIONS				
Bean Burrito	1 (6.5 oz)	387	18	–
Beans Refried	1 serv (9.5 oz)	357	17	–
Beef Burrito	1 (6.5 oz)	449	52	–
Chicken Fajita Burrito	1 (6.25)	370	49	–
Chicken Fajita Salad w/o Dressing	1 serv (12.25 oz)	557	56	–
Chicken Fajita Softshell	1 (4.5 oz)	200	33	–
Chili	1 serv (9.25 oz)	350	56	–
Chimichanga Platter	1 serv (18 oz)	979	59	–
Combination Burrito	1 (6.5 oz)	418	35	–
Crispy Tacos	1 serv (3.25 oz)	182	26	–
Double Enchilada Platter	1 serv (18.25 oz)	967	89	–
Meat & Potato Burrito	1 (7.75 oz)	503	25	–
Mexi Rolls w/ Nacho Cheese	1 serv (9.75 oz)	863	54	–
Mexican Rice	1 serv (8 oz)	567	0	–
Nachos	1 serv (3.5 oz)	333	0	–
Potato Oles Bravo	1 serv (8.88 oz)	579	7	–
Ranch Burrito	1 (7 oz)	447	74	–
Sampler Platter	1 serv (25.5 oz)	1406	126	–
Sierra Chicken Fillet Sandwich	1 (8.5 oz)	534	68	–
Smothered Burrito Platter	1 serv (19.5 oz)	1031	70	–
Softshell Tacos	1 serv (4.25 oz)	230	26	–
Super Burrito	1 (8.5 oz)	465	41	–
Super Nachos	1 serv (13 oz)	919	48	–
Taco Bravo	1 serv (6.25 oz)	346	28	–
Taco Burger	1 (5 oz)	280	32	–
Taco Salad w/o Dressing	1 (12.4 oz)	584	46	–
TACOTIME				
Casita Burrito Meat	1 serv (12 oz)	647	89	16
Cheddar Cheese	1 serv (0.75 oz)	86	22	0

FOOD	PORTION	CALS	CHOL	FIBER
Chicken	1 serv (2.5 oz)	109	33	0
Chips	1 serv (2 oz)	266	0	3
Crisp Burrito Bean	1 (5.25 oz)	427	12	9
Crisp Burrito Chicken	1 (4.75 oz)	422	54	2
Crisp Burrito Meat	1 (5.25 oz)	552	58	7
Crisp Taco	1 (4 oz)	295	48	5
Crustos	1 serv (3.5 oz)	373	0	—
Double Soft Bean Burrito	1 (9.5 oz)	506	22	19
Double Soft Combination Burrito	1 (9.5 oz)	617	63	18
Double Soft Meat Burrito	1 serv (6.5 oz)	726	99	17
Empanada Cherry	1 (4 oz)	250	0	—
Enchilada Sauce	1 serv (1 oz)	12	0	1
Flour Tortilla 10 in	1 (2.75 oz)	213	0	6
Flour Tortilla 7 in	1 (1.75 oz)	88	0	1
Flour Tortilla 8 in	1 (1.25 oz)	107	0	2
Fried Flour Tortilla 10 in	1 (2.75 oz)	318	0	2
Fried Flour Tortilla 8 in	1 (1.35 oz)	205	0	1
Guacamole	1 serv (1 oz)	29	0	1
Hot Sauce	1 serv (1 oz)	10	0	0
Lettuce	1 serv (0.5 oz)	2	0	0
Mexi Fries	1 lg (8 oz)	532	0	—
Mexi Fries	1 reg (4 oz)	266	0	—
Mexican Dressing No Fat	1 serv (2 oz)	20	0	—
Mexican Rice	1 serv (4 oz)	159	0	1
Nachos	1 serv (10.5 oz)	680	78	11
Nachos Deluxe	1 serv (15.25 oz)	1048	109	17
Natural Super Taco Meat	1 (11.25 oz)	627	82	14
Olives	1 serv (0.50 oz)	16	0	0
Quesadilla Cheese	1 serv (3.25 oz)	205	30	1
Ranchero Salsa	1 serv (2 oz)	21	0	1
Refritos	1 serv (2.5 oz)	97	0	6
Refritos	1 serv (7 oz)	326	22	13
Rolled Soft Flour Taco	1 (7 oz)	512	63	12
Soft Taco Chicken	1 (7 oz)	387	48	7
Sour Cream	1 serv (1 oz)	55	19	0

FOOD	PORTION	CALS	CHOL	FIBER
Sour Cream Dressing	1 serv (1.5 oz)	137	8	0
Super Shredded Beef Soft Taco	1 (8 oz)	368	22	7
Taco Cheeseburger	1 (7.5 oz)	633	66	7
Taco Meat	1 serv (2.5 oz)	208	38	5
Taco Salad Chicken w/o Dressing	1 serv (9 oz)	370	48	3
Taco Salad w/o Dressing	1 serv (7.75 oz)	479	63	7
Taco Shell 6 in	1 (1.25 oz)	110	0	2
Thousand Island Dressing	1 serv (1 oz)	160	10	0
Tomato	1 serv (0.5 oz)	3	0	0
Tostada Delight Salad Meat	1 (9.75 oz)	628	82	13
Value Soft Bean Burrito	1 (6.75 oz)	380	15	13
Value Soft Meat Burrito	1 (6.75 oz)	491	56	12
Value Soft Taco	1 (5.25 oz)	316	48	5
Veggie Burrito	1 (11 oz)	491	24	10
Wheat Tortilla 11 in	1 (3.5 oz)	175	0	2
TCBY				
Hand Dipped All Flavors 96% Fat Free	½ cup (3 oz)	140	5	0
Hand Dipped All Flavors Nonfat	½ cup (2.9 oz)	120	0	1
Lowfat Ice Cream All Flavors No Sugar Added	½ cup (2.6 oz)	110	10	0
Nonfat Ice Cream All Flavors	½ cup (2.9 oz)	120	0	1
Soft Serve All Flavors 96% Fat Free	½ cup (3.4 fl oz)	140	15	0
Soft Serve All Flavors No Sugar Added Nonfat	½ cup (2.8 oz)	80	<5	0
Soft Serve All Flavors Nonfat	½ cup (3.4 oz)	110	<5	0

FOOD	PORTION	CALS	CHOL	FIBER
Sorbet All Flavors Nonfat & Nondairy	½ cup (3.4 oz)	100	0	0

TGI FRIDAY'S

FOOD	PORTION	CALS	CHOL	FIBER
Fresh Vegetable Medley w/ Potato	1 serv	470	25	—
Fresh Vegetable Medley w/ Rice	1 serv	407	<2	—
Friday's Gardenburger	1	445	13	—
Garden Dagwood Sandwich	1 serv	375	<2	—
Pacific Coast Chicken	1 serv	415	70	—
Pacific Coast Tuna	1 serv	410	70	—
Pea Salsa	1 serv (6.4 oz)	175	0	—
Salad & Baked Potato	1 serv	250	<2	—
Turkey Burger	1 (9.8 oz)	410	95	—

TOGO'S
SALAD DRESSINGS

FOOD	PORTION	CALS	CHOL	FIBER
1000 Island	1 serv (2.3 oz)	231	30	0
Caesar	1 serv (2.3 oz)	241	20	0
Oriental	1 serv (2.3 oz)	221	5	0
Ranch	1 serv (2.3 oz)	321	15	0
Reduced Calorie Italian	1 serv (2.3 oz)	60	0	0
Reduced Calorie Ranch	1 serv (2.3 oz)	191	25	0

SALADS AND SALAD BARS

FOOD	PORTION	CALS	CHOL	FIBER
Caesar Salad	1 serv	471	72	2
Garden Salad	1 serv	256	214	2
Oriental Salad	1 serv	499	41	3
Taco Salad	1 serv	943	71	11

SANDWICHES

FOOD	PORTION	CALS	CHOL	FIBER
Albacore Tuna	1 sm	701	67	3
Avocado & Turkey	1 sm	675	80	6
Avocado Cucumber & Alfalfa Sprouts	1 sm	637	85	7
Bar-B-Q Beef	1 sm	724	88	3
California Roasted Chicken	1 sm	510	65	3
Cheese Swiss American Provolone	1 sm	859	107	3
Chunky Chicken Salad	1 sm	636	42	3

FOOD	PORTION	CALS	CHOL	FIBER
Egg Salad w/ Cheese	1 sm	728	456	3
Ham & Cheese	1 sm	661	68	3
Hot Pastrami	1 sm	705	72	3
Italian Salami & Cheese	1 sm	770	118	3
Italian Salami Capicolla Mortadella Cotto & Provolone	1 sm	736	85	3
Meatballs w/ Pizza Sauce & Parmesan	1 sm	707	97	4
Pastrami Reuben	1 sm	875	111	2
Roast Beef Hot & Cold	1 sm	552	84	3
Turkey & Cranberry	1 sm	623	49	4
Turkey & Bacon Club	1 sm	667	81	3
Turkey & Cheese	1 sm	638	71	3
Turkey & Ham w/ Cheese	1 sm	670	76	3

TROPIGRILL

FOOD	PORTION	CALS	CHOL	FIBER
Banana Tropical	1 serv (7.55 oz)	498	0	9
Black Beans (combo meal portion)	1 serv (4.78 oz)	153	0	10
Black Beans (side)	1 serv (8.39 oz)	269	0	18
Boiled Yuca	1 serv (12 oz)	334	0	5
Boneless Breast	1 serv (3.14 oz)	140	83	tr
Cheese Potatoes	1 serv (7.42 oz)	177	10	2
Chicken ¼ Dark Meat	1 serv (4.52 oz)	298	187	tr
Chicken ¼ Dark Meat w/o Skin	1 serv (3.42 oz)	170	144	tr
Chicken ¼ White Meat	1 serv (5.09 oz)	295	170	tr
Chicken ¼ White Meat w/o Skin	1 serv (3.82 oz)	167	117	tr
Chicken Caesar Sandwich	1 (6.4 oz)	457	97	tr
Chicken Sandwich	1 (7.92 oz)	442	89	tr
Congri	1 serv (7.08 oz)	439	0	7
Vegetable Kabob	1 (3.07 oz)	106	0	5
White Rice	1 serv (6.82 oz)	341	0	2
Yellow Rice	1 serv (7 oz)	294	0	3
Yucatan Fries	1 serv (5.3 oz)	440	0	3

FOOD	PORTION	CALS	CHOL	FIBER
VILLAGE INN				
French Toast Cinnamon Raisin	1 serv	809	9	–
Fruit & Nut Pancakes Low Cholesterol	1 serv	936	2	–
Omelette Chicken & Cheese	1 serv	721	120	–
Omelette Fresh Veggie	1 serv	704	102	–
Omelette Mushroom & Cheese	1 serv	680	102	–
Turkey & Vegetable Scrambled Sensation	1 serv	726	124	–
WENDY'S				
BEVERAGES				
Cola	11 oz	130	0	0
Diet Cola	11 oz	0	0	0
Frosty Junior	6 oz	170	20	0
Frosty Medium	16 oz	440	50	0
Frosty Small	12 oz	330	35	0
Lemon-Lime Soda	11 oz	130	0	0
CHILDREN'S MENU SELECTIONS				
French Fries Kid's Meal	1 serv (3.2 oz)	270	0	3
Kid's Meal Cheeseburger	1 (4.2 oz)	310	45	2
Kid's Meal Hamburger	1 (3.9 oz)	270	30	1
Kids'Meal Chicken Nuggets	4 pieces (2.1 oz)	190	25	0
MAIN MENU SELECTIONS				
¼ lb Hamburger Patty	1 (2.6 oz)	200	65	0
2 oz Hamburger Patty	1 (1.3 oz)	100	30	0
American Cheese	1 slice (0.6 oz)	70	15	0
American Cheese Jr.	1 slice (0.4 oz)	45	10	0
Bacon	1 strip (4 g)	20	5	0
Baked Potato Chili & Cheese	1 (15.4 oz)	630	40	9
Big Bacon Classic	1 (9.9 oz)	580	100	3
Breaded Chicken Fillet	1 (3.5 oz)	230	50	0

FOOD	PORTION	CALS	CHOL	FIBER
Cheddar Cheese Shredded	2 tbsp (0.6 oz)	70	15	0
Cheddar Shredded	2 tbsp (0.6 oz)	70	15	0
Chicken Breast Filet Sandwich	1 (7.3 oz)	430	56	2
Chicken Club Sandwich	1 (7.6 oz)	470	65	2
Chicken Nuggets	5 pieces (2.6 oz)	230	30	0
Chili	1 lg (12 oz)	310	45	7
Chili	1 sm (8 oz)	210	30	5
Classic Single w/ Everything	1 (7.6 oz)	410	70	2
French Fries Biggie	1 Great (6.7 oz)	570	0	7
French Fries	1 med (5 oz)	420	0	5
French Fries	1 Biggie (5.6 oz)	470	0	6
Grilled Chicken Fillet	1 (2.9 oz)	110	55	0
Grilled Chicken Sandwich	1 (6.6 oz)	300	56	2
Honey Mustard Reduced Calorie	1 tsp (7 g)	25	0	0
Hot Stuffed Baked Potato Plain	1 (10 oz)	310	0	6
Hot Stuffed Baked Potato Bacon & Cheese	1 (12.6 oz)	530	25	7
Hot Stuffed Baked Potato Broccoli & Cheese	1 (14.4 oz)	470	5	9
Jr. Bacon Cheeseburger	1 (5.8 oz)	380	55	2
Jr. Cheeseburger	1 (4.5 oz)	310	45	2
Jr. Cheeseburger Deluxe	1 (6.3 oz)	360	50	2
Kaiser Bun	1 (2.5 oz)	200	0	2
Ketchup	1 tsp (7 g)	10	0	0
Lettuce	1 leaf (0.5 oz)	0	0	0
Mayonnaise	1½ tsp (9 g)	30	5	0
Mustard	½ tsp (5 g)	5	0	0
Nuggets Sauce Barbeque	1 pkg (1 oz)	45	0	0

FOOD	PORTION	CALS	CHOL	FIBER
Nuggets Sauce Honey Mustard	1 pkg (1 oz)	130	10	0
Nuggets Sauce Sweet & Sour	1 pkg (1 oz)	50	0	0
Onion	4 rings (0.5 oz)	5	0	0
Pickles	4 slices (0.4 oz)	0	0	0
Saltines	2 (0.2 oz)	25	0	0
Sandwich Bun	1 (2 oz)	160	0	1
Spicy Chicken Fillet	1 (3.6 oz)	210	60	0
Spicy Chicken Sandwich	1 (7.5 oz)	410	65	2
Tomatoes	1 slice (0.9 oz)	5	0	1
Whipped Margarine	1 pkg (0.5 oz)	70	0	0
SALAD DRESSINGS				
Blue Cheese	1 pkg (2 oz)	360	30	0
French	1 pkg (2 oz)	250	0	0
Hidden Valley Ranch	1 pkg (2 oz)	200	25	0
Hidden Valley Ranch Reduced Fat Reduced Calorie	1 pkg (2 oz)	120	20	0
Italian Reduced Fat Reduced Calorie	1 pkg (2 oz)	80	0	0
Italian Caesar	1 pkg (1.5 oz)	230	25	0
Thousand Island	1 pkg (2 oz)	260	20	0
SALADS AND SALAD BARS				
Bacon Bits	2 tbsp (0.5 oz)	45	10	0
Ceasar Side Salad w/o Dressing	1 (3.2 oz)	110	15	1
Chicken Salad	2 tbsp (1.2 oz)	70	0	0
Deluxe Garden Salad w/o Dressing	1 (9.5 oz)	110	0	4
Grilled Chicken Salad w/o Dressing	1 (11.9 oz)	200	55	4
Side Salad w/o Dressing	1 (5.4 oz)	60	0	2
Soft Breadstick	1 (1.5 oz)	130	5	1
Taco Chips	15 (1.5 oz)	210	0	2
Taco Salad w/o Dressing	1 (16.4 oz)	380	65	8

FOOD	PORTION	CALS	CHOL	FIBER
WHATABURGER				
BAKED SELECTIONS				
Biscuit	1	280	3	–
Blueberry Muffin	1	239	0	–
Cinnamon Roll	1	320	10	–
Cookie Chocolate Chunk	1	247	28	–
Cookie White Chocolate Macadamia Nut	1	269	34	–
Fried Apple Turnover	1	215	0	–
BEVERAGES				
Cherry Coke	1 reg	227	0	–
Coffee	1 sm	5	0	–
Coke Classic	1 reg	211	0	–
Creamer	1 pkg	10	0	–
Diet Coke	1 reg	2	0	–
Dr. Pepper	1 reg	207	0	–
Iced Tea	1 reg	5	0	–
Lemon Juice	1 pkg	1	0	–
Milk 2%	1 serv	113	18	–
Orange Juice	1 serv (10 oz)	140	0	–
Root Beer	1 reg	237	0	–
Shake Chocolate	1 junior	364	36	–
Shake Strawberry	1 junior	352	35	–
Shake Vanilla	1 junior	325	37	–
Sprite	1 reg	211	0	–
Sugar	1 pkg	15	0	–
Sweet And Low	1 pkg	4	0	–
BREAKFAST SELECTIONS				
Biscuit w/ Bacon	1	359	15	–
Biscuit w/ Bacon Egg & Cheese	1	511	213	–
Biscuit w/ Egg & Cheese	1	434	202	–
Biscuit w/ Sausage	1	446	37	–
Biscuit w/ Sausage Egg & Cheese	1	601	236	–
Biscuit w/ Sausage Gravy	1	479	20	–
Breakfast Platter w/ Bacon	1 serv	695	389	–

FOOD	PORTION	CALS	CHOL	FIBER
Breakfast Platter w/ Sausage	1 serv	785	412	—
Breakfast On A Bun w/ Bacon	1	365	210	—
Breakfast On A Bun w/ Sausage	1	455	232	—
Butter	1 pkg	36	11	—
Egg Omelette Sandwich	1	288	198	—
Grape Jelly	1 pkg	45	0	—
Hashbrown	1 serv	150	0	—
Honey	1 pkg	25	0	—
Margarine	1 pkg	25	0	—
Pancake Syrup	1 pkg	180	0	—
Pancakes	3	259	0	—
Pancakes w/ Bacon	1 serv	335	12	—
Pancakes w/ Sausage	1 serv	426	34	—
Srambled Eggs	2	189	374	—
Strawberry Jam	1 pkg	40	0	—
Taquito Bacon & Egg	1	335	286	—
MAIN MENU SELECTIONS				
Bacon	1 slice	38	6	—
Cheese Slice	1 sm	46	12	—
Cheese Slice	1 lg	89	22	—
Chicken Strips	2	120	14	—
Club Crackers	1 pkg	30	0	—
Croutons	1 pkg	30	0	—
Fajita Beef	1	326	28	—
Fajita Grilled Chicken	1	272	33	—
French Fries	1 lg	442	0	—
French Fries	1 reg	332	0	—
French Fries	1 junior	221	0	—
Garden Salad	1	56	0	—
Grilled Chicken Salad	1 serv	150	49	—
Grilled Chicken Sandwich	1	442	66	—
Grilled Chicken Sandwich w/o Bun Oil w/ Mustard	1	300	66	—

FOOD	PORTION	CALS	CHOL	FIBER
Grilled Chicken Sandwich w/o Bun Oil & Dressing	1	358	66	—
Grilled Chicken Sandwich w/o Dressing	1	385	66	—
Jalapeno Pepper	1	3	0	—
Justaburger	1	276	34	—
Ketchup	1 pkg	30	0	—
Onion Rings	1 reg	329	0	—
Onion Rings	1 lg	493	0	—
Peppered Gravy	1 serv (3 oz)	75	0	—
Picante Sauce	1 pkg	5	0	—
Taquito Potato & Egg	1	446	281	—
Taquito Sausage & Egg	1	443	315	—
Texas Toast	1 slice	147	0	—
Whataburger	1	598	84	—
Whataburger Double Meat	1	823	168	—
Whataburger Jr.	1	300	34	—
Whataburger w/o bun oil	1	407	84	—
Whatacatch Sandwich	1	467	33	—
Whatachick'n Sandwich	1	501	40	—
SALAD DRESSINGS				
Low Fat Ranch	1 pkg	66	15	—
Low Fat Vinaigrette	1 pkg	37	0	—
Ranch	1 pkg	320	50	—
Thousand Island	1 pkg	160	15	—
WHITE CASTLE				
Cheeseburger	2 (3.6 oz)	310	30	6
Grilled Chicken Sandwich	2 (4 oz)	250	20	5
Grilled Chicken Sandwich w/ Sauce	2 (4.8 oz)	290	20	5
Hamburger	2 (3.2 oz)	270	20	5
ZUZU				
Beans	1 cup	210	0	—
Cheese Enchilada Platter	1 serv	395	15	—

FOOD	PORTION	CALS	CHOL	FIBER
Chicken Burrito Platter	1 serv	580	60	—
Chicken Taco Platter	1 serv	440	70	—
Chicken Taco w/o Mexican Cream	1	125	35	—
Frozen Yogurt	1 serv	200	0	—
Green Salad w/o Dressing or Avocado	1	20	0	—
Grilled Chicken Salad w/o Dressing	1 serv	305	70	—
Rice	1 cup	150	0	—
Salsa Roja Epazote	¼ cup	8	0	—
Tortilla Corn	1	35	0	—
Tortilla Flour	1	60	0	—